To Mitchell Lewis

With fond and lasting memories

of the ICSH

POLYCYTHEMIA VERA and the MYELOPROLIFERATIVE DISORDERS

POLYCYTHEMIA VERA and the MYELOPROLIFERATIVE DISORDERS

LOUIS R. WASSERMAN, M.D.

Albert A. and Vera G. List Professor of Medicine (Hematology) Emeritus
Distinguished Service Professor Emeritus
Mount Sinai School of Medicine
New York, New York

PAUL D. BERK, M.D.

Lillian and Henry M. Stratton Professor of Molecular Medicine
Professor of Medicine and Biochemistry
Mount Sinai School of Medicine
New York, New York

NATHANIEL I. BERLIN, M.D., Ph.D.

Professor of Medicine Emeritus
University of Miami School of Medicine
Miami, Florida

W. B. SAUNDERS COMPANY

A Division of Harcourt Brace & Company

PHILADELPHIA, LONDON, TORONTO, MONTREAL, SYDNEY, TOKYO

W. B. SAUNDERS COMPANY
A Division of Harcourt Brace & Company

The Curtis Center
Independence Square West
Philadelphia, PA 19106

Library of Congress Cataloging-in-Publication Data

Polycythemia vera / [edited by] Louis R. Wasserman, Paul D. Berk,
Nathaniel I. Berlin.
    p.   cm.
    ISBN 0-7216-4213-6
    1. Polycythemia vera.   I. Wasserman, Louis R.   II. Berk, Paul D.
III. Berlin, Nathaniel I.
    [DNLM: 1. Polycythemia Vera.   WH 180 P7822 1995]
RC647.P63P65 1995
616.1'53—dc20
DNLM/DLC   94-1680

Cover design reproduced with permission of the artist, John Willenbecher, from a poster commissioned by Mrs. Vera List in 1969 for the *American Society of Hematology*.

Polycythemia Vera and the Myeloproliferative Disorders   ISBN   0-7216-4213-6

Printed in the United States of America.

Last digit is the print number: 9   8   7   6   5   4   3   2   1

CONTRIBUTORS

STANLEY P. BALCERZAK, M.D.

Director, Division of Hematology/Oncology, Director, Comprehensive Cancer Center, Ohio State University, Columbus, Ohio

Secondary Polycythemia

PAUL D. BERK, M.D.

Lillian and Henry M. Stratton Professor of Molecular Medicine, Professor of Medicine and Biochemistry, Chief, Division of Liver Diseases, Mount Sinai School of Medicine, New York, New York; Attending Physician, Medical Director, Liver Transplantation, Mount Sinai Hospital, New York, New York

Treatment of Polycythemia Vera: A Summary of Clinical Trials Conducted by the Polycythemia Vera Study Group

NATHANIEL I. BERLIN, M.D., Ph.D.

Teuton Professor of Medicine Emeritus, Northwestern University Medical School, Chicago, Illinois; Professor of Medicine Emeritus, University of Miami School of Medicine, Miami, Florida

Classification of the Polycythemias and Initial Clinical Features in Polycythemia Vera

SHU CHIEN, M.D., Ph.D.

Professor of Bioengineering and Medicine, University of California, San Diego

Rheology in Normal Individuals and Polycythemia Vera

CHRISTINE CHOMIENNE, M.D.

Assistant Professor in Cellular Biology, University Paris VII, Hospital St. Louis, Paris, France

Radioisotope Investigations for the Diagnosis and Follow-up of Polycythemic Patients

EDWARD A. COPELAN, M.D.

Associate Professor of Medicine, Ohio State University College of Medicine, Staff, Ohio State University Hospitals and James Cancer Hospital and Research Institute, Columbus, Ohio

Secondary Polycythemia

CATHERINE DRESCH, M.D.

Research Director, National Institute of Health Research, Paris, France

Radioisotope Investigations for the Diagnosis and Follow-up of Polycythemic Patients

JOHN T. ELLIS, M.D.

David D. Thompson Professor Emeritus of Pathology, Cornell University Medical College, New York, New York; Attending Pathologist, The New York Hospital, Memorial Hospital and New York Downtown Hospital, New York, New York

The Development, Morphology and Function of Normal Bone Marrow: A Review; The Bone Marrow in Polycythemia Vera

ERNEST W. FORDHAM, M.D.

Professor of Radiology and Nuclear Medicine, Rush University, Chicago, Illinois; Director of Nuclear Medicine, Assistant Chairman, Department of Diagnostic Radiology and Nuclear Medicine, Rush University, Chicago, Illinois

Distribution of Erythropoietic Bone Marrow in Polycythemia Vera and Other Myeloproliferative Disorders: Total Body Marrow Imaging with ^{52}Fe

STEVEN M. FRUCHTMAN, M.D.

Assistant Professor of Medicine, Mount Sinai School of Medicine, New York, New York; Director, Bone Marrow Transplantation, The Mount Sinai Hospital, New York, New York

Treatment of Polycythemia Vera: A Summary of Clinical Trials Conducted by the Polycythemia Vera Study Group; Therapeutic Recommendations for Polycythemia Vera

STEPHEN GALLIK, Ph.D.

Associate Professor of Biological Sciences, Mary Washington University, Fredericksburg, Virginia

Rheology in Normal Individuals and Polycythemia Vera

FRANK H. GARDNER, M.D.

Clinical Professor of Medicine, Division of Hematology Oncology, University of Texas Medical Branch, Galveston, Texas; Attending Physician, John Sealy Hospital, Galveston, Texas

Early Approaches in the Treatment of Polycythemia Vera

HARRIET S. GILBERT, M.D.

Clinical Professor of Medicine, Albert Einstein College of Medicine, Bronx, New York; Attending Physician, Mt. Sinai Medical Center, New York, New York; Attending Physician, Montefiore Medical Center, Bronx, New York

Familial Myeloproliferative Disease

JUDITH S. GOLDBERG, Sc.D.

Executive Director, Statistics and Data Management, Medical Research Division, American Cyanamid Company, Pearl River, New York

Treatment of Polycythemia Vera: A Summary of Clinical Trials Conducted by the Polycythemia Vera Study Group

HARRY ILAND, FRACP, FRCPA

Clinical Associate Professor, Department of Medicine, Faculty of Medicine, University of Sydney, Sydney, Australia; Senior Staff Specialist and Clinical Hematologist, The Kanematsu Laboratories, Royal Prince Alfred Hospital, Camberdown, NSW, Australia

Essential Thrombocythemia

WILLIAM H. KNOSPE, M.D.

Professor of Medicine, Rush Medical College; Attending Physician, Presbyterian-St. Luke's Hospital, Chicago, Illinois

Distribution of Erythropoietic Bone Marrow in Polycythemia Vera and Other Myeloproliferative Disorders: Total Body Marrow Imaging with ^{52}Fe

STEPHEN A. LANDAW, M.D., Ph.D.

Associate Chief of Staff, Research and Development, VA Medical Center, Syracuse, New York; Professor of Medicine, SUNY-Health Science Center, Syracuse, New York; Attending in Hematology-Oncology (Internal Medicine), VA Medical Center, University Hospital, Crouse-Irving Memorial Hospital, Syracuse, New York

Acute Leukemia in Polycythemia Vera

JOHN LASZLO, M.D.

National Vice President, Research, American Cancer Society, Atlanta, Georgia

Essential Thrombocythemia

BARUCH MODAN, M.D.

Professor and Head, Department of Clinical Epidemiology, The Chaim Sheba Medical Center, Tel-Aviv University, Tel-Aviv, Israel; Sackler School of Medicine, Tel-Hashomer, Israel

The Epidemiology of Polycythemia Vera

SCOTT MURPHY, M.D.

Professor of Medicine, Cardeza Foundation for Hematologic Research, Jefferson Medical College of Thomas Jefferson University, Philadelphia, Pennsylvania

Megakaryocytes, Platelets, and Coagulation in the Myeloproliferative Diseases; Essential Thrombocythemia

YVES NAJEAN, M.D.

Professor of Hematology, Head of the Department of Nuclear Medicine, Hospital St. Louis, Paris, France

Radioisotope Investigations for the Diagnosis and Follow-up of Polycythemic Patients

POWERS PETERSON, M.D.

Associate Professor of Pathology, Cornell University Medical College, New York, New York; Associate Attending Pathologist, and Director, Laboratory of Clinical Hematology, The New York Hospital, New York, New York; Director of Clinical Laboratories, The New York Hospital, Westchester Division, White Plains, New York

The Development, Morphology and Function of Normal Bone Marrow: A Review; The Natural History of Polycythemia Vera; The Bone Marrow in Polycythemia Vera

ROBERT V. PIERRE, M.D.

Professor of Pathology, University of Southern California School of Medicine, Head, Division of Hematopathology, Los Angeles County Hospital, Los Angeles, California; Professor of Laboratory Medicine and Internal Medicine Emeritus, Mayo Medical School, Rochester, Minnesota

Cytogenetics

ANTHONY V. PISCIOTTA, M.D.

Robert A. Uihlein, Jr. Professor of Hematologic Research, Medical College of Wisconsin, Attending Staff, John L. Doyne Hospital, Froedtert Memorial Hospital, Milwaukee, Wisconsin; Consulting Staff, St. Joseph's Hospital, Mount Sinai Hospital, St. Luke's Hospital and Columbia Hospital, New York, New York

Chronic Myelocytic Leukemia

JEAN-DIDIER RAIN, M.D.

Professor of Hematology, Department of Nuclear Medicine, Hospital St. Louis, Paris, France

Radioisotope Investigations for the Diagnosis and Follow-up of Polycythemic Patients

DAVID S. ROSENTHAL, M.D.

Henry K. Oliver Professor of Hygiene, Harvard University, Associate Professor of Medicine, Harvard Medical School; Director, Harvard University Health Service; Senior Physician, Brigham and Women's Hospital, Boston, Massachusetts

Myeloid Metaplasis with Myelofibrosis (Agnogenic and Postpolycythemia Vera)

JEAN C. SCHULMAN, M.D.

W. O. Boswell Memorial Hospital, Sun City, Arizona

Regulation of Erythropoiesis in Polycythemia Vera

MURRAY N. SILVERSTEIN, M.D.

Professor of Medicine, Mayo Clinic; Chairman Emeritus, Division of Hematology, Mayo Clinic, Rochester, Minnesota

Anagrelide in Myeloproliferative Diseases

LOUIS R. WASSERMAN, M.D.

Albert A. and Vera G. List Professor of Medicine (Hematology) Emeritus, Distinguished Service Professor Emeritus, Mount Sinai School of Medicine; Attending Physician, The Mount Sinai Hospital, New York, New York

The Natural History of Polycythemia Vera; Treatment of Polycythemia Vera: A Summary of Clinical Trials Conducted by the Polycythemia Vera Study Group; Therapeutic Recommendations for Polycythemia Vera

NEAL J. WEINREB, M.D.

Clinical Associate Professor of Oncology, University of Miami School of Medicine, Miami, Florida; Chief of Medical Staff, University Hospital, Tamarac, Florida; Medical Director, Vitas Health Care Corp of Florida

Relative Polycythemia

JACQUELINE WHANG-PENG, M.D.

Professor, Yang-Ming Medical College, Taipei, Taiwan, Republic of China; Director, Cancer Clinical Research Center, Cooperative Ward 191-A, Veterans General Hospital, Taipei, Taiwan, Republic of China

Cytogenetics

TSAI-FAN YU, B.A., M.D.

Research Professor of Medicine Emeritus, Mount Sinai School of Medicine, New York, New York

Urate Metabolism in the Polycythemias

ESMAIL D. ZANJANI, Ph.D.

Professor of Medicine and Physiology, University of Nevada, Reno; Research Career Scientist, VA Medical Center, Reno, Nevada

Regulation of Erythropoiesis in Polycythemia Vera

PREFACE

Some diseases command intensive medical attention because their clinical manifestations, combined with a high incidence and/or prevalence, impose a severe burden of suffering or death on the populace. In the Western world, arteriosclerotic cardiovascular disease, cancer, diabetes, and hypertension are among the major entries in this category, joined in the 1990s by acquired immunodeficiency disease (AIDS) and a resurgence of tuberculosis. Other diseases warrant medical interest not so much because of the public health consequences of the number of cases but because their pathophysiologic manifestations stimulate investigations that greatly enhance our knowledge of human physiology. Polycythemia vera and the myeloproliferative disorders are prime examples of such conditions.

Early descriptions of polycythemia vera focused on the associated and characteristic plethora. Incremental progress, first over centuries, then decades, and most recently measured in months, led to the recognition of an elevated peripheral red blood cell count and hematocrit, hypercellularity of the erythroid components in the bone marrow, low peripheral blood levels and urinary excretion of the hormone erythropoietin, and the presence of abnormal erythroid stem cells in the bone marrow. Indeed, polycythemia was a crucial stimulus to the identification, characterization, and ultimate cloning of erythropoietin. When elevations in the peripheral granulocyte and platelet counts were recognized as a part of the syndrome, studies of derangements of their precursor stem-cell compartments followed. Indeed, polycythemia vera and the other myeloproliferative disorders provided an important model from which developed much of our current understanding of bone marrow stem-cell compartments, lineages, and kinetics.

Similarly, the evolution to acute leukemia, often accompanied by the development of cytogenetically identifiable abnormal clones, stimulated studies of the mechanisms of leukemogenesis. Indeed, studies in patients with polycythemia vera provided important data in support of the theory of the clonal origin of many malignancies. The frequent evolution of polycythemia to myelofibrosis was similarly a goad to investigating the factors that regulate fibroblast proliferation and collagen metabolism within the marrow. Investigations of the delivery of oxygen to the tissues by its release from oxyhemoglobin, the recognition of hereditary high-affinity hemoglobins and of the alteration in the oxyhemoglobin dissociation curve in the presence of carbon monoxide generated by smoking, and the production of erythropoietin in renal cysts and in malignancies such as hepatocellular carcinoma, all these observations led to the construction of physiologically based, logical diagnostic algorithms for correctly classifying patients whose elevated hematocrits may, in fact, result from a myriad of causes. The increased cell turnover in polycythemia leads to hyperuricemia and gout, fostering both basic and clinical studies of this phenomenon. Rheologic studies defined the consequences of blood hyperviscosity when secondary to an elevated hematocrit, while the recognized propensity of polycythemia vera patients both to bleed and to clot greatly advanced studies of both hemostasis and coagulation.

As already implied, it is now recognized that polycythemia vera is a clonal malignancy of the hematopoietic stem-cell compartment. This has led to studies of its therapy with a variety of different classes of myelosuppressive agents, including ionizing radiation in the form of radioactive phosphorus (^{32}P), radiomimetic alkylating agents, and more recently, the nonalkylating marrow suppressant hydroxyurea. The relatively indolent nature of the malignancy in polycythemia vera, at least prior to the sporadic transformation to acute leukemia, has permitted uniquely long-term studies of the effects of these agents, providing striking new observations about the potential of both ionizing radiation and alkylating agents to induce malignant transformation in virtually all the rapidly proliferating tissues of the body: notably the bone marrow, the skin, and the mucosa of the gastrointestinal tract.

The Polycythemia Vera Study Group was organized in the mid-1960s by Louis R. Wasserman to include a group of hematologists with a particular interest in polycythemia vera and the other myeloproliferative disorders. Its expressed goals were to define the natural history of these conditions and determine their optimal therapies. The cooperative study group approach, in which patients at many different institutions were evaluated and treated according to standardized protocols, was adopted. This permitted the acquisition of data in sufficient numbers of cases of these relatively uncommon diseases to reach statistically valid conclusions within time frames that would never have been possible at a single institution. The group initially received support from Dr. Gordon Zubrod of the National Institutes of Health and continued to receive NIH support for more than 20 years, until 1987. Patient follow-up and data acquisition and analysis continue to the present day on some protocols, supported by privately raised funds. Over nearly three decades, the Polycythemia Vera Study Group and its individual members have contributed to virtually every major advance described above and many others. With many of its studies recently completed and with the cutting edge of research in the field passing from the cooperative clinical studies in which the group has excelled to studies of normal and malignant cellular proliferation at the molecular level, conducted by a new generation of investigators, it seemed an appropriate time to summarize the progress of the past three decades. The result is the collection of 23 chapters that follows. In these chapters the reader will find a summary of what is currently known about a fascinating spectrum of interrelated disorders by a unique group of recognized experts in the field, as well as indications of the directions new research must take to answer an entirely new and more fundamental set of questions.

PAUL D. BERK

NATHANIEL I. BERLIN

LOUIS R. WASSERMAN

CONTENTS

1

The Development, Morphology, and Function of Normal Bone Marrow: A Review

POWERS PETERSON *and* JOHN T. ELLIS

The bone marrow is the most widely dispersed and largest organ in the body. An understanding of this organ requires correlation of its embryologic development and function. Earlier studies made largely with conventional light microscopy have been greatly extended by application of new techniques to the study of hematopoietic cell structure and function in human beings and experimental animals, i.e., electron microscopy, immunologic and biochemical procedures, cytogenetics, autoradiography, clonal cultures, transplantation, and recombinant DNA technology.[1, 2] The bone marrow consists of both stromal and hematopoietic elements. We are beginning to understand the functional interrelations between the hematopoietic elements and the matrix that provides the microenvironment for replication, development, and maturation of the cells and their subsequent access to the bloodstream.

DEVELOPMENT

The production center for blood cells is the marrow, but the source of the most primitive ancestral cells involved in cell renewal remained in doubt until recently. Current evidence indicates that the pluripotential cell that gives rise to committed hematopoietic cells requires direct contact with the stromal matrix to survive and propagate.[3-9] In each developing bone, the sequence is the same; i.e., the matrix develops first and then colonization with hemopoietic cells follows. The hematopoietic cells develop from stem cells from the yolk sac, which then migrate via the peripheral blood to the fetal liver and spleen and then later move on to populate the bone marrow matrix. This originates from the perichondral embryonic mesenchyme and migrates into the marrow cavity, i.e., the microenvironment most favorable for growth of the cells. Here maturation of the blood elements occurs outside the vascular compartment, and cells enter the circulating blood through the thin-walled sinusoids which are a part of a closed system. Within the bone marrow, the hematopoietic cells constantly are renewed and then leave, while the stromal cells and vascular system serve as a permanent framework for the cellular proliferation.

Hemopoiesis begins in the extraembryonic mesoblastic tissue; stem cells then migrate via the bloodstream to the intraembryonic tissues. In humans, erythropoiesis is found in the yolk sac as early as the nineteenth day of gestation but decreases by the sixth week and then is found in the liver after 6 weeks, in the spleen by 12 weeks, and in the marrow by 20

1

weeks. Hematopoiesis decreases in the liver and spleen during the second half of intrauterine life while intramedullary blood cell formation progressively increases.[9–11]

At birth and for the first years of life the marrow is completely cellular. Fatty replacement of the active cellular marrow begins by birth in the toes and spreads gradually centripetally. In the adult, hematopoietic marrow is almost exclusively confined to the axial skeleton and the proximal ends of the femur and humerus.[12–14] It is semifluid to gelatinous and varies from yellow to red depending on the proportions of fat cells and active, cellular hematopoietic marrow. With greatly increased demand for blood, blood cell formation may occur in the spleen, liver, and lymph nodes (extramedullary hematopoiesis).

Much of the new morphologic data has come from studies of the marrow of the mouse, rabbit, and other animals. Presumably the marrow structure of humans bears a close resemblance to these experimental animals, but few comparative studies of well-preserved human marrow have been published. At this time, certain rather minor differences have been identified; i.e., human marrow has more trabecular bone and fat cells and the sinuses are thinner and larger.[15, 16]

BONE STRUCTURE

Several observations emphasize the close association of hemopoiesis and osteogenesis.[6–8] The stem cells for these two tissues were once thought to be different.[17, 18] Hemopoiesis in adults is limited to the bony skeleton, which provides a rigid confine for the marrow. There are many vascular connections between the marrow and surrounding bone. In autologous bone-free marrow transplants, the proliferating reticular cells give rise to a lattice of trabecular bone and reconstruct the marrow sinusoids prior to hematopoietic repopulation.[19, 20] After experimental evacuation of the marrow, hemopoietic regeneration is preceded by osteogenesis.[18] In various chronic myeloproliferative conditions, an abnormal hematopoietic clone may be associated with bony proliferation (osteomyelosclerosis) (Fig. 1–1A, B).

The marrow cavities contain hematopoietic tissue, fat, blood vessels, and nerves and are lined by endosteum. The endosteum is composed of reticular cells which cover the walls of the long bones and line the trabeculae of cancellous bone. These cells may develop into osteoblasts, osteoclasts, or osteocytes (Fig. 1–1C). The spongy bone is subdivided by cancellous trabeculae which form a delicate network and surround the hematopoietic marrow (Fig. 1–1D). The marrow has two major anatomic and physiologic compartments, i.e., the vascular and hematopoietic (see below).

VASCULAR COMPARTMENT

As shown in Figure 1–2, the marrow cavity contains an amazingly complicated vascular component.[21–23] The nutrient artery branches repeatedly into arterioles and arteriolar capillaries. The majority of the latter open into a plexus of thin-walled sinusoids that drain into collecting venules and veins. Note the direct connection between the arteriolar capillaries and the venous sinusoids to form a closed system. The vascular supplies of the bone marrow and bone are connected through communication between the endosteal and the periosteal capillaries. Observations in vivo have demonstrated a rhythmic dilatation and emptying of the sinusoids and passage of maturing erythrocytes through the wall via an aperture that closes after cell transit.[24–26] Lymphatic vessels are not present in the marrow. Myelinated and nonmyelinated nerves are found in the vessel walls.[27, 28]

The walls of the sinusoids may be somewhat difficult to define in conventionally stained sections (Figs. 1–3 and 1–7A) but are well demonstrated and have been studied extensively in animals by electron microscopy (Figs. 1–4 through 1–6). Note particularly that the hematopoietic cords are in intimate contact with the sinusoids (Fig. 1–5). With transmission electron microscopy (TEM), the sinus wall has been shown to consist of a thin continuous endothelial layer and a discontinuous adventitial reticular layer. These are separated by an indistinct basal lamina (Fig. 1–6A). The endothelial cells and (to a lesser degree) the macrophages and reticular cells have endocytic functions. Particulate matter is taken up through large bristle-coated pits.[29, 30]

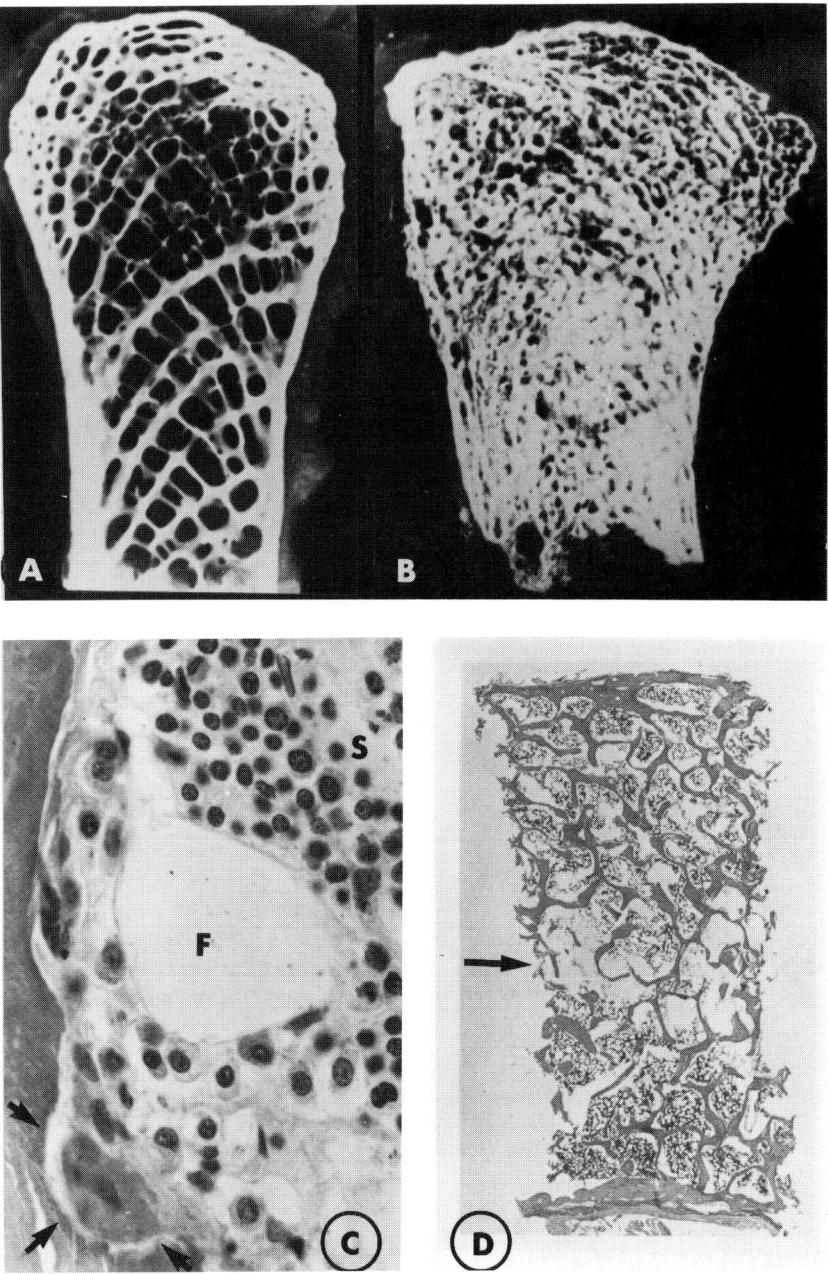

FIGURE 1-1. *A.* Roentgenogram of a coronal section of normal human ileal bone. Note variation in thickness of cortical bone and the cancellous bone density. Marrow cavity is divided by delicate bony trabeculae. (Courtesy of P. G. Bullough, M.D.) *B.* Roentgenogram of a coronal section of ileal bone from a patient with osteomyelosclerosis (myeloid metaplasia). Note the disorganized pattern of the cancellous bone, which also shows increased density due to the formation of reactive bone in the fibrotic marrow cavity. (Courtesy of P. G. Bullough, M.D.) *C.* Photomicrograph of normal, undecalcified human bone marrow embedded in methyl methacrylate. The bony trabecula is lined by osteoblasts and osteoclasts. The surface of the bone trabecula is somewhat irregular and in the lower left is a Howship's lacuna (*arrows*) containing a multinucleate osteoclast. Adjacent marrow contains mainly erythroid islands (*S,* sinusoid; *F,* fat cell) (hematoxylin and eosin stain; × 600). *D.* Low-power photomicrograph of a full-thickness, cortex to cortex, human transileal biopsy. Note that marrow cavity is divided by delicate bony trabeculae which in general connect with each other. Center of bone stains lighter due to increased fat content of marrow (*arrow*). (*From Bullough PG, Vigorita VJ: Atlas of Orthopaedic Pathology with Clinical and Radiographic Correlations, New York, Gower Medical Publishing Ltd, 1984, p. 2, 3. Reproduced with permission.*)

THE MARROW STROMA
AND MICROENVIRONMENT

Many lines of evidence indicate that in the adult the marrow stroma provides a unique, permissive, anatomic, and physiologic envi-

ronment for the lodging of hematopoietic cells and controls their proliferation and differentiation.[4, 15, 31–35] The mechanism for communication between these intertwined cell systems is only now beginning to be elucidated. Morphologically, the microenviron-

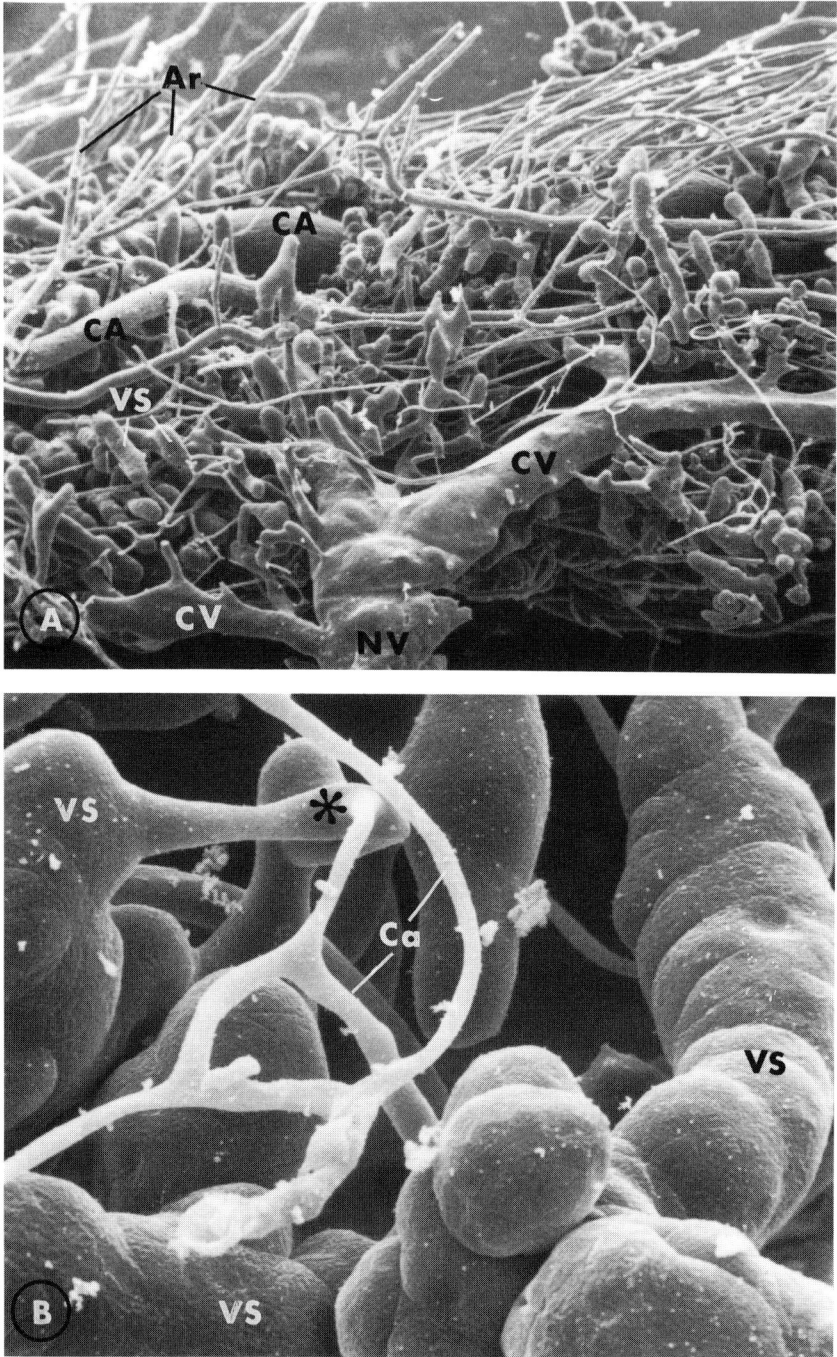

FIGURE 1-2. *See legend on opposite page*

ment includes all the nonhemopoietic elements, i.e., the blood vessel and endothelial cells, the reticular and fat cells, and the nerve tissue.

The hemopoietic cords have a scaffolding of stromal (reticular) cells best visualized by scanning or transmission electron microscopy and immunofluorescence.[33, 36–38] The reticular cells have large numbers of anastomizing cell processes which form a meshwork throughout the hematopoietic cords and on the surface of the sinusoids (Figs. 1–5 and 1–6). It has been estimated that three-fourths of the surface of the developing blood cell may be covered by the stromal cell processes.[36, 39] The reticular cells also produce collagen, which may be demonstrated by electron microscopy and immunologic techniques and may be stained by silver impregnation. The silver staining technique is now known to blacken a glycoprotein associated with the collagen and not the collagen itself.[40, 41] Normal bone marrow contains a fine incomplete network of reticulin fibers continuous with the fibers in the blood vessels, sinusoidal walls, and endosteum. This network serves not only as a framework for the developing hematopoietic cells but also as a binding site for some of the hematopoietic growth factors (HGFs). The HGFs will be discussed further in the following section.

The fat cells are thought to be adventitial reticular cells which have become distended by lipid, and they compose varying percentages of the marrow volume depending on age and the bone sampled.[33] In the adult, fat cells fill about 50 percent of the marrow cavities. Since the volume of the bone is fixed and the cavity is always completely filled, the fatty, inactive marrow is greater near the center (Fig. 1–1D). When there is a change in hematopoietic activity (i.e., red to yellow), the marrow becomes gelatinous, probably due to an increase in water of the adventitial reticular cells.[42] It is interesting and perhaps significant that fat cells are not found when marrow is formed outside bone, i.e., extramedullary hematopoiesis. In long-term culture of human marrow cells, adipocytes are essential for hematopoiesis.[43] Endothelial cells from human umbilical cord produce substances which stimulate granulopoiesis.[44–46]

THE HEMATOPOIETIC CELLS

A totipotent stem cell is the precursor of the cell lines in the marrow.[3, 6–8] These cells lack a known morphology but are identified by other techniques. After irradiation of the bone marrow followed by intravenous injection of bone marrow in mice, discrete hematopoietic colonies, or colony-forming units (CFUs), are found within the spleen and marrow.[47, 48] These colonies of either erythroid or granulocytic or megakaryocytic cells probably develop from a single stem cell.

Hematopoiesis, whether self-renewal of the pluripotential stem cell or differentiation to a specific lineage, requires coordination.[6, 49–52] Cytokines, proteins released by one cell to transmit information to another cell, regulate this complex process and in-

FIGURE 1–2. Scanning electron micrographs (SEM) of the circulation in rat bone marrow. Vascular casts demonstrate the general pattern of circulation present in the bone marrow. The tissue was digested away with a strong alkaline solution, leaving only a polymerized replica of the blood vessels. The arteries are easily distinguished from the veins by the presence of small fusiform depressions on the surface of the cast that correspond to the impressions left by the endothelial cells. Moreover, the arteries are more regular in diameter along their length. These distinguishing features have been observed in casts of every organ of the body that has been prepared for study. The nutrient artery enters the marrow after penetrating the shaft of the bone, and branches to form central arteries (CA) that follow a longitudinal course through the marrow of long bones. The two central arteries near the left in part A originated from a larger nutrient artery. The central arteries give rise to long straight arterioles (Ar) that are much narrower. The arterioles terminate as slender arteriolar capillaries that supply the venous sinuses (VS). In part B, the continuity between an arteriolar capillary and a venous sinus can be observed (*). At the periphery of the marrow, the venous sinuses are supplied by arteriolar capillaries (Ca) originating from haversian arteries that course through the osseous shaft of the bone. The sinusoids anastomose extensively with one another and are highly variable in diameter. They drain into central veins (CV in part A). The central veins converge into a large nutrient vein (NV in part A) that exits the marrow (A, × 80; B, × 700). (From Kessel RG, Kardon RH: Tissues and Organs: A Text-Atlas of Scanning Electron Microscopy, San Francisco, WH Freeman, 1979, p 48. Reproduced with permission.)

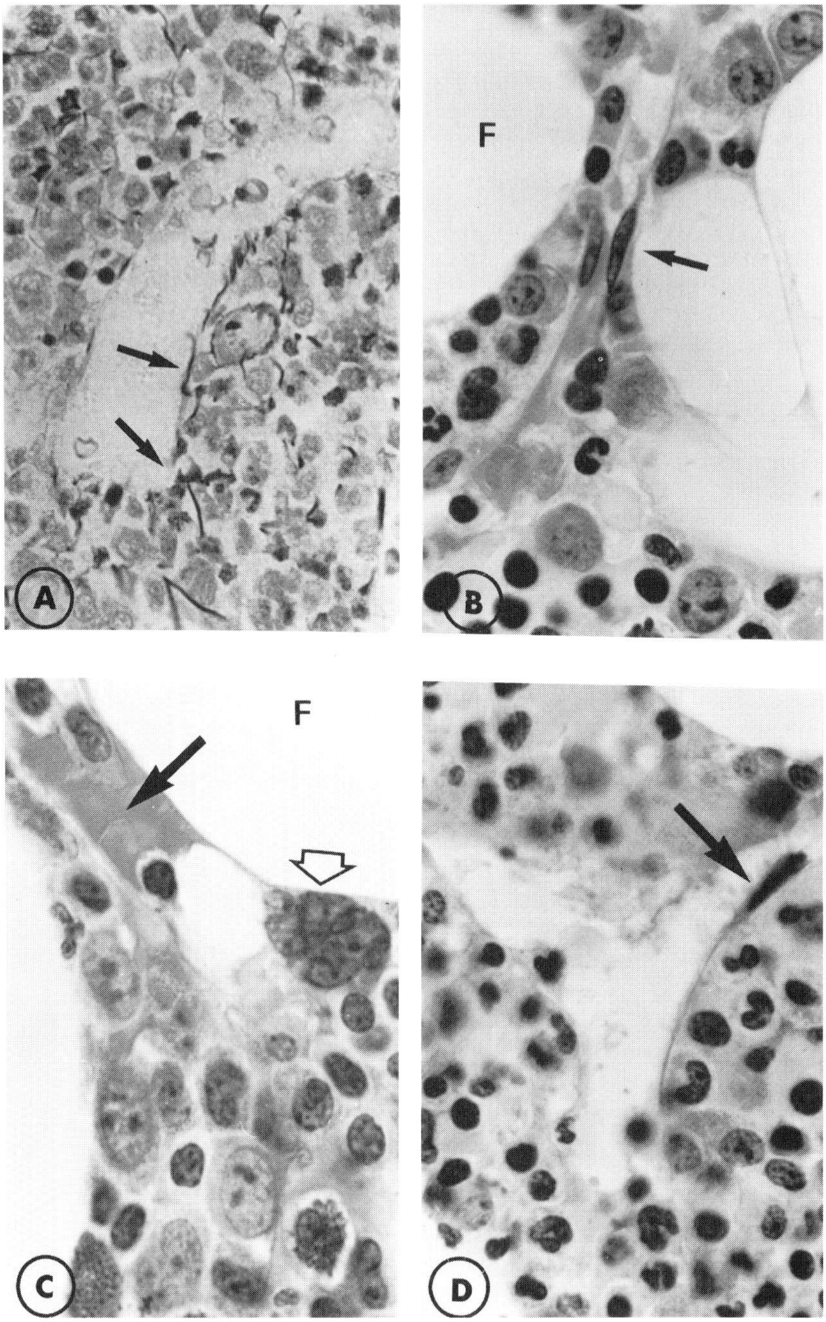

FIGURE 1–3. Photomicrograph of normal human bone marrow. *A*. Fine argyrophilic (*black*) fibers partially outline sinusoidal wall and extend into the adjacent hematopoietic cord (*arrows*) (Foot & Foot silver stain; × 1200). *B*. Thin arteriolar capillary with two endothelial lining cells (*arrow*). Adjacent stroma contains large myelocytes and smaller, dark normoblasts (*F*, fat cell) (hematoxylin and eosin stain; × 1000). *C*. Thin-walled sinusoid (*closed arrow*). A pyknotic megakaryocyte (*open arrow*) abuts the wall of the sinusoid. Adjacent hematopoietic cord contains several large myelocytes (*F*, fat cell) (hematoxylin and eosin stain; × 1200). *D*. Branching sinusoid surrounded by developing marrow cells. Endothelial cell (*arrow*) (hematoxylin and eosin stain; × 800).

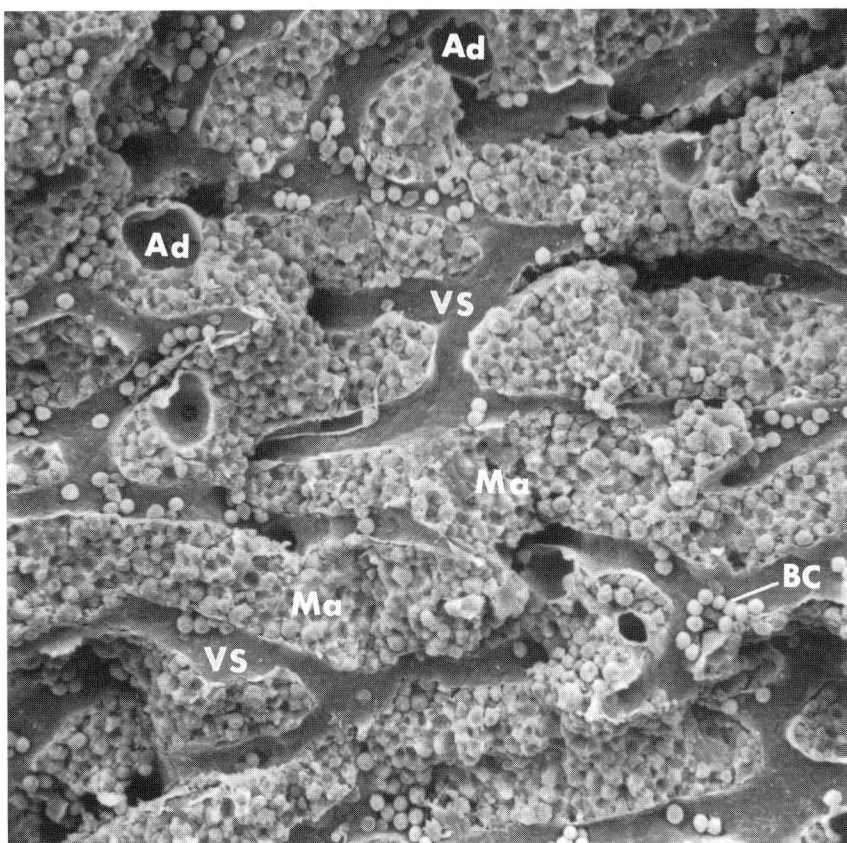

FIGURE 1–4. The bone marrow consists of differentiating blood cells, reticular cells and fibers, many endothelial-lined sinusoids, and fat cells, or adipocytes (*Ad*). This scanning electron micrograph (SEM) of rat marrow was taken after the femur was fractured to expose the marrow shown here. The developing cells of the marrow (*Ma*) are seen to be closely packed in the hematopoietic cords. Networks of channels called venous sinuses (*VS*), or sinusoids, traverse the marrow. In the living state, blood with mature blood cells (*BC*) flows through the sinuses and is segregated from the surrounding immature blood cells of the marrow by endothelial cells of the sinusoidal wall. (From Kessel RG, Kardon RH: Tissue and Organs: A Text-Atlas of Scanning Electron Microscopy, San Francisco, WH Freeman, 1979, p. 46. Reproduced with permission.)

clude the HGFs. HGFs "control" the proliferation and differentiation of progenitor cells, affect a broad range of target cells, and are produced by numerous cell types of both hematopoietic and nonhematopoietic origin.[35, 51, 52] Table 1–1 lists some of the known cytokines and their effects on marrow cells and their progeny.

Two families of HGFs are the colony-stimulating factors (CSFs) and the interleukins (ILs). CSFs are produced by fibroblasts, endothelial cells, stromal cells, macrophages, and lymphocytes. Their primary function is to maintain the marrow's cell populations by stimulating and sustaining hematopoietic cell proliferation. They also induce commitment to differentiation. ILs are multifunc-

tional cytokines that act within the lympho-hematopoietic system. Their actions include mimicking the functions of CSFs (e.g., IL-3 and IL-6).[53–56]

In addition to these two families of glycoproteins, there are other cytokines whose functions are often more inhibitory than permissive. These include tumor necrosis factor (TNF), transforming growth factor β (TGF-β), macrophage inflammatory protein 1α (MIF-1α), and the interferons (IFNs). IFNs are glycoproteins produced in response to viral infection.[57] The acid-stable group includes the α and β IFNs; the acid-labile group includes the γ IFNs. IFN-α is also known as *leukocyte IFN*, IFN-β as *fibroblast IFN*, and IFN-γ as *immune IFN*. All

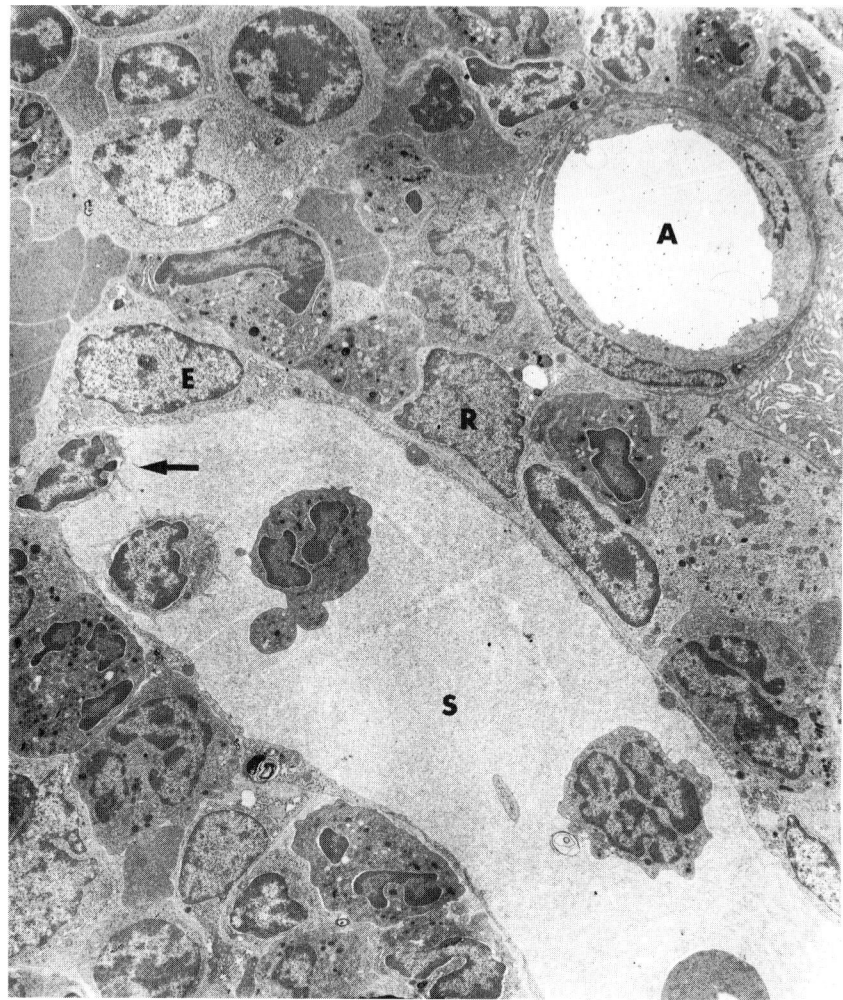

FIGURE 1–5. Transmission electron micrograph (TEM) of a venous sinus (sinusoid) of rat bone marrow. The endothelial lining is in several places extremely attenuated but remains continuous. A blood cell is seen in passage through the endothelium (*arrow*) (*R*, adventitial reticular cell; *A*, arteriole; *E*, endothelial cell; *S*, sinusoid). (From De Bruyn PHH: Semin Hematol 18:180, 1981. Reproduced with permission.)

exhibit potent effects (stimulatory and inhibitory) with many different cells within the lymphohematopoietic system.

A newer category of cytokines includes the genetically engineered fusion proteins. An example is PIXY 321, a fusion of granulocyte-macrophage CSF and IL-3.[58] At the marrow level, PIXY 321 enhances cycling of multipotential CFU-granulocyte-erythroid-macrophage-monocyte (GFU-GEMM) cells.[59]

The hematopoietic cords in human beings have localized areas of proliferation of the various cell lines, but this may be difficult to appreciate in routine sections. Mega-karyopoiesis usually occurs adjacent to the sinusoidal wall, erythropoiesis occurs in islands, and granulopoiesis occurs in less well defined foci[60] (Fig. 1–7). Perhaps these are similar to the hematopoietic colonies found in experimental animals that were irradiated and given intravenous injections of bone marrow. Lymphocytes are usually found in small nodules.[61] Macrophages are located along the sinusoidal wall and in the center of the erythroblastic islands. Plasma cells are located along capillary walls, consistent with their origin from adventitial reticular cells; fat cells often are parasinal.

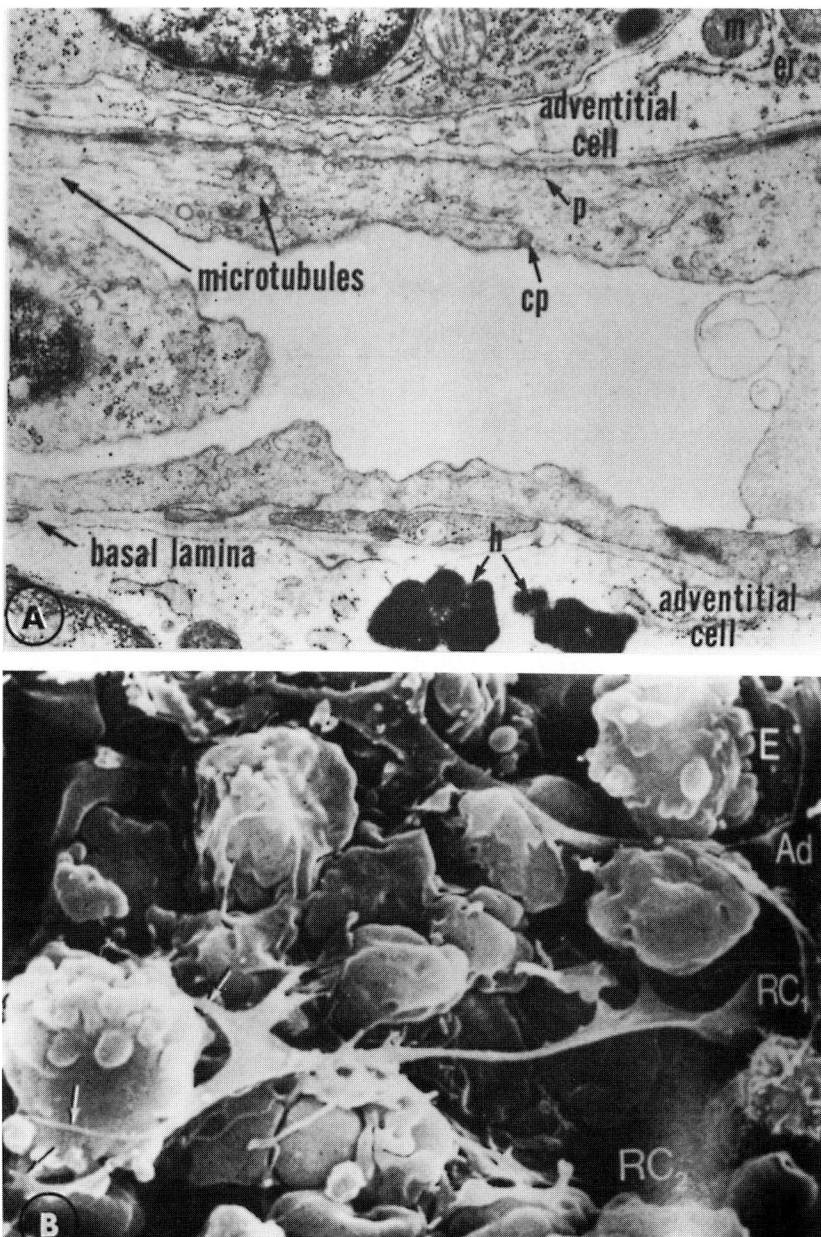

FIGURE 1-6. A. Transmission electron micrograph (TEM) of mouse marrow to show sinusoidal adventitial cells, basal lamina, and endothelial lining cells. The adventitial reticular cells contain mitochondria (*m*), rough surfaced endoplasmic reticulum (*er*), and hemosiderin (*h*). The nucleus (*N*), microtubules, coated pits (*cp*), and uncoated pits (*p*) of the endothelial lining cell are illustrated ($\times$ 20,500). (From Campbell FR: Am J Anat 135:527, 1972. Reproduced with permission.) B. Scanning electron micrograph (SEM) of rat bone marrow. A sinus runs vertically along the right margin, its outside surface on view. The basal endothelial surface (*E*) is exposed in places. Elsewhere reticular cells in an adventitial position on the wall (*AD*) are present and branch into the surrounding hematopoietic cords. Several other reticular cells are present. RC_1 extends from the sinus wall and branches across the cord, tightly enclosing a myelocyte (*arrows*) on the left. A third cell (RC_2) is in the background ($\times$ 4275). (From Weiss L: Anat Rec 186:180, 1976. Reproduced with permission.)

TABLE 1–1. HEMATOPOIETIC CYTOKINES: EFFECTS ON MARROW CELLS
AND THEIR PROGENY

	Factors Involved with Cycling of Progenitors
IL-1α, β	Pleiotropic; synergistic with IL-3, G-CSF
IL-3	Multipotent for early erythroid, G-M, megakaryocyte progenitors
IL-4	Enhance/suppress multilineage colony formation by progenitors
IL-6	Pleiotropic; synergistic with IL-3
IL-11	Synergistic with IL-3 in megakaryocyte colony formation
IL-12	Synergistic with IL-3
G-CSF	Synergistic with IL-3 to trigger proliferation of cell cycle
	Lineage-Nonspecific Factors
IL-3	Proliferation of multipotential progenitors; mast cell growth factor
IL-4	Proliferation of multipotential progenitors: mast cells, erythroid cells, granulocytes, megakaryocytes
IL-6	Potentiates stimulatory activity of multilineage GFs; influences differentiation of T and B cells
GM-CSF	Interacts with late-acting GFs in production of PMNs, eosinophils, and GFs that initiate cycling of dormant progenitor populations
kit ligand	Potentiates stimulatory activity of multilineage GFs
	Lineage-Specific Factors
IL-1	Megakaryopoiesis, platelet production; activation of T- and B-cell precursors; lymphocyte proliferation
IL-3	Megakaryopoiesis, platelet production
IL-5	Proliferation, maturation of eosinophil progenitors
IL-6	Megakaryopoiesis; growth, differentiation of T and B cells
IL-9	Megakaryocyte proliferation; early erythroid
IL-11	Megakaryopoiesis, platelet production
IL-13	Differentiation of macrophages
G-CSF	Proliferation, maturation of neutrophil progenitors
M-CSF	Proliferation, maturation of monocyte/macrophage progenitors
GM-CSF	Megakaryopoiesis, platelet production
EPO	Later-stage erythropoiesis
LIF	Megakaryopoiesis, platelet production
bFGF	Megakaryopoiesis, platelet production
	Inhibitory Cytokines
IFN-α	Lineage nonspecific; antiproliferative throughout range
TNF-α	Lineage nonspecific; cytotoxic for many cells
TGF-β	Inhibition of early progenitors
MIP-1α	Antagonizes early acting cytokines

Note: IL, interleukin; G, granulocyte; CSF, colony-stimulating factor; M, monocyte; EPO, erythropoietin; LIF, leukemia inhibitory factor; bFGF, basic fibroblast growth factor; IFN, interferon; TNF, tumor necrosis factor; TGF, transforming growth factor; MIP, macrophage inflammatory protein.
Source: Derived from refs. 1, 6, and 49–57.

Despite the marrow's large size and wide distribution, a single biopsy has been shown to be generally representative of the entire marrow if one discounts known variations in fat content.[62] Figure 1–1D illustrates a large biopsy of the posterior iliac crest, the most frequent biopsy site.

RELEASE OF BLOOD CELLS FROM THE MARROW

Much has been learned in recent years about how the vast numbers of the various hematopoietic cells that develop outside the vascular system gain access to the blood. The passage must be a remarkably selective one, since under normal conditions only mature cells enter the blood, while immature ones remain outside the vessels. The endothelium appears to be the morphologic basis for the selectivity of the marrow-blood barrier, but the regulatory mechanism is not clear at this time.

The movement of cells, proteins, hormones, etc. across the marrow-blood barrier is bidirectional. The exchange is thought to occur in the thin-walled vascular sinusoids which are lined by a single cell layer of continuous endothelium separated by a poorly defined ground substance from the discontinuous adventitial cell layer. (See Figs. 1–5

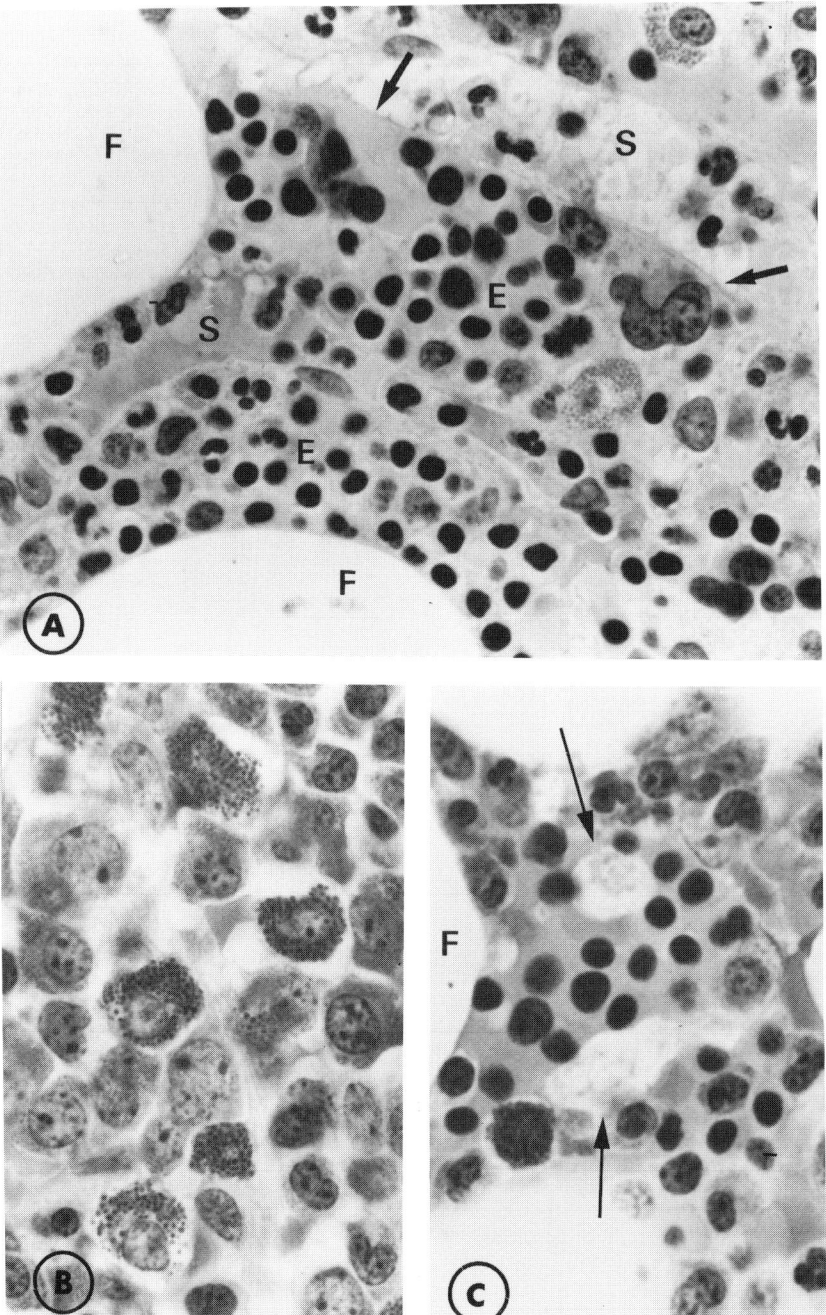

FIGURE 1-7. Photomicrograph of undecalcified human bone marrow. *A.* Two sinusoids (*S*) with adjacent hematopoietic cords. Note characteristic parasinusoidal location of megakaryocytes (*arrows*). Erythroid islands (*E*) are present (*F*, fat cell) (hematoxylin and eosin stain; × 900). *B.* Focus of granulopoiesis contains mainly eosinophilic and neutrophilic myelocytes (hematoxylin and eosin stain; × 900). *C.* Erythropoietic island containing mainly normoblasts. Note pale-staining cytoplasm of centrally located histiocytes (*arrows*) (*F*, fat cell) (hematoxylin and eosin stain; × 1000).

and 1–6). In rats and rabbits, from 30 to 60 percent of the external surface of the sinusoid is covered by adventitial reticular cell cytoplasm. The passage of cells (see Fig. 1–5) is thought to be transcellular (transendothelial) rather than intercellular, since there are no preformed pores and any new pore is closed after cellular transit.[34,63–65] Recent studies have shown that the apertures described by early workers were artifacts. Only cells that are deformable are capable of transit, and this is not the case with nucleated red cells, which normally lose their nuclei in transit.[66,67] The pores are usually 2 to 3 μm in diameter, but some must be of a size sufficient to allow passage of megakaryocytes (6 μm). The endothelial cells contain filaments which probably are related to the contraction of the sinusoids.

REFERENCES

1. Metcalf D: The Hemopoietic Colony Stimulating Factors. Amsterdam, Elsevier Biomedical, 1984
2. Tavassoli M, Yoffey JM: Bone Marrow Structure and Function. New York, Alan R Liss, 1983
3. Moore MAS, Metcalf D: Ontogeny of the haemopoietic system: Yolk sac origin of in vivo and in vitro colony forming cells in the developing mouse embryo. Br J Haematol 18:279–296, 1970
4. Fliedner TM, Calvo W: Hematopoietic stem-cell seeding of a cellular matrix: A principle of initiation and regeneration of hematopoiesis. In Clarkson B, Marks PA, Till JE (eds): Differentiation of Normal and Neoplastic Hematopoietic Cells, book B. Cold Spring Harbor, NY, Cold Spring Harbor Laboratory, 1978, pp 757–773
5. Weissman I, Papaioannou V, Gardner R: Fetal hematopoietic origins of the adult hematolymphoid system. In Clarkson B, Marks PA, Till JE (eds): Differentiation of Normal and Neoplastic Hematopoietic Cells, book A. Cold Spring Harbor, NY, Cold Spring Harbor Laboratory, 1978, pp 33–47
6. Eaves CJ, Eaves AC: Fundamental control of hematopoiesis. In Fisher JW (ed): Biochemical Pharmacology of Blood and Blood-Forming Organs. Berlin, Springer-Verlag, 1992, pp 5–32
7. Dexter TM, Spooncer E: Growth and differentiation in the hemopoietic system. Annu Rev Cell Biol 3:423–441, 1987
8. Campbell AD, Wicha MS: Extracellular matrix and the hematopoietic microenvironment. J Lab Clin Med 112:140–146, 1988
9. Zamboni L: Electron microscopic studies of blood embryogenesis in humans: II. The hemopoietic activity in the fetal liver. J Ultrastruct Res 12:525–541, 1965
10. Bloom W, Bartelmez, GW: Hematopoiesis in young human embryos. Am J Anat 67:21–44, 1940
11. Chen L-T, Weiss L: The development of vertebral bone marrow of human fetuses. Blood 46:389–408, 1975
12. Emery JL, Follett GF: Regression of bone-marrow haemopoiesis from the terminal digits in the foetus and infant. Br J Haematol 10:485–489, 1964
13. Piney A: The anatomy of the bone marrow: With special reference to the distribution of the red marrow. Br Med J 2:792–795, 1922
14. Russell WJ, Yoshinaga H, Antoku S, et al: Active bone marrow distribution in the adult. Br J Radiol 39:735–739, 1966
15. Lichtman MA: The ultrastructure of the hemopoietic environment of the marrow: A review. Exp Hematol 9:391–410, 1981
16. Samson JP, Hulstaert CE, Molenaar I, et al: Fine structure of the bone marrow sinusoidal wall in idiopathic and drug-induced panmyelopathy. Acta Haematol 48:218–226, 1972
17. Amsel S, Dell ES: Bone formation by hemopoietic tissue: Separation of preosteoblast from hemopoietic stem cell function in the rat. Blood 39:267–273, 1972
18. Tavassoli M, Khademi R: The origin of hemopoietic cells in ectopic implants of spleen and marrow. Experientia 36:1126–1127, 1980
19. Tavassoli J, Crosby WH: Transplantation of marrow to extramedullary sites. Science 161:54–56, 1968
20. Tavassoli M, Crosby WH: Bone marrow histogenesis: A comparison of fatty and red marrow. Science 17:291–293, 1970
21. De Bruyn P, Breen PC, Thomas TB: The microcirculation of the bone marrow. Anat Rec 168:55–63, 1970
22. Kessel RG, Kardon RH: Tissues and Organs: A Text-Atlas of Scanning Electron Microscopy. San Francisco, WH Freeman, 1979, pp 46–50
23. Zamboni L, Pease DC: The vascular bed of red bone marrow. J Ultrastruct Res 5:65–85, 1961
24. Bronemark P-I: Bone marrow microvascular structure and function. Adv Microcirc 1:1–65, 1968
25. Bronemark P-I: Vital microscopy of bone marrow in rabbit. Scand J Clin Lab Invest 11(suppl 38):1–82, 1959
26. Kinosita R, Ohno S: Studies on bone marrow biodynamics: Observations on microcirculation in rabbit bone marrow in situ. Bibl Anat 1:106–109, 1960
27. Miller MR, Kasahara M: Observations on the innervation of human long bones. Anat Rec 145:13–23, 1963
28. Miller ML, McCuskey RS: Innervation of bone marrow in the rabbit. Scand J Haematol 10:17–23, 1973
29. De Bruyn PPH, Michelson S, Becker RP: Endocytosis, transfer tubules, and lysosomal activity in myeloid sinusoidal endothelium. J Ultrastruct Res 53:133–151, 1975
30. Hudson G, Yoffey JM: Ultrastructure of reticuloendothelial elements in guinea-pig bone marrow. J Anat 103:515–525, 1968
31. Bentley SA: Bone marrow connective tissue and the haemopoietic microenvironment. Br J Haematol 50:1–6, 1982
32. Trenton JJ: Hemopoietic microenvironments. Transplant Proc 10:77–82, 1978

33. Weiss L: The hemopoietic microenvironment of the bone marrow: An ultrastructural study of the stroma in rats. Anat Rev 186:162–184, 1976

34. De Bruyn PPH: Structural substrates of bone marrow function. Semin Hematol 18:179–193, 1981

35. Metcalf D: The Molecular Control of Blood Cells. Cambridge, MA, Harvard University Press, 1988, pp 19–25

36. Shaklai M, Tavassoli M: Cellular relationship in the rat bone marrow studied by freeze fracture and lanthanum impregnation thin-sectioning electron microscopy. J Ultrastruct Res 69:343–361, 1979

37. Bentley SA, Foidard J-M, Kleinman HK: Connective tissue elements in rat bone marrow: Immunofluorescent visualization of the hematopoietic microenvironment. J Histochem Cytochem 32:114–116, 1984.

38. Bentley SA, Alabaster O, Foidart J-M: Collagen heterogeneity in normal human bone marrow. Br J Haematol 48:287–291, 1982

39. Tavassoli M, Yoffey JM: Bone Marrow Structure and Function. New York, Alan R Liss, 1983, p 60

40. Irvin EA, Tomlin SG: Collagen, reticulum and their argyrophilic properties. Proc R Soc Lond (Biol) 142:113–125, 1954

41. Tomlin SG: Reticulin and collagen (letter). Nature 171:302, 1953

42. Tavassoli M, Eastlund DT, Yam LT, et al: Gelatinous transformation of bone marrow in prolonged self-induced starvation. Scand J Haematol 16:311–319, 1976

43. Gartner S, Kaplan HS: Long-term culture of human bone marrow cells. Proc Natl Acad Sci USA 77:4756–4759, 1980

44. Knudtzon S. Mortensen BT: Growth stimulation of human bone marrow cells in agar culture by vascular cells. Blood 46:937–943, 1975

45. Quesenberry PJ, Gimbrone MA, McDonald MJ: Endothelial derived colony-stimulating activity. Exp Hematol 6:4a, 1978

46. Brennan JK, Lichtman MA, DiPersio JF, et al: Chemical mediators of granulopoiesis: A review. Exp Hematol 8:441–464, 1980

47. Till JE, McCulloch EA: A direct measurement of the radiation sensitivity of normal mouse bone marrow cells. Radiat Res 14:213–222, 1961

48. Calvo W, Fliedner TM, Herbst E, et al: Regeneration of blood-forming organs after autologous leukocyte transfusion in lethally irradiated dogs: II. Distribution and cellularity of the marrow in irradiated and transfused animals. Blood 47:593–601, 1976

49. Clark S, Kamen R: The human hematopoietic colony stimulating factors. Science 236:1229–1238, 1987

50. Metcalf D: The molecular control of cell division, differentiation, commitment and maturation in hematopoietic cells. Nature 339:27–30, 1989

51. Ogawa M: Differentiation and proliferation of hematopoietic stem cells. Blood 81:2844–2853, 1993

52. Testa U, Pelosi E, Gabbianelli M, et al: Cascade transactivation of growth factor receptors in early human hematopoiesis. Blood 81:1442–1456, 1993

53. Ishibashi T, Kimura H, Uchida T, et al: Human interleukin 6 is a direct promoter of maturation of megakaryocytes in vitro. Proc Natl Acad Sci USA 86:5953–5957, 1989

54. Asano S, Okano A, Ozawa K, et al: In vivo effects of recombinant human interleukin 6 in primates: Stimulated production of platelets. Blood 75:1602–1605, 1990

55. Bruno E, Cooper RJ, Wilson EL, et al: Basic fibroblast growth factor promotes the proliferation of human megakaryocyte progenitor cells. Blood 82:430–435, 1993

56. McKenzie ANJ, Culpepper JA, deWaal Malefyt R, et al: Interleukin 13, a T-cell derived cytokine that regulates human monocyte and B-cell function. Proc Natl Acad Sci USA 90:3735–3739, 1993

57. Pestka S, Langer JA, Zoon KC, Samuel CE: Interferons and their actions. Annu Rev Biochem 56:727–777, 1987

58. Williams DE, Park LS: Hematopoietic effects of a granulocyte-macrophage colony-stimulating factor/interleukin 3 fusion protein. Cancer 67 (suppl):27705–27707, 1991

59. Broxmeyer HE, Benninger L, Cooper S, et al: Effects of treatment of patients with sarcoma with PIXY 321 (a genetically engineered fusion protein) on proliferation kinetics of bone marrow and blood myeloid progenitor cells. Blood 80:87a, 1992

60. Mohandas N, Prenant M: Three-dimensional model of bone marrow. Blood 51:633–643, 1978

61. Rywlin AM, Ortega RS, Dominguez CJ: Lymphoid nodules of bone marrow: Normal and abnormal. Blood 43:389–400, 1974

62. Bartl R, Frisch B, Burkhardt R: Bone Marrow Biopsies Revisited: A New Dimension for Haematologic Malignancies. Basel, Karger, 1982, pp 9–13

63. Tavassoli M: The marrow-blood barrier. Br J Haematol 41:297–302, 1979

64. Aoki M, Tavassoli M: Dynamics of red cell egress from bone marrow after blood letting. Br J Haematol 49:337–347, 1981

65. Tavassoli M, Yoffey JM: Bone Marrow Structure and Function. New York, Alan R Liss, 1983, pp 85–104

66. Lichtman M, Weed RI: Alteration of the cell periphery during granulocyte maturation: Relationship to cell function. Blood 39:301–316, 1972

67. Lichtman M, Chamberlain JK, Simon W, et al: Parasinusoidal location of megakaryocytes in marrow: A determinant of platelet release. Am J Hematol 4:303–312, 1978

ACKNOWLEDGMENTS: The authors gratefully acknowledge the expert technical assistance of Mr. Emilio Campo.

2

The Natural History
of Polycythemia Vera

POWERS PETERSON *and* LOUIS R. WASSERMAN

HISTORY OF POLYCYTHEMIA VERA

Polycythemia vera (PV) has been known since antiquity; Hippocrates noted "plethora vera."[1] Yet it was centuries later before Von Haller recognized the increase in the red cells; he perhaps was the first to associate thrombosis with gangrene as a frequent occurrence in polycythemia.[2] Not until approximately one hundred years ago, however, did PV enter the medical literature. In 1892, Vaquez described PV as an autonomous erythrocytosis.[3] Nine years later, Sir William Osler eloquently delineated PV as a specific disease, one in which the "clinical picture is very distinctive, the symptoms somewhat indefinite, and the pathology quite obscure."[4] Neither Vaquez nor Osler, however, recognized PV as more than an erythrocytosis; both failed to recognize the truly generalized nature of the myeloproliferation, as evidenced by concomitant hyperplasia of both the granulocytic and megakaryocytic lines. The following year Turk noted the peculiar peripheral blood picture that accompanies the extramedullary hematopoiesis in PV.[5] Slightly over 30 years later, Hirsch described the marrow fibrosis and sclerosis that may occur in later-stage PV.[6] Rosenthal and Bassen's 1938 paper reviewed the natural history and course of PV. Stating that "primary polycythemia is remarkable chiefly for its chronicity and the unusual variations which occur in its course and terminal phases,"[7] they divided the disease into the asymptomatic phase, followed by the polycythemic, or symptomatic, phase. The highly variable final phase they termed the anemic, or spent, phase, and they specifically recognized that acute leukemic and fibrotic terminations occurred. The seriousness of this disorder is emphasized by the fact that a symptomatic patient with untreated PV historically had a median life expectancy of 6 to 18 months from diagnosis.[8]

Although radiation therapy had been in clinical use since the early part of the twentieth century, Lawrence introduced radioactive phosphorus (^{32}P) in 1938 as an effective treatment modality, adding an easily administered, highly effective drug to the limited armamentarium.[9] Since radiation leukemogenesis was well documented,[10, 11] this inevitably led to questions regarding the development of acute leukemia (AL) in irradiated PV patients.[12–18] The debate centered around the question of a therapy-induced process versus an additional manifestation resulting from a previously unattainable, prolonged survival.

The introduction of a number of chemotherapeutic agents [nitrogen mustard, thiotriethylenephosphoramide (Thiotepa), busulfan (Myleran), chlorambucil (Leukeran), cyclophosphamide (Cytoxan), melphalan (Alkeran)] in the following decades offered alternatives to either phlebotomy or radiation therapy with what was initially thought to be a much lower risk of AL. In addition, these agents had the added advantages over phlebotomy of controlling not only the erythrocytosis but also the thrombocytosis, leukocytosis, and spleen size.[19]

Thirty years after PV's initial description in the literature, Minot and Buckman[20] recognized the "intimate" relation between PV and chronic myelogenous leukemia (CML) as "varying degrees of primary pathological activity of the myeloid tissue." Their conceptual advance was that of a shared origin in disordered growth of the hematopoietic precursor cell. What separated PV from CML was the predominant cell line, which in PV was the red cell. Nearly thirty years later, Rosenthal[21] expanded this concept to include thrombocytosis and some leukemias. It was Dameshek,[22] however, who stated the unified theory as we know it today, classifying PV as one of a group of related hematopoietic syndromes, the myeloproliferative disorders (MPDs). His initial schema also included chronic granulocytic leukemia, idiopathic myeloid metaplasia of the spleen, megakaryocytic leukemia, and erythroleukemia. Osgood[23] and Ward and Block[24] interpreted PV as benign. Others—notably Minot and Buckman[20] and Wasserman[13,25]—disagreed, favoring interpretation as a neoplastic process.

The experiments of Adamson and colleagues[26] nearly a quarter century later resolved the question of a benign versus malignant cellular proliferation. Their studies of two black female patients with PV who also were heterozygous for the enzyme glucose-6-phosphate dehydrogenase (G6PD) confirmed the clonal, or unicellular, nature of PV. Confirmation of these data has included cytogenetic analyses and clonogenic assays. The presumed neoplastic clonal cell is the multi- or pleuripotential stem cell.

Now recognized as a stem-cell disorder, PV is a panhyperplastic, malignant, and neoplastic marrow disorder. The *sine qua non* of the diagnosis is an absolute increase in the red cell mass, a result of increased production of red blood cells. Among the now discarded theories of the pathogenesis of PV were the proliferation of normal stem cells in response to some abnormal stimulus[27,28] and increased sensitivity of the marrow cells to normal regulatory factors, i.e., erythropoietin.[29] Normal stem cells are present in patients with PV, and the relationship of the normal stem cells to the clonal stem cells in PV is interesting. Erythroid colony-forming units (CFU-E) in marrow cell culture will form without exogenous erythropoietin in patients with PV,[30,31] whereas marrow cell cultures from normal patients require the addition of an exogenous erythopoietin for CFU-E formation.[32] Presumably the growth and proliferation of the normal stem cells are either suppressed or interfered with by the PV clone. Available evidence indicates that an unregulated neoplastic proliferation is the etiology of the panmyelosis. Still unanswered, however, is the question of what accounts for the malignant transformation.

CLINICAL FEATURES

PV is a relatively rare disorder with an estimated annual incidence rate of 0.6 to 1.6 per 1 million population.[33-35] It has no sex predilection, although there are slightly more males than females in most studies. Although some investigators originally thought there were ethnic predilections, specifically Jewish, many studies have documented that this is not the case. Indeed, PV occurs in all populations. Its peak incidence is in persons aged 50 to 70 years, but it occurs in all age groups, including early adulthood and (rarely) childhood.

The symptomatology varies considerably, depending on the stage of the disease and other factors, and the diagnosis may be confused with other erythematous conditions, specifically secondary and relative polycythemias. In a fully developed case, there is little difficulty in making the diagnosis. The accepted diagnostic criteria are given in Table 2–1.[36] Figure 2–1 graphically charts the course of PV, as discussed below.

The onset is insidious, and symptoms frequently precede a diagnosis of PV by several years. Accordingly, the duration of the *developmental* phase is not precise. Asymptomatic patients may have only an elevated hemoglobin level, hepatosplenomegaly, or thrombocytosis as an indicator of the latent PV. At this stage, the marrow is presumably hypercellular, but the typical red cell mass elevation is not yet present.

The *erythrocytotic* phase may be either symptomatic or asymptomatic. It ranges from 5 to 20 years in duration and is characterized by obvious panmyelosis, an increased red cell mass, and an expanded blood volume. Symptoms include headaches, dizziness, tinnitus, visual disturbances, erythro-

TABLE 2-1. DIAGNOSTIC CRITERIA FOR POLYCYTHEMIA VERA

Category A:	A1.	Increased red cell mass: males ≥ 36 ml/kg, females ≥ 32 ml/kg
	A2.	Normal arterial oxygen saturation: ≥ 92 percent
	A3.	Splenomegaly
Category B:	B1.	Thrombocytosis: platelets ≥ 400,000/μl
	B2.	Leukocytosis: white cell count ≥ 12,000/μl (in the absence of fever or infection)
	B3.	Elevated leukocyte alkaline phosphatase score: >100 in the absence of fever or infection
	B4.	Elevated serum B_{12} or unbound B_{12}-binding capacity: B_{12} > 900 pg/ml; $UB_{12}BC$ > 2200 pg/ml.

Source: Adapted from Berlin NI, Semin Hematol 12:342, 1975; reproduced with permission.

melalgia, paresthesias, pruritus, intermittent claudication, gout, and peptic ulcer. These largely reflect the excess hematopoietic cell production with hyperviscosity, resulting in tissue hypoxia. In addition, hemorrhagic and thrombotic events (epistaxis, gastrointestinal hemorrhage, myocardial and cerebral infarcts, mesenteric insufficiency, venous thromboembolism[37]) are very common.

With time, hematopoietic activity wanes, the red cell mass and volume stabilize, and the patient is said to have entered the *stable*, or *spent*, phase. Also known as *postpolycythemic myeloid metaplasia* (PPMM), this stage is characterized by varying degrees of anemia, leukopenia, and thrombocytopenia and a leukoerythroblastic peripheral blood picture.[38] Blood cell production shifts to extramedullary sites, the marrow becomes progressively

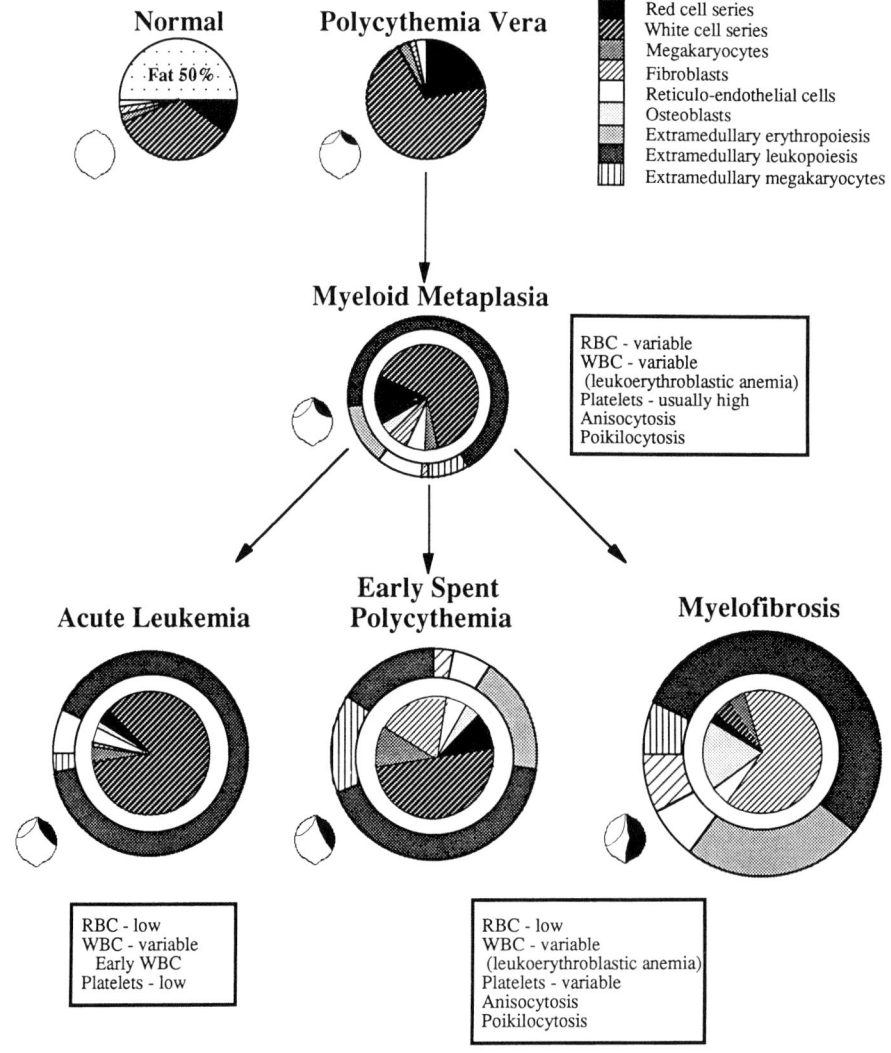

FIGURE 2-1. *See legend on opposite page*

fibrotic, and hepatosplenomegaly becomes massive and more problematic. Estimates of the number of patients with this complication range from between 6 and 15 to 20 percent.[16, 39–41] The true incidence of PPMM has been difficult to ascertain because of variations in diagnostic criteria, in length of patient survival, in associated therapy, and in patient follow-up. More important, however, has been the lack of controlled studies.

As mentioned earlier, similar difficulties confounded attempts to ascertain the relationship of therapy to the evolution into AL, which was invariably fatal. The problem of elucidating the complications of differing therapeutic modalities reflected in part the difficulty in comparing patients with variable criteria for the diagnosis of both PV and AL. Furthermore, comparable groups of patients had not been treated by different methods. Lastly, "it was impossible to establish from any previous reports the true incidence of AL in an unselected group of unirradiated patients."[42]

THE POLYCYTHEMIA VERA STUDY GROUP

Because it had been so difficult to ascertain the natural history of PV, Louis R. Wasserman instituted a multinational cooperative group study, the Polycythemia Vera Study Group (PVSG), in 1967. Under the auspices of the National Cancer Institute, this prospective, randomized study was intended to resolve the many dilemmas confronting the physician treating a patient with PV. The questions to be answered were (1) What is the natural course of the disease in untreated or phlebotomy-only treated patients? (2) What is the incidence of complications such as hemorrhage and thrombosis in phlebotomy-treated as contrasted with myelosuppression-treated patients? (3) Does chemical and/or radiation treatment increase the incidence of myeloid metaplasia and myelofibrosis and of acute leukemia independent of any effect on increasing survival?[43] The PVSG established diagnostic criteria; documented the natural

---

FIGURE 2–1. Hypothetical concept of the course of polycythemia vera. The blood, bone marrow, and extraosseous potential marrow, considered the "blood tissue," reflect simultaneous changes occurring during the course of polycythemia vera. In polycythemia vera, the hyperplastic marrow expands to encompass the total marrow space at the expense of the fat cells. There is a neoplastic panmyelosis with stimulation of all hematic cellular derivatives of the primitive reticulum cell. Blood examination reveals an erythrocytosis and usually a granulocytic leukocytosis, thrombocytosis, and immature red and white cells. Splenomegaly and hepatomegaly are frequently present, initially due to the increase in blood volume and subsequently associated with reticulum cell hyperplasia and heteroplastic blood formation. With continued hyperactivity, the dormant extraosseous potential marrow becomes functionally active and the site of extramedullary hematopoiesis (stage of myeloid metaplasia) as the spleen and liver enlarge (outer circle designates extramedullary blood formation). The bone marrow shows diminution in erythrogenesis and secondary proliferation of the fixed reticulum cells and the fibroblasts. The peripheral blood mirrors the marrow changes with usually a mild to moderate anemia, although normal values (a compensated state) may prevail for many years. Thrombocytosis is common, as is a leukoerythroblastic blood picture. With time, progressive changes in cellular composition of the marrow occur (stage of early spent polycythemia). Fibroblastic or osteoblastic proliferation may encroach on hematic cell activity with the reduction most particularly in erythropoiesis. Megakaryocytes appear more plentiful due either to increased proliferative activity or to a quantitative decrease in other hematic cells. The liver and spleen, the site of extramedullary hematopoiesis, are not encased in bone and hence can expand markedly. There is now a leukocytosis and thrombocytopenia or thrombocytosis and leukoerythroblastic anemia with morphologically bizarre red cells. Further fibroblastic or osteoblastic proliferation may obliterate the marrow cavity with all blood formation occurring in the extraosseous marrow (stage of myeloid metaplasia). Note that nonhematic cell proliferation occurs in the liver and spleen also. The anemia becomes more severe, with usually a leukopenia, thrombopenia, and a marked leukoerythroblastic blood picture. Hepatosplenomegaly may be tremendous. This phase of myelofibrosis (myeloid metaplasia) may be a terminal picture in polycythemia vera. Other lines of proliferation may gain ascendency, e.g., the white cells, with development of an acute leukemia occasionally preceded by a stage similar to chronic myelogenous leukemia; megakaryocytic hyperactivity may result in so-called megakaryocytic myelosis, etc. Acute leukemia, spent polycythemia, and myelofibrosis are all depicted as stemming from a common stage of myeloid metaplasia. Variation in proliferative activity of any combination of cellular categories may produce complex clinical and pathologic syndromes. Thus well-developed myelofibrosis may frequently show large numbers of myeloblasts and myelocytes in the blood, and similarly, a terminal acute blastic leukemia may show extensive fibroblastic proliferation. (The area represented for any specific cellular series is only approximate and merely represents an attempt to demonstrate graphically a few of the multiple developmental potentialities in polycythemia vera.) (Adapted from Wasserman LR: Bull NY Acad Med 30:354, 1954. Reprinted with permission of The New York Academy of Medicine.)

evolution of PV, including hemorrhagic and thrombotic events, causes of death, the incidence of both AL and PPMM, and complications of therapy; and attempted to define optimal therapy. For the major protocol, protocol 01, the therapeutic agents chosen were the alkylating agent chlorambucil and ^{32}P. Patients randomized to these therapies were compared with the control group of patients treated with phlebotomy only.

THERAPY AND COMPLICATIONS OF THERAPY

The chronicity and undulating course of PV provide a challenge both in the selection of an optimal form of therapy and in the recognition of the numerous complications. The goal of therapy in the erythrocytotic phase is reduction of the red cell mass, whether accomplished by removal of the end product (phlebotomy), control of production (myelosuppression), or some combination thereof. Table 2–2 lists some of the treatments administered in the past and currently.[44] To date, only phlebotomy, ^{32}P, and chemotherapy have proven acceptable, but each modality has its own hazards and limitations.

The PVSG studies have shown that the mode of therapy decidedly and markedly influences the complications and the causes of death. Although there were no statistically significant differences in survival among the groups after 20 years of study, patients treated with phlebotomy alone have an excess mortality within the first 2 to 4 years, principally because of thrombotic complications.[16,45,46] The most susceptible patients were those over 70 years of age and those with a history of prior thrombosis. In retrospect, this is not surprising. Phlebotomy does not suppress the marrow and so does not control the associated leuko- and thrombocytosis, nor the blood viscosity, as well as the other modalities.

While not so susceptible to thrombotic complications as the phlebotomy-treated group, patients treated by myelosuppression also suffer increased risks, albeit different. The first is an increased risk of AL.[14–16,18,47–49] As mentioned earlier, the literature is fraught with contradictions as to the role of therapies and dosages in inducing AL in treated PV patients. In this regard, the PVSG protocol 01 study has unquestionably established the following.[45,50,51] First, transition to AL is part of the natural history of PV, but it occurs in only 1 to 2 percent of patients treated with phlebotomy only. Second, there is a strikingly increased incidence of AL in patients

TABLE 2–2. METHODS OF TREATMENT OF POLYCYTHEMIA VERA: VARIATIONS ON BLOODLETTING

General or topical:	Phlebotomy
	Cupping
	Iatrogenic hookworm infection
Miscellaneous	Gastric lavage (to remove Castle's intrinsic factor)
	Gastrectomy to remove intrinsic factor
	Diet (iron-free, high-fat, low-purine)
	Liver extracts
Chemical	Benzol and derivatives
	Phenylhydrazine: acetylphenhydrazine
	Onions (onion oil, N-propyldisulfide)
	Arsenic: Fowler's solution
	Oxygen inhalation (for bone marrow anoxia)
Radiation	Total body, splenic, long bones, stomach
	Radium, thorium X, Grenzstrahlen
	Radioactive phosphorus (^{32}P), sodium, gold, zirconium, yttrium
Chemotherapy:	Nitrogen mustard, thiotriethylenephosphoramide, busulfan, triethylene-melamine, pyrimethamine, melphalan, chlorambucil, cyclophosphamide, procarbazine, pipobroman, hydroxyurea, anagrelide, interferon-α

Source: Adapted from Wasserman, LR, Semin Hematol 23:184, 1986; reprinted with permission.

treated with myelosuppression compared with patients treated with phlebotomy only. Among patients treated with chlorambucil, the risk is 2.3 times that of patients treated with phlebotomy alone.[45] The risk among patients treated with ^{32}P approaches that of chlorambucil-treated patients and may eventually be even greater.[45, 51] One of the major differences between the two agents is the time to onset of AL. Over half the chlorambucil-treated patients who developed AL did so within 5 years of randomization to therapy, suggesting that this is a drug-related effect rather than a consequence of prolonged survival. The ^{32}P-treated patients who developed AL did so much later in the study, with half occurring more than 11 years after randomization. Because survival in all three treatment groups is similar, the implication is that ^{32}P is an inherently leukemogenic drug.

Myelosuppression is also associated with an increased risk of malignancies other than AL, although the mechanisms remain to be elucidated and dose-response relationships are unclear. A different subset of chlorambucil-treated patients developed non-Hodgkin's (large cell) lymphoma (NHL).[52] In contrast to the ALs in the chlorambucil-treated patients, none of the NHLs occurred until at least 5 years after randomization to therapy. In essence, one of five patients treated with the alkylating agent chlorambucil developed a second hematologic malignancy, either AL or NHL. Patients treated with chlorambucil or ^{32}P also have an increased incidence of neoplasms of the gastrointestinal tract and skin as compared with patients treated by phlebotomy alone.[53]

The PVSG protocol 01 study has shown that regardless of the type of therapy administered, evolution to PPMM, or the spent phase, occurs in 9 percent of patients, confirming that this complication is an integral part of the natural history of PV and its incidence is not related to or altered by therapy.[50] Still to be explained, however, is the pathogenesis of myelofibrosis in PV, since the fibroblasts are not a part of the clonal proliferation.[54–57] Furthermore, anecdotal literature reports have documented that AL occurs in the setting of myelofibrosis (MF), but an unequivocal relationship was more problematic.[39, 40, 48, 58, 59] After 11 years on study, the risk of AL in myelosuppressed spent-phase patients has been shown to be 15 times that in non-spent-phase patients.[60] At least in PV, the spent phase is a risk factor for the development of AL, regardless of mode of therapy. Whether these conclusions can be extrapolated to other MPDs or even to other conditions with MF is debatable.

SUMMARY

Although the symptoms remain somewhat indefinite and the perfect therapy for PV has yet to be devised, neither the pathology nor the pathophysiology of PV is as obscure as in Osler's time. Through the efforts of many intellectually curious and dedicated physicians and scientists, much more is now known about the natural history of this clonal hematopoietic stem-cell disorder. The complications of the disease itself and its various treatments have been well documented. Therapeutic recommendations have been revised accordingly to reflect our greater understanding of both PV and the agents used to treat it.[61–63] Currently, the drug of choice in younger patients who require myelosuppression is hydroxyurea (Hydrea) and in older patients remains [32]P. During the last few years, two additional therapeutic agents, anagrelide and interferon-α, have been used in treating PV and other myeloproliferative diseases. Anagrelide is discussed in Chapter 22 in this volume and interferon-α in Chapter 23. Which of these agents is or are of greater value in the therapy of the PV must be determined over time. The knowledge from the Polycythemia Vera Study Group has been translated into greater longevity with fewer complications for the patient with PV. Although not all the questions about PV have been answered and new questions will arise, some of the dilemmas confronting the physician treating a patient with PV have been solved.

REFERENCES

1. Hippocrates: De humoribus, Chap. 1
2. von Haller A: Elementa Physiologiae Corporis Humani, vol 2, Lausanne, Switzerland, 1757, p 34
3. Vaquez HM: Sur une forme speciale de cyanose s'accompagnant d'hyperglobulie excessive et persistante. C R Soc Biol (Paris) 44:384–388, 1892
4. Osler W: Chronic cyanosis with polycythemia and enlarged spleen: A new clinical entity. Am J Med Sci 126:187–201, 1903

5. Turk W: Beitrage zur Kenntnis des Symptomenbildes Polyzythamie mit Milztumor und Zyanose. Wein Klin Wochenschr 17:153–160, 189–193, 1904

6. Hirsch R: Generalized osteosclerosis with chronic polycythemia vera. Arch Pathol 19:91–97, 1935

7. Rosenthal N, Bassen FA: Course of polycythemia. Arch Intern Med 62:903–917, 1938

8. Chievitz E, Thiede T: Complications and causes of death in polycythaemia vera. Acta Med Scand 172:513–523, 1962

9. Lawrence JH: Nuclear physics and therapy: Preliminary report on a new method for the treatment of leukemia and polycythemia. Radiology 35:51–60, 1940

10. Cronkite EP, Moloney W, Bond VP: Radiation leukemogenesis: An analysis of the problem. Am J Med 28:673–682, 1960

11. Bizzozero OJ, Johnson KG, Ciocco A: Radiation-related leukemia in Hiroshima and Nagasaki, 1946–1964. N Engl J Med 274:1095–1101, 1966

12. Schwartz SO, Ehrlich L: The relationship of polycythemia vera to leukemia: A critical review. Acta Haematol 4:129–147, 1950

13. Wasserman LR: Polycythemia vera—Its course and treatment: Relation to myeloid metaplasia and leukemia. Bull NY Acad Med 30:343–375, 1954

14. Modan B, Lilienfeld AM: Leukaemogenic effect of ionising-irradiation treatment in polycythemia. Lancet 2:439–441, 1964

15. Perkins J, Israels MCG, Wilkinson JF: Polycythaemia vera: Clinical studies on a series of 127 patients managed without radiation therapy. Q J Med 33:499–518, 1964

16. Modan B, Lilienfeld AM: Polycythemia vera and leukemia—The role of radiation treatment. Medicine 44:305–344, 1965

17. Halnan KE, Russell MH: Polycythemia vera: Comparison of survival and causes of death in patients managed with and without radiotherapy. Lancet 1:760–763, 1965

18. Lawrence JH, Winchell HS, Donald WG: Leukemia in polycythemia vera: Relationship to splenic myeloid metaplasia and therapeutic radiation dose. Ann Intern Med 70:763–771, 1969

19. Gilbert HS: Problems relating to control of polycythemia vera: The use of alkylating agents. Blood 32:500–505, 1968

20. Minot GR, Buckman TE: Erythremia (polycythemia rubra vera): The development of anemia; the relation to leukemia; consideration of the basal metabolism, blood formation and destruction and fragility of the red cells. Am J Med Sci 166:469–489, 1923

21. Rosenthal MC: Extramedullary hematopoiesis: Myeloid metaplasia. Bull N Engl Med Center 12:154–160, 1950

22. Dameshek W: Some speculations on the myeloproliferative syndromes. Blood 6:372–375, 1951

23. Osgood EE: Polycythemia vera: Age relationships and survival. Blood 6:243–256, 1965

24. Ward HP, Block M: The natural history of agnogenic myeloid metaplasia (AMM) and a critical evaluation of its relationship with the myeloproliferative syndrome. Medicine 50:357–420, 1971

25. Krauss S, Wasserman LR: Leukemia in patients with polycythemia vera treated with radioisotopes. In Atomic Energy Commission Symposium No. 20, Medical Radionuclides: Radiation Dose and Effects, USAEC Div Tech Info, 1970

26. Adamson JW, Fialkow PJ, Murphy S, et al: Polycythemia vera: Stem cell and probable clonal origin of the disease. N Engl J Med 295:913–916, 1976

27. Ward HP, Robinson WA: Presence of a myelostimulatory factor in polycythemia vera (PV) and agnogenic myeloid metaplasia (AMM). J Clin Invest 51:100, 1972

28. Ward HP, Vautrin R, Kurnick J: Presence of a myeloproliferative factor in patients with polycythemia vera and agnogenic myeloid metaplasia: I. Expansion of the erythopoietin-responsive stem cell compartment. Proc Soc Exp Biol Med 147:305–308, 1974

29. Zanjani ED: Hematopoietic factors in polycythemia vera. Semin Hematol 13:1–12, 1976

30. Prchal JF, Axelrad AA: Bone-marrow responses in polycythemia vera. N Engl J Med 290:1382, 1974

31. Weinberg RS, Worsley A, Gilbert HS, et al: Comparison of erythroid progenitor cell growth in vitro in polycythemia vera and chronic myelogenous leukemia: Only polycythemia vera has endogenous colonies. Leukemia Res 13:331–338, 1988

32. Eaves CJ, Eaves AC: Erythropoietin (Ep) dose-response curves for three classes of erythroid progenitors in normal human marrow and in patients with polycythemia vera. Blood 52:1196–1210, 1978

33. Modan B: An epidemiologic study of polycythemia vera. Blood 26:657–667, 1965

34. Silverstein MN, Lanier AP: Polycythemia vera, 1935–1969: An epidemiologic survey in Rochester, Minnesota. Mayo Clin Proc 46:751–753, 1971

35. Berglund S, Zettervall O: Incidence of polycythemia vera in a defined population. Eur J Haematol 48:20–26, 1992

36. Berlin NI: Diagnosis and classification of the polycythemias. Semin Hematol 12:339–351, 1975

37. Wanless IR, Peterson P, Das A, et al: Hepatic vascular disease and portal hypertension in polycythemia vera and agnogenic myeloid metaplasia: A clinicopathologic study of 145 patients examined at autopsy. Hepatology 12:1166–1174, 1990

38. Silverstein MN: Postpolycythemia myeloid metaplasia. Arch Intern Med 134:113–115, 1974

39. Bouroncle BA, Doan CA: Myelofibrosis: Clinical, hematologic and pathologic study of 110 patients. Am J Med Sci 243:697–715, 1962

40. Silverstein MN, Brown Al, Linman JW: Idiopathic myeloid metaplasia: Its evolution to acute leukemia. Arch Intern Med 132:709–712, 1973

41. Silverstein MN: The evolution into and the treatment of late stage polycythemia vera. Semin Hematol 13:79–84, 1976

42. Szur L, Lewis SM: The haematological complications of polycythaemia vera and treatment with radioactive phosphorus. Br J Radiol 39:122–130, 1966

43. Wasserman LR: The treatment of polycythemia vera. Semin Hematol 13:57–78, 1976

44. Wasserman LR: The treatment of polycythemia vera. Semin Hematol 23:183–187, 1986

45. Berk PD, Goldberg JD, Silverstein MN, et al: Increased incidence of acute leukemia in polycythemia vera associated with chlorambucil therapy. N Engl J Med 304:441–447, 1981

46. Wasserman LR, Goldberg JD, Balcerzak SP, et al: Influence of therapy on causes of death in polycythemia vera. Clin Res 29:573, 1981

47. Nand S, Messmore H, Fisher SG, et al: Leukemic transformation in polycythemia vera: Analysis of risk factors. Am J Hematol 34:32–36, 1990

48. Rosenthal DS, Moloney WC: Occurrence of acute leukaemia in myeloproliferative disorders. Br J Haematol 36:373–382, 1977

49. Cervantes F, Tassies D, Salgado C, et al: Acute transformation in nonleukemic myeloproliferative disorders: Actuarial probability and main characteristics in a series of 218 patients. Acta Haematol 85:124–127, 1991

50. Ellis JT, Peterson P, Geller SA, et al: Studies of the bone marrow in polycythemia vera and the evolution of myelofibrosis and second hematologic malignancies. Semin Hematol 23:144–155, 1986

51. Landaw SA: Acute leukemia in polycythemia vera. Semin Hematol 23:156–165, 1986

52. Peterson P, Ellis JT, Geller SA, Rappaport H: Occurrence of non-Hodgkin's lymphoma in treated polycythemia vera. Lab Invest 52:51, 1985

53. Berk PD, Goldberg JD, Balcerzak SP, et al: Non-hematologic malignancies in patients receiving myelosuppressive treatment for polycythemia vera. Clin Res 30:558, 1982

54. de la Chappelle A, Vuopio P, Borgstrom GH: The origin of bone marrow fibroblasts. Blood 41:783–787, 1973

55. Golde DW, Hocking WG, Quan SG, et al: Origin of human bone marrow fibroblasts. Br J Haematol 44:183–187, 1980

56. Adamson JW, Fialkow PJ: The pathogenesis of myeloproliferative syndromes. Br J Haematol 38:299–303, 1978

57. Buschle M, Janssen JWG, Drexler H, et al: Evidence for pluripotent stem cell origin of idiopathic myelofibrosis: Clonal analysis of a case characterized by a N-*ras* mutation. Leukemia 2:658–660, 1988

58. Rosenthal DR, Moloney WC: Myeloid metaplasia: A study of 98 cases. Postgrad Med 45:136–142, 1969

59. Varki A, Lottenberg R, Griffith R, Reinhard E: The syndrome of idiopathic myelofibrosis: A clinicopathologic review with emphasis on the prognostic variables predicting survival. Medicine 62:353–371, 1983

60. Peterson P, Ellis JT, Geller SA, et al: Increased incidence of acute leukemia in spent polycythemia vera following myelosuppressive therapy. Lab Invest 54:49, 1986

61. Kaplan ME, Mack K, Goldberg JD, et al: Long-term management of polycythemia vera with hydroxyurea: A progress report. Semin Hematol 23:167–171, 1986

62. Fruchtman SM, Wasserman LR, Berk PD: Polycythemia rubra vera. *In* Brain MC, Carbone PP (eds): Current Therapy in Hematology Oncology 3. Philadelphia, Decker, 1988, pp 46–52

63. Fruchtman SM, Kaplan ME, Peterson P, et al: Hydroxyurea (HU) in the management of polycythemia vera (PV): Analysis of long-term leukemogenic potential. Clin Res 40:281, 1992

ACKNOWLEDGMENTS: We are indebted to fellow members of the Polycythemia Vera Study Group, without whose collaboration this work would not have been possible: W. R. Arrowsmith, M.D., S. P. Balcerzak, M.D., R. Berger, M.D., N. I. Berlin, M.D., E. C. Besa, M.D., M. H. Block, M.D. (deceased), J. Brière, M.D., L. H. Brubaker, M.D., E. W. Campbell, M.D., M. Coleman, M.D., M. R. Cooper, M.D., A. A. Cooperberg, M.D., P. B. Donovan, M.D., C. Dresch, M.D., J. T. Ellis, M.D., G. B. Faguet, M.D., S. M. Fruchtman, M.D., F. H. Gardner, M.D., R. D. Goldman, M.D., K. Goldstein, M.D., G. L. Holcomb, M.D., P. Jacobs, M.D., M. E. Kaplan, M.D., D. B. Kimball, M.D., W. H. Knospe, M.D., E. H. Kraut, M.D., S. A. Landaw, M.D., J. H. Lawrence, M.D. (deceased), V. Loeb, Jr., M.D., R. O. Lundy, M.D., O. Ross McIntyre, M.D., L. M. Meyer, M.D., B. Modan, M.D., S. Murphy, M.D., W. D. Noyes, M.D., M. C. Perry, M.D., P. Peterson, M.D., R. M. Petitt, M.D., R. V. Pierre, M.D., J. Poindexter, M.D., K. Rai, M.D., H. Rapapport, M.D., D. S. Rosenthal, M.D., Y. Sacks, M.D., A. Sawitsky, M.D., R. F. Schilling, M.D., E. B. Silberstein, M.D., R. T. Silver, M.D., M. N. Silverstein, M.D., Ph.D., C. L. Spurr, M.D., H. L. Stauffer, M.D., A. P. Tartaglia, M.D., I. Tatarsky, M.D., R. O. Wallerstein, M.D., J. K. Weick, M.D., N. J. Weinreb, M.D., J. Whang-Peng, M.D., and D. Wurster-Hill, Ph.D.

Additional thanks go to the statistical, administrative, and secretarial staffs: Judith Goldberg, Sc.D., Karen Mack, M.A., Bernard Pasternack, Ph.D., Helen Walton, and Ruth Wittman, M.S.

3

Classification of the Polycythemias and Initial Clinical Features in Polycythemia Vera

NATHANIEL I. BERLIN

That polycythemia vera is a rare disease is well known, but not until Prochazka and Markowe summarized the published data and reported their data from England and Wales was there epidemiologic data based on a large population.[1] The previously reported incidence varied from 0.2 cases per million per year in Japan to a high of 22.2 cases per million per year in Rochester, Minnesota. Most of the reports indicate an incidence between 5 and 10 cases per million per year.[1] The age-specific mortality calculated by Prochazka and Markowe shows a very sharp increase beginning in the early 40s (Fig. 3–1), with the age-specific mortality reaching a maximum in the 75- to 84-year age group. This figure also shows the age-specific registration (incidence). In Prochazka and Markowe's study, the male/female ratio was 1:3. This is close to that of patients in the Polycythemia Vera Study Group (PVSG) and in other large series of patients.

The descriptions of polycythemia vera by Vasquez,[2] Osler,[3] and Weber and Watson[4] between 1892 and 1904 clearly recognized an entity characterized by ruddy cyanosis, splenomegaly, and an increased red cell count and which was not associated with (secondary to) some form of congenital heart disease. Later (in 1992), Gaisbock[5] described an entity he called "polycythemia hypertonica" that fits well with what has come to be known as stress polycythemia, also designated as *stress erythrocytosis, spurious polycythemia, Gaisbock syndrome*, etc. (see Chap. 18). These early publications set the stage for the classification of the polycythemias into three categories:

1. Polycythemia vera
2. Secondary polycythemias
3. Relative polycythemia

The latter term described a condition in which the concentration of red cells (hematocrit) was increased but the total circulating red cell volume was not. Osler recognized that this could be a long-standing condition without obvious cause. The relationship to Gaisbock's polycythemia is not clear, since Gaisbock did not report blood volume measurements and proof of the existence of relative polycythemia requires a total red cell volume determination, preferably with isotopically labeled red cells. Today this structural base for the classification of the polycythemias remains. Polycythemia vera is a distinct entity and is a clonal disorder of stem cells.[6] The secondary polycythemias are disorders in which the concentration of red cells in peripheral blood and the total circulating red cell volume are increased as a result of increased production of erythropoietin, the hormone that regulates erythropoiesis. In some instances, the increase in erythropoietin production is the appropriate physiologic response, e.g., in a right-to-left cardiac shunt

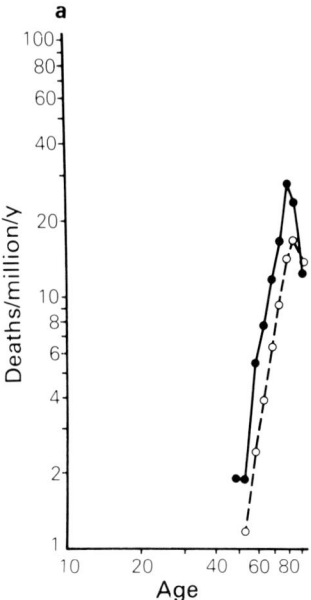
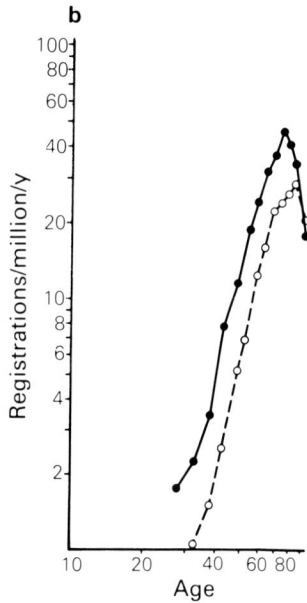

FIGURE 3-1. Age-specific death rate and registration (incidence) of polycythemia vera in England and Wales. (From Prochazka AV, Markowe HLJ: Br J Cancer 53:59–64, 1986.)

and in those living at high altitude. In others, the increased production is not physiologically appropriate, e.g., in the polycythemia produced in patients with cerebellar hemangioblastomas—a neoplasm in which Waldman and colleagues[7] demonstrated the production of erythropoietin by the tumor. Until recently, these two groups of patients with a secondary polycythemia were designated as either physiologically appropriate or physiologically inappropriate, but presently, the terminology favored is appropriate or inappropriate erythropoietin production. The following outline lists the entities in these two classes that lead to secondary polycythemia:

I. Polycythemia vera

II. Secondary polycythemia (increased erythropoietin production)
    A. Physiologically appropriate
        1. High altitude
        2. Chronic obstructive pulmonary disease
        3. Postural hypoxemia
        4. Cardiovascular shunt (right to left)
        5. Pickwickian syndrome (massive obesity)
        6. High oxygen affinity hemoglobulinopathy
        7. Congenital decreased red cell 2–3DPG (diphosphoglycerate)
        8. Smokers' polycythemia
    B. Physiologically inappropriate
        1. Tumor
            a. Renal carcinoma
            b. Cerebellar hemangioblastoma
            c. Hepatoma
            d. Uterine fibroid
            e. Adrenal cortical adenoma (and/or hyperplasia)
            f. Ovarian carcinoma
        2. Renal
            a. Cysts
            b. Hydronephrosis
            c. Bartter's syndrome
            d. Transplantation
        3. Cobalt
    C. Recessive familial polycythemia

III. Relative polycythemia (also called stress polycythemia, spurious polycythemia, pseudopolycythemia, and Gaisbock's syndrome)

The third major group is relative polycythemia. For purposes of discussion, the group of patients in this chapter (and in Chap. 18) does not include patients with a temporary elevation, such as would occur in transient dehydration, but only those with an elevated hematocrit of long duration. It was not until the measurement of the total circulating red cell volume by isotopically labeled red cells that definitive evidence for the existence of this syndrome was possible.[8]

From time to time, other descriptions have been used, such as benign erythrocytosis (Modan[9]), pure erythrocytosis (Najean et al.[10]), idiopathic erythrocytosis (Pearson and Wetherley-Mein,[11] Dudley et al.[12]), and unclassified polycythemia with endogenous erythroid colomes (EECs) (Lemoine et al.[13]).

Benign erythrocytosis is defined as erythrocytosis (an elevated total red cell volume) without splenomegaly, leukocytosis, or thrombocytosis and with no "overt underlying condition."

Najean et al.[10] have used the term *pure erythrocytosis* in different ways: (1) an elevated total red cell volume with no splenomegaly, granulocytosis, or thrombocytosis, normal arterial oxygen saturation, normal intravenous polycythemia (IVP), and a quest for other tumors (this is *pure primary erythrocytosis*) and (2) an elevated total red cell volume in the absence of the criteria for polycythemia vera (these are the secondary polycythemias). *Idiopathic erythrocytosis* is applied to patients with an elevated total red cell volume who do not satisfy criteria for polycythemia vera but there is no cause for secondary polycythemia.

In *unclassified polycythemia* with EEC (endogenous erythroid colome), there is an elevated total red cell volume, but these patients do not satisfy the PVSG "standard" criteria. They have a bone marrow and serum erythropoietin similar to polycythemia vera and an active course of the disease.

While it is not difficult to differentiate most patients with an increased hematocrit (increased red count and hemoglobulin concentration) on the basis of a history, physical examination, and peripheral blood counts, a number of patients require additional diagnostic laboratory tests and x-ray or other imaging techniques before a definitive diagnosis can be made. The principal laboratory test is a measurement of the total volume of circulating red cells with isotopically labeled cells. Nielson and Rodbro[14] compared a measured total red cell volume with that predicted from a measured plasma volume and the peripheral hematocrit corrected by an *f* factor:

$$f = \frac{\text{Hct total body}}{\text{Hct venous}}$$

Figure 2 of their paper indicates a very wide spread (± 500 ml for 2 standard deviations) in the difference between a measured total red cell volume (TRCV) and the predicted TRCV. Hence the prediction of TRCV from a measured plasmic volume should not be used for diagnostic purposes. However, in a subsequent paper, a more complex statistical approach is used to separate the normal patients from those with an elevated total red cell volume.[14, 15] The measurement of total red cell volume separates patients who have an elevated hematocrit and an increased total circulating red cell volume and are therefore truly polycythemic (absolute polycythemia) from those with a relative polycythemia, in whom the elevated hematocrit represents increased (hemo) concentration of red cells but not an increased total volume of circulating red cells (relative polycythemia). Relative polycythemia is a much more common condition than polycythemia vera or secondary polycythemia, but how common is not known.

On the basis of a number of studies of the total red cell volume in the normal male and normal female with isotopically labeled cells, the upper bounds for a normal total red cell volume are generally considered to be 32 ml/kg for women and 36 ml/kg for men.[16] However, it must be recognized that while these upper bounds are the generally accepted index used, the interpretation of the volume of red cells per kilogram of body weight is subject to some uncertainty because of variation in body composition.[17] Lean individuals will tend to have a higher value in terms of total red cell volume than obese individuals. This is so because it is generally held that the total red cell volume correlates better with lean body mass and that increments of fat affect the total red cell volume to a lesser degree. A measurement of lean body mass is not a simple procedure and is best carried out by measuring both total-body water and body density; neither is simple or widely available. Measurement of lean body mass is not held to be necessary for differential diagnosis of the polycythemias.

When the total red cell volume is elevated, the measurement of blood oxygen saturation identifies those patients whose polycythemia is secondary to a decreased blood oxygen saturation and thus is a secondary polycythemia. This group includes patients with congenital cardiac abnormalities, those with chronic obstructive pulmonary disease, and those who reside at high altitudes.

Most of the reported measurements of blood oxygen saturation in polycythemia vera were done in the late 1940s[18] and early 1950s[19] and do not include data on whether or not the individual was a cigarette smoker. Cigarette smoking does cause an increase in carboxyhemoglobin concentration, and that alone is sufficient in some instances to cause an increase in the total circulating red cell volume and an increase in the hematocrit without a concomitant increase in total red cell volume,[20] an entity that Smith and Landow have designated as "smokers polycythemia." The lower bound for normal blood oxygen saturation has been set at 92 percent, but a small number of patients with polycythemia vera (on the order of 10 percent) have a blood oxygen saturation that is lower than this, in the range of 88 to 92 percent. Considering the wide prevalence of cigarette smoking at the time these studies were done, it is entirely possible that most of these patients with polycythemia vera were smokers and that they had an increased carboxyhemoglobin concentration and, at the same time, chronic obstructive pulmonary disease. Hence, when all other evidence indicates that the patient has polycythemia vera, a blood saturation below 92 percent leads to the conclusion that the observed polycythemia is mixed in its origin. The $P500_2$ laboratory test measures the partial pressure of oxygen at which the hemoglobin is 50 percent saturated. This test identifies patients with a polycythemia due to increased hemoglobin affinity for oxygen and who, in a sense, are anoxic because the red cell oxygen is not as readily given up to the tissues as in the normal individual. Thus the polycythemia is physiologically appropriate.

The original description by Charache, Westherall, and Clegg[21] of a polycythemia associated with Chesapeake hemoglobin has been followed by observations of polycythemia in other high oxygen affinity hemoglobinopathies, of which there are at least 40.[22]

An intravenous pyelogram (IVP) will identify patients with some of the renal abnormalities that lead to polycythemia. These include renal tumors, renal cysts, and obstructive uropathies. Most, if not all, of the observations of polycythemia associated with renal disease were diagnosed with an IVP. Today, an ultrasound examination may be sufficient or even better for this purpose than an IVP, without the risk of allergic reaction to the contrast medium.

The measurement of carboxyhemoglobin is necessary only in smokers and is apparently not widely carried out. The measurement of either a serum or urinary erythropoietin level for diagnostic purposes is also not widely applied because initially it was a time-consuming, labor-intensive biologic assay that was not sufficiently sensitive. Today there is a radioimmunoassay that makes this determination more widely available. Patients with secondary polycythemia have increased serum or urinary erythropoietin, while it is normal or below normal in polycythemia vera.[23-26]

The most recent laboratory test to be used is a bone marrow culture.[27] The bone marrow from patients with polycythemia vera can be put into culture without additional erythropoietin, unlike bone marrow from all other entities studied. This separates patients with polycythemia vera from those with the other polycythemias. While this observation has been confirmed,[12, 13, 28] it is not a widely available laboratory test, and it may be necessary in only a few instances.

Chapter 16 describes in detail the secondary polycythemias; the rare polycythemias are described in Chap. 17, and a description of relative polycythemia is found in Chap. 16.

Given the history, physical examination, peripheral blood counts, and laboratory determinations as described, it is possible to assign most patients with an increased hematocrit to a specific diagnosis. From time to time, even this scheme presents difficulties, e.g., a patient with polycythemia vera and a large renal cyst in whom the renal cyst has been shown to contain erythropoietin.

A decision tree (algorithm) has been developed for describing the flow of information necessary to make the differential diagnosis[29, 30] (Fig. 3–2). That part of the decision tree beyond the IVP is not often used, nor is it often necessary.

Where in this diagnostic scheme do the patients fall who have an elevated total red cell volume but no splenomegaly, a white blood cell count less than 12,000, and a normal platelet count (less than 30,000), a normal IVP, and no other evidence of a secondary polycythemia?

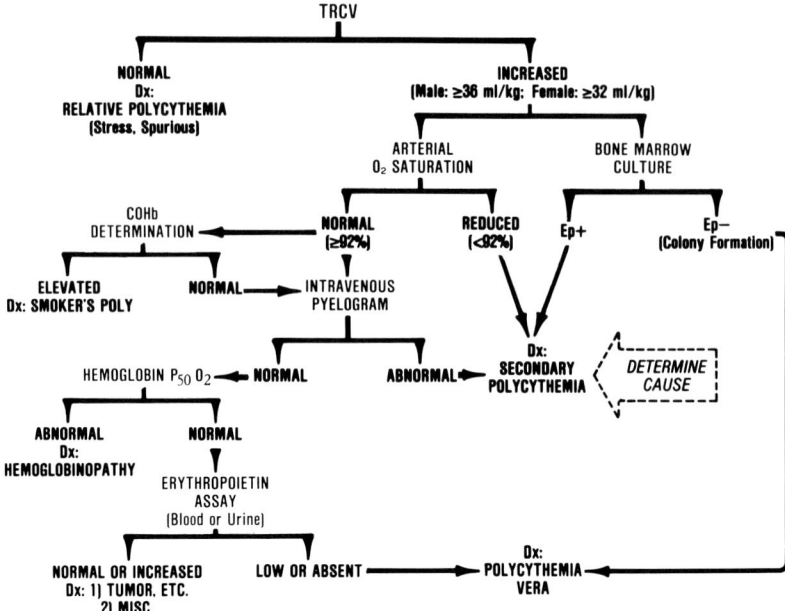

FIGURE 3-2. A decision tree (algorithm) for the evaluation of an elevated hematocrit.

It has been reported that about 10 percent of patients with polycythemia vera do not have splenomegaly, leukocytosis, or thrombocytosis.[31] These data were obtained before the measurement of erythropoietin was available and before the existence of a high oxygen affinity hemoglobinopathy and some of the other rare causes of a physiologically appropriate polycythemia were recognized. These patients have been put into the classification of "pure erythrocytosis" (Najean, Triebel, and Dresch[10]), benign erythrocytosis (Modan[9]), or idiopathic erythrocytosis (Pearson and Wetherly-Mein[11]). Najean et al.[10] described 51 cases of pure erythrocytosis in 350 patients referred to them.

In the PVSG major protocol, there were only two patients entered who could be considered by these criteria to have "pure erythrocytosis." This is undoubtedly a result of the criteria used for entry into that study. These criteria included a history and physical examination in which splenomegaly was an important characteristic, a white blood count and platelet count, and the measurement of B_{12} binding capacity and leukocyte alkaline phosphate. These criteria are shown in Table 3-1. This was done in order to create a group of patients that was as homogeneous as possible for a randomized, controlled trial of the comparative merits of radioactive phos-

TABLE 3-1. PVSG DIAGNOSTIC CRITERIA

CATEGORY A		CATEGORY B
1. Increased red cell mass Male $\geq$ 36 ml/kg Female $\geq$ 32 ml/kg	1.	Thrombocytosis Platelet count > 4,000,000/mm³
2. Normal art. 02 sat. $\geq$ 92%	2.	Leukocytosis > 12,000/mm³ (no fever or infection)
3. Splenomegaly	3.	Leukocyte alkaline phosphatase (>100) (no fever or infection)
	4.	Serum B_{12} (>900 pg/ml) or unbound B_{12} binding capacity (>220 pg/ml)

Patient eligible if following combinations are present:

A1 + A2 + A3

A1 + A2 + any two from category B

Patient eligible for special randomization category:

A1 + A3 if A2 between 88 and 92%

phorus (^{32}P), chlorambucil, and phlebotomy in the treatment of polycythemia vera (see Chap. 15). These diagnostic criteria have become known in the literature as the "standard criteria" and, since their publication in 1975,[21] have been cited 247 times (Science Citation Index) as of May 1993.

In order to demonstrate that this was a progressive disease, each patient in the PVSG study was phlebotomized sufficiently to reduce the hematocrit to the normal level at the time of initial evaluation; before entry into the therapeutic part of the study, it was required that there be a subsequent rise in the hematocrit or hemoglobin. These criteria thus define the group of patients who were included in the PVSG major protocol.

It is entirely possible that patients with polycythemia vera were excluded from the study, since there was at that time no single criterion on which the diagnosis of polycythemia vera could be made, while the constellation of criteria used made it possible for the group to enroll only those patients who met the most rigorous diagnostic criteria available in 1965–1966.

The principal features of patients with polycythemia vera have been reported from several large series,[19,31,32] the largest from the PVSG. There are no major differences between these groups of patients; in fact, the essential features are very well described in Osler's paper in 1908.[3] The PVSG patients can be used as an example. The male/female ratio was 1.2:1. The principal value of this information is that relative polycythemia (stress polycythemia, spurious polycythemia, Gaisbock's syndrome) is almost exclusively a disorder of males. The mean age at diagnosis of the patients in the PVSG is 60 years, but as reported previously, this represents a substantial and impressive increase from 1912, when the average age at diagnosis was 44.3 years.[29] The interval between onset and diagnosis is difficult to determine but may be on the order of 12 to 18 months and perhaps longer.

Table 3–2 lists the symptoms reported by patients in the PVSG in order of decreasing frequency—headaches, weakness, and pruritus being the most common symptoms. Most patients report the ruddy cyanosis.

The principal findings on physical examination are ruddy cyanosis (67 percent), injection of the conjunctival small vessels (59 percent), engorgement of the veins of the fundus (46 percent), enlarged liver (40 percent), and an enlarged spleen (70 percent). In fact, the enlarged spleen can be a major factor in differentiating, early in the evaluation of patients with an elevated hematocrit, between those with polycythemia vera and those with other disorders with an elevated hematocrit, since splenomegaly is not a characteristic finding in any of the other polycythemias. A substantial number (77 percent) of patients with polycythemia vera have hypertension according to the criterion of a systolic pressure greater than 140 mmHg and/or a diastolic pressure greater than 90 mmHg (32 percent).

Figures 3–3, 3–4 and 3–5 show the hematocrit, white blood count and platelet counts at the time of entry into the PVSG major (01) protocol.

The leukocyte alkaline phosphate level is elevated and, as previously shown, cannot be correlated with the white blood count (Fig. 3–6). The blood oxygen saturation is 92 percent or greater. However, approximately 10 percent of patients in the PVSG had a blood oxygen saturation between 88 and 92 percent, and an even smaller number had less than 88 percent, for which there is no simple explanation. It is entirely possible that these patients had polycythemia vera upon which was superimposed some degree of secondary polycythemia due to emphysema (e.g., chronic bronchitis due to cigarette smoking). It should be pointed out that these data were collected before there was a marked decrease in cigarette smoking in males over age 40.

Additional laboratory findings reflect a reticulocyte count greater than 1.5 percent in 48 percent of the patients, and the leukocyte alkaline phosphates score was greater than 100 in 71 percent of the patients. The total bilirubin was greater than 1.0 percent in 35 percent of the patients, with a mean value of 0.89 mg/dl. This is close to the expected value based on the increased total circulating red cell volume. Of particular interest is the serum iron determination, as shown in Table 3–3.

It is often held that the serum iron level is reduced in patients with polycythemia vera,

TABLE 3–2. SYMPTOMS

Headache	48%
Weakness	47%
Pruritus	43%
Dizziness	43%
Sweating	33%
Visual	31%
Weight loss	29%
Paresthesias	29%
Dyspnea	26%
Joint symptoms	26%
Epigastric distress	24%

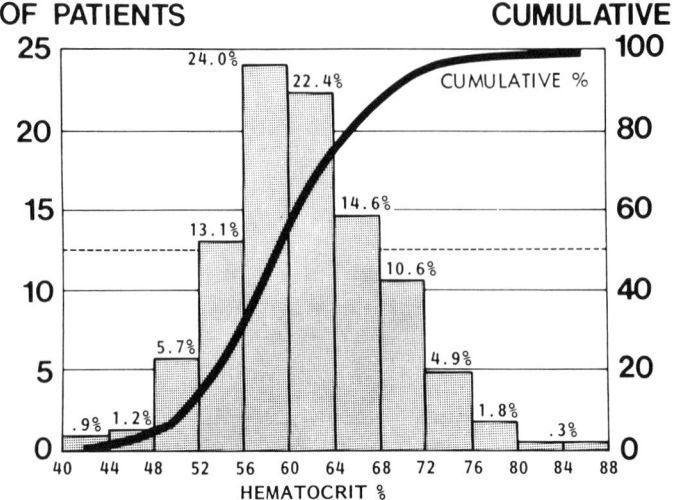

FIGURE 3–3. The hematocrit in PVSG patients.

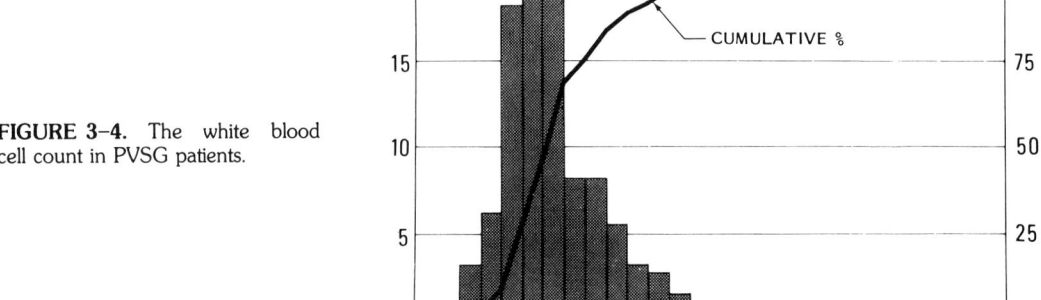

FIGURE 3–4. The white blood cell count in PVSG patients.

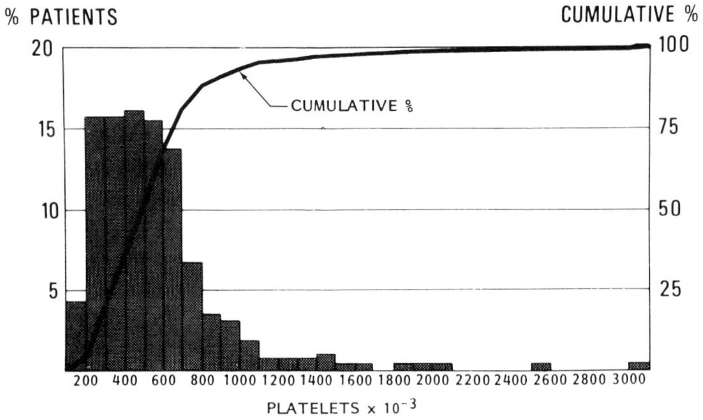

FIGURE 3–5. The platelet count in PVSG patients.

but when the patients in the PSVG were divided into three groups, (1) those without a previous phlebotomy, (2) those with a phlebotomy in the year before the initial evaluation, and (3) those phlebotomized more than 1 year before initial evaluation, it became apparent in both men and women that there was a distinct decrease in the serum iron level in the phlebotomized patients. In males, there was a strong tendency for the serum

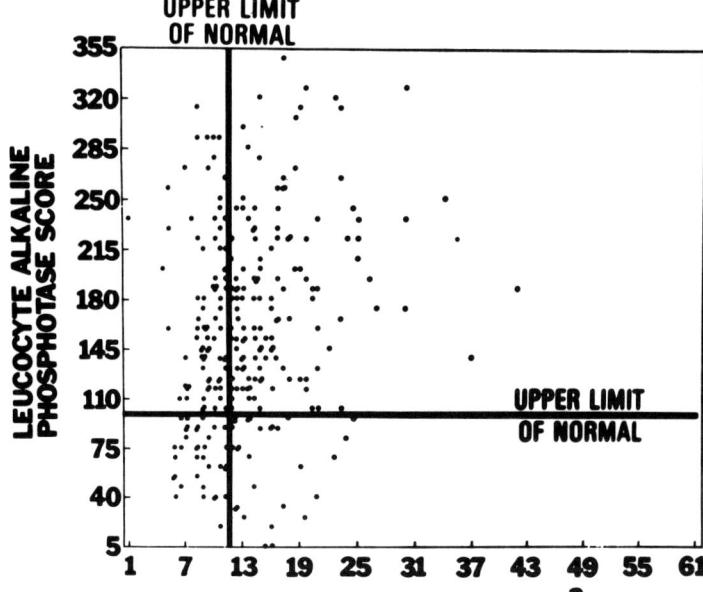

FIGURE 3-6. The leukocyte alkaline phosphatase score as a function of the white blood cell count in PVSG patients.

iron level to be lower in those phlebotomized more than 1 year before initial evaluation. The presumption is that these patients had more phlebotomies than patients phlebotomized in the year before initial evaluation by the PVSG. Clearly, phlebotomy reduces total-body iron stores that are not rapidly repleted, and this decrease in total-body iron is reflected in a decreased serum iron. Other measurements of total-body iron stores, such as a serum ferritin determination, were not carried out in these patients.

In summary, polycythemia vera is a disease principally of the elderly. During the 100 years in which it has been recognized as a disease entity, the average age of onset has increased substantially. There are slightly more male patients than female patients. Patients present with a number of symptoms, of which headache and fatigue are prominent, and often friends and family have commented that the patient has a red face or ruddy complexion. On physical examination, hyperten-

sion and splenomegaly are common findings. In the laboratory, an elevated hematocrit, white blood cell count, and platelet count are, with some exceptions, the rule. The differential diagnosis can be made on the basis of a history, a physical examination, and several key laboratory investigations. These include measurement of the total volume of circulating red cells, blood oxygen saturation, and hemoglobin P500$_2$ and an intravenous polygram or ultrasound examination of the kidneys. With the possible exception of a bone marrow culture, other laboratory determinations are of lesser value for the differential diagnosis, but a carboxyhemoglobin determination may be necessary in smokers. However, it must be recognized that bone marrow culture is not widely available. Finally, it must be noted that the principal features of this disease were described 90 years ago by Osler, and some 30 years to 40 years ago, large groups of patients were described by Lawrence, Berlin, and Huff,[19] Calabresi and Meyer,[32] and Wasserman and Bassen.[33]

TABLE 3-3. SERUM IRON DETERMINATION IN PVSG PATIENTS

	SERUM IRON (mg/dl)	
	Male	Female
Without previous phlebotomy	93 ± 6	73 ± 5
Phlebotomy in previous year	62 ± 7	56 ± 9
Phlebotomy more than 1 year before evaluation by PVSG	44 ± 8	53 ± 8

REFERENCES

1. Prochazka AV, Markowe HLJ: The epidemiology of polycythemia rubra vera in England and Wales 1968–1982. Br J Cancer 53:59, 1986
2. Vazquez MH: Concerning a special form of cyanosis with accompanying excessive and persistent hyperglobulia. C R Soc Biol 44:384, 1892

3. Osler W: Chronic cyanosis, with polycythemia and enlarged spleen: A new entity. Am J Med Sci 126:187, 1903

4. Weber FP, Watson JH: Chronic polycythemia with enlarged spleen, probably a disease of the bone marrow. Br Med J 1:729, 1904

5. Gaisbock F: Die polycythemia. Ergeb Inn Med Kinderheilk 21:234, 1922

6. Adamson JW, Fiakow PJ, Murphy S, et al: Polycythemia vera: Stem-cell and probable clonal origin of the disease. N Engl J Med 295:913, 1976

7. Waldman TA, Levin EH, Baldwin M: The association of polycythemia with a cerebellar hemangioblastoma. Am J Med 31:318, 1961

8. Berlin NI, Lawrence JH, Gartland J: Blood volume in polycythemia as determined by ^{32}P-labeled red cells. Am J Med 9:474, 1950

9. Modan B: Polycythemia: A review of epidemiological and clinical aspects. J Chron Dis 18:605, 1965

10. Najean Y, Triebel F, Dresch C: Pure erythrocytosis: Reappraisal of a study of 51 cases. Am J Hematol 10:129, 1981

11. Pearson TC, Wetherley-Mein G: The course and complications of idiopathic erythrocytosis. Clin Lab Haematol 1:189, 1979

12. Dudley JM, Westwood N, Leonard S, et al: Primary polycythaemia: Positive diagnosis using the differential response of primitive and mature erythroid progenitors to erythropoietin, interleukin 3 and alpha-interferon. Br J Haematol 75:188, 1990

13. Lemoine F, Najman A, Baillou C, et al: A prospective study of bone marrow erythroid progenitor cultures in polycythemia. Blood 68:996, 1986

14. Nielsen S, Rodbro P: Validity of rapid estimation of erythrocyte volume in the diagnosis of polycythemia vera. Eur J Nucl Med 15:32, 1989

15. Landsfeldt U, Nielsen EM, Mathiassen B, Rodbro P: Comments on validity of rapid estimation of erythrocyte volume in the diagnosis of polycythemia vera. Eur J Nucl Med 17:96, 1990

16. Belcher EH, Berlin NI, Eernisse JG, et al: Standard techniques for the measurement of red-cell and plasma volume. Br J Haematol 25:801, 1973

17. Nathan DG: Comments on the interpretation of measurements of total red cell volume in the diagnosis of polycythemia vera. Semin Hematol 3:216, 1966

18. Wasserman LR, Dobson RL, Lawrence JH: Blood oxygen studies in patients with polycythemia and in normal subjects. J Clin Invest 28:60, 1949

19. Lawrence JH, Berlin NI, Huff RL: The nature and treatment of polycythemia. Medicine 32:288, 1953

20. Smith JR, Landaw SA: Smokers' polycythemia. N Engl J Med 298:6, 1978

21. Carache S, Weatherall DJ, Clegg JB: Polycythemia associated with a hemoglobulinopathy. J Clin Invest 45:813, 1966

22. Erslev AJ, Williams WJ, Beutler E, Lichtman MA: Hemoglobulinopathies producing erythrocytosis. In Hematology, 4th ed, New York, McGraw-Hill, 1990, pp 717–721

23. Koeffler HP, Goldwasser E: Erythropoietin radioimmunoassay in evaluating patients with polycythemia. Ann Intern Med 94:44, 1981

24. Cotes MP, Dore CJ, Liu Yin JA, et al: Determination of serum immunoreactive erythropoietin in the investigation of erythrocytosis. N Engl J Med 315:283, 1986

25. Birgegård G, Wide L: Serum erythropoietin in the diagnosis off polycythaemia and after phlebotomy treatment. Br J Haematol 81:603, 1992

26. Najean Y, Schlageter M-H, Toubert M-E, Podgorniak M-P: Radioimmunoassay of immunoreactive erythropoietin as a clinical tool for the classification of polycythaemias. Nouv Rev Fr Hematol 32:237, 1990

27. Zanjani ED, Lutton JD, Hoffman R, Wasserman LR: Erythroid colony formation by polycythemia vera bone marrow in vitro: Dependence on erythropoietin. J Clin Invest 59:841, 1977

28. Partanen S, Juvonen E, Ikkala E, Ruutu T: Spontaneous erythroid colony formation in the differential diagnosis of erythrocytosis. Eur J Haematol 42:327, 1989

29. Berlin NI: Diagnosis and classification of the polycythemias. Semin Hematol 12:338, 1975

30. Berk PD, Goldberg JD, Donovan PB, et al: Therapeutic recommendations in polycythemia vera based on polycythemia vera study group protocols. Semin Hematol 23:132, 1986

31. Berlin NI: Differential diagnosis of the polycythemias. Semin Hematol 3:209, 1966

32. Calabresi P, Meyer OO: Polycythemia vera: I. Clinical and laboratory manifestations. Ann Intern Med 50:1182, 1959

33. Wasserman LR, Bassen F: Polycythemia. J Mt Sinai Hosp 26:1, 1959

4

The Bone Marrow in Polycythemia Vera

POWERS PETERSON *and* JOHN T. ELLIS

This chapter summarizes the current status of the histologic studies of the bone marrow and lymph nodes of patients randomized to the Polycythemia Vera Study Group (PVSG).[1-3] Even though this study has been underway since 1967, many of the morphologic studies must still be considered preliminary because one-fifth of the patients are alive and on study. Large numbers of patients with sequential biopsies covering the entire long course from diagnosis to death are essential to appreciate the full spectrum of tissue changes of this disease.

The literature contains many studies of the bone marrow in polycythemia vera (PV), but none of these is prospective, randomized, or contains large numbers of patients. Previously reported bone marrow abnormalities in PV consist of increases in marrow cellularity,[4-7] increases in the number or size of megakaryocytes,[4,6-9] increases in the number of eosinophils,[7] increases in the amount of reticulin and/or myelofibrosis,[10-20] depletion of marrow iron pigment,[2-4,7] and increases in the volume of the venous sinuses.[20,21]

METHODS AND MATERIALS

An international Polycythemia Vera Study Group was organized in 1967 to answer questions concerning the natural history of the disease and the optimal form of therapy in patients with well-documented PV. After screening by strict diagnostic criteria,[22] 432 patients were randomized to one of three treatment regimens differing in their modes of action, *viz.*, phlebotomy, chlorambucil (Leukeran, Burroughs-Wellcome, Research Triangle Park, N.C.), and radioactive phosphorus (^{32}P). Patients randomized must have had PV of recent onset, with a history not exceeding 4 years, and must not have received previous treatment other than phlebotomy. The bone marrow was biopsied before treatment was instituted and usually every 2 years thereafter.

The details of the biopsy techniques, preparation of sections, biopsy evaluation, and statistical methods have been described previously[1,2] and were based on standard methodologies employed by ourselves and others. Such methods of evaluation yielded reproducible results when the biopsies were reexamined as unknowns.

Reticulin was evaluated in a fashion similar to that employed by others[14,22-24] and was graded as follows (Fig. 4-1):

Normal	No fibers, occasional individual fibers, or focal areas with a fine fiber network.
Slight increase	Fine fiber network throughout much of section; no coarse fibers demonstrated.
Moderate increase	Diffuse fiber network with focal collections of thick, coarse fibers arranged in bundles.

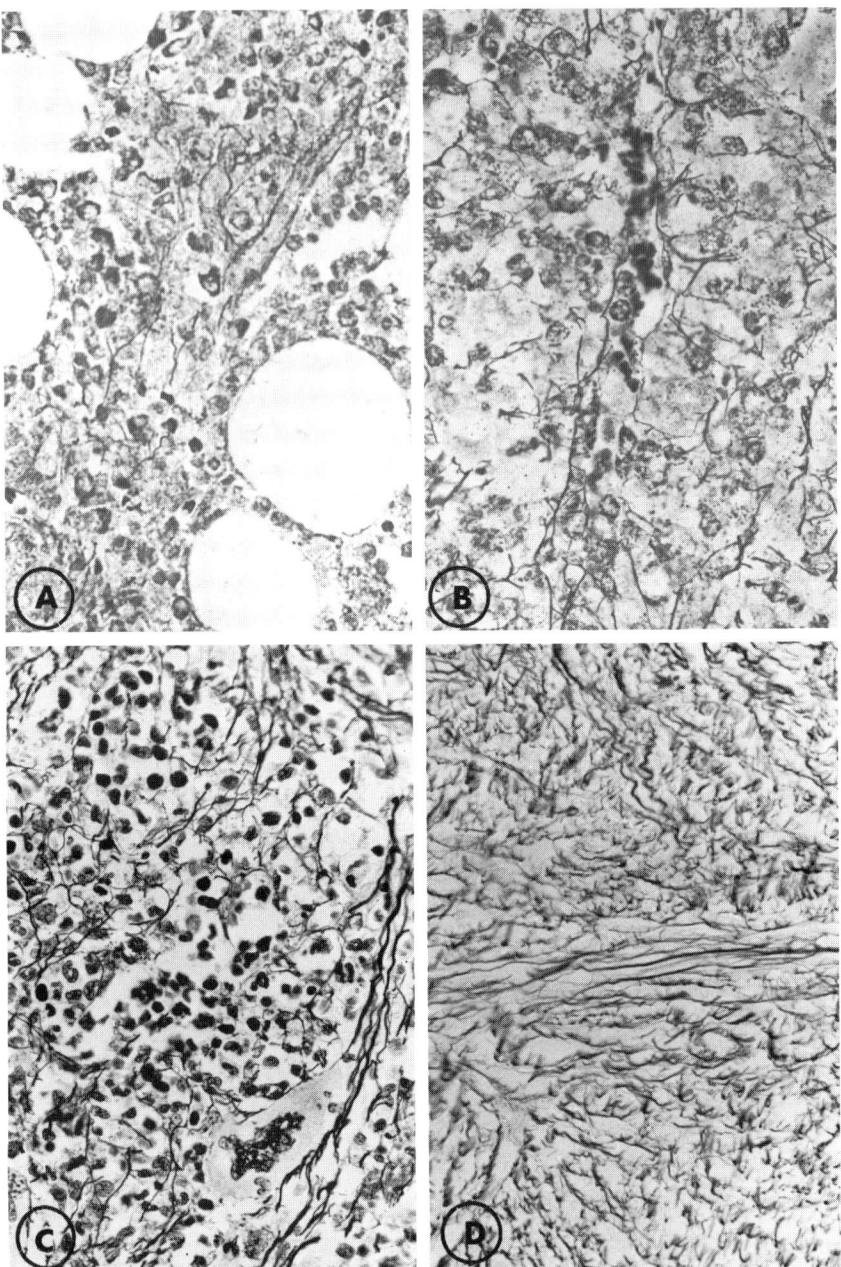

FIGURE 4–1. Photomicrographs of representative fields of four biopsies showing variation in reticulin content in PV. See text for description (Foot & Foot silver stain; × 330). (A) Normal reticulin content. (B) Slight increase in reticulin content. (C) Moderate increase in reticulin content. (D) Marked increase in reticulin content.

Marked increase Diffuse, often coarse, long fibers usually arranged in bundles.

Individual coarse reticulin fibers are generally positive for collagen in properly stained Mallory-Azan or other trichrome preparations.

CELLULARITY AND MEGAKARYOCYTES IN PRETREATMENT BIOPSIES

It has long been known that biopsies from patients with untreated PV have an increase in the content of the erythroid, granulocytic, and megakaryocytic precursors in the bone marrow, as illustrated in Fig. 4–2. Prior to the PVSG study, it was not appreciated that there is a wide variation in cellular elements among individual cases, as is shown in the histograms of the 191 patients studied quantitatively (Figs. 4–3 and 4–4). The cellularity ranged from 37 to 100 percent, with a mean of 82 percent. Figure 4–4 shows the distribution of megakaryocytes per square millimeter. The values for whole marrow ranged from 12 to 145 megakaryocytes per square millimeter, with a mean of 62 per square millimeter. Qualitative observations corre-

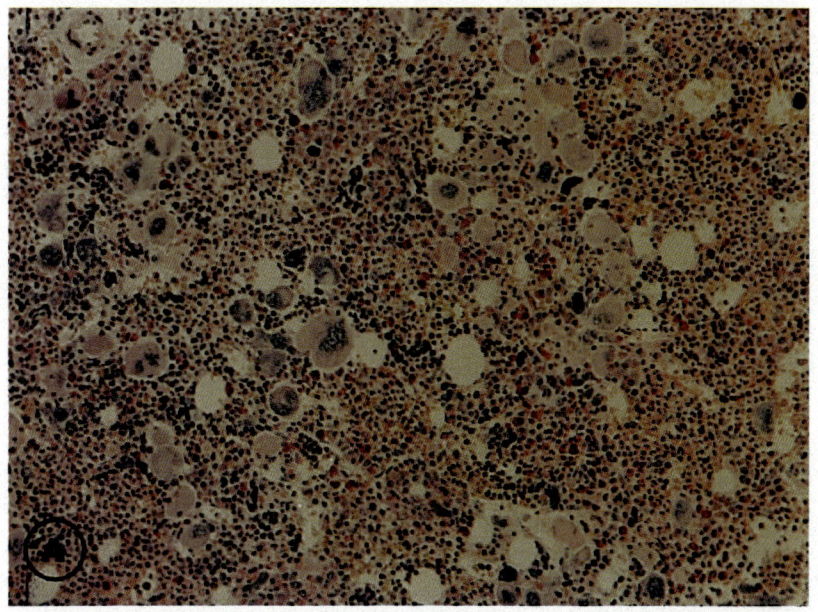

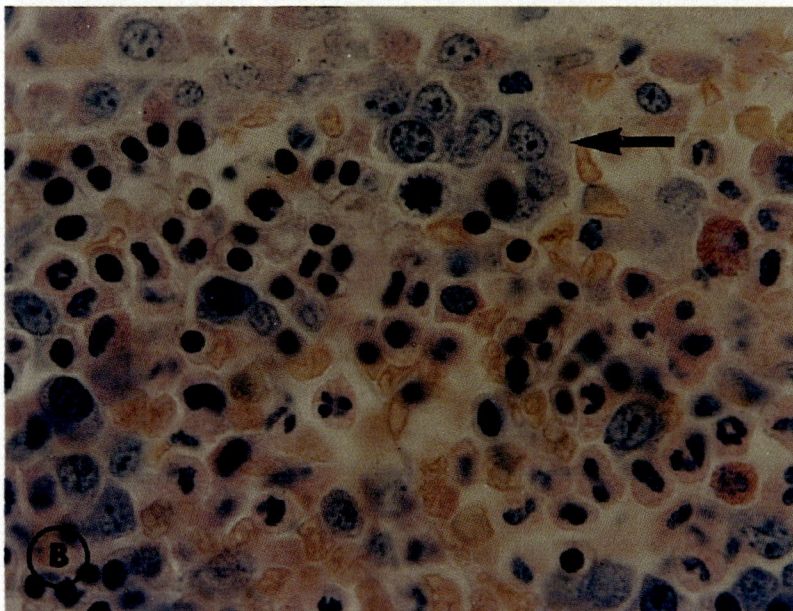

FIGURE 4–2. (A) Photomicrograph of pretreatment biopsy in PV showing marked marrow hypercellularity due to panhyperplasia. Note variations in megakaryocytic size and nuclei (Giemsa stain; × 125). Parts B, C, and D are different fields from same case. (B) Erythroid hyperplasia. Note clusters of basophilic erythroblasts (*arrow*) with adjacent pyknotic normoblasts (× 1000).

Illustration continued on following page

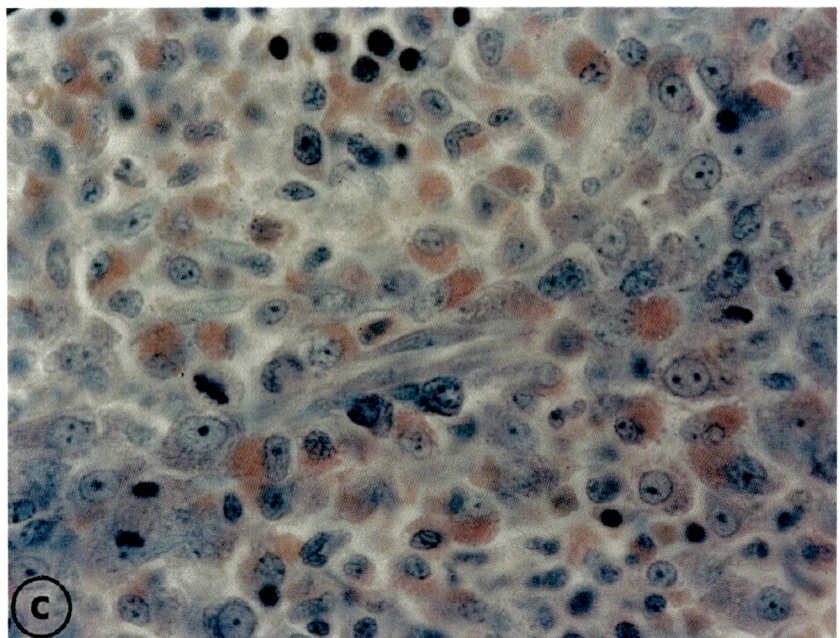

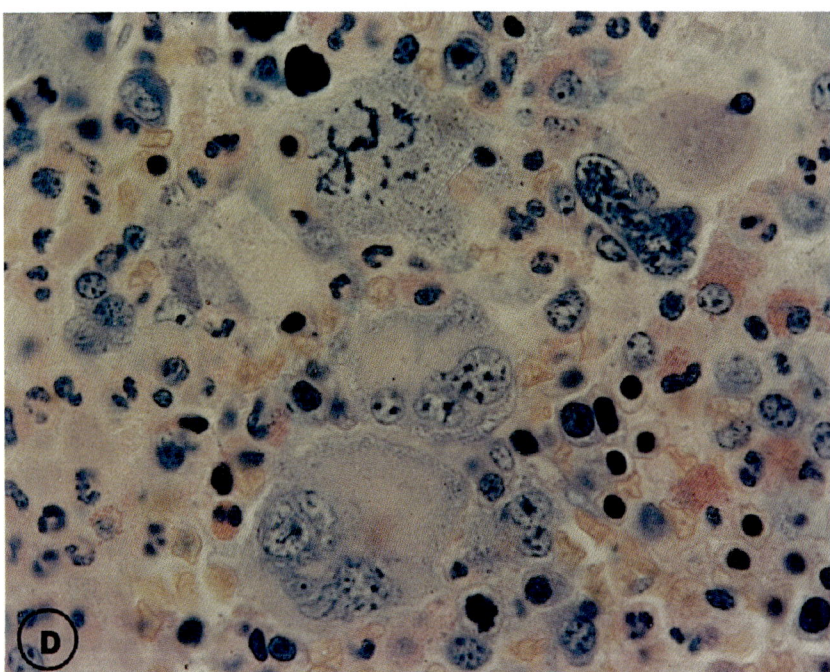

FIGURE 4–2 *Continued (C and D)* (C) Granulocytic hyperplasia. Focus of neutrophilic and eosinophilic myelocytes surrounding vessel (× 1000). (D) Megakaryocytic hyperplasia. Cluster of megakaryocytes in varying stages of development from mitosis to degranulation and pyknosis (× 1000).

lated well with the quantitative evaluations of the marrows.

Since marked hypercellularity of the bone marrow was to be expected in PV, it was surprising that of the 281 pretreatment biop-

sies, 36 (13 percent) demonstrated initial marrow cellularity of less than 60 percent and therefore appeared relatively normal (Fig. 4–5). This group of patients was studied to determine whether the diagnosis of PV

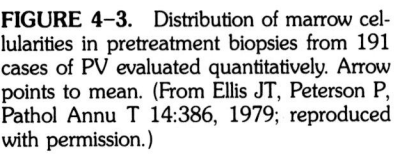

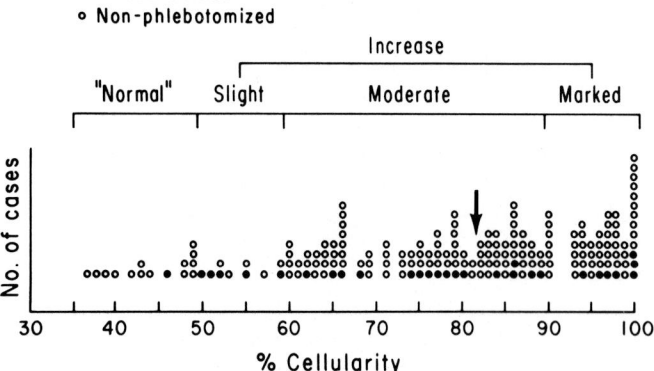

FIGURE 4-3. Distribution of marrow cellularities in pretreatment biopsies from 191 cases of PV evaluated quantitatively. Arrow points to mean. (From Ellis JT, Peterson P, Pathol Annu T 14:386, 1979; reproduced with permission.)

was valid and if the group constituted a subset of PV. No unique clinical or laboratory features distinguished this group of patients, whose ages ranged from 42 to 83 years. Each of the patients met the PVSG strict criteria for diagnosis, and 35 of the 36 patients required continuous therapy to control their disease. Thirteen patients had a normal megakaryocytic concentration on pretreatment biopsy but later showed a significant increase in cellularity and/or megakaryocytes on subsequent biopsies. This was considered additional morphologic evidence indicative of PV.

For these reasons, it has been concluded that no particular prognostic or biologic significance can be attached to the occurrence of cellularities of less than 60 percent or of normal concentrations of megakaryocytes in pretreatment biopsies of this small and interesting group of PV patients. Whether or not

these initial biopsies were representative of the marrow in general cannot be decided from the data.

Other investigators[26,27] have proposed that increased numbers of megakaryocytes per square millimeter in PV, chronic myelogenous leukemia (CML), and essential thrombocythemia (ET) are related to the development of myelofibrosis and to decreased median survival. Unfortunately, the data on the PVSG patients cannot be closely compared with these data in terms of diagnostic criteria, randomization to different therapies, numbers and sequence of posttreatment biopsies, clinical and laboratory data, etc.

BONE MARROW HEMOSIDERIN

Absence of iron pigment is to be expected in PV, and this finding may be diagnostically useful.[1-4,7] Iron pigment was present in only

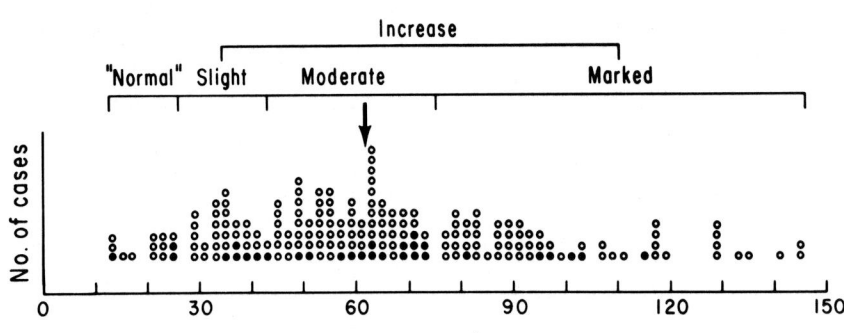

FIGURE 4-4. Distribution of megakaryocytes per square millimeter of whole marrow in pretreatment biopsies of 191 cases of PV evaluated quantitatively. Arrow points to mean. (From Ellis JT, Peterson P, Pathol Annu T 14:387, 1979; reproduced with permission.)

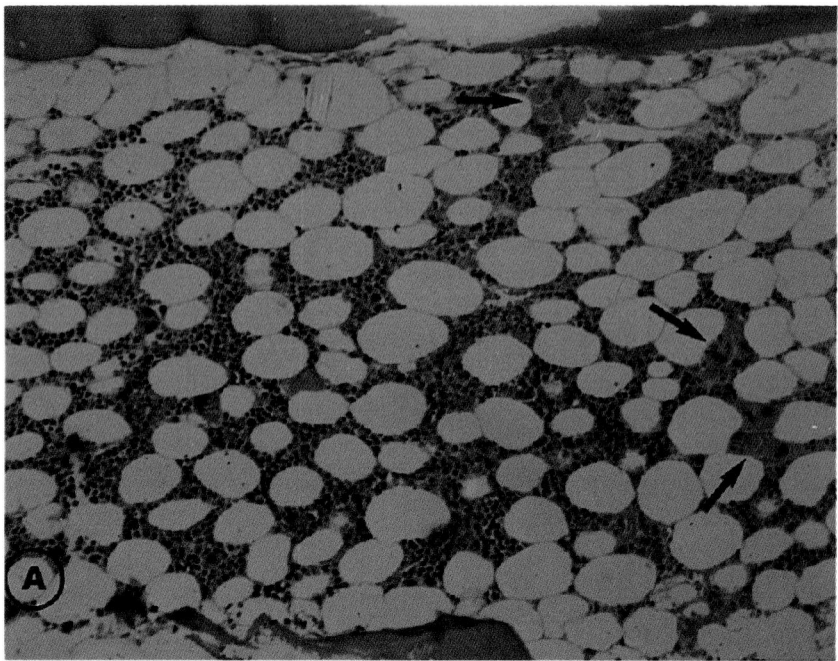

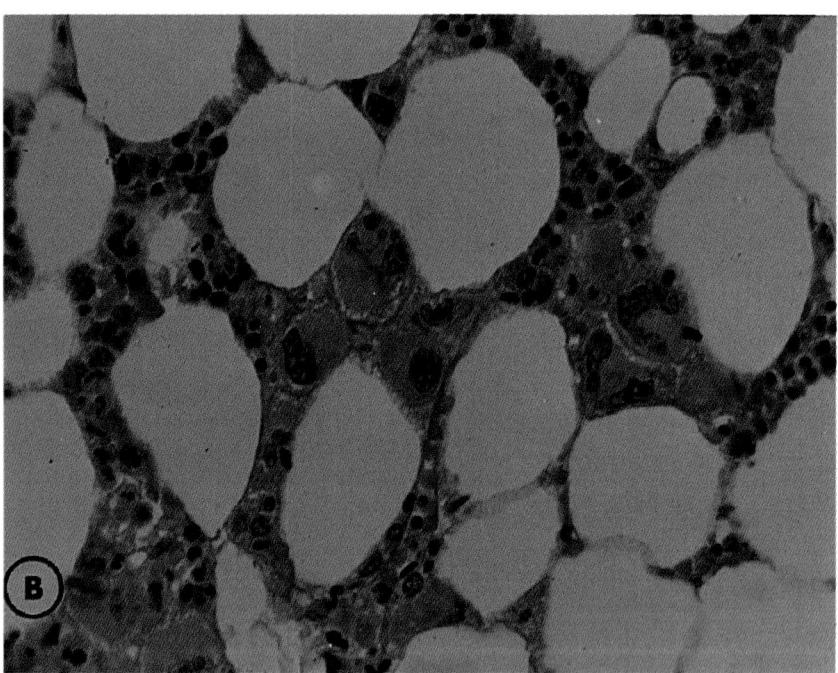

FIGURE 4–5. (A) Photomicrograph of pretreatment biopsy in PV with 40 percent cellularity. Compare with Fig. 2A. Note clusters of megakaryocytes (*arrows*), suggestive of a diagnosis of PV (hematoxylin and eosin stain; × 120). (B) Higher magnification of one of the megakaryocytic clusters (× 450).

17 of 256 (6.6 percent) pretreatment PVSG biopsies in which stained material was available for evaluation. Depletion of iron pigment in marrow histiocytes in PV is generally

thought to be secondary to expansion of the blood volume or to iron deficiency caused by chronic bleeding.

In the staining of histiocytes in marrow

sections by the Prussian blue reaction, ferritin gives a diffuse blue reaction and hemosiderin has a granular form.[28] Caution should be employed in interpretation of iron content of marrow based on sections alone. Sections fixed or stored in acidic solutions for long periods and then decalcified with acids may lose appreciable amounts of iron-containing pigment into the solution.[29] The preceding statements are not true of marrow aspirates, since they are air-dried, do not require decalcification, and are not fixed in acidic solutions. Similarly, undecalcified (methacrylate) sections are the equal of aspirates in assessing iron stores.

NATURE OF RETICULIN AND TYPES OF MARROW FIBROSIS

The supporting network of the bone marrow is composed of branched fibroblastic (reticular) cells that elaborate delicate fibers termed *reticulin*. These fine fibers are blackened by silver impregnation but do not take histochemical stains for collagen. In contrast, *collagen* fibers are coarser, stain with the usual trichrome stains, and do not usually blacken with silver impregnation. Earlier workers[30,31] incorrectly considered reticulin and collagen fibers as different entities, but both have the same cross-striations by electron microscopy,[32,33] and biochemical methods and immunofluorescent staining indicate that the fine fibers are mainly type III collagen and the coarse fibers are type I collagen.[34,35] Both type I and type III collagen are thought to be synthesized by individual reticular cells.[36-39] Currently, it is thought that the blackening of the fibers by silver impregnation is due to staining of a glycoprotein or proteoglycan matrix admixed with the collagen fibers.[32,40] The biologic significance of these various types of collagen in the bone marrow is not fully understood at this time.

The terms *reticulin fibrosis* and *collagen fibrosis* are well established in the literature. In bone marrow fibrosis, sequential biopsies indicate that initially there is a diffuse or patchy increase in reticulin fibers admixed with abundant hematopoietic elements (reticulin fibrosis). In later biopsies, the marrow is replaced by coarse collagen fibers with a paucity of hematopoietic cells (collagen fibrosis).[18,41] This progression from reticulin fibrosis to collagen fibrosis in the marrow may be analogous to the similar progression occurring in experimental dermal wound healing, in which collagen composition changes as time passes (type III is replaced by type I).[42-44]

Cytogenetic studies, isoenzyme markers, and gene mutation studies by polymerase chain reaction (PCR) have shown the hematopoietic cells to be of clonal origin and presumably neoplastic in idiopathic myelofibrosis (IMF) and the other chronic myeloproliferative disorders (PV, ET, and CML).[45-53] These studies also indicate that marrow fibroblasts are not a part of the abnormal clone; therefore, marrow fibrosis is now generally considered to be a secondary response.[54,55] At this time, the precise mechanisms by which the cells of the abnormal clone stimulate the host's fibroblasts to produce the excessive amounts of collagen are unknown. Megakaryocytes,[56] mast cells,[57] autoimmune reactions,[58] autoimmune complexes,[59] and platelet-derived growth factor[60-63] have been suggested as possibly being of importance in mediating the fibrosis.

STUDIES OF BONE MARROW RETICULIN IN PV

Clinical experience has shown that the course of PV can be divided into developmental, erythrocytotic, stable, and spent phases. Progression between the phases is gradual over the long course and should be anticipated if the patient does not die of complications of PV or of unrelated causes. The developmental phase is usually clinically silent and of unknown duration. The erythrocytotic phase is of long duration and requires therapy because of marrow overproduction, while in the stable/spent phase the converse is present, and the patient may require therapy for marrow failure. *Postpolycythemic myeloid metaplasia* (PPMM) refers to both clinical and morphologic abnormalities and is characterized by increasing splenomegaly, teardrop poikilocytes, a normal or decreasing red cell volume, and fibrosis of the marrow.[11,14-16] In common usage, the syndrome of PPMM is synonymous with the spent phase of PV.

Use of the term *myeloid metaplasia* is not entirely satisfactory, since it implies a knowledge, which may be quite imperfect, of the formation of hematopoietic elements outside the marrow cavities of the bony skeleton, i.e., in the spleen, liver, lymph nodes, and other sites. Unfortunately, the histologic proof of myeloid metaplasia is often lacking, since these tissues frequently are studied only at the time of splenectomy or death. The clinical diagnosis of myeloid metaplasia is not precise, since enlargement of the liver and spleen may be due to causes other than myeloid metaplasia, and even the size of these organs may be difficult or impossible to determine accurately by physical examination alone.

There are many difficulties in elucidating the precise sequence of the bone marrow findings in relation to the clinical course of PV. The true onset of the disease may be impossible to determine, since the disease may be present for an indeterminate period before symptoms occur. PV is a rare disease, and it is extremely difficult to obtain sequential marrow biopsies from significant numbers of patients except in a research setting. The course of PV is very long, and prolonged follow-up is difficult but is essential to appreciate the natural history of the disease. Finally, many patients die of other conditions and thus do not live long enough to show progressive marrow changes.

As will be shown by the PVSG data, the relationship of reticulin content to the clinical activity of PV is not entirely clear, but an isolated finding of reticulin fibrosis is not synonymous with nor indicative of the imminent development of spent-phase PV (PPMM); significant increase of reticulin may be present in pretreatment biopsies early in the course of PV and also during therapy for marrow overproduction.

Reticulin and collagen stains were carefully evaluated in the PVSG patients, and the results were correlated with the activity of the disease, the need for therapy, and manifestations of PPMM.

Pretreatment Biopsies

Of the 226 pretreatment biopsies from patients in the PVSG that were graded for reticulin, 64 percent were normal, 25 percent showed only a slight increase in reticulin, and 11 percent showed a moderate to marked increase in reticulin fibers. It was surprising to find that 11 percent of patients had a moderate to marked increase in reticulin content, since the biopsies were taken early in the course of the disease and prior to any cytotoxic therapy.[1,2]

The course of these 25 patients following therapy was quite varied, but the presence of increased reticulin on a pretreatment biopsy was not indicative of the imminent development of PPMM. The mean length of follow-up was 85 months, with a range of 8 to 134 months. The findings were as follows (Table 4–1):

1. In 7 patients (cases 1 to 7), the increased reticulin content was unchanged in the first posttreatment biopsy taken from 11 to 53 months later. Case 7 progressed to spent-phase PV approximately 6 years after the initial diagnosis of PV (Fig. 4–6).

2. In 10 patients (cases 8 to 17), the first posttreatment biopsies were normal. These biopsies were taken from 24 to 51 months later. In case 15, the first posttreatment biopsy (2 years later) was normal, but two subsequent biopsies taken at $4^{1}/_2$ and 5 years later showed a moderate increase in reticulin. In case 17, the reticulin fibrosis apparently reverted to normal, as evidenced by three biopsies with a normal reticulin content over 4 years. Three and one-half years thereafter, the patient entered the spent phase, and the marrow biopsy showed a moderate increase in reticulin content. Three of these 10 patients later progressed to AL (cases 10, 13, and 16). In case 16, there was clinical evidence of spent-phase PV 5 months prior to the diagnosis of AL.

3. Eight patients (cases 18 to 25) with an initially significant increase in reticulin did not have a second biopsy performed. Six of these patients have died, one of AL.

Of the 17 patients who had repeat biopsies, 7 had been treated with chlorambucil, 8 with ^{32}P, and 2 by phlebotomy alone. All 10 patients who apparently showed a decrease in the reticulin content on posttreatment biopsies were treated with myelosuppressive agents (chlorambucil or ^{32}P). Of the 7 patients in whom the moderate to marked increase in reticulin was confirmed on repeat posttreatment biopsies, 2 were treated by phlebotomy alone and 5 with myelosuppressive agents.

TABLE 4-1. ANALYSIS OF 25 CASES OF PV SHOWING A MODERATE OR MARKED INCREASE IN RETICULIN CONTENT PRIOR TO THERAPY

CASE NO.		RETICULIN CONTENT*				
		Pretreatment	Posttreatment			
1		+ + +	+ + +			
2		+ + +	+ + +			
3	▲	+ + +	+ + +			
4		+ + + +	+ + +			
5		+ + +	+ + +	+ +		
6		+ + + +	+ + +	+ + +	+ +	+ + +
7	■	+ + + +	+ + + +	+ + +	+ + + +	+ + + + (×3)
8	▲	+ + +	+			
9		+ + +	+			
10	★	+ + +	+			
11		+ + +	+	+		
12	▲	+ + +	+	+		
13	★	+ + + +	+	+ +		
14	▲	+ + +	+	+ +		
15		+ + + +	+	+ + +	+ + +	
16	■★	+ + +	+	+ +	+ + +	
17	■▲	+ + +	+	+	+	+ + +
18–25	1▲; 1★	+ + +/+ + + +	No repeat biopsies			

* + = normal; + + = slight increase; + + + = moderate increase; + + + + = marked increase; ■ = spent PV/PPMM; ★ = acute leukemia; ▲ = alive.

Source: Modified from Ellis JT, Peterson P, Semin Hematol 23:147, 1986; reproduced with permission.

Posttreatment Biopsies with Reticulin Fibrosis from Patients in the Active Phase of PV

After randomization and following the inception of therapy, a moderate to marked increase in reticulin content developed in 31 patients prior to any clinical symptoms or laboratory evidence of spent-phase PV. Currently, 15 of these patients have developed spent-phase PV and will be discussed in the next subsection, while 16 remain in the active phase of PV (Table 4–2).

The course of these 16 patients is similar to that of the patients in the previous subsection, in whom reticulin fibrosis was found prior to therapy and strengthens the observation that reticulin fibrosis may be present long before other evidence of spent-phase PV. The mean length of follow-up was 78 months, with a range of 26 to 117 months. Thirteen of these patients had a normal or slightly increased reticulin level on pretreatment biopsy (cases 26 to 38), and in the other three instances there were no pretreatment biopsies (cases 39 to 41). In the 13 patients with pre- and posttreatment biopsies, a moderate to marked increase in reticulin content has been present for periods ranging from a few months to 6½ years. Nine patients have died while in the active phase of PV; none of these 9 developed spent-phase PV or AL. Therapy administered in the 16 patients was as follows: 7, phlebotomy alone; 6, chlorambucil; and 2, ^{32}P. One other patient randomized to treatment by phlebotomy alone was later given ^{32}P.

Of the 16 patients with increased reticulin content in posttreatment biopsies, 13 had multiple biopsies which provide documentation as to the progression or regression of the marrow fibrosis. In 3 patients (cases 39 to 41), progression of the fibrosis could not be evaluated because there were no pretreatment biopsies. In 13 patients (cases 26 to 38), the pretreatment biopsies showed reticulin content that was essentially normal. Each of these later had posttreatment biopsies in which the reticulin content was either moderately or markedly increased. Ten of these patients (cases 26 to 32 and 39 to 41) had only a single posttreatment biopsy which demonstrated the reticulin fibrosis. In 3 patients (cases 33 to 35), there were multiple posttreatment biopsies which reconfirmed the reticulin fibrosis. In 3 patients (cases 36 to 38), an apparently normal reticulin content was present in the next sequential biopsy. Additional biopsies will be required to fully evaluate this issue. These patients were treated as follows: 1, phlebotomy alone; 1, chlorambucil; 1, ^{32}P.

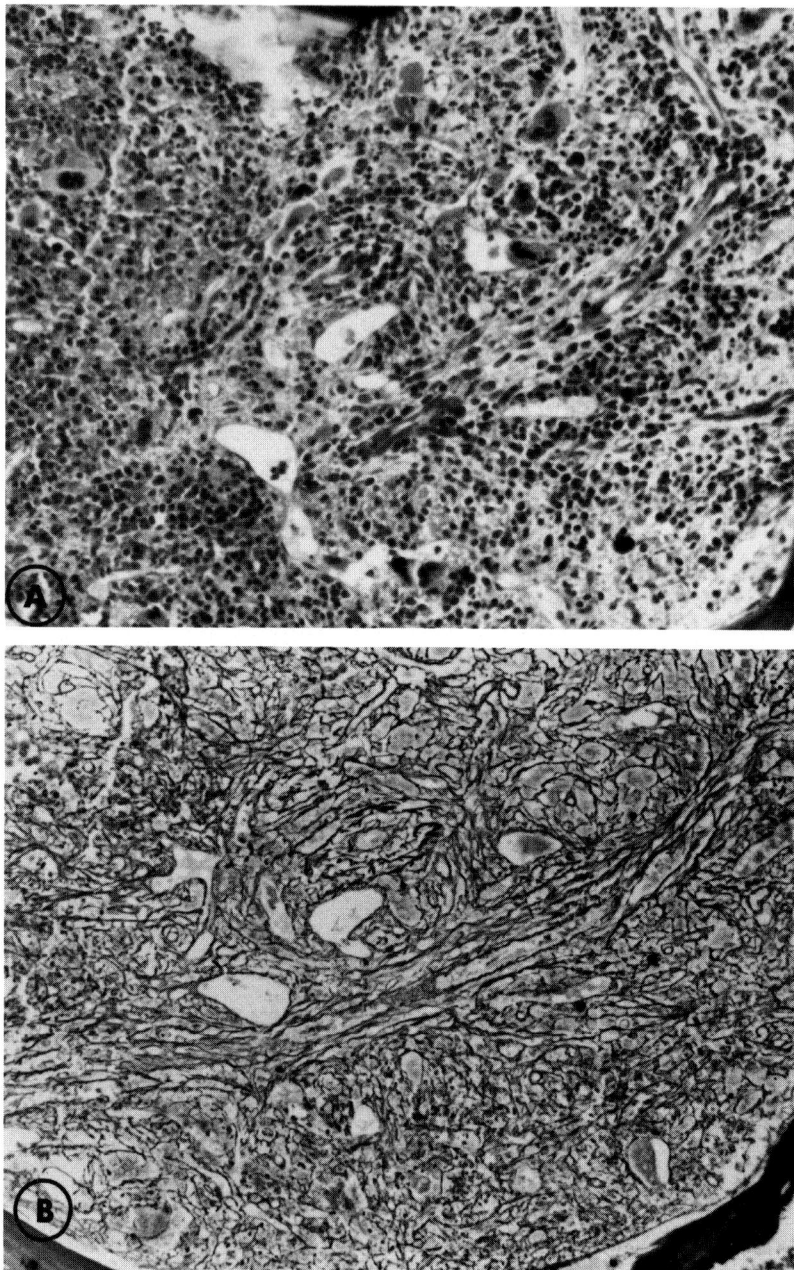

FIGURE 4–6. Photomicrographs of posttreatment biopsy in spent-phase PV (PPMM). This 69-year-old woman had been treated with ^{32}P and progressed to the spent phase 6 years after randomization. The pretreatment biopsy showed a marked increase in reticulin (case 7, Table 4–1). (A) The moderately cellular marrow contains many megakaryocytes (hematoxylin and eosin stain; × 170). (B) Serial section of same biopsy demonstrating marked increase in reticulin fibers. Note the parallel arrangement of coarse reticulin fibers to form bundles (Foot and Foot silver stain; × 170). (From Ellis JT, Peterson P, Semin Hematol 23:149, 1986; reproduced with permission.)

TABLE 4-2. ANALYSIS OF 16 CASES OF ACTIVE PV
WITH INCREASED RETICULIN CONTENT ON POSTTREATMENT
BIOPSIES

		RETICULIN CONTENT*					
CASE NO.		Pretreatment	Posttreatment				
26		+	+ + +				
27		+	+ + +				
28		+	+ + +				
29	▲	+ +	+ + +				
30	▲	+	+	+ + +			
31	▲	+	+	+ + +			
32		+	+	+	+ + +		
33		+	+ + + +	+ +	+ + + +		
34		+ +	+ + +	+ +	+ + +		
35		+ +	+ +	+ +	+ + +	+ + + +	+ + +
36	▲	+	+ + +	+			
37	▲	+	+	+ + +	+		
38	▲	+	+ + +	+	+ +	+ +	
39	▲	No biopsy	+ + +				
40		No biopsy	+ + + +				
41		No biopsy	+ + + +				

* + = normal; + + = slight increase; + + + = moderate increase; + + + + = marked increase;
▲ = alive.
Source: Modified from Ellis JT, Peterson P, Semin Hematol 23:147, 1986; reproduced with permission.

Spent-Phase Polycythemia (PPMM)

PPMM is characterized by increasing splenomegaly, teardrop poikilocytes, a normal or decreasing red cell volume, and fibrosis of the marrow[11,14,16] and in common usage is synonymous with the spent phase of PV. Thirty-eight (8.7 percent) of the 432 randomized patients met these criteria. The typical marrow histology is shown in Fig. 4–6, and examples of the progression of marrow findings are shown in Fig. 4–7.

The marrow biopsies from every case of spent-phase PV have shown a moderate to marked increase in reticulin. The time (mean) between randomization and onset of spent-phase PV was 7 years and 10 months, with a range of 39 to 144 months. These ranges constitute the minimum time intervals because patients may have had untreated PV for as long as 4 years prior to randomization to this protocol. The patients were divided among the three treatment arms as follows: phlebotomy, 15; chlorambucil, 11; and ^{32}P, 12. Attempts were made to correlate the onset of reticulin fibrosis with the clinical status. Fifteen of these 38 patients showed increases in reticulin while in the active phase and long before the clinical change to spent-phase PV. In each of these, the reticulin increase was documented from 2 to 6 1/2 years prior to the clinical onset of PPMM. An example is case P 138 in Fig. 4–7. In 8 additional instances, biopsies were not taken reg-

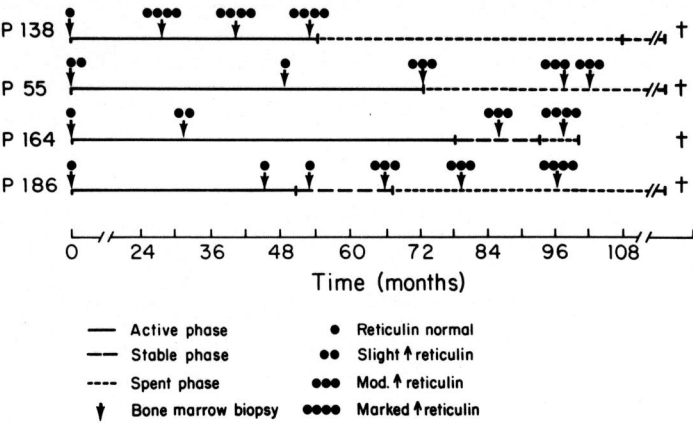

FIGURE 4-7. Correlation of marrow reticulin and the spent phase of PV. The clinical course of four patients who developed spent-phase PV (PPMM) is correlated with the reticulin content of their sequential marrow biopsies (see text for description). Note that all these cases showed progression of the fibrosis. (From Ellis JT, Peterson P, Semin Hematol 23:150, 1986; reproduced with permission.)

ularly during the active phase of the disease; therefore, the reticulin content was not determined prior to the clinical onset of the spent phase. An example is case P 164 in Fig. 4–7. In 11 instances in which biopsies were obtained regularly during the active phase, the reticulin fibrosis was documented either simultaneously or within a year before or after the clinical change. Examples of this are cases P 55 and P 186 in Fig. 4–7. Four (of the 38) patients have been excluded from this analysis. In 2 patients, the transition to AL was so close to the onset of the spent phase that the two processes could not be temporally separated. Two patients were lost to follow-up for almost 10 years each, and therefore, the onset of the spent phase could not be properly documented.

Of the 38 patients with spent-phase PV, 35 had pretreatment and multiple posttreatment biopsies which provide documentation as to the progression or regression of the marrow fibrosis. Frequent biopsies over long periods of time are essential for evaluation of the change in reticulin. The distribution of the number of biopsies evaluated in the 35 patients is shown in Table 4–3. Seven patients had three sequential biopsies, while 20 patients had five or more sequential biopsies. A tabulation of the change in the reticulin content is shown in Table 4–4. Each of the pretreatment biopsies showed an essentially normal reticulin content, while the posttreatment biopsies showed reticulin fibrosis. The most frequent pattern observed was a normal reticulin content progressing to a marked increase in 21 of the 35 patients. In none of these 35 patients was there evidence of regression of the marrow fibrosis (i.e., decrease in reticulin content), as determined by these sequential biopsy studies of silver-stained preparations.

TABLE 4–3. DISTRIBUTION OF SEQUENTIAL MARROW BIOPSIES IN 35 CASES OF SPENT-PHASE PV

NO. OF BIOPSIES PER CASE	NO. OF CASES
3	7
4	8
5	10
6	8
7	2

Source: Modified from Ellis JT, Peterson P, Semin Hematol 23:150, 1986; reproduced with permission.

TABLE 4–4. PROGRESSION OF RETICULIN FIBROSIS IN 35 CASES OF SPENT-PHASE PV

RETICULIN CONTENT*		
Pretreatment Biopsy	Posttreatment Biopsy	NO. OF CASES
+ to	+ + +	7
+ to	+ + + +	21
+ + to	+ + +	1
+ + to	+ + + +	6

* + = normal reticulin content; + + = slight increase in reticulin content; + + + = moderate increase in reticulin content; + + + + = marked increase in reticulin content.
Source: Modified from Ellis JT, Peterson P, Semin Hematol 23:150, 1986; reproduced with permission.

Evidence for Change in Reticulin Fiber Content

In the literature, myelofibrosis has been considered to be a more or less irreversible process and to be either stable or slowly progressive in the majority of patients. This was true of the reticulin fibrosis that occurred in the PV patients reported in the preceding subsection and illustrated in Fig. 4–5.

The question of progression and/or regression of the reticulin content in the biopsy groups still in the erythrocytotic phase is less clear. For example, 10 of the 25 patients with a moderate to marked increase in reticulin content prior to therapy showed an apparent decrease in reticulin in the first posttreatment biopsy (Table 4–1, cases 8 to 17). In addition, in biopsies from 3 of the 16 patients who developed reticulin fibrosis in the active stage of the disease, the reticulin content of the next sequential biopsy was apparently normal (Table 4–2, cases 36 to 38). At this time it is difficult or impossible to evaluate the apparent regression until additional biopsies are studied during the further course of these patients.

The usual course of marrow fibrosis in various myeloproliferative diseases (except CML) is indicated by another group of patients who were studied by the PVSG to evaluate the effect of treatment on marrow fibrosis.[64] In these prospective studies, serial needle biopsies were procured. Twenty-four previously treated patients had either demonstrable reticulin or collagen fibrosis initially and were treated with fluoxymesterone (Halotestin, Upjohn, Kalamazoo, Mich.) or transfusions. In the 10 patients on whom sequential biopsies were performed (13 to 38 months later), all showed no change or progression of the fibrosis. In only 1 patient did collagen fibrosis revert to normal; this occurred simultaneously with blastic transformation. There was a similar experience in patients with myelofibrosis, who were randomized to a separate protocol (protocol 07) to assess the potential antifibrosing activity of potassium p-aminobenzoate (Potaba, Glenwood, Tenafly, N.J.). Posttreatment biopsies obtained in 19 of these patients continued to show marked reticulin and collagen fibrosis, and many showed progression of the fibrosis (PVSG, unpublished data).

Spent-Phase PV and Acute Leukemia

Nine of the 38 patients with spent-phase PV later terminated in AL,[65] and a more detailed discussion follows in the next section. One of these patients was treated with phlebotomy, 5 with chlorambucil, and 3 with ^{32}P. In 3 patients, the transition to AL occurred within 6 months of the onset of spent-phase PV. In the other 6 patients, the onset of the spent phase preceded the development of AL by 1 to 3 years.

Summary of Studies of Marrow Reticulin Content

Unless serial biopsies are taken throughout the course of the disease, it is impossible to elucidate the sequence of marrow changes, to determine how long reticulin fibrosis has been present, or to correlate changes in reticulin with the clinical course of the disease. Regression or progression cannot be evaluated adequately on the basis of a single biopsy.

A significant increase in bone marrow reticulin (i.e., a moderate or marked increase) was present in 11 percent of pretreatment biopsies from recently diagnosed cases of PV. Follow-up data did not show this to be indicative of the imminent development of spent-phase PV. In addition to the pretreatment biopsies, the subsequent biopsies taken during the period when therapy was required to control symptoms showed that a moderate to marked increase in reticulin content may be present for months to years before the onset of spent-phase PV. In bone marrow biopsies taken when the activity of the disease changes from the erythrocytotic to the stable or spent phase, a moderate to marked increase in re-

ticulin was found either simultaneously or within a year following the clinical change. This was present in all patients.

Thirty-eight (8.7 percent) of randomized patients developed spent-phase PV an average of 8 years after randomization. Thirty-five of these had sequential pre- and posttreatment biopsies. The posttreatment biopsies uniformly showed a progressive increase in the reticulin content. The question of regression of marrow fibrosis was considered,[26, 66–70] but we have found no convincing evidence of this in three separate PVSG protocol studies (protocols 01, 04, and 07). Once established, the marrow fibrosis continued unchanged or increased in severity.

The incidence of the spent phase is equal in the three treatment arms, i.e., phlebotomy, ^{32}P, and chlorambucil.[3, 65] These data differ from those of earlier investigators, who suggested an increased incidence of fibrosis of the bone marrow in PV treated by radioactive phosphorus.[16, 71, 72]

An increased reticulin content may be found in pretreatment biopsies or during the active phase of the disease; it is not indicative of the imminent onset of the spent phase. However, at this time, 50 percent of those patients who have had a significantly increased reticulin content documented at some time during their clinical courses have progressed to the spent phase.

Patients who develop spent-phase PV are at increased risk of developing AL.[65] Of the 38 patients with spent-phase PV, 9 progressed to AL within 3 years (see next section).

ACUTE LEUKEMIA

As is shown in Table 4–5, of the 42 secondary hematologic malignancies that have occurred in PV, the great majority (37) have been AL (blastic transformation). The leukemias may manifest either de novo or following the spent phase (PPMM)[65] (see below). Previously published reports from the PVSG[73–75] have documented that the incidence of AL was much greater following myelosuppressive therapy (chlorambucil or ^{32}P) than following therapy by phlebotomy alone. The risk of developing AL is approximately equal whether treatment is an alkylating agent or radiation. The major difference appears to be in the "lag time" to the development of AL, those cases secondary to chlo-

TABLE 4–5. SECONDARY HEMATOLOGIC MALIGNANCIES
IN POLYCYTHEMIA VERA

	PHLEBOTOMY	CHLORAMBUCIL	[32]P	TOTAL
Randomized	135	141	156	432
AL*	3	19	15	37
No spent-phase PV	2	14	12	28
Spent-phase PV	1	5	3	9
NHL[†]	—	5	—	5
TOTAL	3	24	15	42

* Acute leukemia.
† Non-Hodgkin's lymphoma.

rambucil generally occurring some years earlier (on average) than those cases secondary to [32]P. The incidence of AL in the phlebotomy arm—2 percent—represents the natural, albeit low, incidence of acute leukemia in PV unmodified by therapeutic agents. Five of the 42 hematologic malignancies were non-Hodgkin's lymphomas (NHL) and are discussed in the next section.

Histopathology

To date, AL has evolved in 37 (8.6 percent) of the 432 randomized patients in the PVSG protocol 01. Figure 4–8 shows a typical example of a marrow biopsy and aspirate. With one exception, the leukemias occurring in PV have been nonlymphocytic. Many of these cases occurred prior to the availability of cell markers and other immunocytochemical techniques, such that only conventional morphologic assessment of the type of AL was carried out.[76–79] In the one exceptional case, the blast cells exhibited terminal deoxynucleotidyl transferase (TdT) activity and contained classic Auer rods; this leukemia was considered biphenotypic.[3, 75]

The bone marrow biopsies, aspirate smears, and peripheral blood smears from patients who developed AL were reviewed as unknowns to determine if this group of patients had distinctive features. There were no morphologic features of the pretreatment biopsies or smears that allowed prediction of which patients would progress to AL. The biopsies taken immediately prior to the development of leukemia also were studied as unknowns. In 8 of the 37 patients, biopsies had been obtained within 6 months preceding the leukemic transformation and in 10 other patients between 7 and 12 months before. Even these biopsies obtained immediately prior to the development of leukemia failed to show myelodysplasia or other morphologic features predictive of blastic transformation.

Spent-Phase PV as a Risk Factor for AL

As previously reported,[65] those PV patients who progressed to AL were not homogeneous and could be divided into two large groups. Of the 37 cases of AL, 28 arose without a preceding spent phase, or de novo, and 9 arose following the spent phase (see Table 4–5). These 9 patients with AL constituted 23.7 percent of the 38 patients with a preceding spent phase, defined as myeloid metaplasia and biopsy-proven marrow fibrosis. This is in striking contrast to the 7.1 percent of patients without spent-phase PV (i.e., 28 of 394) who progressed to de novo AL. The difference in incidence of AL between the two groups (i.e., 23.7 versus 7.1 percent) is statistically significant.[65, 75] These data indicate that the spent phase (PPMM) is an independent risk factor for the development of AL in PV.

Time Intervals from Randomization to Diagnosis of AL

Previously published reports from the PVSG have shown that the time intervals from randomization to the diagnosis of AL were different in the three treatment arms.[73, 75] The three leukemias occurring in the patients treated by phlebotomy alone occurred within the first 5 years. In the 19 chlorambucil-treated patients, the leukemias occurred from 2 to 15 years following randomization, with slightly over half the cases occurring within the first 5 years and the others occurring after 6 years. In the [32]P-

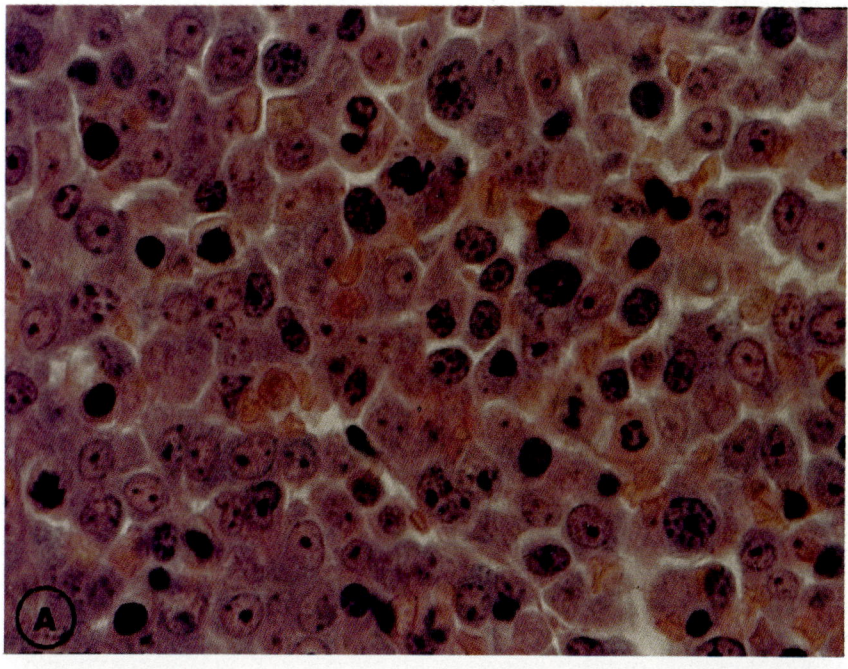

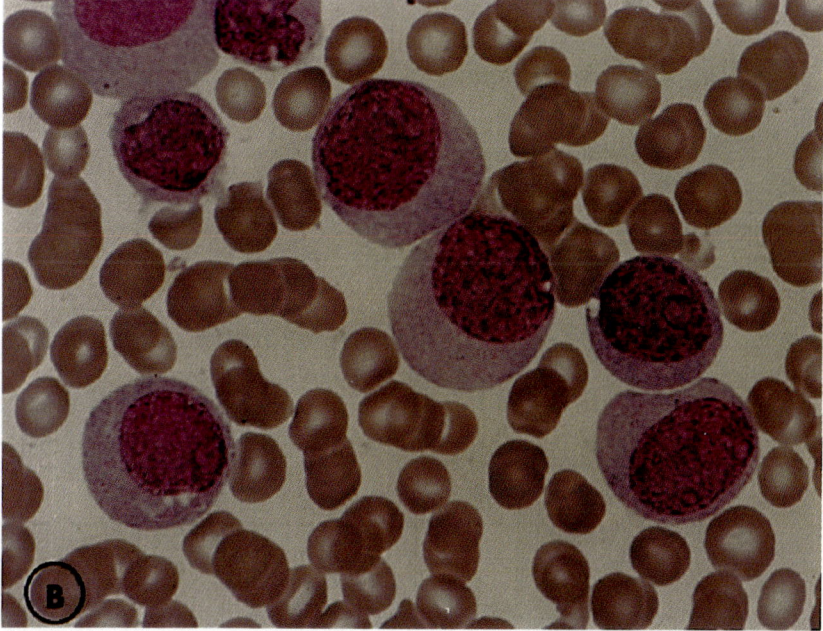

FIGURE 4–8. Acute leukemia (blastic transformation) in PV. (A) Photomicrograph of marrow biopsy from a patient treated with chlorambucil who developed AL 3 years after randomization. Note the uniformity of the proliferating myeloblasts and the absence of normal hematopoietic cells (hematoxylin and eosin stain; × 1000). (B) Photomicrograph of marrow aspirate from the same patient showing numerous myeloblasts with one to two prominent nucleoli. The blasts stained positively with peroxidase and chloroacetate esterase (Wright-Giemsa stain; × 1300).

treated patients, two-thirds of the 15 leuke-mias occurred after 6 years.

The time intervals from randomization to biopsy-proven AL in the de novo cases ranged from 2.1 to 12.7 years. For those cases of AL occurring following spent-phase PV, the time from randomization to AL ranged from 3.4 to 14.7 years. At this time, these slight differences are not considered to be significant.

Sex Ratio

The sex distribution in the 37 cases of AL paralleled the sex distribution by treatment groups. In patients randomized to chloram-bucil, the male-to-female ratio was 2 : 1. In those chlorambucil-treated patients with AL, the sex ratio was also 2 : 1. In patients randomized to ^{32}P and to phlebotomy alone, the male-to-female ratio (in each group) was 1 : 1. In those ^{32}P-treated patients with AL, the sex ratio was identical, 1 : 1. Since so few patients (three patients: two males, one female) in the phlebotomy alone group progressed to AL, the ratio (2 : 1) may be misleading. Statistical analysis of these ratios by treatment arm fails to show any significant differences. These analyses do not stratify the leukemic patients by presence or absence of the spent phase, as will be explored in the Cox model in the next subsection.

If the male-to-female ratio is examined in terms of presence or absence of antecedent spent phase in the myelosuppressed patients, there are striking differences in the sex ratio in patients with spent-phase PV. Among the 274 randomized patients without antecedent spent-phase PV, the incidence of AL (26 patients) was approximately equal in males and females: 10 versus 8.8 percent (Table 4–6). Among the 23 spent-phase patients, there were nearly twice as many females as males, but many more males progressed to AL: 5 of 8 males (62.5 percent) as compared with 3 of

15 females (20 percent). Because the total number of patients in this spent-phase group is only 23, statistical conclusions regarding sex as an independent risk factor may not be valid.

Therapy

Myelosuppression (chlorambucil or ^{32}P) has been shown to be an important risk factor for the development of AL. The data were examined to see if myelofibrosis (MF) was an independent risk factor for the development of AL in those cases which followed the spent phase.

The distribution of the leukemic cases according to therapy is as follows (see Table 4–5): In the de novo cases of AL, 2 patients had been treated by phlebotomy alone, 14 patients had been treated with chlorambucil, and 12 patients had received ^{32}P. Eight cases of AL developed in the 23 spent-phase patients who received myelosuppressive therapy. Twenty-six cases of AL developed in the 274 non-spent-phase patients who also received myelosuppressive therapy. Statistical analyses of these data comparing the incidence of AL in these two groups (spent phase versus no spent phase) indicate that myelosuppression greatly enhances the risk of AL in spent-phase PV ($p = 0.039$).[65]

In summary, myelosuppression is not a risk factor for the development of spent-phase PV. In contrast, in patients receiving myelosuppressive therapy, the development of spent-phase PV further increases the risk of AL.[65]

To explore possible relationships among factors predictive of AL, numerous variables were examined using a Cox regression model.[80] This analysis excluded the 135 patients randomized to phlebotomy alone. Because there was only 1 patient with both spent-phase PV and AL in the phlebotomy-

TABLE 4–6. INCIDENCE OF ACUTE LEUKEMIA IN 297 MYELOSUPPRESSED PATIENTS WITH PV BY SEX AND SPENT PHASE

	WITHOUT SPENT PHASE		SPENT PHASE	
	Male	Female	Male	Female
Randomized cases	160	114	8	15
Acute leukemia	16	10	5	3
Percent developing AL	10	8.8	62.5	20

treated group, statistical analysis was probably not valid. Some of the variables included in the analysis were (1) age at time of randomization to PVSG protocol 01, (2) sex, (3) pretreatment hematologic data, including hemoglobin, hematocrit, white blood cell and platelet counts, mean corpuscular volume, serum iron and total iron binding capacity, serum leukocyte alkaline phosphatase (LAP) level, and serum vitamin B_{12} and folate levels, (4) spleen size, (5) pretreatment cytogenetic studies, (6) progression to the spent phase, and (7) therapy. The three variables predictive for the development of AL were treatment modality, sex, and presence of the spent phase[65] (Table 4–7).

For the 296 patients randomized to chlorambucil or ^{32}P, the relative risk of developing AL is 1.7 times greater for the chlorambucil-treated patients than for the ^{32}P-treated patients. If the analysis is restricted to only those patients alive and on study for 7 years or more, the risk of AL is approximately equal in both groups (relative risk 1.04). For patients on study for 9 years or more, the relative risk is 1.37 times greater for chlorambucil-treated patients. The reason for the changing relative risks is that half the leukemias occurring with chlorambucil occurred within the first 5 years after randomization; therefore, these patients are not included in the Cox analyses of patients on study for 7 or more and for 9 or more years.

As discussed earlier, the presence of the spent phase itself increases the risk of developing AL. In the Cox model, the relative risk is 2.4 times greater for myelosuppressed spent-phase patients than for similarly myelosuppressed patients without spent-phase PV for total time on study. This risk rises with increasing length of time on study; for patients on study 9 years or more, the relative risk is 12 times greater.

With regard to sex ratios, there is only a very slight increase in the relative risk of AL for males versus females for total time on study. However, for patients on study 7 years or more, the relative risk of AL for males is nearly three times that for females and rises to 4.5 times greater for patients on study 9 years or more.

The Cox model analysis further confirms that myelosuppressive therapy and the presence of the spent phase of PV are both risk factors for development of AL. As noted in the first paragraph of this section, sex has not been implicated previously as a risk factor for AL in PV. However, this Cox model indicates that among myelosuppressed patients with spent-phase PV, male sex may be an important risk factor for AL.

Discussion

Both radiation and alkylating agents are recognized as leukemogenic and also may be associated with other neoplasias in various organs.[81–90] Blastic transformation occurs in PV treated by phlebotomy alone, although the incidence is low. It is well known that AL occurs as a terminal event in several nonleukemic hematologic disorders not treated by cytotoxic agents.[91] It has been postulated that bone marrow damage, chromosomal abnormalities, or an altered immune system may contribute to blastic transformation in the already abnormal clone. The pathogenesis of secondary hematologic malignancies in PV is entirely speculative. Since the marrow fibrosis in PV is now considered a secondary phenomenon, its occurrence presumably reflects a basic change in the biology of the abnormal hematopoietic clone. Perhaps the change from the erythrocytotic to the spent phase and blastic transformation are also manifestations of the underlying biologic change.

To date, the incidence of the spent phase is equal among the three PVSG treatment arms. Since only one patient randomized to phle-

TABLE 4–7. RELATIVE RISKS OF ACUTE LEUKEMIA IN PV PATIENTS RECEIVING MYELOSUPPRESSIVE THERAPY

RISK FACTOR	TIME ON STUDY		
	Total	≥7 Years	≥9 Years
Chlorambucil versus ^{32}P	1.70	1.04	1.37
Spent phase versus no spent phase	2.42	4.86	12.12
Male versus female	1.46	2.89	4.47
p Value	0.0390	0.0349	0.0005

botomy alone developed both spent-phase PV and AL, statistical analysis is probably not valid. However, among patients receiving either chlorambucil or ^{32}P, the spent phase does increase the risk of developing AL.

Although some authors[92] have suggested that male sex may be an independent risk factor for AL in PV, these current analyses, as well as other studies,[72,93,94] fail to support the assertion. This statement is true when the patients are not stratified according to presence or absence of the spent phase. However, in myelosuppressed male patients in the spent phase, the risk of AL is significantly increased, and this risk rises with lengthening time on study.

NON-HODGKIN'S LYMPHOMA

In addition to the leukemias, there also have been 5 cases of non-Hodgkin's lymphoma (NHL) in the 432 randomized patients[95] (see Table 4–5). Each of these cases of NHL followed therapy with chlorambucil, there being no cases on either the phlebotomy alone or ^{32}P arms. Each was classified as a diffuse large cell malignant lymphoma (LCML) in the working formulation.

Clinical Setting

These 5 patients, 3 females and 2 males, did not differ from the other 427 randomized patients with respect to sex distribution or age (Table 4–8). Their ages ranged from 39 to 68 years, with a mean of 55 years. Four of the 5 presented with intraabdominal tumors requiring exploratory laparotomy. Each of these four tumors involved extensive segments of bowel, frequently appearing to originate near the cecum. The fifth patient presented with a nonhealing lower leg ulcer

requiring amputation. The time from randomization to the diagnosis of LCML ranged from 5.3 to 9.9 years, with a mean time of 7.3 years. Each patient died within 4 months of diagnosis of LCML, regardless of whether or not the lymphoma was treated.

Histopathology

Although each was called an LCML, there was considerable histologic variation among these five tumors. Because of the nature of the study and the numerous institutions participating, histologic review of these cases often occurred many months after the diagnostic biopsies, and there was no opportunity for more sophisticated studies, such as markers, immunohistochemistry, and gene rearrangement. One case was initially called a granulocytic sarcoma (chloroma). This diagnosis was changed when electron microscopy of that tumor failed to show primary or secondary myeloid granules and the tumor was chloroacetate esterase negative. Three of the 5 patients had marrow biopsies obtained 1 to 5 weeks after the diagnosis of LCML; in none was there evidence of acute myelogenous leukemia (AML) or of LCML.

The pre- and posttreatment marrow biopsies and smears and diagnostic biopsies from all these patients were examined as unknowns. Similar to our observations in the leukemia patients, there were no morphologic features predictive of evolution into NHL.

Role of Chlorambucil Therapy

This series of 5 patients represents the first series of documented cases of NHL following single-agent chemotherapy, in this case chlorambucil. The difference in the incidence of LCML observed among the three different arms is statistically significant ($p = 0.001$).[95]

TABLE 4–8. NON-HODGKIN'S LYMPHOMA IN PV TREATED WITH CHLORAMBUCIL

CASE	SEX	AGE*	CLINICAL PRESENTATION	TIME FROM RANDOMIZATION TO NHL (YEARS)
1	M	43	Small bowel obstruction	8.4
2	F	68	Intermittent obstruction with cecal mass	5.3
3	F	64	Weight loss, abdominal pain, cecal mass	9.9
4	M	61	Small bowel obstruction	6.8
5	F	39	Nonhealing leg ulcer	6.1

* Age at randomization.

Therefore, chlorambucil, in addition to increasing the risk of AL, also increases the risk of NHL.

OTHER HEMATOLOGIC CONDITIONS

To date, three additional randomized patients have developed other lymphoproliferative disorders, two malignant and one probably so. This is not surprising since PV has been reported previously in association with chronic lymphocytic leukemia (CLL),[96-99] plasma cell myeloma,[97,100,101] and lymphoma.[26,97] One patient developed Hodgkin's lymphoma, nodular sclerosis type, 7 years after randomization and treatment with [32]P. He has subsequently died. A second patient developed CLL 10 years after randomization to therapy with chlorambucil. He is alive 18 months after the diagnosis of CLL. A third developed angioimmunoblastic lymphadenopathy (AILD), or immunoblastic lymphadenopathy (IBL), 6 years after randomization to therapy with [32]P. He died soon after diagnosis; his clinical course was more typical of IBL-like lymphoma.

Because myelosuppressive therapy increases the risk of both AL and NHL in PV patients, the question of the role of therapy in the induction of second malignancies in these three patients arises. However, the number of patients is too small to draw any meaningful or valid conclusions.

DIFFERENTIAL DIAGNOSIS

The diagnosis of PV and the various other chronic myeloproliferative diseases is generally not made on morphologic changes alone. The results of the bone marrow biopsy were not included in the PVSG criteria for randomization to the original polycythemia protocol.[22,102] Even so, the study of the bone marrow is important in understanding the disease and may be a helpful adjunct in diagnosis.[27] In the setting of an elevated red cell mass, a finding of increased cellularity due to hyperplasia of erythroid, granulocytic, and megakaryocytic precursors together with an increase in size of megakaryocytes and absence of iron pigment is diagnostic of PV and can be confused with few other conditions. Relative and secondary polycythemias, es-

sential thrombocythemia (ET), the cellular phase of myelofibrosis, and chronic myelogenous leukemia may offer problems in diagnosis.

In relative and secondary polycythemias, the marrow hyperplasia is almost exclusively limited to the erythroid elements. In general, the cellularity is lower than in PV. The megakaryocytes are of normal size, and the concentration of megakaryocytes in relative and secondary polycythemias parallels that of normal individuals. Reticulin content is usually normal in all these conditions.

The changes in the bone marrow in PV share many common features with ET. The clinical diagnosis of PV can be masked by chronic occult gastrointestinal bleeding, so the clinical presentation may be that of thrombocythemia.[103] Marrow iron content may be helpful in differentiating the two conditions; patients with ET have demonstrable iron in the marrow, while 94 percent of patients with PV do not. If iron cannot be demonstrated in a case of suspected thrombocythemia, the marrow should be rebiopsied and the peripheral blood findings reevaluated after adequate iron therapy. In a PVSG protocol study of 37 previously untreated patients with ET,[104] over 90 percent of patients had a pretreatment marrow cellularity greater than 50 percent, but only 11 percent had cellularities greater than 90 percent. Two-thirds of biopsies showed marked megakaryocytic hyperplasia with bizarre, atypical megakaryocytes. Reticulin content was essentially normal in 90 percent of these pretreatment biopsies.

In typical cases of CML, the replacement of the normal marrow by mature granulocytic elements may be very helpful. In 90 percent of cases, the Philadelphia (Ph[1]) chromosome is positive and of practical importance, since its presence is also diagnostic. In an additional 5 to 8 percent of patients, there is a *bcr* (breakpoint cluster region) on chromosome 22 that identifies another subset of CML patients. At times, the differentiation on morphologic grounds between CML and PV may be difficult, since in both conditions marrow fibrosis and increased numbers of megakaryocytes may be present. In some of these cases, the morphology of the megakaryocytes may be of help in differentiating the two conditions. In PV there is great variation in size of the megakaryocytes, and they are hypertrophied, while in CML they are more likely uniform and distinctly small.[8,105]

Postpolycythemic marrow fibrosis cannot be differentiated from idiopathic myelofibrosis on morphologic grounds alone.

SUMMARY

The PVSG study is unique in that it is prospective and provides the opportunity for studies of numerous sequential biopsies in this rare condition. Pretreatment biopsies revealed considerable variation in hematopoietic elements among individual cases, although panhyperplasia was the usual finding. The occurrence of cellularities of less than 60 percent and of relatively normal levels of megakaryocytes did not appear to be of prognostic or biologic significance. Reticulin fibrosis occurred in 11 percent of pretreatment biopsies, but this was not indicative of the imminent development of spent-phase PV. The incidence of spent-phase PV at this time is 9 percent and is the same irrespective of whether the patient was treated by phlebotomy alone, chlorambucil, or ^{32}P. After treatment and during the active phase of PV, reticulin fibrosis was documented in 15 of 38 patients who much later developed spent-phase PV. Reticulin fibrosis also has been documented in 16 patients currently in the active phase of the disease. Since about 50 percent of patients with a significant increase in reticulin content at some time in their clinical course developed spent-phase PV, presumably many of these remaining patients also would develop spent-phase PV, provided they did not first die of other complications of PV or of unrelated causes.

The 37 patients who have developed AL represent 8.6 percent of the 432 randomized patients. The incidence of AL in patients treated with phlebotomy alone is low and is significantly increased after treatment with chlorambucil or ^{32}P. There were no morphologic features predictive of blastic transformation in the pre- and posttreatment biopsies. The spent phase increases the risk of developing AL, even though the incidence of the spent phase is the same in all three treatment arms. Myelosuppressed males in the spent phase have a much higher incidence of AL than do females in the spent phase. In addition to the leukemias, there have been 5 cases of diffuse large cell lymphoma, all of which occurred in patients randomized to chlorambucil.

REFERENCES

1. Ellis JT, Silver RT, Coleman M, et al: The bone marrow in polycythemia vera. Semin Hematol 12:433–444, 1975
2. Ellis JT, Peterson P: The bone marrow in polycythemia vera. Pathol Annu 14:383–403, 1979
3. Ellis JT, Peterson P Geller SA, et al: Studies of the bone marrow in polycythemia vera and the evolution of myelofibrosis and second hematologic malignancies. Semin Hematol 23:144–155, 1986
4. Franzén S: The bone marrow punctate in polycythaemia vera before and after treatment with ^{32}P. Acta Med Scand 145:311–314, 1953
5. Block M, Bethard WF: Bone marrow studies in polycythemia. J Clin Invest 31:618a, 1952
6. Lundin PM, Ridell B, Weinfeld A: The significance of bone marrow morphology for the diagnosis of polycythaemia vera. Scand J Haematol 9:271–282, 1972
7. Kurnick JE, Ward HP, Block MH: Bone marrow sections in the differential diagnosis of polycythemia. Arch Pathol 94:489–499, 1972
8. Franzén S, Strenger G, Zajicek J: Microplanimetric studies on megakaryocytes in chronic granulocytic leukaemia and polycythaemia vera. Acta Haematol 26:182–193, 1961
9. Kutti J, Ridell B, Weinfeld A, et al: The relation of thrombokinetics to bone marrow megakaryocytes and to the size of the spleen in polycythaemia vera. Scand J Haematol 10:88–95, 1973
10. Burston J, Pinniger JL: The reticulin content of bone marrow in haematological disorders. Br J Haematol 9:172–184, 1963
11. Ikkala E, Rapola J, Kotilainen M: Polycythaemia vera and myelofibrosis. Scand J Haematol 4:453–464, 1967
12. Nelson B, Kniseley RM: Marrow fibrosis in myeloproliferative disorders. In Clarke WJ, Howard EB, Hackett PL (eds): Myeloproliferative Disorders of Animals and Man. US Atomic Energy Commission Symposium Series 19. 1970, pp 533–555
13. Pitcock JA, Reinhard EH, Justus BW, et al: A clinical and pathological study of seventy cases of myelofibrosis. Ann Intern Med 57:73–84, 1962
14. Roberts BE, Miles DW, Woods CG: Polycythaemia vera and myelosclerosis: A bone marrow study. Br J Haematol 16:75–85, 1969
15. Roberts BE, Woods CG, Miles DW, et al: Bone changes in polycythaemia vera and myelosclerosis. J Clin Pathol 22:696–700, 1969
16. Silverstein MN: Postpolycythemia myeloid metaplasia. Arch Intern Med 134:113–115, 1974
17. Szur L, Lewis SM: The haematological complications of polycythaemia vera and treatment with radioactive phosphorus. Br J Radiol 39:122–130, 1966
18. Ward HP, Block MH: The natural history of agnogenic myeloid metaplasia (AMM) and a critical evaluation of its relationship with the myeloproliferative syndrome. Medicine 50:357–420, 1971
19. Bouroncle BA, Doan CA: Myelofibrosis: Clinical, hematologic and pathologic study of 110 patients. Am J Med Sci 243:697–715, 1962

20. Demmler K: Die Histopathologie des Gefäβ-systems im spongiösen Knochen: Ihrklinische und funktionelle Bedeutung bei Osteopathien und Myelopathien. Munich, Habilitations-schrift, 1974

21. Thiele J, Rompcik V, Wagner S, Fischer R: Vascular architecture and collagen type IV in primary myelofibrosis and polycythaemia vera: An immunomorphometric study on trephine biopsies of the bone marrow. Br J Haematol 80:227–234, 1992

22. Berlin NI: Diagnosis and classification of the polycythemias. Semin Hematol 12:339–351, 1975

23. Bauermeister DE: Quantitation of bone marrow reticulin-a normal range. Am J Clin Pathol 56:24–31, 1971

24. Burston J, Pinniger JL: The reticulin content of bone marrow in haematological disorders. Br J Haematol 9:172–184, 1963

25. Foot NC, Foot EB: A technique of silver impregnation for general laboratory purposes. Am J Pathol 8:245–254, 1932

26. Bartl R, Frisch B, Burkhardt R: Bone Marrow Biopsies Revisited: A New Dimension for Haematologic Malignancies. Basel, Karger, 1982, pp 15–33

27. Bartl R, Frisch B, Wilmanns W: Potential of bone marrow biopsy in chronic myeloproliferative disorders (MPD). Eur J Haematol 50:41–52, 1993

28. Richter GW: The iron-loaded cell—The cytopathology of iron storage. Am J Pathol 91:361–369, 1978

29. Lillie RD: Experiments on the solubility of hemosiderin in acids and other reagents during and after various fixations. Am J Pathol 15:225–239, 1939

30. Mall FP: Reticulated tissue, and its relation to the connective tissue fibril. Johns Hopkins Hosp Rep 1:171–208, 1896

31. Mallory FB, Parker F: Reticulum. Am J Pathol 3:515–526, 1927

32. Irving EA, Tomlin SG: Collagen, reticulum and their argyrophilic properties. Proc R Soc Lond [Biol] 142:113–125, 1954

33. Kramer H, Little K: Nature of reticulin. In Randall JT, Jackson SF (eds): Nature and Structure of Collagen. New York, Academic Press, 1953, pp 33–50

34. Charron D, Robert L, Couty MC, et al: Biochemical and histological analysis of bone marrow collagen in myelofibrosis. Br J Haematol 41:151–161, 1979

35. Gay S, Gay RE, Prchal JT: Immunohistological studies of bone marrow collagen. In Berk PD, Castro-Malaspina H, Wasserman LR (eds): Myelofibrosis and the Biology of Connective Tissue. New York, Alan R. Liss, 1984, pp 291–306

36. Bentley SA: Collagen synthesis by bone marrow stromal cells: A quantitative study. Br J Haematol 50:491–497, 1982

37. Castro-Malaspina H, Gay RE, Jhanwar SC, et al: Characteristics of bone marrow fibroblast colony-forming cells (CFU-F) and their progeny in patients with myeloproliferative disorders. Blood 59:1046–1054, 1982

38. Bentley SA, Foidart J-M, Kleinman HK: Connective tissue elements in rat bone marrow: Immu-nofluorescent visualization of the hematopoietic microenvironment. J Histochem Cytochem 32:114–116, 1984

39. Bentley SA, Alabaster O, Foidart J-M: Collagen heterogeneity in normal human bone marrow. Br J Haematol 48:287–291, 1982

40. Tomlin SG: Reticulin and collagen (letter). Nature 171:302, 1953

41. Lennert K, Nagai K, Schwarze E-W: Pathoanatomical features of the bone marrow. Clin Haematol 4:331–351, 1975

42. Hunt TK, Van Winkle W Jr: Normal repair. In Hunt TK, Dunphy JE (eds): Fundamentals of Wound Management. New York, Appleton-Century-Crofts, 1979, pp 2–67

43. Miller EJ: Chemistry, structure and function of collagen. In Menaker L (ed): Biologic Basis of Wound Healing. Hagerstown, Md, Harper and Row, 1975, pp 244–257

44. Ross R, Benditt EP: Wound healing and collagen formation: I. Sequential changes in components of guinea pig skin wounds observed in the electron microscope. J Biophys Biochem Cytol 11:677–700, 1961

45. Maniatis AK, Amsel S, Mitus WJ, et al: Chromosome pattern of bone marrow fibroblasts in patients with chronic granulocytic leukaemia. Nature 222:1278–1279, 1969.

46. Van Slyck EJ, Weiss M, Dully M: Chromosomal evidence of the secondary role of fibroblastic proliferation in acute myelofibrosis. Blood 36:729–735, 1970

47. Hentel J, Hirschhorn K: The origin of some bone marrow fibroblasts. Blood 38:81–86, 1971

48. de la Chapelle A, Vuopio P, Borgström GH: The origin of bone marrow fibroblasts. Blood 41:783–787, 1973

49. Adamson JW, Fialkow PJ, Murphy S, et al: Polycythemia vera: Stem-cell and probable clonal origin of the disease. N Engl J Med 295:913–916, 1976

50. Fialkow PJ, Jacobson RJ, Papayannopoulou T: Chronic myelocytic leukemia: Clonal origin in a stem cell common to the granulocyte, erythrocyte, platelet and monocyte/macrophage. Am J Med 63:125–130, 1977

51. Jacobson RJ, Salo A, Fialkow PJ: Agnogenic myeloid metaplasia: A clonal proliferation of hematopoietic stem cells with secondary myelofibrosis. Blood 51:189–194, 1978

52. Golde DW, Hocking WG, Quan SG, et al: Origin of human bone marrow fibroblasts. Br J Haematol 44:183–187, 1980

53. Fialkow PJ, Faguet GB, Jacobson RJ, et al: Evidence that essential thrombocythemia is a clonal disorder with origin in a multipotent stem cell. Blood 58:916–919, 1981

54. Wang JC, Lang H-D, Lichter S, et al: Cytogenetic studies of bone marrow fibroblasts cultured from patients with myelofibrosis and myeloid metaplasia. Br J Haematol 80:184–188, 1992

55. Buschle M, Janssen JWG, Drexler H, et al: Evidence for pluripotent stem cell origin of idiopathic myelofibrosis: Clonal analysis of a case characterized by a N-ras gene mutation. Leukemia 2:658–660, 1988

56. Hickling RA: Chronic non-leukaemic myelosis. Q J Med 6:253–275, 1937

57. Udoji WC, Razavi SA: Mast cells and myelofibrosis. Am J Clin Pathol 63:203–209, 1975

58. Lewis CM, Pegrum GD: Immune complexes in myelofibrosis: A possible guide to management. Br J Haematol 39:233–239, 1978
59. Caligaris-Cappio F, Vigliani R, Novarino A, et al: Idiopathic myelofibrosis: A possible role for immune-complexes in the pathogenesis of bone marrow fibrosis. Br J Haematol 49: 17–21, 1981
60. Burke JM, Ross R: Collagen synthesis by monkey arterial smooth muscle cells during proliferation and quiescence in culture. Exp Cell Res 107:387–395, 1977
61. Ross R, Vogel A: The platelet-derived growth factor. Cell 14:203–210, 1978
62. Scher CD, Shepard RC, Antoniades HN, et al: Platelet-derived growth factor and the regulation of the mammalian fibroblast cell cycle. Biochim Biophys Acta 560:217–241, 1979
63. Kaplan DR, Chao FC, Stiles CD, et al: Platelet alpha granules contain a growth factor for fibroblasts. Blood 53:1043–1052, 1979
64. Brubaker LH, Brière J, Laszlo J, et al: Treatment of anemia in myeloproliferative disorders: A randomized study of fluoxymesterone (Halostestin) vs transfusions only. Arch Intern Med 142:1533–1537, 1982
65. Peterson P, Ellis JT, Geller SA, et al: Increased incidence of acute leukemia in spent polycythemia vera following myelosuppressive therapy. Lab Invest 54:49a, 1986
66. Bentley SA, Herman CJ: Bone marrow fibre production in myelofibrosis: A quantitative study. Br J Haematol 42:51–59, 1979
67. Myelofibrosis (editorial). Lancet 1:127–129, 1980
68. Crosby WH: Fibrosis of the marrow is not cast in cement (editorial). JAMA 246:1940–1941, 1981
69. Wolf BC, Neiman RS: Myelofibrosis with myeloid metaplasia: Pathophysiologic implications of the correlation between bone marrow changes and progression of splenomegaly. Blood 65: 803–809, 1985
70. Duhamel G, Stachowiak J: La fibrose de la moelle osseuse dans les hémopathies malignes et les cancers: Étude histologique de 2786 biopsies. Semin Hop Paris 57:111–116, 1981
71. Silverstein MN: Myeloproliferative diseases. Postgrad Med 61:206–210, 1977
72. Modan B, Lilienfeld AM: Polycythemia vera and leukemia: The role of radiation treatment. Medicine 44:305–344, 1965
73. Berk PD, Goldberg JD, Silverstein MN, et al: Increased incidence of acute leukemia in polycythemia vera associated with chlorambucil therapy. N Engl J Med 304:441–447, 1981
74. Berk PD, Goldberg J, Ellis JT, et al: Malignant complications of long term myelosuppression with ^{32}P or chlorambucil in polycythemia vera. Blood 66:194a, 1985
75. Landaw SA: Acute leukemia in polycythemia vera. Semin Hematol 23:156–165, 1986
76. Bennett JM, Catovsky D, Daniel M-T, et al: Proposals for the classification of the acute leukaemias. Br J Haematol 33:451–458, 1976
77. Bennett JM, Catovsky D, Daniel M-T, et al: Proposed revised criteria for the classification of acute myeloid leukemia. Ann Intern Med 103:620–625, 1985
78. First MIC Cooperative Study Group: Morphologic, immunologic and cytogenetic (MIC) working classification of acute lymphoid leukemia. Cancer Genet Cytogenet 28:189–197, 1986
79. Second MIC Cooperative Study Group: Morphologic, immunologic and cytogenetic (MIC) working classification of the acute myeloid leukemias. Br J Haematol 68:487–494, 1988
80. Cox DR: Regression models and life-tables. J R Soc Surg [B] 34:187–220, 1972
81. Cronkite EP, Moloney W, Bond VP: Radiation leukemogenesis: An analysis of the problem. Am J Med 28:673–682, 1960
82. Bonnadonna G, DeLena M, Banfi A, et al: Secondary neoplasms in malignant lymphomas after intensive therapy. N Engl J Med 88: 1242–1243, 1973
83. Reimer RR, Hoover R, Fraumeni JF, et al: Acute leukemia after alkylating-agent therapy of ovarian cancer. N Engl J Med 297:177–181, 1977
84. Casciato DA, Scott JL: Acute leukemia following prolonged cytotoxic agent therapy. Medicine 58:32–47, 1979
85. Pui C-H, Behm FG, Raimondi SC, et al. Secondary acute myeloid leukemia in children treated for acute lymphoid leukemia. N Engl J Med 321:136–142, 1989
86. Kaldor JM, Day NE, Pettersson F, et al: Leukemia following chemotherapy for ovarian cancer. N Engl J Med 322:1–6, 1990
87. Kaldor JM, Day NE, Clarke A, et al: Leukemia following Hodgkin's disease. N Engl J Med 322:7–13, 1990
88. Coltman CA Jr, Dahlberg S. Treatment-related leukemia. N Engl J Med 322:52–53, 1990
89. Nand S, Messmore H, Fisher SG, et al: Leukemic transformation in polycythemia vera: Analysis of risk factors. Am J Hematol 34:32–36, 1990
90. Cervantes F, Tassies D, Salgado C, et al: Acute transformation in nonleukemic chronic myeloproliferative disorders: Actuarial probability and main characteristics in a series of 218 patients. Acta Haematol 85:124–127, 1992
91. Bloomfield CD, Brunning RD: Acute leukemia as a terminal event in nonleukemic hematopoietic disorders. Semin Oncol 3:297–317, 1976
92. Rosenthal DS, Moloney WC: Occurrence of acute leukemia in myeloproliferative disorders. Br J Haematol 36:373–382, 1977
93. Weinfeld A, Westin J, Ridell B, et al: Polycythaemia vera terminating in acute leukaemia. Scand J Haematol 19:255–272, 1977
94. Donovan PB, Landaw SA, Dresch C, et al: Resistance to therapy of acute leukemia developing in the course of polycythemia vera. Nouv Rev Fr Hematol 23:187–192, 1981
95. Peterson P, Ellis JT, Block MH, et al: Occurrence of non-Hodgkin's lymphoma in treated polycythemia vera. Lab Invest 52:51a, 1985
96. Bethard WF, Block MH, Robson M: Coexistent chronic lymphatic leukemia with polycythemia vera: Morphologic and clinical studies with particular reference to unusual iron metabolism. Blood 8:937–942, 1953
97. Heinle EW Jr, Sarasti HO, Carcia D, et al: Polycythemia vera associated with lymphomatous diseases and myeloma. Arch Intern Med 118: 351–355, 1966

98. Vianna NJ, Essman LJ: Suppression of chronic lymphocytic leukemia by polycythemia vera. Cancer 27:1337–1341, 1971

99. Taberner DA, Chang J, Otridge BW: Co-existent chronic lymphatic leukaemia with polycythaemia vera. Postgrad Med J 53:222–223, 1977

100. Lawrence JH, Rosenthal RL: Multiple myeloma associated with polycythemia: Report of four cases. Am J Med Sci 218:149–152, 1949

101. Maeda K, Abraham J: Polycythemia associated with myeloma. Am J Clin Pathol 82:501–505, 1984

102. Wasserman LR: The management of polycythaemia vera. Br J Haematol 21:371–376, 1971

103. Iland HJ, Laszlo J, Case DC, et al: Differentiation between essential thrombocythemia and polycythemia vera with marked thrombocytosis. Am J Hematol 25:191–201, 1987

104. Iland HJ, Laszlo J, Peterson P, et al: Essential thrombocythemia: Clinical and laboratory characteristics at presentation. Trans Assoc Am Physicians 96:165–174, 1983

105. Lagerlöf B, Franzén S: The ultrastructure of megakaryocytes in polycythaemia vera and chronic granulocytic leukaemia. Acta Pathol Microbiol Scand 80:71–83, 1972

5

Regulation of Erythropoiesis in Polycythemia Vera

JEAN C. SCHULMAN *and* ESMAIL D. ZANJANI

In normal animals and human beings, changes in the number of circulating blood cells promptly lead to compensatory adjustments in the proliferative rate of hematopoietic progenitors, resulting in the restoration of normal peripheral blood cell levels. A number of regulatory signals operate to control this complex series of events. It is now well established that the glycoprotein hormone erythropoietin (Ep), produced by the kidney in the adult,[1] is the primary regulator of erythropoiesis.[2,3] The production of Ep is regulated by the relative amounts of oxygen available to the tissues involved in its synthesis. In general, decreased oxygen availability induced by hypoxia or anemia leads to elevated Ep levels, which, in turn, result in enhanced formation of red blood cells.[4,5] When tissue oxygen supply is increased by exposure to a hyperoxic environment[6] or hypertransfusion,[7–9] Ep production and erythropoiesis are suppressed.

This direct association between Ep levels and red cell production explains some but not all clinical disorders of erythropoiesis. Increased Ep production occurs in patients with erythrocytosis secondary to tissue hypoxia in such conditions as cyanotic heart disease, pulmonary insufficiency, high-affinity hemoglobins, and high-altitude residence,[10–15] as well as in erythrocytotic conditions associated with certain tumors such as renal and hepatic carcinomas and uterine leiomyomas.[16–18] In these patients, the hematopoietic abnormality is limited to the red cell compartment, since it represents an appropriate response to elevated Ep levels, and is alleviated by correction of the underlying cause. Similarly, the anemia of renal failure has been associated with decreased Ep formation[19,20] and can be alleviated by administration of Ep.[21,22] However, clinical states exist in which a direct correlation between Ep levels and erythropoiesis cannot be established.

Polycythemia vera (PV) is a myeloproliferative disorder characterized by overproduction of red blood cells and occasionally of leukocytes and platelets in the absence of any identifiable physiologic demand. The mechanism underlying the increased production of erythrocytes in PV is not understood. In contrast to the elevated levels of Ep present in patients with secondary erythrocytoses, generally below-normal levels of Ep have been found in urine and plasma of PV patients.[10,11,23–28] The decrease in Ep levels is appropriate for the level of hematocrit and resembles that seen in hypertransfused subjects,[5] suggesting that the regulation of Ep production remains sensitive to physiologic stimuli. This is supported by the fact that in response to hypoxia, increased iron turnover and reticulocytosis occur in PV.[29] Similarly, in most[5,23] but not all[11] PV patients, a reduction in circulating red cell mass induced by phlebotomy or ^{32}P treatment results in increased Ep production and reticulocytosis. The fact that elevated red cell mass is maintained in the presence of low Ep levels, however, suggests that the regulatory defect in PV must reside at the level of the hematopoietic progenitors. Considerable in vivo and in vitro evidence supports this contention and further suggests that this defect is not restricted to the erythroid compartment. In this regard, a number of in vitro studies have identified a unique class of erythroid progenitors in PV.

The development of in vitro semisolid culture techniques that facilitate the proliferation and differentiation of animal and human hematopoietic progenitors has refined our concepts of the regulation of hematopoiesis by permitting the operational identification of different classes of hematopoietic precursors and their growth requirements. These techniques have provided evidence that the proliferation and differentiation of hematopoietic progenitors along different pathways depend on the presence of environment influences that allow these cells to survive, amplify, and reach a stage from which commitment to terminal differentiation occurs. Numerous studies have provided evidence for the appropriateness of using these in vitro clonal assay systems to obtain data relevant to the regulation of hematopoiesis. Both multipotent progenitors and precursors with highly restricted lineage commitments can be detected routinely in these in vitro clonal assays. A family of well-defined factors (e.g., Ep, granulocyte-macrophage colony-stimulating factor, interleukin 3, stem-cell factor, etc.) has been shown to control the proliferation of the hematopoietic progenitors in animals and humans.[30–36]

Erythropoietin is an important regulator of erythropoiesis in vitro. The more mature erythroid progenitors, CFU-Es (colony-forming units–erythroid), from normal adult human marrow will develop erythroid colonies in vitro only in the presence of Ep.[35, 36] The primitive erythroid progenitors, BFU-Es (burst-forming units–erythroid), can begin to develop colonies in the absence of Ep, but these will not form mature hemoglobinized cells unless Ep is present.[36, 37] Interleukin 3 (IL-3), granulocyte-macrophage colony-stimulating factor (GM-CSF), and a factor designated as burst-promoting activity (BPA) influence BFU-E development.[33–40]

Analysis of the in vitro proliferative behavior of erythroid progenitors from patients with PV has helped better define the regulatory defect in these patients. Unlike normal erythroid progenitors, which produce colonies only when exogenous Ep has been ad-

ded to cultures, bone marrow cells from these patients behaved abnormally and formed erythroid colonies in the absence of added Ep[41–45] (Fig. 5–1). These "endogenous" colonies arising from a population of mature erythroid progenitors, designated as *endogenous erythroid colony-forming units* (eCFU-Es), tend to be small and poorly hemoglobinized. They represent approximately 20 percent of all erythroid progenitors present[42, 43, 45, 46] (Fig. 5–2). Although endogenous erythroid colony formation has been described in other myeloproliferative disorders such as myelofibrosis, chronic myelogenous leukemia, and essential thrombocythemia,[25, 44, 47] recent reports limit their presence to PV and essential thrombocythemia.[48, 49]

The possibility that the elevated numbers of circulating red cells in PV result from the proliferation and differentiation of a clone of erythroid progenitors not under the usual regulatory influences of Ep was initially proposed by Krantz,[50] who described an abnormal erythropoietic response to Ep by PV marrow in suspension cultures. Subsequent studies utilizing the semisolid culture systems confirmed this possibility but also provided evidence for the existence of erythroid progenitors that responded normally to Ep. This was demonstrated by the fact that while PV bone marrow formed significant numbers of erythroid colonies in the absence of an exog-

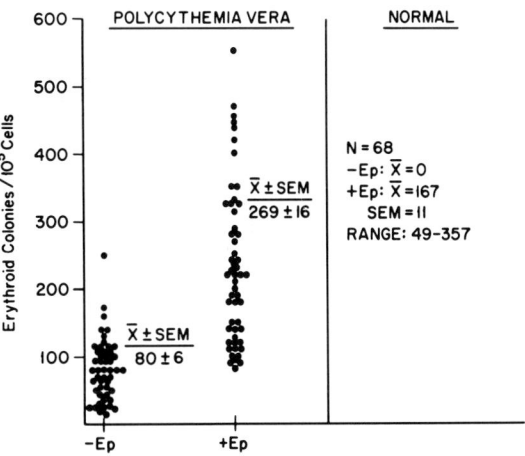

FIGURE 5–1. Erythroid colony formation by normal and PV bone marrow cells in vitro. Results from 51 patients with confirmed diagnosis of PV and 68 normal donors are presented. Bone marrow mononuclear cells were cultured in the presence or absence of erythropoietin in plasma clot cultures,[42] and CFU-E–derived colonies were enumerated on day 7 of culture.

Polycythemia Vera:

Endogenous Erythroid Colonies: % of Total Colonies

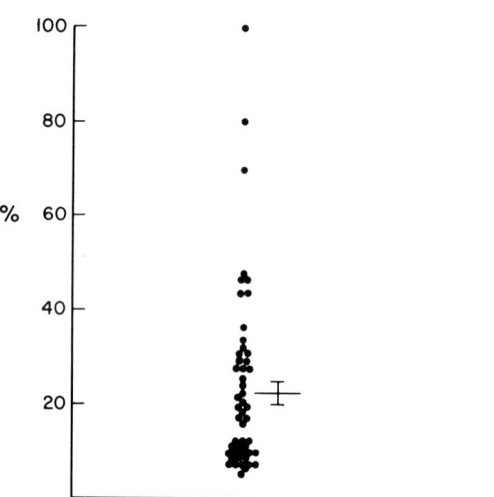

FIGURE 5–2. Formation of endogenous erythroid colonies by bone marrow cells obtained from patients with PV as a percentage of total CFU-E–derived colonies. Percent values shown here were derived from data presented in Fig. 5–1.

enous source of Ep, greater numbers of erythroid colonies could be produced when Ep was added to culture[41–43,45] (see Fig. 5–1).

Definitive evidence for the existence of both normal and abnormal clones of erythroid progenitors in PV was provided by Adamson et al.[46,51] in studies involving two female PV patients heterozygous for glucose-6-phosphate dehydrogenase (G6PD). In normal G6PD heterozygotes, peripheral blood cells are a mixture of types A and B; in two PV patients, all circulating erythrocytes, granulocytes, and platelets were of type A only, although skin fibroblasts were a mixture of both types,[52] indicating the clonal origin of the three hematopoietic cell lines in PV. Analysis of G6PD isoenzyme patterns of colonies derived from hematopoietic progenitors of these patients revealed the presence of both type A and type B colonies. All endogenous erythroid colonies (about 20 percent of the erythroid progenitors) were type A and hence derived from the abnormal clone. However, significant numbers of type B colonies were produced in the presence of exogenous Ep.[46,51] In a G6PD heterozygote, nonclonal colonies would be expected to be 50 percent type A and 50 percent type B. Although one patient grew only one G6PD

type CFU-E and BFU-E regardless of the amount of Ep present, the other patient grew solely type A CFU-Es and BFU-Es only when little Ep was present in culture; when Ep was added 1 of 47 CFU-Es and 14 of 128 BFU-Es were of type B, as were 20 percent of CFU-C–derived colonies.[46,51] Since only type A blood cells were found in this patient's circulation, these findings provide direct evidence that the proliferation and/or differentiation of the normal hematopoietic progenitors is suppressed in PV.

Additional evidence in support of this possibility was obtained by the examination of the relative changes in the proportions of CFU-Es during the course of the disease in 13 PV patients (Fig. 5–3). Although in four patients the relative proportions of eCFU-Es (as a percentage of the total CFU-E population: eCFU-E + CFU-E) remained relatively unchanged over the 3-year study period (see Fig. 5–3), in the remaining patients, a gradual but significant increase in the eCFU-E population was detected over time (Figs. 5–3 and 5–4). In none of the patients did the ratio decrease, and no correlations were noted between changes in the ratio and duration of disease, mode of therapy, and the level

Polycythemia Vera:

Endogenous Erythroid Colony Formation

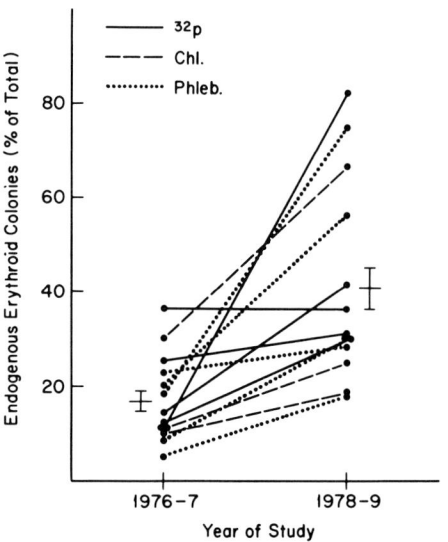

FIGURE 5–3. Formation of endogenous erythroid colonies as a percentage of total CFU-E–derived colonies in 13 patients with PV over a 2-year study period. Patients had been treated with either phlebotomy (Phleb.), ^{32}P, or chlorambucil (Chl.).

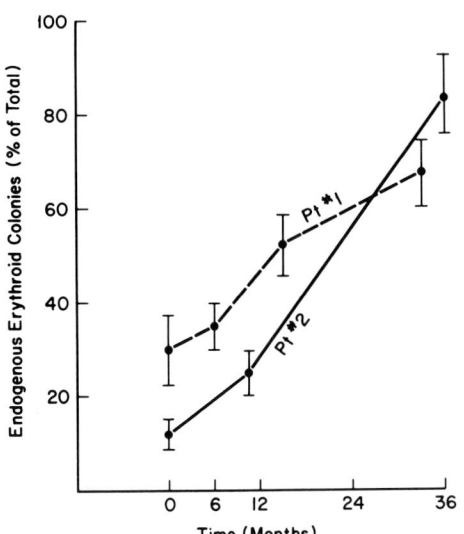

Polycythemia Vera:

Increase in Endogenous Erythroid Colony Formation with Time

FIGURE 5–4. Increase in endogenous erythroid colony formation in two patients with PV over time. Patient 1 had received ³²P, and patient 2 had been treated with chlorambucil.

of eCFU-E activity at the time of initial study. These results can be interpreted to mean that at least in some patients with PV, either a progressive expansion of the abnormal clone of erythropoietic progenitors occurs or the increased relative eCFU-E expression is a reflection of decreased activity of the normal erythroid progenitors.

The mechanism(s) by which the abnormal erythroid progenitors participate in red cell production in PV is not understood. Clearly, despite the presence of normal erythroid progenitors, the abnormal progenitors appear to represent the major red cell–producing elements in these patients. The eCFU-Es differ from CFU-Es by having a higher sedimentation velocity (Fig. 5–5) and in some studies exhibiting a greater sensitivity to ³H-thymidine (³H-TdR) suicide than normal human CFU-Es.[53] There are indications that the proliferative activity of eCFU-Es is regulated by Ep but that these progenitors have developed a significantly greater sensitivity to the hormone than CFU-Es.[42,54] Thus, when steps were taken to ensure that the cultures were devoid of Ep, either by the direct addition of anti-Ep to cultures or by

the use of anti-Ep–treated culture components, endogenous erythroid colony formation was effectively, albeit not completely, suppressed.[42] Moreover, bone marrow cells obtained from patients with PV and cultured in defined serum-free media failed to produce endogenous colonies.[54] Dose-response studies involving the addition of Ep to cultures of PV bone marrow established with anti-Ep–treated media revealed an area of response in the low Ep dose ranges not detected with normal human bone marrow (Fig. 5–6). Such an increased sensitivity to Ep would be compatible with the elevated production of red cells in the presence of low in vivo levels of Ep in PV.

Other studies, however, have raised doubts about the Ep-dependent nature of eCFU-Es.[55] Working with Ep concentrations below those needed to support erythroid colony formation by normal human CFU-Es, Eaves and Eaves[56] were unable to detect a significant change in the numbers of endogenous erythroid colonies produced by PV bone marrow in vitro when Ep levels were raised from 2 to 50 mIU/ml. Although the absence of a significant response to higher Ep doses may be explained by the possibility that all available eCFU-Es may have been activated by the lower Ep concentrations, further studies by this group[55] suggest that the proliferative activity of the abnormal erythroid progenitor may not be under the control of

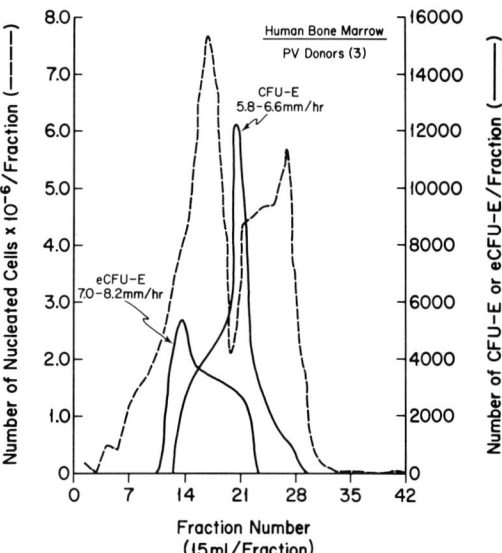

FIGURE 5–5. Sedimentation profile of PV bone marrow CFU-Es determined at unit gravity.

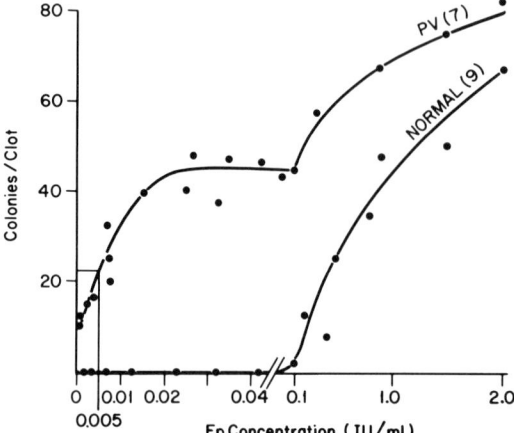

FIGURE 5-6. Dose-response study of the effect of erythropoietin on CFU-E–derived erythroid colony formation by normal human and PV bone marrow cells in vitro.

Ep. Using a monospecific anti-Ep antibody preparation raised against pure natural human Ep, Eaves et al.[55] found that PV bone marrow produced significant numbers of endogenous erythroid colonies even in the total absence of Ep in culture. It is interesting to note, however, that the erythroid colony-forming cells in PV exhibit Ep receptors structurally similar to Ep receptors present on normal human erythroid precursor cells.[57,58]

It is possible that factors other than Ep known to affect hematopoietic progenitor cell growth in vitro may play a role in the development of endogenous erythroid colonies in vitro. Fetal calf serum or other sera used in most cultures are suspected to contain significant amounts of these non-Ep factors which may help support the growth of eCFU-Es. The fact that endogenous colonies did not form in serum-free cultures unless Ep was added[54] may thus reflect the absence of these factors. While some studies indicate that the abnormality of the PV erythroid progenitors is evident only at the level of CFU-Es,[58] other studies demonstrate that this abnormality may be expressed at both CFU-E and BFU-E levels.[59–61] This was evident from the formation of endogenous BFU-E–derived colonies by PV bone marrow and peripheral blood erythroid progenitors in the absence of Ep. In this regard, BFU-Es from PV patients were found to exhibit increased sensitivity to IL-3 and GM-CSF[59–61]; IL-3 and GM-CSF are potent regulators of BFU-E activity.

Because CFU-Es are more likely to form endogenous erythroid colonies than BFU-Es (BFU-Es generally require higher Ep concentrations for optimal development in vitro),[46,56] the possibility exists that the low Ep levels in vivo may select out the relatively Ep-independent erythroid subclones. Arguing against this are the observations that the percentage of endogenous erythroid colonies does not necessarily correlate with time since diagnosis, stage of disease, or mode of therapy. Moreover, it has been shown that individual BFU-Es from patients with PV produce both normal (Ep-dependent) and abnormal (endogenous erythroid colony-producing) progenitors,[62] and the fact that CFU-Es from PV patients grown without Ep usually produce small colonies, whereas CFU-Es cultured in the presence of Ep form large, well-hemoglobinized colonies suggests that individual erythroblasts within an erythroid colony may differ in their sensitivity to Ep. Hypersensitivity to Ep, therefore, does not appear to represent an intrinsic property of the abnormal clone and cannot by itself explain the erythroid hyperproliferation characteristic of the disease.

The increased production of erythrocytes, granuylocytes, and platelets in PV could reflect an increase in the numbers and/or proliferative activity of hematopoietic progenitors. Whether these changes result from a fundamental change in these cells compatible with neoplastic transformation or from loss of response to normal physiologic regulatory forces (stimulatory and/or inhibitory) is not known. Fauser and Messner[63] reported that both endogenous and Ep-dependent peripheral blood multipotent progenitors (CFU-Mix) in PV patients, in contrast to normal controls, were more likely to be undergoing DNA synthesis, as measured by decreased colony formation after exposure to ^{3}H-TdR. Some PV patients appeared to also have increased numbers of CFU-Mix.[64] The numbers of peripheral blood or bone marrow BFU-Es and/or CFU-Es have been reported to be increased,[44,45,65] decreased,[46] or normal.[25,53] The percentage of erythroid progenitors (both abnormal and Ep-dependent) actively cycling, as assessed by ^{3}H-thymidine suicide technique, was found not to be increased in peripheral blood[45] or marrow,[53] although in two G6PD heterozygotes clonal CFU-GMs were selectively killed by exposure to high-specific-activity ^{3}H-TdR.[53] Other authors[55] have found CFU-GMs and BFU-Es from both blood and bone marrow from PV patients to be far more susceptible to ^{3}H-TdR suicide than those from normal controls or patients with secondary polycythemias. It is interesting to note that the ratio of myeloid/erythroid hematopoietic progenitors in patients with PV has been found to be similar to that observed in normal controls.[25,46] This would argue against the possibility, suggested by the predominance of increased red cell mass in these patients, that erythroid differentiation may be favored over myelopoiesis.

Evidence for increased proliferative activity of hematopoietic progenitors in PV also has been obtained in long-term bone marrow cultures. In these cultures, normal primitive progenitors in the adherent layer cycle actively after their weekly feeding with fresh media and then return to a quiescent state. Cells in the nonadherent layer cycle continuously. Long-term cultures of PV marrow show continuous cycling in both the adherent and nonadherent layers.[55] Whether insensitivity to inhibitory signals produced in culture plays a role in this phenomenon will have to be determined.

The underlying cause(s) of the abnormality of hematopoietic progenitors in PV is not known. Chromosomal abnormalities have been detected in a number of cases of PV, both before and after treatment. Unlike chronic myelogenous leukemia, however, these changes are quite heterogeneous; a mixture of deletions, translocations, and aneuploidy have been reported,[66,67] involving essentially all chromosomes. It does not seem likely, therefore, that these chromosomal abnormalities could be important in the pathogenesis of the disease.

Some interesting similarities exist between fetal erythropoiesis and erythropoiesis in PV. Extramedullary hematopoiesis is a feature of PV, and the involved organs, liver and spleen, are those responsible for hematopoiesis in the fetal state. Endogenous erythroid colonies are produced by fetal spleen, liver, and marrow cells in vitro[68]; as in PV, they comprise approximately 20 percent of the total CFU-E population. The fetal eCFU-Es possess some of the characteristics exhibited by endogenous erythroid colony-forming units of PV. These include an apparent hypersensitivity to Ep, increased

susceptibility to ^{3}H-TdR suicide, and a higher sedimentation velocity.[69,70] Endogenous erythroid colonies in PV produce substantial amounts of fetal hemoglobin (HbF), although HbF levels are not increased in vivo.[71] The production of HbF was not clonal; within single colonies, both HbA- and HbF-producing cells could be detected. In a study of 50 PV patients, 20 percent were found to have HbF in as many as 45 percent of their circulating erythrocytes.[72] Although eCFU-Es are present during the early neonatal periods,[70] no endogenous erythroid colony-forming progenitors can be detected in normal adults. It is interesting to note that the circulating levels of red cells in the fetus and newborn in most mammalian species, including humans, is higher than in the normal adult. Whether this physiologically appropriate increased red cell mass in the normal fetus/newborn is associated with the proliferative activity of eCFU-Es is not known.

The applications of in vitro clonal assays for human hematopoietic progenitors to the study of the regulation of hematopoiesis in PV has helped confirm the clonal nature of the disease and has provided direct evidence for the existence of hematopoietic progenitors with altered regulatory responses in PV. The exact nature of the regulatory defect in PV remains unclear. Although endogenous erythroid colony-forming cells also have been detected in other myeloproliferative disorders,[25,44,47] they are absent in the marrow of patients with secondary erythrocytoses, and hence they provide a valuable diagnostic tool[73] in cases of PV that do not readily fulfill the clinical criteria established by the Polycythemia Vera Study Group.[74]

REFERENCES

1. Jacobson LO, Goldwasser E, Fried W, et al: Role of the kidney in erythropoiesis. Nature 179:633, 1957
2. Erslev AJ: Humoral regulation of red cell production. Blood 8:349, 1953
3. Erslev AJ: Erythropoietin function of the kidney. In Wesson LG (ed): Physiology of the Human Kidney. New York, Grune and Stratton, 1969, p 521
4. Carmena A, Garcia de Testa N, Frias FL: Urinary erythropoietin in men subjected to acute hypoxia. Proc Soc Exp Biol Med 125:441, 1967
5. Adamson JW: The erythropoietin/hematocrit relationship in normal and polycythemic man: Implication of marrow regulation. Blood 32:597, 1968

6. Linman JW, Pierre RV: Studies on the erythropoietic effects of hyperbaric hyperoxia. Ann NY Acad Sci 149:25, 1968

7. Adamson JW, Finch CA: Mechanism of erythroid marrow activation. Trans Assoc Am Physicians 79:419, 1966

8. Jacobson LO, Goldwasser E, Plzack L, et al: Studies on erythropoiesis: IV. Reticulocyte response of hypophysectomized and polycythemic rodents to erythropoietin. Proc Soc Exp Biol Med 94:243, 1957

9. Zanjani ED, Mann LI, Burlington H, et al: Evidence for a physiologic role of erythropoietin in fetal erythropoiesis. Blood 44:285, 1974

10. Koeffler HP, Goldwasser E: Erythropoietin radioimmunoassay in evaluation patients with polycythemia. Am J Med 94:44, 1981

11. Napier JAF, Janowsko-Wieczorck A: Erythropoietin measurements in the differential diagnosis of polycythemia. Br J Haematol 48:393, 1981

12. Adamson JW, Stamatoyannopoulos G: Erythrocytosis associated with abnormal hemoglobins: Aspects of marrow regulation. Blood 30:848, 1967

13. Charache S, Weatherall DJ, Clegg JB: Polycythemia associated with hemoglobinopathy. J Clin Invest 45:813, 1966

14. Novy MJ, Edwards MJ, Metcalfe J: Hemoglobin Yakima: II. High blood oxygen affinity associated with compensatory erythrocytosis and normal hemodynamics. J Clin Invest 46:1848, 1967

15. Siri WE, Van Dyke DC, Winchell HS, et al: Early erythropoietin, blood and physiological responses to severe hypoxia in man. J Appl Physiol 21:73, 1966

16. Ossias AL, Zanjani ED, Zalusky R, et al: Studies on the mechanism of erythrocytosis associated with a uterine fibromyoma. Br J Haematol 25:179, 1973

17. Hewlett JS, Hoffman GC, Senhauser DA, et al: Hypernephroma with erythrocythemia: Report of a case and assay of tumor for erythropoietic stimulating substance. N Engl J Med 262:1058, 1960

18. Nahao K, Kimura K, Miura Y, et al: Erythrocytosis associated with carcinoma of the liver (with erythropoietin assay of tumor extract). Am J Med Sci 251:161, 1966

19. Brown R: Plasma erythropoietin in chronic uremia. Br Med J 2:1036, 1965

20. Eschbach JW, Fush D, Admanson JW, et al: Erythropoiesis in patients with renal failure undergoing chronic dialysis. N Engl J Med 276:653, 1967

21. Winearls CG, Oliver DO, Pippard MJ, et al: Effect of human erythropoietin derived from recombinant DNA on the anaemia of patients maintained by chronic hemodialysis. Lancet 2:1175, 1986

22. Eschbach JW, Egrie JC, Downing MR, et al: Correction of the anemia of end-stage renal disease with recombinant human erythropoietin: results of a combined phase I and II clinical trial. N Engl J Med 316:73, 1987

23. Adamson JW, Finch CA: Erythropoietin and the polycythemia. Ann NY Acad Sci 149:560, 1968

24. Erslev AJ, Caro J, Kansoe E, et al: Plasma erythropoietin in polycythemia. Am J Med 66:243, 1979

25. Eaves AC, Henkelman DH, Eaves CJ: Abnormal erythropoiesis in the myeloproliferative disorders: An analysis of underlying cellular and humoral mechanisms. Exp Hematol 8(suppl 8):235, 1980

26. deKlerk G, Rosengarten PCJ, Vet RJWM, et al: Serum erythropoietin (ESF) titers in polycythemia. Blood 59:1171, 1981

27. Rege AB, Brookins J, Fisher JW: A radioimmunoassay for erythropoietin: Serum levels in normal human subjects and patients with hemopoietic disorders. J Lab Clin Med 100:829, 1982

28. Birgegard G, Miller O, Caro J, et al: Serum erythropoietin levels by radioimmunoassay in polycythemia. Scand J Haematol 29:161, 1982

29. Bomchil G, Carmena A, Segade A, et al: Studies on the response to hypoxia and relative hyperoxia in two polycythemia vera patients. Ind J Med Res 55:540, 1967

30. Fauser AA, Messner HA: Granuloerythropoietic colonies in human bone marrow, peripheral blood, and cord blood. Blood 52:1243, 1978

31. Messner HA, Fauser AA: Culture studies of human pluripotent hemopoietic progenitors. Blut 41:327, 1980

32. Ash RC, Detrick RA, Zanjani ED: Studies of human pluripotential hemopoietic stem cells (CFU-GEMM) in vitro. Blood 58:309, 1981

33. Metcalf D: The molecular biology and functions of the granulocyte-macrophage colony stimulating factors. Blood 67:257, 1986

34. Hoffman R, Yang HH, Bruno E, et al: Purification and particular characterization of a megakaryocyte colony-stimulating factor from human plasma. J Clin Invest 75:1174, 1985

35. Gregory CJ, Eaves AC: Human marrow cells capable of erythropoietic differentiation in vitro: Definition of three erythroid colony responses. Blood 49:855, 1977

36. Lipton JM, Kudisch M, Nathan DG: Response of three classes of human erythroid progenitors to the absence of erythropoietin in vitro as a measure of progenitor maturity. Exp Hematol 9:1035, 1981

37. Tsang RW, Aye MT: Evidence for proliferation of erythroid progenitor cells in the absence of added erythropoietin. Exp Hematol 7:383, 1977

38. Aye MT: Erythroid colony formation in cultures of human marrow: Effect of leukocyte conditioned medium. J Cell Physiol 91:69, 1977

39. Ascensoa JL, Vercellotti GM, Jacob HS, et al: Role of endothelial cells in human hematopoiesis: Modulation of mixed colony growth in vitro. Blood 63:553, 1984

40. Fukamachi H, Urabe A, Saito T, et al: Burst-promoting activity in anemia and polycythemia. Int J Cell Cloning 4:74, 1986

41. Prchal JF, Axelrad AA: Bone marrow response in polycythemia vera. N Engl J Med 290:1382, 1974

42. Zanjani ED, Lutton JD, Hoffman R, et al: Erythroid colony formation by polycythemia vera bone marrow in vitro: Dependence on erythropoietin. J Clin Invest 59:841, 1977

43. Lacombe C, Casadevall N, Varet B: Polycythemia vera: In vitro studies of circulating erythroid progenitors. Br J Haematol 44:189, 1980

44. Lutton JD, Levere RD: Endogenous erythroid colony formation by peripheral blood mononuclear cells from patients with myelofibrosis and polycythemia vera. Acta Haematol 62:94, 1979

45. Mladenovic J, Adamson JW: Characteristics of circulating erythroid colony forming cells in nor-

mal and polycythemic man. Br J Haematol 51: 377, 1982

46. Adamson JW, Singer JW, Catalano P, et al: Polycythemia vera: Further studies of hematopoietic regulation. J Clin Invest 66:1363, 1980

47. Eridani S, Batten E, Sawyer B: Erythroid colony formation in primary thrombocythemia: Evidence of hypersensitivity to erythropoietin. Br J Haematol 55:157, 1983

48. Florensa L, Besses C, Almarcha J, et al: Circulating erythroid and megakaryocytic progenitors in polycythemia vera and essential polycythemia. Eur J Haematol 43:417, 1989

49. Weinberg RS, Worsley A, Gilbert HS, et al: Comparison of erythroid progenitor cell growth in vitro in polycythemia vera and chronic myelogenous leukemia: Only polycythemia vera has endogenous colonies. Leukemia Res 13:331, 1989

50. Krantz SB: Response of polycythemia vera marrow to erythropoietin in vitro. J Lab Clin Med 71: 999, 1968

51. Prchal JF, Adamson JW, Murphy S, et al: Polycythemia vera: The in vitro response of normal and abnormal stem cell lines to erythropoietin. J Clin Invest 61:1044, 1978

52. Adamson JW, Fialkow PJ, Murphy S, et al: Polycythemia vera: Stem cell and probably clonal origin of the disease. N Engl J Med 295:913, 1976

53. Singer JW, Fialkow PJ, Adamson JW, et al: Polycythemia vera: Increased expression of normal committed granulocytic stem cell in vitro after exposure to tritiated thymidine. J Clin Invest 64:1320, 1979

54. Casadevall N, Vainchenker W, Lacombe C, et al: Erythroid progenitors in polycythemia vera: Demonstration of their hypersensitivity to erythropoietin using serum free cultures. Blood 59:447, 1982

55. Eaves AC, Krystal G, Cashman JD, Eaves CJ: Polycythemia vera: In vitro analysis of regulatory defect. In Zanjani ED, Tavassoli M, Ascensao JL (eds): Regulation of Erythropoiesis. New York, PMA Publishing Corporation, 1988, p 523

56. Eaves CJ, Eaves AC: Erythropoietin (Ep) dose-response curves for three classes of erythroid progenitors in normal human marrow and in patients with polycythemia vera. Blood 52:1196, 1978

57. Means RT, Krantz SB, Sawyer ST, et al: Erythropoietin receptors in polycythemia vera. J Clin Invest 84:1340, 1989

58. Fibach E, Rachmilewitz EA: Proliferation and differentiation of erythroid progenitors in liquid culture: Analysis of progenitors derived from patients with polycythemia vera. Am J Hematol 35:151, 1990

59. de Wolf JT, Beentjes JA, Esselink MT, et al: In polycythemia vera human interleukin 3 and granulocyte-macrophage colony-stimulating factor enhance erythroid colony growth in the ab-

sence of erythropoietin. Exp Hematol 17:981, 1989

60. Dai CH, Krantz SB, Means RT, et al: Increased sensitivity of polycythemia vera blood burst-forming units-erythroid to interleukin 3. Trans Assoc Am Physicians 103:249, 1990

61. Dai CH, Krantz SB, Means RT, et al: Polycythemia vera blood burst-forming units-erythroid are hypersensitive to interleukin 3. J Clin Invest 87:391, 1991

62. Cashman J, Henkelman D, Humphries K, et al: Individual BFU-E in polycythemia vera produce both erythropoietin dependent and independent progeny. Blood 61:876, 1983

63. Fauser AA, Messner HA: Pluripotent hematopoietic progenitors (CFU-GEMM) in polycythemia vera: Analysis of erythropoietin requirement and proliferative activity. Blood 58:1224, 1981

64. Ash RC, Detrick RA, Zanjani ED: In vitro studies of human pluripotential hematopoietic progenitors in polycythemia vera: Direct evidence of stem cell involvement. J Clin Invest 69:1112, 1982

65. Golde DW, Bersch N, Cline MJ: Polycythemia vera: Hormonal modulation of erythropoiesis in vitro. Blood 49:399, 1977

66. Kay HEM, Lawler SD, Millard RE: The chromosomes in polycythemia vera. Br J Haematol 12:507, 1966

67. Wurster-Hill D, Whang-Peng J, McIntyre OR, et al: Cytogenetic studies in polycythemia vera. In Berlin NI, Jaffe ER, Miescher PA (eds): Polycythemia. New York, Grune and Stratton, 1976, p 123

68. Zanjani ED, Poster J, Mann LI, et al: Regulation of erythropoiesis in the fetus. In Fisher JW (ed): Kidney Hormones: Erythropoietin. New York, Academic Press, 1977, p 463

69. Zanjani ED, Weinberg RS, Nomdedeu B, et al: In vitro assessment of similarities between erythroid precursors of fetal sheep and patients with polycythemia vera. In Murphy MJ (ed): In Vitro Erythropoiesis. New York, Springer-Verlag, 1978, p 208

70. Roodman DG, Zanjani ED: Endogenous erythroid colony forming cells in the fetus and newborn sheep. J Lab Clin Med 94:699, 1979

71. Papayannopoulou T, Buckley J, Nahamoto B, et al: HbF production in endogenous colonies of polycythemia vera. Blood 53:446, 1979

72. Hoffman R, Papayannopoulou T, Landaw S, et al: Fetal hemoglobin in polycythemia vera: Cellular distribution in 50 unselected patients. Blood 53:1148, 1979

73. Lemoine F, Njmn A, Baillou C, et al: A prospective study of the value of bone marrow erythroid progenitor cultures in polycythemia. Blood 68:996, 1986

74. Wasserman LR: The management of polycythemia vera. Br J Haematol 21:371, 1971

6

Distribution of Erythropoietic Bone Marrow in Polycythemia Vera and Other Myeloproliferative Disorders: Total-Body Marrow Imaging with ^{52}Fe

WILLIAM H. KNOSPE *and* ERNEST W. FORDHAM

Atrophy of central bone marrow (axial skeleton) with extension of active hematopoiesis into the long bones and myeloid metaplasia of liver and spleen constitute the classic pattern of marrow distribution in myelofibrosis. Variations on this pattern or the same pattern may occur in myeloproliferative disorders other than myelofibrosis, but their frequency is not known.[1-4]

Other investigators, including Van Dyke et al.[5] and McNeil et al.,[7] have reported scanning studies of the distribution of marrow and other hematopoietic tissues in the myeloproliferative disorders. These authors have emphasized that scanning agents defining the distribution of reticuloendothelial tissue do not correspond consistently with erythropoietic tissue.[5-7] Although indium-111 (^{111}In) has been recommended as an agent metabolized similarly to iron, binding to transferrin, others have reported that it does not enter into the pathways of hemoglobin synthesis.[8-10]

The present studies utilizing total-body marrow scanning with iron-52 (^{52}Fe) were undertaken to better define the patterns of distribution of erythropoietic bone marrow and hematopoietic tissue in patients with polycythemia vera (PV), myelofibrosis (MF),

essential thrombocytosis (ET), and chronic granulocytic leukemia (CGL). These disorders are generally accepted as being closely related neoplastic diseases with similarities in clinical findings, course, and pathogenesis. We were particularly interested in determining the frequency of central marrow atrophy, expansion of marrow into the long bones, and extramedullary hematopoiesis in the spleen in these several different myeloproliferative disorders.

PATIENT SELECTION

Polycythemia vera patients met the diagnostic criteria set by the Polycythemia Vera Study Group: (1) an elevated red cell mass, (2) splenomegaly, and (3) an O_2 saturation greater than 92 percent or the first two of these criteria plus two of the following: (1) elevated platelet count, (2) elevated leukocyte count, (3) increased leukocyte alkaline phosphatase (LAP) score, and (4) elevated serum vitamin B_{12} level or increased serum unbound vitamin B_{12} binding capacity[11] (see also Chap. 15). Myelofibrosis patients all had a positive bone marrow biopsy for fibrosis, and most had splenomegaly, elevated leukocyte and platelet counts, and increased LAP scores. Chronic granulocytic leukemia patients met accepted diagnostic criteria, including the presence of a Philadelphia chromosome, splenomegaly, and increased leukocyte and platelet counts (see Chap. 21). Essential thrombocytosis patients all had elevated platelet counts greater than 500,000 per microliter in the absence of any conditions associated with thrombocytosis (see Chap. 20).

Twenty-two patients with PV, 22 patients with MF, 16 patients with CGL, and 6 patients with ET were studied with ^{52}Fe total-body marrow imaging. Twenty-six of these patients were rescanned after intervals of 1 to 8 years.

PREPARATION OF ^{52}FE AND TECHNIQUE OF MARROW SCANNING

^{52}Fe was produced at Argonne National Laboratory using ^{52}Cr(^{3}He, 3n)^{52}Fe[1] and at Brookhaven National Laboratory using ^{55}Mn(p,4n)^{52}Fe[2,12]. In both cases, the product was purified by anion exchange chromatography, converted into the chloride, and formulated into ^{52}Fe(II)citrate by ascorbic acid reduction and citric acid addition. The final product was passed through a 0.22-μm filter. Radiochemical purity and assay measurements were performed using a Ge(Li)-4096 system.

Aseptic techniques were used in both cases throughout formulation of ^{52}Fe(II)citrate. Each preparation was checked for the absence of bacteria using tryptic soy broth and thioglycolate growth media, and alternate batches were checked for apyrogenicity.

In both methods, ^{55}Fe levels were measured to be about 0.7 percent at the end of bombardment (EOB). Up to 500 μCi was administered to each patient within 10 to 16 hours after EOB. The internal radiation to the red marrow and whole body for a 500-μCi dose due to ^{52}Fe + ^{52m} + ^{52}Mn + ^{55}Fe was calculated to be about 5.5 and 0.55 rad, respectively, at 16.4 hours after EOB.[13]

Following a complete explanation of the procedure to the patient, approximately 500 μCi of ^{52}Fe was incubated with patient's plasma for 30 minutes, to permit binding by transferrin, and then administered intravenously. Scanning was performed 4 to 16 hours later on Ohio Nuclear 84D dual 5-in probe rectilinear scanners fitted with over-size tables and additional probe shielding. High-energy coarse collimation (38H−19 hole) was employed to give highest possible information densities. A relatively narrow (10 percent) window was centered on the 0.51-MeV peak; while lowering information densities, the narrow window also was useful in sharply lowering unwanted scatter. Minimal background suppression (5 percent) was used with no contrast enhancement. With x-axis scanning speeds of 750 cm/min and y-axis increments of 0.3 cm, whole-body imaging required approximately 1 hour while yielding information densities of 30 to 50 counts/cm^2. At these information densities, 5 : 1 minification yielded images acceptable for interpretation.

EVALUATION OF THE ^{52}FE SKELETAL DISTRIBUTION

Skull, spine, ribs, and pectoral and pelvic girdles were separately evaluated for degrees of radioactivity, which were graded as normal or decreased by comparison with normal marrow in the same patient and in other normal subjects. Decreased central marrow activity was classified as none (0), minimal (−1), moderate (−2), or markedly decreased with only minimal or no activity present (−3). Extension of marrow into parts of the peripheral skeleton normally occupied by inactive yellow marrow also was evaluated and quantitated as slight (1+), moderate (2+), or marked (3+). 1+ expansion was defined as barely perceptible radioactivity in the femora or humeri of extremities at sites normally without erythropoietic activity. Expansion into proximal sites of long bones was designated P and at distal sites D. 2+ expansion indicated activity in radii, ulnae, tibiae, or fibulae, in addition to more proximal activities at sites designated as 1+. 3+ expansion included sites designated under 1+ and 2+ as well as activity in hands or feet. Splenomegaly was graded as 1+ (slight splenomegaly), 2+ (moderate enlargement to the level of the iliac crests), or 3+ (enlargement into the pelvic cavity). Intensity of splenic ^{52}Fe uptake was designated by "normal"—no ^{52}Fe activity; "A"—slight ^{52}Fe activity but less than in intramedullary marrow sites; "B"—activity equivalent to normal intramedullary mar-

TABLE 6–1. RESULTS OF SCANNING IN PATIENTS WITH PV

PATIENT	DATE OF DIAGNOSIS	AGE AT DIAGNOSIS	DATE OF SCANS	WBC	HGB/HCT	PLTS.	THERAPY	PV DISEASE ACTIVITY AT TIME OF SCAN	52IRON ACTIVITY AND DISTRIBUTION — Central Marrow Atrophy	Distal Marrow Expansion	Spleen	STATUS
E.A.	1973	63 ♀	5/22/73		19.2/58.6		Venesection	Active	0	0	0	Lost to follow-up
			6/21/77				Venesection		0	1 P-A	0	
J.B.	1961	40 ♂	1/23/75	8,400	15.7/51.0	482,000	Venesection	Active	-1	1 D-B	1 A	Alive 1985
			5/12/77						-1	1 D-B	0	
G.B.	1969	67 ♂	12/16/81	9,400	12.3/37.3	318,000	Venesection + uracil mustard	Spent	-1	1 D-B	0	Died 1985
			4/30/75	22,500	10.1/36.7	595,000		Active	-1	2 P-A	1 A	
			7/11/78	27,500	11.3/37.5	920,000		Active	-2	2 D-C	1 A	
F.B.	1979	71 ♂	4/4/79	16,300	12.8/39.3	890,000	Venesection + 32P	Active	-1	1 P-A	0	Alive/well 1985
			6/16/82						-1	1 P-A	0	
E.B.	1974	42 ♂	4/8/75	11,000	12.3/40.2	1,014,000	Venesection + hydroxyurea	Active	0	0	0	Alive/well 1985
S.C.	1967	62 ♂	10/23/73	20,600	13.1/42.4	1,057,500	Venesection + uracil mustard	Active	-1	1 P-A	0	Lost to follow-up
S.D.	1969	55 ♂	5/23/73	12,000	13.3/44.0	767,500	Venesection + uracil mustard	Active	0	1 D-A	0	Acute leukemia 1980, died 1980
			3/15/79	8,000	13.5/45.0	882,000			-1	2 P-A	0	
V.F.	1972	73 ♂	8/21/73	22,400	13.9/48.5	682,000	Venesection + uracil mustard	Active	-1	0	None	Lost to follow-up 1980
			6/28/77	29,500	13.9/46.3	715,000			-1	1 D-A	1 A	
H.H.	1967	68 ♀	9/11/73	4,100	12.9/37.9	101,500	Venesection	Active	0	1 D-A	1 A	Evolution to acute leukemia + myelofibrosis 1976, died 1976
			2/5/76	4,900	11.0/35.5	101,000			-2	1 D-A	1 B	
S.K.	1976	55 ♂	8/8/78	17,500	14.5/48.4	492,000	Venesection	Spent	-1	2 P-A	0	Myelofibrosis, alive/well 1985
L.L.	1975	43 ♂	8/8/78	7,400	16.3/46.1	320,000	Venesection	Active	0	0	0	Died of lung cancer 1982
			12/16/80	6,300	15.9/45.7	260,000			0	0	0	
V.M.	1973	69 ♀	10/22/74	26,700	10.0/36.0	208,000	Venesection + 32P	Spent	-2	2 D-B	1 A	Died of breast cancer 1981
			7/11/78	67,400	12.6/41.3	330,000			-2	3 B	2 B	
J.N.	1973	56 ♀	4/9/75	5,200	11.9/34.0	510,000	Venesection, chlorambucil, uracil mustard, hydroxyurea	Spent	0	1 P-A	0	Alive/well 1985
			7/11/78	7,600	13.5/41.4	615,000			0	1 D-A	0	
D.P.	1974	67 ♀	2/14/74	12,300	15.7/50.9	712,000	Venesection + uracil mustard	Spent	-1	1 P-A	0	Alive/well 1985
			8/8/78	5,600	14.5/40.2	247,000			-1	1 P-A	0	
R.R.	1970	53 ♀	8/21/73	25,200	14.5/43.5	597,500	Venesection, uracil mustard, hydroxyurea	Active	-1	1 P-A	2 A	Evolution to acute leukemia and myelofibrosis 1983–84, died 1984
			6/28/77	26,400	16.2/49.3	625,000			-1	2 P-B	3 A	
			11/7/79	36,800	13.5/42.2	440,000			-2	2 D-A	3 C	
			12/16/81	35,300	12.5/39.1	250,000			-3	2 D-A	3 C	
H.R.	1974	74 ♀	10/22/74	4,600	13.3/39.7	235,000	Venesection, hydroxyurea	Spent	0	1 P-A	1 A	Lost to follow-up 1984
			6/28/77	8,600	13.6/41.2	542,000			-1	1 P-A	1 A	
W.R.	1973	52 ♂	10/22/74	13,500	15.0/57.0	260,000	Venesection	Active	-1	2 P-C	1 A	Alive 1985
			7/11/78	10,200	15.0/49.0	520,000			-2	2 P-C	2 A	
J.W.	1974	80 ♂	2/5/76	8,100	11.9/37.1	760,000	Venesection + uracil mustard	Active	0	0	0	Died 1975

row sites; and "C"—exceeding ^{52}Fe activity at normal intramedullary marrow sites and the dominant activity in the total-body scan.

RESULTS IN THE VARIOUS MYELOPROLIFERATIVE DISORDERS

Polycythemia Vera

Eighteen patients were studied (Table 6–1). When first scanned, 7 of these had a normal central marrow pattern (Fig. 6–1), and 11 showed evidence of central marrow atrophy. Fourteen of these patients were studied after intervals varying from 10 months to 6 years. Six of these showed progressive marrow failure, although in only 1 was the failure marked, and this occurred over a 4-year period.

Expansion of erythropoietic marrow into

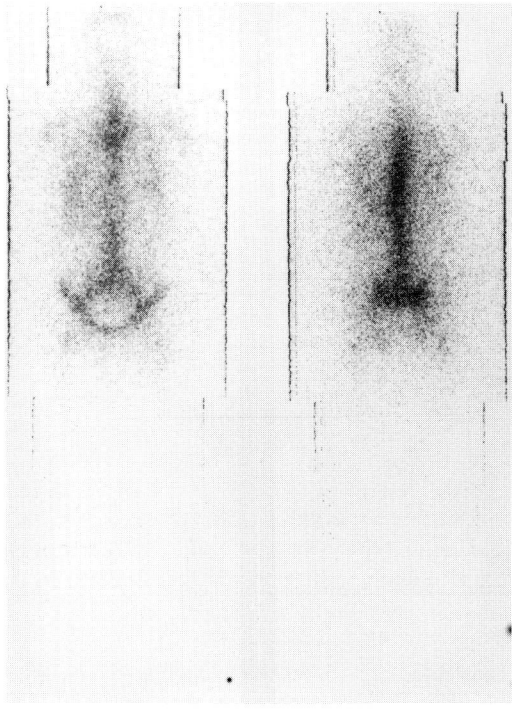

FIGURE 6–1. The ^{52}Fe scan of this 43-year-old man (L.L.) with stable PV demonstrates a *normal* marrow distribution. Maximum activity is seen on the anterior view in the sternum and anterior pelvis (and lumbar spine in this slender individual). The spine and posterior pelvis are the dominant sites posteriorly. Note minimal normal ^{52}Fe uptake in skull and the most proximal portions of humeri and femora. Note also the lack of any hematopoietic activity in the more distal portions of the extremities.

the long bones was a very common finding and was present in 16 of the 18 patients at some point in their course (Fig. 6–2). The expansion was only slight in 9 of these patients and was confined to the proximal parts of the long bones (femora and humeri). In 5 patients, the expansion was more marked and involved the tibiae and/or the radii/ulnae. One patient had extensive involvement of the long bones into the feet and/or hands. In only 5 of these did the intensity of extramedullary erythropoiesis appear to equal or exceed that of normal central marrow (Fig. 6–3D). Splenic erythropoiesis was seen in 8 of these patients; in 3 of them the amount of activity appeared moderate to marked.

Fourteen patients were rescanned one or more times after intervals of 2 to 8 years. Ten patients showed evolutionary changes typical of spent-phase PV, usually with atrophy of central marrow and/or progressive expansion into the long bones and/or increased splenomegaly with increasing erythropoiesis (see Fig. 6–3). Four patients showed no changes over intervals of 2, 4, 4½, and 6 years (see Fig. 6–2).

Six of 12 patients had a normal marrow biopsy, and 6 showed evidence of increased collagen and/or reticulin (Table 6–2).

Polycythemia Vera with Myelofibrosis Present at Time of Diagnosis (Intermediate Myeloproliferative Syndrome)

Four patients presented with myelofibrosis at the time polycythemia was diagnosed (Table 6–3). All these patients had central marrow atrophy; in 2 it was marked, but in 2 others it was only minimal (Fig. 6–4).

Expansion of erythropoietic marrow into the long bones was present in all 4, and in 3 of the 4 the involvement was extensive, including the tibiae and/or radii/ulnae. In 1 patient the expansion was marked and involved all the long bones, including the feet.

Splenomegaly was marked to massive, and spleens were much larger than in most of the patients with PV. Two patients showed no splenic erythropoiesis when first scanned, even though splenomegaly was present (see Fig. 6–4).

The intensity of the extramedullary erythropoiesis was variable. In 3 of the 4 patients,

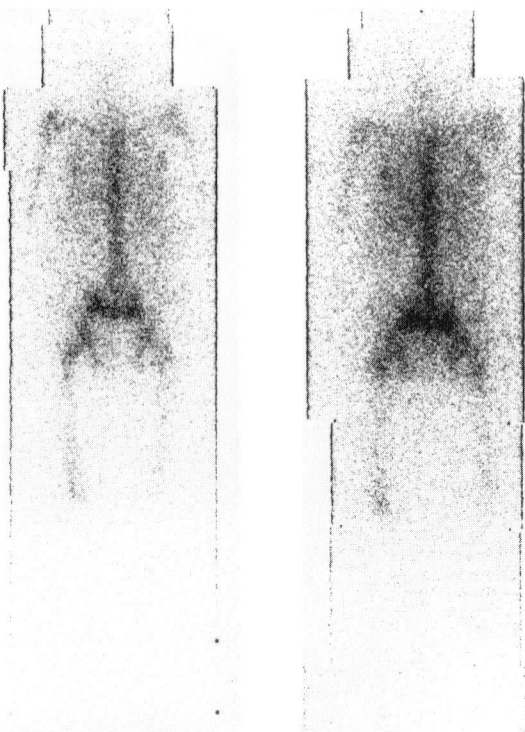

FIGURE 6–2. Single posterior views from ^{52}Fe scans performed 6 years apart on this 40-year-old man (J.B.) with stable PV show no demonstrable change. Unchanged expansion of hematopoietic marrow down much of the length of the humeri and femora (right greater than left) is apparent. The difference in intensity of the uptake between the two scans is due to technical scanning factors and is not related to any real difference in marrow function.

the intensity of ^{52}Fe uptake in the long bones was only slight and clearly less than the intensity in normal central marrow sites. In 1 patient erythropoietic activity in the expanded marrow sites was equivalent to ^{52}Fe activity in central marrow sites. Two patients showed markedly increased ^{52}Fe uptake in the spleen, and this exceeded that visible throughout the central marrow sites (Fig. 6–5). One patient, followed for over 16 years, showed remarkable stability of the extent of marrow expansion as well as splenomegaly. Although splenomegaly was marked (to the umbilicus) and stable throughout this period, ^{52}Fe uptake progressed from 0 to 2B over 11 years, and some central marrow atrophy occurred (see Fig. 6–4).

Two patients were rescanned after intervals of 5 and 7 years, and both showed progressive expansion into the long bones and increasing splenomegaly with increasing erythropoiesis in the spleen. One showed no change in a slight atrophy of central marrow,

and one progressed from slight to moderate central marrow atrophy.

Myelofibrosis

Twenty-two patients with myelofibrosis were studied (Table 6–4). Central marrow atrophy was present in all but 1 of these patients from first diagnosis. In 7 patients this was moderate to marked, and in 10 patients it was extreme, with virtually no central marrow activity present (Figs. 6–6 and 6–7). Five of these patients with extreme central marrow atrophy had low hemoglobin levels and a transfusion requirement, and 3 had only minimal erythropoietic activity in the spleen (see Fig. 6–7).

Marrow expansion into long bones was present in 15 of these 22 patients but surprisingly was not present at all in 5 patients, 3 of whom had very severe myelofibrosis with transfusion requirements (see Fig. 6–6).

Splenomegaly and splenic erythropoiesis

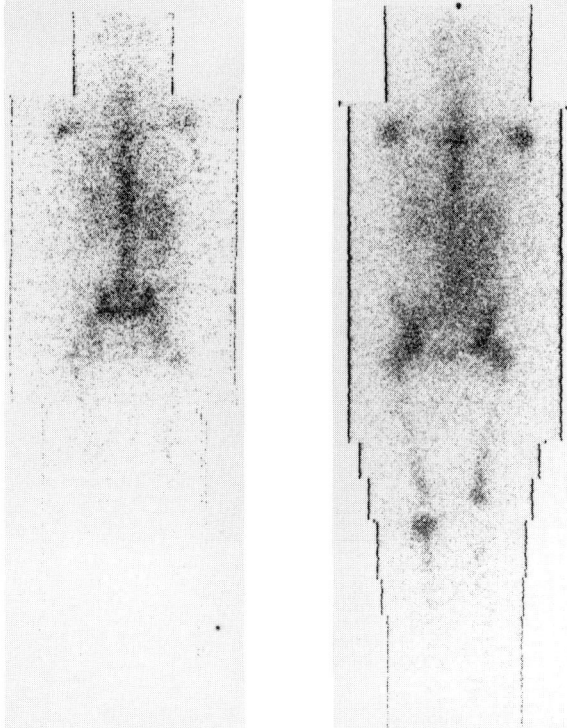

FIGURE 6–3. In contrast to Fig. 6–2, this series of scans of a 53-year-old woman (R.R.) with PV shows marked progression of disease over a 6-year period. The initial scan (A) shows irregular central marrow, implying some central failure with minimal peripheral expansion and subtle uptake in the minimally enlarged spleen. Four years later, peripheral expansion is impressive (B), with uptake in the proximal right tibia equaling the intensity of the central marrow. Subtle uptake continues to be apparent in a spleen which is enlarged to reach the pelvis.

Illustration continued on following page

TABLE 6–2. CORRELATION OF MARROW BIOPSIES AND ^{52}Fe SCANS IN PATIENTS WITH PV

						DATE	^{52}Fe SCAN
Positive Biopsy							
H.H.	Slightly	↑ Collagen	+	↑	Reticulin	2/2/76	Spleen 3 +, liver 2 +
V.F.	Slightly	↑ Collagen	+	↑	Reticulin	3/27/77	Spleen 1 +
G.B.				↑	Reticulin	12/14/77	Spleen 1 +
F.B.				↑	Reticulin	1/3/78	Spleen negative
R.R.	Normal			↑	Reticulin	12/26/73	Spleen 1 +
				↑	Reticulin	7/20/82	Spleen 3 +
S.K.		↑ Collagen	+	↑	Reticulin	1/5/82	Spleen negative
Negative Biopsy							
J.W.						2/2/76	Liver 1 +
S.D.						12/6/73	Negative (liver trace)
S.C.						1/17/74	Spleen 1 +, liver 1 +
L.L.	Occasional osteoid seams and osteoblastic activity					11/20/78	Spleen negative
J.N.						2/28/75	Spleen negative
H.R.						9/13/78	Spleen 1 +

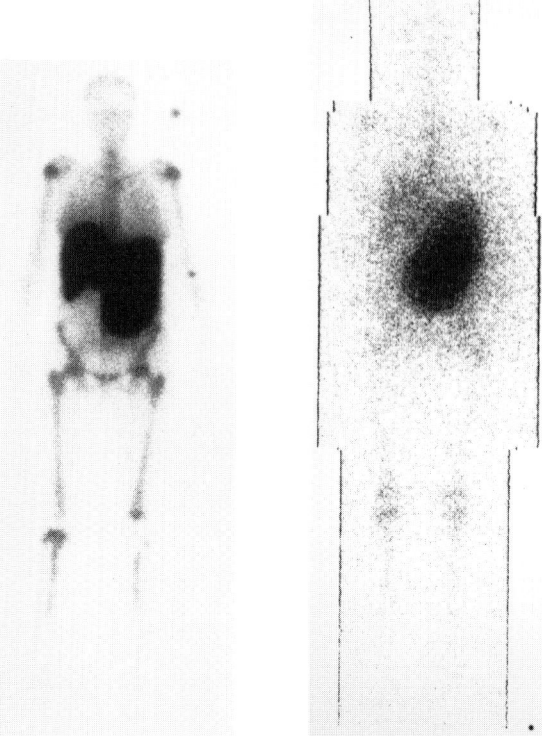

FIGURE 6–3 *Continued (C* and *D)*   RE marrow imaging *(C)* on the same occasion demonstrates a distribution of RE marrow identical to hematopoietic marrow if better defined (inherent to the larger doses of ^{99m}Tc sulfur colloid with ideal imaging characteristics). Note the markedly enlarged and clearly defined spleen. The final scan *(D)* shows marked change with near-complete failure of central marrow, reduction in activity of expanded marrow, and dominant uptake by the large spleen, implying that it is now the major erythropoietic organ.

were present in all but 2 patients (see Figs. 6–6 and 6–7). The splenic enlargement was marked in 9 patients and massive in 3 patients. The intensity of ^{52}Fe uptake was equivalent to or exceeded the level of intramedullary erythropoiesis in 11 patients.

Five patients were rescanned after intervals of 2 to 4 years, and none of them showed evolutionary changes in central or peripheral marrow or spleen (see Fig. 6–7).

Chronic Granulocytic Leukemia

Sixteen patients with CGL were scanned with ^{52}Fe (Table 6–5). Central marrow showed a normal pattern without atrophy in 4 patients. Twelve patients showed central atrophy; 6 had slight, 4 had moderate, and 2 had severe atrophy of the central marrow (Figs. 6–8 and 6–9).

Thirteen patients had expansion of erythropoietic marrow into the long bones. In 4 patients, this was slight, involving only the femora or humeri. In 6 patients the expansion was moderate to marked, involving femora, tibiae, humeri, radii, and ulnae, and in 3 patients the expansion also involved the feet (see Figs. 6–8 and 6–9).

Splenic ^{52}Fe activity was absent in 6 patients and present in 9 patients. The spleen was moderately enlarged in 7 patients and massively enlarged in only 1 patient. The intensity of ^{52}Fe uptake was equivalent to normal central marrow sites in 5 patients and more intense than normal marrow sites in only patient N.B. (see Table 6–4).

Three patients were rescanned after intervals of 1 to 6 years. One of these patients showed no change after an interval of 6 years, one showed an improvement after 2 years (a patient with severe busulfan marrow suppression), and one patient showed striking changes after an interval of less than 1 year with marked central marrow atrophy,

TABLE 6-3. RESULTS OF SCANNING IN PATIENTS WITH PV AND MF

PATIENT	DATE OF DIAGNOSIS	AGE AT DIAGNOSIS	DATE OF SCANS	WBC	HGB/HCT	PLTS.	THERAPY	PV DISEASE ACTIVITY AT TIME OF SCAN	52IRON ACTIVITY AND DISTRIBUTION			STATUS
									Central Marrow Atrophy	Distal Marrow Expansion	Spleen	
J.F.	1968	48 ♀	8/21/73	11,900	12.8/42.6	495,000	Venesection	Active	−1	2 P-B	0	Evolution to acute leukemia, died December 1984
			7/11/78	15,600	12.4/41.0	485,000		Active	−1	2 D-B	2 A	
M.G.	1970	47 ♀	3/15/79	28,600	9.8/32.5	378,000	Venesection	Active	−3	3 A	3 C	Myelofibrosis 1970, alive/well 1985
A.G.	1974	48 ♂	2/5/74	10,400	11.4/36.1	598,000	Venesection	Active	−3	2 P-A	3 C	Alive/well 1985
C.Mc.	1967	50 ♂	8/28/73	8,000	15.1/45.3	397,000	Venesection	Active	−1	0	0	
			5/11/77	9,700	15.4/44.2	450,000		Active	−1	1 P-A	2 A	
			12/16/80	8,900	12.6/38.6	330,000		Active	−2	1 D-A	2 B	

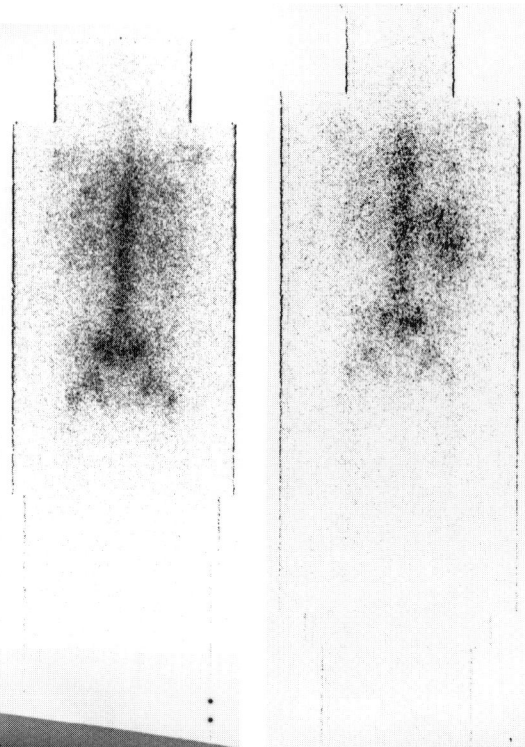

FIGURE 6–4. Posterior views from scans 7 years apart show significant interval changes in hematopoietic activity in this 50-year-old man (C.Mc.) with PV and MF. The initial scan shows only subtle central marrow irregularity without demonstrable peripheral expansion or splenic activity. The second scan shows greater loss of central marrow activity, minimal activity (better seen in originals than in reproductions) in long bones, and the level of activity in the moderately enlarged spleen equaling that in central marrow.

marked expansion into the long bones, and increasing splenomegaly.

Essential Thrombocytosis

Six patients with ET were scanned (Table 6–6). Central marrow activity was normal in 2 of these patients. Slight central atrophy was present in 3 patients, and moderate atrophy was seen in 1 patient (Fig. 6–10).

Expansion of erythropoietic marrow was present in 3 patients and involved only the femora and/or humeri. In 3 patients there was no evidence of expansion into the long bones (see Fig. 6–10).

Splenic uptake of ^{52}Fe was not observed, and in only one patient was splenomegaly present. Two patients were rescanned after intervals of 3 years. One of these patients showed no change. The other patient developed minimal central marrow atrophy but also showed an improvement in a minimal degree of expanded marrow.

CONCURRENT SCANNING WITH ^{52}FE AND TECHNETIUM-99M (^{99M}TC) SULFUR COLLOID

^{99m}Tc sulfur colloid total body reticuloendothelial scans were done concurrently with the ^{52}Fe total-body scans in 34 of these scans. There was essentially identical distribution of ^{99m}Tc in reticuloendothelial marrow compared with ^{52}Fe erythropoietic marrow in these concurrently scanned patients.

INTERPRETATION AND DISCUSSION

These studies indicate similarities between PV and the other disorders with a common pattern of central marrow atrophy, extension of active erythropoiesis into the peripheral skeleton of arms and legs, and myeloid metaplasia of the spleen. This pattern was seen to a greater or lesser degree in all categories of

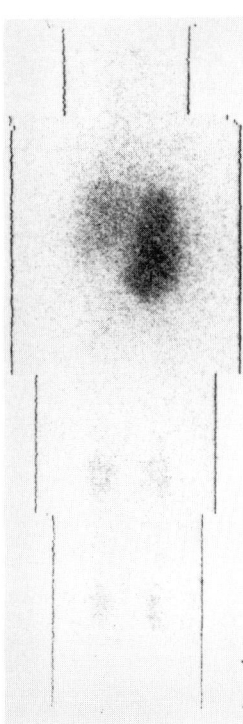

FIGURE 6–5. ⁵²Fe imaging of this 47-year-old woman (M.G.) with PV and MF shows a distribution of hematopoietic activity very similar to that seen in Fig. 6–3. Central marrow is almost completely atrophied; minimally functioning peripheral marrow can be identified as far peripherally as the feet. The striking feature is dominant hematopoietic activity in the markedly enlarged spleen.

myeloproliferative disorders studied. However, this pattern was not present in all the patients in any of the disease categories, although it was most frequent in the MF group. The complete pattern was observed in the four patients with PV who had concurrent erythrocytosis, myelofibrosis, and myeloid metaplasia, and these patients all required phlebotomy to control excessive red cell production. This group could be assigned to either category—PV or MF—and represented an overlap syndrome. Several patients have been followed for periods of 4 to 15 years without hematopoietic failure developing. One of these patients died unexpectedly of pulmonary emboli after several years of clinical observation and treatment for erythrocytosis. In two of these patients, exuberant red cell production continued over many years in the presence of extensive MF.

Pettit et al.[14] have recently described 11 patients with PV and MF and have reported that such patients may remain in a stable and nonprogressive state for periods up to 10 years. These patients did not evolve into classic MF with marrow failure, hypersplenism, etc. We are able to confirm the observations of Pettit et al. that the development of a transitional myeloproliferative syndrome does not necessarily indicate an inexorable progression to MF and marrow failure.

Evidence of splenic myeloid metaplasia without MF occurred in 8 of 14 patients with PV, as reflected by ⁵²Fe uptake in the spleen. All these patients had easily aspirable bone marrow. Although marrow biopsies were not done on all these patients, in 6 of 12 patients, some evidence of marrow fibrosis was seen, significantly so in only 1 patient. This is a much higher incidence than that of 8.6 percent of 150 patients reported by Wasserman.[3] The ⁵²Fe marrow scanning studies support the abundant documentation referred to by Dameshek,[2] Wasserman,[3] Ward and Block,[4] and others that myeloid metaplasia in spleen, liver, and peripheral marrow is coexistent with hyperplasia of the erythropoietic and total marrow organ. Such evidence argues against a simplistic theory of compensatory marrow hyperplasia.

Analysis of scans in spent-phase PV revealed no features that set these patients apart from those with active PV or patients with MF. Similar patterns of central marrow atrophy, peripheral expansion and degree of splenomegaly, and intensity of splenic erythropoiesis were observed. One of the patients (E. B.) who rapidly evolved from a diagnosis of PV to MF and death in 4 years had no unique clinical or scanning features. Progression to the spent phase of PV did not necessarily herald a rapid development of MF or bone marrow failure.

Scanning intensities observed in the spleen were usually of slight or moderate degree. Markedly increased and dominant degrees of splenic erythropoiesis were observed only in patients with MF. Information derived from ⁵²Fe total-body imaging could be useful in assessing the extent of splenic hematopoiesis, particularly in situations where transfusion-dependent anemia develops and where splenectomy is being considered.

There was no correlation between the degree of splenomegaly and the degree of ⁵²Fe uptake. This raises a question as to the cause

TABLE 6-4. RESULTS OF SCANNING IN PATIENTS WITH MF

PATIENT	DATE OF DIAGNOSIS	AGE AT DIAGNOSIS	DATE OF SCANS	WBC	HGB/HCT	PLTS.	THERAPY	52IRON ACTIVITY AND DISTRIBUTION — Central Marrow Atrophy	Distal Marrow Expansion	Spleen	STATUS
G.A.	1955	55 ♀	9/11/73	26,300	10.2/30.1	710,000		−2	0	1 C	Died 1974
E.B.	1973	62 ♂	5/11/77 3/7/73	40,100	14.6/46.3	690,000	Busulfan	−2	2 D-B	2 C	Previous history of PV, died February 1, 1977
J.B.	1973	36 ♀	8/28/73	4,600	11.1/33.0	92,500	Busulfan	0	0	0	Alive/well 1985
L.D.	1967	66 ♀	10/22/74	4,300	7.6/26.0	198,000	Hydroxyurea	−2	3 B	1 C	Prior PV, died 1977
			7/7/76	6,600	12.8/39.7	95,000		−2	1 D-A	0	
			10/17/78	6,000	9.5/30.5	305,000		−2	2 D-A	1 B	
C.D.	1974	68 ♀	4/16/74	12,400	11.2/34.6	76,000	Busulfan	−1	2 P-A	2 B	Alive/well 1984
J.D.	1968	44 ♂	1/23/73	1,400	8.5/25.0	150,500		−3	2 D-A	3 C	Died 1975
H.E.	1974	37 ♂	7/22/74	8,500	9.6/28.3	490,000	Transfusions	−2	0	1 A	Evolution to acute leukemia 1978, died 1978
			2/5/76	14,700	8.9/26.4			−3	0	1 A	
			3/11/76	10,500	10.1/30.7			−3	0	1 A	
S.E.	1976	55 ♀	4/4/79	36,200	13.2/42.9	601,000	Busulfan	−2	2 P-B	2 B	Died 1982
			12/16/81	25,900	11.9/37.5	323,000		−2	2 P-B	2 B	
C.F.	1969	48 ♀	3/3/82	10,000	9.4/29.9	880,000	Transfusions	−3	2 D-A	3 C	Lost to follow-up
B.G.	1974	53 ♂	5/11/77	10,500	6.9/20.4	425,000	Busulfan	−3	3 C	1 A	Died December 1977
J.H.	1976	52 ♀	3/24/76	11,500	13.9/43.7			−2	2 P-A	2 C	Alive with gastric ulcer, massive splenomegaly in 1985
B.K.	1975	60 ♂	6/16/82	6,500	14.3/43.1	47,000	Androgen	−3	3 A	2 C	Previous history of PV, Alive/well 1985
E.K.	1974	57 ♂	7/24/73	12,500	8.2/28.2	850,000	Busulfan, transfusions	−2	2 D-B	0	Died 1978
			3/24/76	29,900	9.8/34.0	3,500		−1	2 D-B	0	
L.K.		58 ♂	7/11/78	3,600	11.9/33.1	95,000	Busulfan, transfusions	−2	2 D-A	0	Died 1978
R.L.	1974	46 ♀	4/5/79	7,300	7.2/23.1	275,000	Transfusions, hydroxyurea	−3	3 A	2 C	Began as thrombocytosis, evolution to myelofibrosis 1978, lost to follow-up 1979
M.L.	1970	55 ♀	4/16/74	3,600	9.6/28.6	104,000	Busulfan, transfusions	−2	0	2 B	Died 1974
H.M.	1973	68 ♀	7/24/73	26,800	6.3/20.6	500,000	Transfusions, busulfan	−1	2 P-A	0	Died 1974
A.M.	1966	52 ♀	11/6/79	12,000	10.8/31.7	8,000	Transfusions, busulfan	−3	0	1 A	Died 1983
			12/16/81	1,800	9.1/26.1			−3	0	1 A	
D.N.	1982	49 ♀	3/3/82	4,000	12.3/36.0	213,000		−3		3 C	Lost to follow-up
K.O.	1980	66 ♂	3/3/82	7,300	9.8/31.1	299,000	Androgens, transfusions	−1	2 P-A	2 A	Lost to follow-up
J.S.	1981	72 ♀	3/3/82	26,200	11.6/35.0	53,000		−3	2 D-A	2 A	Died August 1982
M.U.	1974	66 ♀	8/14/74	8,400	11.5/35.7	800,000	Uracil mustard	−1	0	1 A	Alive/well 1985

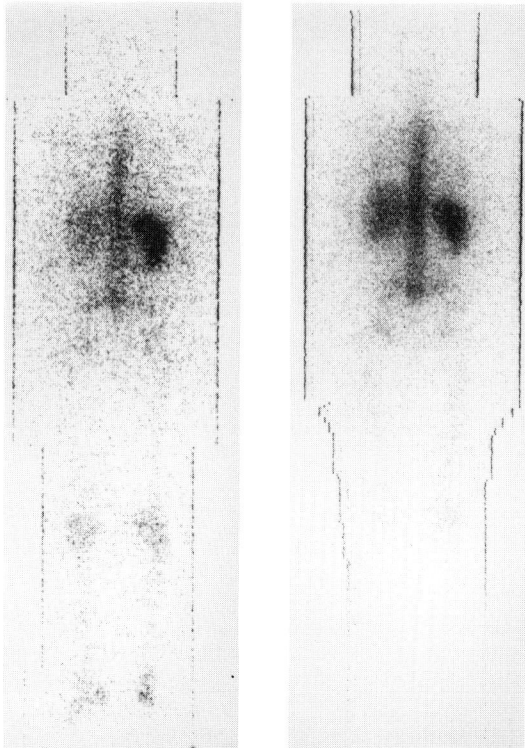

FIGURE 6–6. ^{52}Fe scans of this 73-year-old woman (L.D.) with MF at a 4-year interval show an unusual change in our series of the myeloproliferative disorders. In addition to marked retraction of peripheral marrow activity and diminished activity in the mildly enlarged spleen (relative to spine), there is distinct improvement in the level of central activity, except for pelvis, where marrow remains atrophic.

of the splenomegaly. A recent study of splenic aspiration with cytologic study of the aspirate revealed a hypertrophy of splenic reticulum and little or no erythropoiesis.[15]

Although most of these patients showed evidence of hematopoietic expansion into peripheral skeletal sites, the amount of activity at these sites compared with overall erythropoiesis in the central marrow was not large. Expanded sites of hematopoiesis in long bones, including liver or spleen, do not usually seem to contribute significantly to the overall economy of hematopoiesis in humans.[16]

^{52}Fe total-body marrow imaging may be helpful in evaluating a patient suspected of having a myeloproliferative disorder but who does not fulfill diagnostic criteria needed for a firm diagnosis. Examples of such patients might be a patient with only elevated red cells or obscure leukocytosis or obscure thrombocytosis. The presence of central marrow atrophy and/or expansion of marrow into the long bones and/or splenic erythropoiesis may

make a myeloproliferative syndrome more likely.

Hepatic uptake of ^{52}Fe does not necessarily indicate hepatic erythropoiesis because the liver is the site of primary iron localization when there is complete hematopoietic failure, as in aplastic anemia or when iron stores are saturated. There is no way to distinguish by isotope scanning techniques between hepatic uptakes due to extramedullary erythropoiesis in the liver and the nonhematopoietic uptake that occurs in the absence of extramedullary erythropoiesis in the liver.

Myelofibrosis may accompany CGL and has been considered an unfavorable clinical sign with respect to prognosis. It may be a harbinger of blastic transformation or an unresponsive terminal phase of the disease.[17] Two of our patients with CGL were in the accelerated phase of CGL, and both had increased peripheral marrow activity and signs of myeloid metaplasia of liver and spleen. One patient in the early phase of his CGL

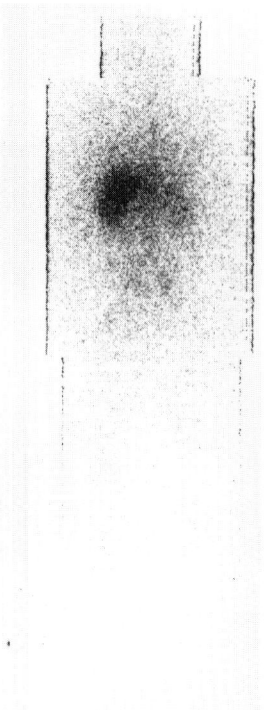

FIGURE 6-7. ^{52}Fe scans of this 37-year-old man (H.E.) with MF show profound central marrow atrophy without demonstrable compensatory activity in the peripheral marrow and only minimal activity in a spleen of relatively normal size. Dominant ^{52}Fe uptake by the liver does not necessarily imply hematopoietic activity in this organ, since iron not utilized at usual sites will be taken up by the liver.

showed significant central marrow depression and myeloid metaplasia of liver and spleen, although he appeared to be sensitive to chemotherapy and without evidence of blastic transformation.

Gralnick et al.[17] investigated the incidence of MF in patients with CGL. Two groups of patients were identified. One group with survival characteristics identical to the usual patients with CGL developed MF in the terminal phases of their disease. In these patients, once MF established itself, survival was short (mean 4.9 months) and blastic transformation frequent. A small group of patients developed MF early in the course of their disease. In these patients, survival was short, with a mean of 8.8 months after diagnosis, and blastic transformation was frequent. These authors performed marrow scanning with ^{99m}Tc sulfur colloid, and three patterns of marrow distribution were observed: (1) a pattern of marrow expansion into long bones with normal or increased marrow activity in central adult sites, (2) a pattern of central marrow depression in adult sites with extension into juvenile sites in long bone, and (3) a pattern of generalized depression in both central adult sizes and juvenile long bone sites.[17]

Patients with pattern 1 had hypercellular marrow without MF or increased reticulin, while patients with patterns 2 and 3 had extensive MF. These authors raised the possibility that busulfan might be involved in the pathogenesis of the MF, although 5 of 39 patients developed MF who never received busulfan.[17]

Most of our patients with CGL could be fit into pattern 1 or 2 of Gralnick et al. Nine patients showed evidence of extramedullary hematopoiesis in the spleen or liver. Only one of our patients showed pattern 3. Extramedullary trilineal hematopoiesis in the spleen or liver of patients with CGL has been described by Rappaport.[18]

The present studies confirm the long-established principle that all the myeloproliferative disorders are related diseases with common pathogenetic mechanisms.[2] Central marrow atrophy, extension into long bones,

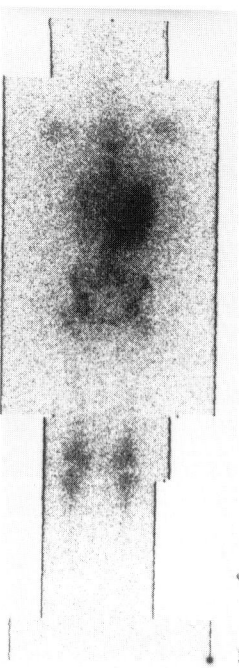

FIGURE 6-8. In the face of rather mild central atrophy, the ^{52}Fe scan of this 30-year-old woman (V.P.) with CGL demonstrates fairly marked peripheral expansion and rather intense uptake by the moderately enlarged spleen.

TABLE 6–5. RESULTS OF SCANNING IN PATIENTS WITH CGL

PATIENT	DATE OF DIAGNOSIS	AGE AT DIAGNOSIS	DATE OF SCANS	WBC	HGB/HCT	PLTS.	Central Marrow Atrophy	Distal Marrow Expansion	Spleen	STATUS
J.A.	1978	37 ♂	10/17/78	39,300	14.7/42.7	230,000	−2	3 D-B	2 B	Died 1981
L.A.	1967	47 ♂	12/3/74	8,500	14.0/42.4	198,000	−1	2 P-A	0	Alive/well 1985
			6/28/78	8,100	13.2/	229,000	−1	2 P-A	0	
			12/16/80	16,800	12.9/38.5	238,000	−1	2 P-A	0	
N.B.	1976	44 ♀	3/11/76	19,100	12.0/36.0	465,000	−3	2 P-A	2 C	Died 1979
W.D.	1971	60 ♂	11/5/74	1,100	11.0/32.3	108,000	−2	3 B	2 A	Died
R.F.	1976	40 ♀	12/16/81	6,000	13.3/39.9	486,000	0	0	0	Died 1984
J.G.	1976	53 ♂	11/19/74	231,200	11.0/28.0	880,000	−1	1 D-A	1 B	Died March 1976
L.H.	1976	56 ♂	12/16/81	7,700	15.9/45.7	210,000	−1	1 D-A	0	Died December 1983
H.K.	1975	61 ♂	4/8/75	7,500	14.8/43.0	114,000	−1	0	0	Died May 1977
C.K.		♀	2/5/76				−1	2 P-B		Died
T.M.	1974	28 ♂	10/17/78	14,800	13.5/40.7	730,000	0	1 P-A	2 B	Died 1979
			4/4/79	49,400	10.0/31.3	235,000	−3	2 D-B	3 B	
R.M.	1967	18 ♂	3/11/76	1,200	12.6/35.7	4,500	−2	0	1 A	Myleran toxicity, alive/well 1985
			8/8/78	10,000	15.3/46.4	250,000	−1	0	0	
A.M.	1980	47 ♂	12/16/81	28,800	14.3/42.0	242,000	−1	2 P-B	0	Blast crisis 1984, alive February 1985
V.P.	1974	20 ♀	4/8/75	6,300	12.0/34.7	797,000	−1	2 P-B	2 B	Lost to follow-up 1978
			7/11/78				−2	3 B	0	
J.R.	1974	20 ♂	4/8/75	7,200	11.1/34.8	121,000	0	1 D-A	2 A	Died 1975
O.R.	1973	44 ♀	12/3/74	5,200	13.3/38.9	235,000	0	1 D-A	0	Died 1978
A.S.	1962	8 ♂	10/19/74	14,400	8.6/26.4	1,802,500	0	2 P-B	2 B	Died 1975

The Central Marrow Atrophy, Distal Marrow Expansion, and Spleen columns fall under the heading **52IRON ACTIVITY AND DISTRIBUTION**.

TABLE 6–6. RESULTS OF SCANNING IN PATIENTS WITH ESSENTIAL THROMBOCYTOSIS

PATIENT	DATE OF DIAGNOSIS	AGE AT DIAGNOSIS	DATE OF SCANS	WBC	HGB/HCT	PLTS.	^{52}I IRON ACTIVITY AND DISTRIBUTION			STATUS
							Central Marrow Atrophy	Distal Marrow Expansion	Spleen	
I.A.	1975	83 ♀	3/11/76	8,400	9.9/32.1	705,000	−1	0	0	Lost to follow-up 1980
			3/14/79	4,100	11.3/33.9	N	0	0	0	
C.C.	1978	46 ♀	8/8/78	6,100	11.9/35.2	659,000	−1	1 D-A	0	Lost to follow-up 1979
S.F.	1978	62 ♂	3/14/79	4,900	12.5/39.2	409,000	0	1 P-A	0	Alive/well 1985
			3/3/82	6,400	13.4/40.0	540,000	−1	0	0	
M.G.	1974	35 ♀	11/19/74	7,500	11.5/33.8	657,000	0	1 P-A	0	Lost to follow-up 1975
J.P.	1972	77 ♂	1/25/75	6,300	14.7/43.9	302,500	0	0	0	Died 1974
M.T.	1978	50 ♀	8/8/78	6,900	13.8/41.5	888,000	−2	0	0	Lost to follow-up 1979

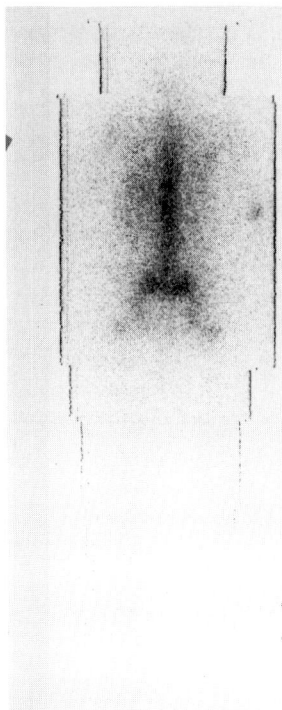

FIGURE 6-9. The ⁵²Fe scan of this 60-year-old man (W.D.) with CGL demonstrates severe central marrow atrophy, far distant expansion of peripheral marrow to include the feet, with only moderate uptake of ⁵²Fe. Note mild uptake by the moderately enlarged spleen. Note that hepatic uptake of ⁵²Fe does not necessarily imply hematopoietic function in that organ.

yellow marrow organ or spleen or liver are unknown. Tavassoli and Crosby[19] have suggested that red marrow and yellow marrow have different regenerative capacities, suggesting autosomal genetic differences in the two types of marrow tissue. If such differences were present, the tissues could respond differently to hematopoietic stimuli. Dameshek's concepts of myeloid metaplasia in the myeloproliferative syndromes postulated that the extramedullary hematopoiesis and MF were neoplastic in nature and autonomous and not subject to regulatory influences.

We have reported studies of marrow distribution using ⁵²Fe scanning in patients with lymphoma treated with local radiotherapy. Following extensive radiotherapy (usually total nodal irradiation), increased erythropoietic activity was observed in the marrow of the long bones, usually within a few months of irradiation. This expanded marrow activity usually regressed 1 to 2 years after irradiation. We interpreted these events to mean that inactive yellow marrow is responsive to

and myeloid metaplasia of the liver and spleen occurred frequently in all the myeloproliferative disorders investigated. These changes were least prominent in the six patients with ET, but the numbers of patients are too few to make any firm conclusions. These three types of changes were frequently concurrently present within hematopoietic tissues, but they were not invariably associated. Some patients showed only central atrophy or only extension into long bones or only myeloid metaplasia of the liver and/or spleen. We could not identify any sequence in these changes, nor could they be related to the stage of the disease. Any or all these phenomena occurred early in the disease in some patients.

The pathogenesis of changes within the hematopoietic tissues in patients with myeloproliferative disorders remains obscure. The factors causing MF in the central organ or activation of hematopoiesis in the peripheral

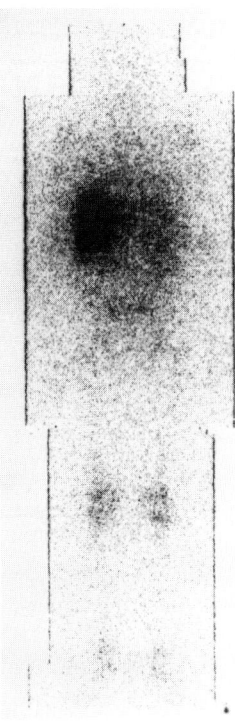

FIGURE 6-10. A near-normal ⁵²Fe scan is apparent in this 46-year-old woman (C.C.) with ET. Central marrow may show mild irregularity. Minimal marrow expansion is apparent in the femora. No splenic ⁵²Fe uptake is apparent in the absence of splenomegaly.

activation by large ablative doses of irradiation, perhaps through the mediation of humoral stimuli.[20] Ward and Block[4] have reported extensive clinical and laboratory studies of patients with MF, and these authors postulated that the patterns of MF and marrow expansion and myeloid metaplasia of the liver and spleen are compatible with the hypothesis that humoral factors mediate these varying patterns of hematopoietic activity. These varying patterns of hematopoietic activity in the myeloproliferative syndromes suggest complex interactions of normal and neoplastic tissues with variable responsiveness to humoral agents. ^{52}Fe total-body marrow scanning represents a useful investigative tool to assess function in the total erythropoietic organ.

SUMMARY

Sixty-six patients with PV and other myeloproliferative disorders were studied using ^{52}Fe total-body marrow imaging. Patients with myeloproliferative disorders frequently show a pattern of central marrow atrophy, expansion of erythropoietic activity into the normally inactive long bones, and extramedullary hematopoiesis of the spleen and liver.

REFERENCES

1. Hashimoto M: The distribution of active marrow in the bones of normal adult. Kyushu J Med Sci 11:103–111, 1960
2. Dameshek W: Some speculations on the myeloproliferative syndromes. Blood 6:372–375, 1952
3. Wasserman LR: Polycythemia vera. Its course and treatment: Relation to myeloid metaplasia and leukemia. Bull NY Acad Med 30:343–375, 1954
4. Ward HP, Block MH: The natural history of agnogenic myeloid metaplasia (AMM) and a critical evaluation of its relationship with the myeloproliferative syndrome. Medicine 50:357–420, 1971
5. Van Dyke D, Anger HO: Patterns of marrow hypertrophy and atrophy in man. J Nucl Med 6:109–120, 1965
6. Raich PC, Sorenson JA, Tyson IB, Korst DR: Linear profile scanning of marrow in myelofibrosis. J Reticuloendothel Soc 16:282–288, 1974
7. McNeil BJ, Holman BL, Button LN, Rosenthal DS: Use of indium chloride scintigraphy in patients with myelofibrosis. J Nucl Med 15:647–651, 1974
8. Farrer PA, Saha GB, Katz M: Further observations on the use of ^{111}In-transferrin for the visualization of bone marrow in man (abstract). J Nucl Med 14:394–395, 1973
9. Lilien DL, Bennett LR: A comparison of the uptake and disposition of radioiron and ^{111}In-chloride in human erythrocytes (abstract). J Nucl Med 13:786–787, 1972
10. McIntyre PA, Larson SM, Scheffel U, et al: Comparisons of metabolism of iron-transferrin and indium-transferrin by the erythropoietic marrow (abstract). J Nucl Med 14:425–426, 1973
11. Wasserman LR: Annotation: The management of polycythaemia vera. Br J Haematol 21:371–376, 1971
12. Saha GB, Farrer PA: Production of ^{52}Fe by the ^{55}Mn$(p,4n)^{52}$Fe reaction for medical use. Int J Appl Radiat Iso 22:495–498, 1971
13. Richards P, Ku T, Sodd VJ: Personal communication, May 1978
14. Pettit JE, Lewis SM, Nicholas AW: Transitional myeloproliferative disorder. Br J Haematol 43:167–184, 1979
15. Berg B, Ståhl E, Söderström N: The cytology of spleen aspiration in uncomplicated polycythaemia vera. Scand J Haematol 10:59–61, 1973
16. Njoku OS, Lewis SM, Catovsky D, Gordon-Smith EC: Anaemia in myelofibrosis: its value in prognosis. Br J Haematol 54:79–89, 1983
17. Gralnick HR, Harbor J, Vogel C: Myelofibrosis in chronic granulocytic leukemia. Blood 37:152–162, 1971
18. Rappaport H: Tumors of the hematopoietic system. *In* Atlas of Tumor Pathology, sec III, fasc 8. Washington, Armed Forces Institute of Pathology, 1966, p F8-266
19. Tavassoli M, Crosby WH: Bone marrow histogenesis: A comparison of fatty and red marrow. Science 169:291–293, 1970
20. Knospe WH, Rayudu VMS, Cardello M, et al: Bone marrow scanning with ^{52}iron (^{52}Fe): Regeneration and extension of marrow after ablative doses of radiotherapy. Cancer 37:1432–1442, 1976

ACKNOWLEDGMENTS: We gratefully acknowledge the assistance of Mary L. Ogrinc, R.N., M.S., who aided in the collection of clinical data. We also thank Mary Ann Cardello, M.T. (ASCP), and Joan Walasek, M.T. (ASCP), who provided technological assistance in the injection of ^{52}Fe, and Patricia G. Konieczny for secretarial assistance in the preparation of the manuscript. We also gratefully acknowledge the assistance of Garimella V. Rayudu, Ph.D., in the radiochemical preparation of ^{52}Fe.

7

Radioisotope Investigations for the Diagnosis and Follow-Up of Polycythemic Patients

YVES NAJEAN, CATHERINE DRESCH,
JEAN-DIDIER RAIN, *and* CHRISTINE CHOMIENNE

Radioisotope techniques occupy an important place among the laboratory investigations necessary for the diagnosis and follow-up of polycythemia vera (PV). The precise diagnosis, determination of prognosis, and follow-up of PV depend on the measurement of blood volume (red cell, plasma, and total blood volumes). Other isotope methods such as bone marrow scintigraphy, blood flow measurement, and studies of cell kinetics provide additional and often important data in certain circumstances. The measurement, interpretation, and significance of each of these in vivo methods will be discussed in this chapter. Various in vitro methods using radioisotopes also have been shown to be useful in PV and will be described.

The measurement of red cell mass (red cell volume) is an essential element in establishing the diagnosis of PV, and in fact, demonstration of an increased total red cell volume is a critical criterion for making this diagnosis. Our own experience has shown us, however, that three major points have to be discussed:

1. The method used
2. The interpretation of the results
3. The practical use of red cell and plasma volumes measurements in the diagnosis and follow-up of the disease

MEASUREMENT OF BLOOD VOLUME

Determination of Red Cell Volume

The measurement of red blood cell and plasma volumes is based on the principle of dilution. This measurement was performed initially with various dyes but not with radioactive isotopes, the main advantages of which are their ability to label red cells and plasma proteins in vitro and the relative ease of their measurement. Although ^{51}Cr-labeled sodium chromate is the reference label, other red cell markers such as ^{32}P sodium phosphate, ^{11}C-carbon monoxide and technetium-99m have specific advantages. A recent suggestion has been to use nonradioactive ^{52}Cr chromate and its measurement by absorption spectrophometry.[29]

Choice of Label

The reference method for the measurement of total red cell volume is the in vitro labeling of autologous erythrocytes with ^{51}Cr sodium chromate, as described by the International Committee for Standardization in Hematology,[37] and subsequent measurement of the volume of dilution in the patient. No significant modification of the method has been suggested over the years following publication of this document. The usual dose of ^{51}Cr infused is 5 to 10 μCi (2 to 4 kBq) to an adult patient.

The diisopropylfluoro-32-phosphate technique referred to in the ICSH document[37] is a reference method that is no longer used. ^{11}C-carbon monoxide,[27] a hemoglobin marker, has the advantage of a very low radiation dose to the patient but is technically very difficult to use because of the short half-life of [11]C (20 minutes) and the need for access to a cyclotron for its production.

At the time the ICSH document was written,[37] the use of ^{99m}Tc for red cell labeling was new. Now, some 10 years later, it can be evaluated more effectively. The in vitro preparation time is longer, and the error due to the elution of the marker or to cell injury is greater than with [51]Cr. The elution rate of ^{99m}Tc, approximately 6 to 10 percent per hour,[20] can be reduced to about 4 percent per hour by pretreating the red cells with tin chloride instead of the usual postlabeling treatment.[38] The short half-life of [99m]Tc (6 hours) reduces the radiation dose administered to the patient and also makes it possible to repeat the measurement at comparatively short intervals. These two advantages are of little consequence in patients with PV. In contrast, ^{99m}Tc labeling is particularly useful in intensive care procedures (in which repetition of the examination is useful) and in cardiology (since ^{99m}Tc is a radioisotope particularly well adapted to the use of the gamma camera).

The red cell volume (RCV) is calculated from three quantitative measurements: (1) the amount A of radioactivity injected, (2) the radioactivity contained in 1 ml of blood B after the interval necessary for equilibration within the vascular system, and (3) the venous hematocrit H. RCV (ml) = $A/B \times H$.

Hematocrit Determination

The measurement of red cell volume implies that the true venous hematocrit H (i.e., after correction for the trapped plasma) is known. Different correction factors have been developed to calculate the true hematocrit from the measured hematocrit,[15, 16, 55, 97, 98] depending on the technique used (Wintrobe's tube, microhematocrit method, the usual factor, when using this last method, is 0.985), the speed and the duration of centrifugation,

and the hematocrit itself (indeed, much more plasma is trapped when the hematocrit is increased). Microcytosis or spherocytosis also increases the amount of trapped plasma. This could explain why, in many cases of PV, the microhematocrit method (centrifugation) yields a higher value than the Coulter counter measurement.[18, 65, 89] On the other hand, the hematocrit, as measured by the Coulter counter method, also may be inaccurate if the mean red cell volume is altered by prolonged presence of red cells in the saline medium used for the measurement.[6] Recent studies, including our own, show that the most recent machines give hematocrit values lower by 2 percent in comparison with centrifugation up to a value of 50 percent, but their underestimation may increase to 5 percent between hematocrits of 50 and 55 percent and even higher beyond this value (sometimes 10 percent beyond hematocrits of 60 percent). Such an underestimation may be important in the follow-up of PV patients.

Timing of Blood Samples

The splenic red cell pool may be large[5] in the patients with a very enlarged spleen, and in this case, equilibration within the vascular system may take 15 to 30 minutes or even longer because of the large splenic pool. A substantial error in the calculated red cell volume might therefore exist if the total red cell volume were calculated from the circulating radioactivity measured after 5 to 10 minutes as compared with that calculated from a sample obtained 30 minutes after injection.[85] The "circulating" red cell volume can be calculated by extrapolation to t_0 of the measurements obtained at 10, 20, and 30 minutes.

The red cell and plasma volume determinations have to be done in a patient at rest (at least half an hour) because a fall in plasma volume due to increased capillary pressure and a shift from the intravascular to the interstitial space.[74] The patient will be studied nonfasting ("European" breakfast). Smoking is not allowed for at least 1 hour before the study.

Determination of Plasma Volume

The measurement of *plasma volume* is based on the dilution of a labeled protein, usually albumin, but occasionally ^{59}Fe-labeled transferrin. The use of macroglobulins has been suggested because of their slow exchange with the extravascular space, but they are of no practical use. ^{125}I is generally chosen as the tracer because of its convenient $t_{1/2}$ (50 days), which permits long storage, and because of the easy discrimination between ^{51}Cr and ^{125}I, allowing simultaneous measurement of the red cell and plasma volumes.

Plasma volume PV is calculated by the formula

$$PV = \frac{A}{B}$$

where A is the amount of isotope injected, and B is the amount of isotope per milliliter of plasma.

Like all proteins used for the measurement of plasma volume,[80] albumin leaves the circulating pool for an exchangeable pool (the interstitial space). To obtain a correct measurement of the dilution space, the radioactivity must be measured on at least three plasma samples taken from 15 to 60 minutes after the injection, which allows one to extrapolate the B value to time zero.

No commercially available automatic apparatus is reliable for plasma volume measurement, and as early as 1973, the ICSH advised against the use of such apparatuses.[37]

Determination of Total Blood Volume

The total blood volume is simply calculated by the sum of the red cell and plasma volumes. The problem currently raised in clinical practice is whether it may be calculated reliably from a measurement of only one of the two volumes (red cell or plasma) using the hematocrit to deduce the total blood volume from a measured red cell volume or from a measured plasma volume. However, the measurement of venous hematocrit is not a true measure of the body hematocrit[24,32,75] (Table 7–1). If the ratio of body hematocrit to venous hematocrit (the so-called f ratio) were constant (or nearly so) from one patient to another,[58] it would be possible to deduce the total blood volume from only one measured fractional volume by using an a priori correction for the venous hematocrit (in normal subjects, the mean of ratio is 0.91–0.92, to be multiplied by the correction factor for plasma trapping—0.985). This correction factor f is, however, extremely variable in pathologic states,[17,33,45,61,75] which has led some authors to claim that "it is time to abandon entirely the use of the 'f-cell ratio' for calculating blood volume."[98]

We have studied 329 patients in which the hematocrit was measured by the microhematocrit method and the total red cell and plasma volumes were measured by ^{51}Cr-labeled red blood cells and ^{125}I-labeled albumin.[58] Table 7–1 shows that, in fact, the statistical variation in the total-body versus venous hematocrit ratio is slight in PV patients when the spleen is not enlarged and that, in these patients, the error arising from a systematic correction of the venous hematocrit would be minimal and of no clinical consequence. In the absence of splenomegaly or of another concomitant disease, it is possible to calculate the blood volume from a

TABLE 7–1. BODY/VENOUS HEMATOCRIT RATIO AND POSSIBLE ERROR IN CALCULATING TOTAL BLOOD VOLUME WITH A FIXED RATIO

	POLYCYTHEMIA VERA WITHOUT SPLENOMEGALY (83 CASES)	PURE ERYTHROCYTOSIS (122 CASES)	NORMAL SUBJECTS (66 CASES)	DYSPROTEINEMIA* (59 CASES)	SPLENOMEGALY† (36 CASES)
Body/venous hematocrit ratio (mean value)	0.864	0.865	0.858	0.819	0.850
Standard deviation	0.030	0.032	0.030	0.067	0.085
Error of total blood volume (if calculated with a fixed f value)					
5 to 10%	16.5% of the cases	15%		52%	61%
>10%	1.1% of the cases	1.5%		24%	31%

* Multiple myeloma, Waldenström's disease.
† Patients with myelofibrosis or spent-phase polycythemia.

measurement of *either* the total red cell volume *or* the plasma volume if one accepts a 10 percent error.

Expression of the Results

The results of blood volume measurements are generally reported in milliliters per kilogram.[9] This is open to criticism for underweight and chiefly for overweight patients. In the latter group, the excess of fat, poorly vascularized, leads to an underestimation of the degree of PV. We therefore can not accept the opinion of those,[34] including the Polycythemia Vera Study Group (PVSG),[9] who consider the expression of volume per kilogram as sufficient in clinical practice.

Numerous equations have been proposed to calculate an "ideal" volume from the subject's weight and height to which the observed results would be compared. Some of these are presented in Table 7–2. However, several criticisms can be made concerning these equations:

The linearity of the equations is only true within rather large limits.[25,36,55]

The methods used in the published papers are not always adequate; for example, the calculation of total blood volume is based exclusively on a direct measurement of plasma[52] or red cell[62,100] volumes.

Finally, the measurements used to establish such equations are generally obtained in young male volunteers and not on a wide spectrum of subjects of all ages and both sexes. It is not surprising, therefore, that Pearson et al.[63] considered as abnormal only those values which exceeded by more than 25 percent the theoretical "normal" volume.

Reference data are more scarce in children and newborn babies. Although in these cases there is, of course, no risk of PV, measurements of red cell volume may sometimes be required in emergency situations (i.e., neonatal erythrocytosis). Some reference data may be found in the literature.[12,44]

APPLICATION OF BLOOD VOLUME MEASUREMENTS TO DIAGNOSIS

Why is the red blood cell volume measurement considered to be essential[9] for the diagnosis of PV? Is the level of hematocrit not sufficient? The following data will show that to differentiate PV from primary thrombocythemia, pure erythrocytosis, spurious polycythemia, and the secondary polycythemias, the simultaneous measurement of red cell and plasma volumes is more reliable than either the hematocrit measurement or the measurement of one single volume alone.[57]

As we showed earlier, a fairly close relationship is observed in PV patients between venous hematocrit and red cell volume (Fig. 7–1). However, it may be disturbed by a number of factors, namely, a disproportionate increase or decrease in plasma volume.[11,33] Furthermore, for a hematocrit value over 56 percent in males and 52 percent in females, the increase in red cell volume with hematocrit is not linear, owing to a progressive decrease of plasma volume for the highest values of hematocrit.[8]

When writing the first version of this chapter in 1984, we reviewed our own results, obtained during the previous 6 months. In 66 normal subjects (hematocrit lower than 50 percent in males and 48 percent in females), the mean red cell volume was 28.7 ± 2.6 ml/kg in males and 25.5 ± 3.3 ml/kg in females. No

TABLE 7–2. NORMAL VALUES OF RED CELL AND TOTAL BLOOD VOLUMES ACCORDING TO SOME PARAMETERS REPORTED IN THE LITERATURE

		RED CELL VOLUME (ML)	TOTAL BLOOD VOLUME (ML)
In ml/kg	Men	29.6	70.4
	Women	24.2	65.1
In ml/m² of surface area	Men	1100	2530
	Women	850	2350
Single function of height (cm)	Men	8.6 H + 18.6 W − 830	38.5 H + 31.7 W − 2830
and weight (kg)	Women	7.5 H + 14.3 W − 600	16.5 H + 38.4 W − 1370
Cubic function of height (m)	Men	—	36.7 H³ + 32.2 W + 604
and single function	Women	—	35.6 H³ + 33.0 W = 183
of weight (kg)			

* Data from references 8, 13, 53, and 100.

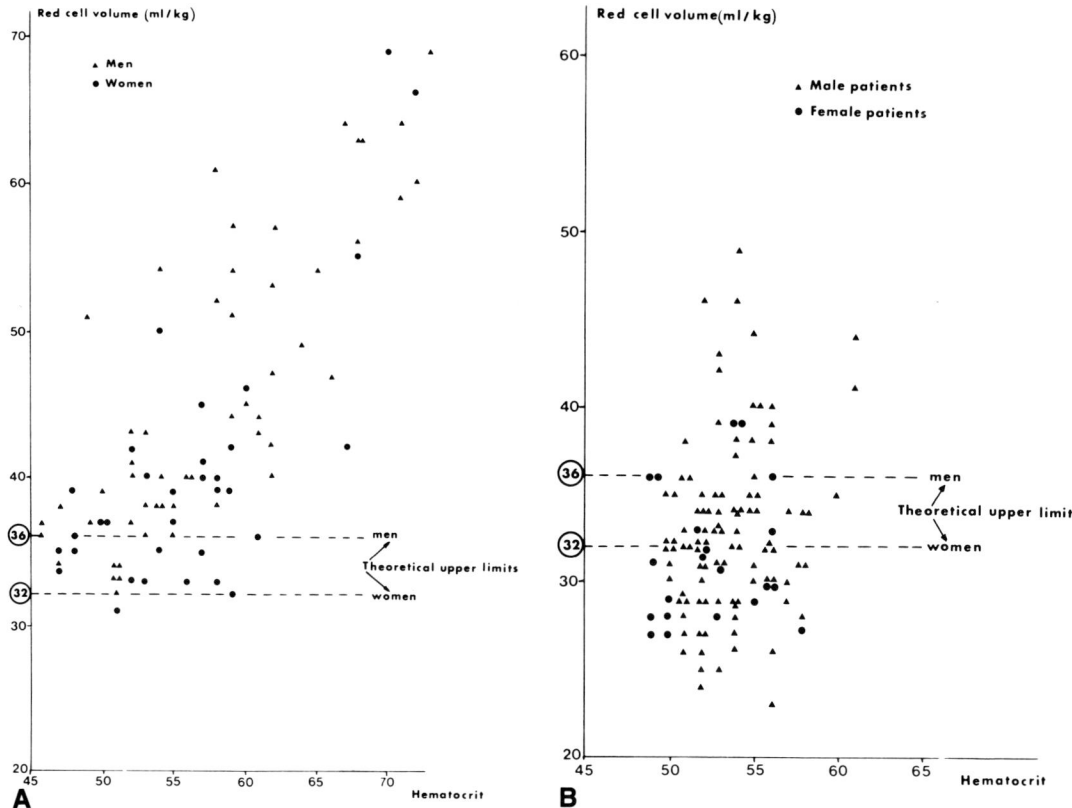

FIGURE 7–1. (A) Red cell volume at initial evaluation and during clinical remission in PV patients. (B) Results observed in pure erythrocytosis.

male subject had a red cell volume exceeding 35 ml/kg, and no female subject had a red cell volume exceeding 31 ml/kg. These data confirm that the upper limits used by the PVSG[9] remain valid. In 83 PV patients (studied at the time of diagnosis or in relapse), the cell volume was remarkably well correlated with the hematocrit ($r = 0.76$).

In contrast, the 122 patients with pure erythrocytosis form a heterogeneous group (Fig. 7–1) in which the red cell volume was poorly correlated with hematocrit ($r = 0.20$). Despite a hematocrit greater than 50 percent, 34 men but no women had a red cell volume less than 30 ml/kg and so could be classified as spurious polycythemia[60,64,96] due to hemoconcentration which was sometimes explained by a prolonged diuretic treatment or by androgen therapy, but in most of our patients no explanation was found for this anomaly, frequently observed in middle age, hypertensive, well-living and -drinking men.[7,23] Another 39 men and 13 women had an increased red cell volume (ac-

cording to the limits set by the PVSG); these cases corresponded to true erythrocytosis, which needed further study. In these patients, the criteria of PVSG are clearly inadequate; the dosage of erythropoietin and the in vitro culture of stem cells seem really useful for the classification of these patients into or out of the group of autonomous (malignant?) myeloproliferative diseases, and perhaps have to be treated as other, primary, myeloproliferative diseases. The remaining patients in this group had only a slight increase in hematocrit and red cell volume with no apparent cause; when followed over the long term, they remained remarkably stable. These patients were principally middle-aged men (30 to 50 years of age) and may be considered as normal subjects at the upper limit of the normal range.

Hume and Goldberg,[34] on the basis of a small study of patients suffering from bronchitis, reported that the hematocrit was not a good reflection of the total red cell volume in cardiopulmonary disease. Congestive heart failure in chronic obstructive lung disease may generate hemodilution and conceal an excessive red cell volume.[14] In contrast, in a study of 22 smokers published by Smith and Landaw,[78] the total red cell volume was greater than 36 ml/kg in half the subjects, but plasma volume was reduced in all but 4, making the hematocrit a poor indicator of the true increase in red cell volume. Several other papers also demonstrate the heterogeneity of the so-called erythrocytosis and the need for simultaneous red cell and plasma measurements.[40,42,79]

In brief, extremely variable data from one study to another and from one patient to another imply that the measurement of both red cell and plasma volumes should be performed in clinical studies evaluating patients for a diagnosis of PV, at least when the hematocrit does not exceed 60 percent.

Microcytic Polycythemias

Patients with a raised red blood cell count, with small red blood cells, generally correspond to heterozygous thalassemias, which may sometimes only be discovered in adulthood. The total red cell volume is always normal in these patients, as is the hematocrit and hemoglobin concentration. Sometimes, however, microcytic polycythemia may correspond to true polycythemia in which blood loss (e.g., postoperative or after phlebotomies) has occurred before the blood volume measurement. In these patients, the red cell volume may be increased despite a normal hematocrit due to an increase in the plasma volume.

Values Observed in Thrombocytosis

In thrombocythemias, normal red cell volume (after correction of a possible hyposideremia) is a necessary parameter for diagnosis.[95] As a matter of fact, some patients with only slightly increased hematocrit may have an excess of red cell volume and have to be considered and treated as having PV.

From the data summarized earlier, *it may be concluded* that:

The measurement of red cell volume is necessary before including patients with a moderately increased hematocrit in the group of PV. This is not just a casual remark, since we have seen patients with only a slightly increased hematocrit

"treated" by chemotherapy without proof of myeloproliferative disease, which constitutes an inappropriate and even a possibly dangerous decision.

When the increase in hematocrit is moderate, measurement of both the red cell *and* plasma volumes is necessary to classify a patient into one of the groups of polycythemias—true erythrocytosis or pseudopolycythemia—and to guide appropriately further diagnostic studies.

The measurement of red cell volume is also necessary in apparent cases of idiopathic thrombocytosis and in some rare cases of hypochromic, microcytic, nonthalassemic polycythemias.

PROGNOSTIC VALUE OF BLOOD VOLUME MEASUREMENT

Vascular accidents are the main clinical risks in polycythemia: chiefly arterial thrombosis of the brain, heart, and iliac arteries. In fact, in the context of this chapter, the practical question is to know whether this risk is linked to the degree of red cell volume excess.

The ratio between blood viscosity, on the one hand, and hematocrit and blood volume, on the other, is not clearly defined.[71,87] Nevertheless, experience shows, for cerebral vascular lesions, in congenital heart disease[66] and in polycythemia vera (PVSG data) that maintenance of the hematocrit (and thus of the red cell volume) at a normal level is the major determinant of the prognosis. Some data suggest that an increase in total blood volume by simultaneous expansion of both red cell and plasma volumes also could be a vascular risk factor. If this is true, the measurement of both fractional volumes, even when hematocrit is normal or only slightly increased, would be important to ascertain the quality of remission. Our personal data, however, do not demonstrate that the risk of thrombosis is clearly increased in these patients who have an excessive blood volume despite a normal hematocrit (patients in the spent phase, or chronically phlebotomized patients without any large excess of the platelet count). As far as the short-term prognosis is concerned, it seems that the hematocrit is a sufficient parameter to decide the use of phlebotomies, whatever the decision about further therapy; a value of 55 percent, and possibly lower in the patients with vascular risk (age, antecedents, diabetes) could be accepted for such an urgent blood depletion, since radiotherapy or chemotherapy only give delayed results.

RED CELL AND PLASMA VOLUME MEASUREMENTS IN THE FOLLOW-UP OF PV

In the absence of complications, namely, the development of splenic enlargement and myelofibrosis, the clinical monitoring of a treated PV patient consists of regular measurements of the hemoglobin concentration, hematocrit, and platelet count. The frequent measurement of blood volume is not necessary.

Patients treated with myelosuppressive agents (radiotherapy or chemotherapy) are efficiently monitored by repeated hematocrit measurements. In patients treated by phlebotomies alone, an excess of both the red cell and plasma volumes may be observed despite a normal hematocrit; this could be the first symptom of a spent phase (myelofibrosis), which appears very early in many patients treated by phlebotomies.

STUDIES OF CELL KINETICS IN ACTIVE PV AND ESSENTIAL THROMBOCYTOPENIA (ET)

Ferrokinetic studies in uncomplicated PV are not relevant in clinical practice. There is no difference in the erythrokinetics between primary and secondary polycythemias: accelerated clearance of radioiron from the plasma and no sign of dyserythropoiesis, hemolysis, or splenic erythroid metaplasia. In this uncomplicated phase, patients with PV have a qualitatively normal erythropoiesis, at normal sites, which is simply quantitatively increased.[22,72,81]

In ET, the platelet life span shows normal or only slightly increased platelet destruction.[28] The direct measurement of platelet production using ^{75}Se-methionine only showed the expected increased production.[1] Excessive splenic blood flow and splenic platelet pool have been observed in the case of splenomegaly.[67] In vitro kinetic studies of blood and bone marrow stem cells, as well as the effects of the growth factors, are discussed in another chapter of this book.

USE OF RADIOISOTOPIC METHODS FOR THE EVALUATION OF COMPLICATIONS IN PV

With the improvement in the treatment and monitoring of patients with PV, late hematologic complications are being observed more and more frequently.[73,86,93,94] These complications include development of splenomegaly resistant to therapy in a patient remaining in the polycythemic phase, development of spent-phase polycythemia, development of myelofibrosis with myeloid metaplasia, and development of acute leukemia. The role of the Nuclear Medicine Department in the detection and evaluation of these complications is discussed below.

Polycythemia with Development of Significant Splenomegaly

Blood volume measurements in these patients show that despite the normal or slightly increased hematocrit, the red cell volume is increased beyond the accepted limits and the plasma volume is also increased (Table 7–3). In this group there is no correlation between the hematocrit and the red cell volume. The absence of myelofibrosis and myeloid metaplasia can be clearly shown by a ferrokinetic study, which typically demonstrates increased plasma clearance, red cell radioiron

TABLE 7–3. BLOOD VOLUME IN PATIENTS WITH ACTIVE PV WITH SPLENOMEGALY DURING THE SPENT PHASE AND IN POST-PV MYELOFIBROSIS

	ACTIVE PHASE WITH SPLENOMEGALY (18 CASES)	SPENT PHASE (19 CASES)	MYELOFIBROSIS (26 CASES)
Hematocrit	46.6 (30 to 55)	35.5 (20 to 48)	35.0 (20 to 42)
Red cell volume (ml/kg)	38.2 (30 to 47)	35.5 (23 to 43)	30.2 (20 to 41)
Plasma volume (ml/kg)	44.7 (32 to 61)	60.5 (48 to 82)	60.0 (46 to 73)

incorporation in excess of 80 percent, and a low uptake into the spleen at 24 hours. However, this study is long, costly, and cumbersome for the patient.[20] Bone marrow scintigraphy using ^{111}In-labeled transferrin may be used in this case instead of a traditional ferrokinetic study. It shows that the bone marrow remains hyperactive with increased uptake of ^{99m}Tc colloid, ^{111}In chloride, or [52]Fe, with extension into the long bones[41] and the absence of any obvious splenic uptake of ^{111}In-labeled transferrin. Bone marrow biopsy would confirm that there is not (or at least not yet) any collagen fibrosis. The serum procollagen III amino-terminal peptide level does not differ from the values usually observed in the active phase of PV (no or low increase).

Spent Phase

This phase corresponds to the next step of increasing severity and is characterized by weakness, a very large spleen, a normal or reduced hematocrit, and generally a thrombocytopenia.[54] In this stage, the total blood volume is greater than in the previous phase due to a large excess of the plasma volume (see Table 7–3). In this group of patients there is only myelofibrosis, with no myelosclerosis. Bone marrow scintigraphy shows the permanent uptake into the axial skeletal bone marrow with, however, a moderate splenic uptake of ^{111}In and an abnormal uptake of the radioactive isotope into the knees, shoulders, and elbows. Procollagen III values are generally increased at this stage of the disease.

Postpolycythemia Myeloid Metaplasia (PPMM)

In the different series reported in the literature,[51,67,76,77] 6 to 28 percent of patients with PV develop myeloid metaplasia as a terminal event in the course of their disease. In fact, in our own series (results in Brit J Haemol, 86:233, 1994), 40 percent of the ^{32}P-treated patients still living and followed at the twentieth year after diagnosis and more than 80 percent of the patients treated at long term by phlebotomies alone are in the spent phase or have developed PPMM. Such a "complication" actually appears to constitute the natural course of very long-standing PV. The clinical status of the patients at this stage is similar to primary myeloid metaplasia, although the long-term prognosis is certainly better in these post-PV users than in the primary myelofibrosis.[83,92]

Diagnosis of PPMM is confirmed by bone marrow biopsy and the splenic uptake of ^{111}In transferrin.[2] Raised procollagen III values may have prognostic significance,[3,31,58a] and very excessive values suggest a malignant evolution.

Isotope studies have a prognostic value.[50,54] The degree of true anemia (i.e., red cell volume) and of blood volume dilution (i.e., excess of plasma volume) may be useful for indicating blood transfusion. Our own experience suggests that a remaining ^{111}In uptake into the bone marrow axis, with diffusion of active bone marrow to limbs, indicates a better prognosis than a pure splenic uptake. On the other hand, radioiron kinetics may show a severe dyserythropoiesis (high plasma clearance, low incorporation into the red blood cells), which is a bad prognostic index. As far as splenectomy is discussed, the degree of hypersplenism (excess of plasma volume, platelet sequestration) and the degree of hemolysis (red cell life span) are other useful parameters.[4,50,56,62,68,73a]

Leukemic Transformation

Leukemic transformation may present in two ways: as a "classic" acute myelogenous or undifferentiated leukemia (M1 or M3, according to the FAB classification, sometimes M4, in the context of evolutive myelofibrosis) with total bone marrow invasion or, more frequently encountered in this clinical context, as pancytopenia or refractory anemia with slight blast excess (myelodysplasia).[58a] In either of these two clinical presentations, isotope methods are of little practical value, except for in vitro kinetic studies of stem cells (labeling index of blasts and suicide rate may be of prognostic value).

OTHER IN VIVO AND IN VITRO TESTS USING RADIOTRACERS

In Vitro Studies

Some interesting pathophysiologic observations have been made in PV patients using in vivo radioisotope methods. Cerebral blood flow,[35,84] measured by the ^{133}Xe method, is clearly decreased as a function of the hematocrit increase both in primary and secondary PV. It has been given as an argument for resuming active therapy when the hematocrit exceeds 50 percent.

Splenic blood flow also may be measured by the clearance of ^{133}Xe. However, the method proposed by Peters et al.,[67] based on the equilibration of the circulating and the splenic pools of labeled platelets, is easier to perform. The splenic blood pool also may be measured by quantitative isotope scanning.[30,49] The pool measured is not correlated with the total circulating red cell volume but related to the size of the spleen. Another interesting finding is that with an equal spleen size, the splenic pool is twice as large in primary as in secondary polycythemia.[5,49] Blood flow measurements[43] are, however, of doubtful practical value.

Among the isotope methods, spleen scintigraphy may be used to quantify splenomegaly, but physical examination is in fact nearly always sufficient, and when necessary, ultrasonography gives the same information as scintigraphy without the injection of a radioactive agent. Another indication for spleen scintigraphy is the search for a splenic infarct in case of splenic pain in patients with spent-phase polycythemia or myelofibrosis.

In Vitro Studies

Vitamin B_{12} plasma concentration is presently assayed by competition methods using radioactive vitamin B_{12} and intrinsic factor as a binder. The clinical value of this test as a criterion of PV seems very poor; sensitivity is 36 percent, specificity is 70 percent, according to recent data. A French consensus conference recently (June 1993) decided to exclude this dosage from the list of criteria required at the initial evaluation of the PV.

Erythropoietin (EPO) was studied initially by using in vivo or in vitro biologic assays, with low sensitivity, high cost, and great time expense. Since obtaining a recombinant protein, the radioimmunologic dosage, then other immunoassays (ELISA, IRMA), are easily used. Some personal results are given in Table 7–4. Schematically, the use of the dosage could be:

> The cases with pure erythrocytosis, in which a high EPO titer (more than 20 mU/ml) practically excludes the diagnostic of myeloproliferative disease.

> And the cases of suspected PV, without the usual criteria, in which a low EPO value (less than 10 mU/ml) is a very good argument for the diagnosis of primary myeloproliferative disease.[75a]

No biologic test seems presently useful for predicting the thrombotic risk in PV, in which hematocrit, and so the blood viscosity, remains the only significant parameter (with the patient's age and vascular antecedents). The dosage of platelet factor 4 and beta-thromboglobulin[46,47] did not demonstrate any predictive value. During the last few years, considerable progress has been made in characterizing hypercoagulable states, but the predictive value of these new tests has not yet been evaluated in PV patients.[101]

TABLE 7–4. STATISTICAL COMPARISON OF EPO CONCENTRATION (UNITS PER LITER) IN POLYCYTHEMIA VERA AND IN PURE ERYTHROCYTOSIS

	PV	DIFFERENCE	PE
Ht < 50% (i.e., treated cases)	$n = 59$ $m = 8.24$ U/liter ± 3.72	$F = 39.22$ $p < 0.001$	$n = 40$ $m = 30.55$ U/liter ± 27.06
Ht = 50 to 60%	$n = 58$ $m = 6.58$ U/liter ± 2.58	$F = 14.17$ $p < 0.001$	$n = 131$ $m = 21.67$ U/liter ± 26.91
Ht > 60%	$n = 35$ $m = 5.04$ U/liter ± 3.01	$F = 29.22$ $p < 0.001$	$n = 19$ $m = 16.16$ U/liter ± 11.69

Note: PV is defined as an excess of red cell volume and either splenomegaly or excess of granulocytes and/or platelets. These patients were studied at diagnosis, in remission, or in relapse. Pure erythrocytosis (PE) is defined as an excess of red cell volume without any excess of leukocytes or platelets and no splenomegaly.

The serum concentration of the amino-terminal peptide of procollagen III, which is measured by radioimmunoassay, has been proposed as a parameter indicative of the course of fibrosis. From a 6-year personal experience with about 600 dosages in PV patients,[58a] the following conclusions may be drawn:

A low discriminative value between PV and pure erythrocytosis.

A predictive value of progression toward myelofibrosis and of evolution of my-elofibrosis, when instituted.

A possible drop in myelofibrotic patients treated by hydroxyurea, which could be a useful indication for the efficiency of the treatment.

REFERENCES

1. Ardaillou N, Najean Y, Eberlin A: Study of platelet kinetics using 75 Seselonomethionine. *In* Paulus JM (ed): Platelet Kinetics. Amsterdam, North Holland, 1971, p 131–142.
2. Arrago JP, Rain JD, Vigneron N, et al: Diagnostic value of bone marrow imaging with ^{111}In transferrin and [99m]technetium colloids in myelofibrosis. Am J Hematol 18:275–282, 1985
3. Arrago JP, Najean Y, Poirier O: Utilisation du dosage du procollagene III pour la surveillance de l'évolution vers la myélofibrose des polyglobulies. Presse Med 13:2429–2432, 1984
4. Barosi G, Cazzola H, Frassoui F, et al: Erythropoïesis in myelofibrosis with myeloid metaplasia: Recognition of different classes of patients by erythrokinetics. Br J Haematol 48:263–272, 1981
5. Bateman S, Lewis SM, Nicholas A, Zaafran A: Splenic red cell pooling: A diagnostic feature in polycythaemia. Br J Haematol 40:389–396, 1978
6. Beautyman W, Bills T: Osmotic error in erythrocyte volume determination. Am J Hematol 12:383–389, 1982
7. Bealer SL: Central nervous system control of plasma volume. Fed Proc 69:2461–2464, 1986
8. Bentley SA, Lewis SA: The relation-ship between total red cell volume, plasma volume and venous haematocrit. Br J Haematol 33:301–307, 1976
9. Berlin NI: Diagnosis and classification of the polycythemias. Semin Hematol 12:5–17, 1975
10. Birgerard G, Miller O, Caro J, Erslev I: Serum erythropoïetin levels by radio-immuno assay in polycythaemia. Scand J Haematol 29:161–167, 1982
11. Bowdler AJ: Plasma volume and splenomegaly in polycythaemia vera. Br J Haematol 22:331–339, 1972
12. Brans YW, Shaunon DL, Ramamurthy RS: Neonatal polycythemia: Plasma, blood and red cell volume estimates in relation to hematocrit levels. Pediatrics 68:175–182, 1981
13. Brassinne A: Le volume sanguin de l'homme normal: Recherche de formules de prédiction. Pathol Biol 16:257–271, 1968
14. Burton RR, Smith AH: The effect of chronic erythrocytic polycythemia and high altitude upon plasma and blood volume. Proc Soc Exp Biol Med 140:920–923, 1972
15. Chaplin H, Mollison PL: Correction for plasma trapping in the red cell column of the hematocrit. Blood 7:1227–1233, 1952
16. Chaplin H, Mollison PL, Vetter H: The body/venous hematocrit ratio: Its constancy over a wide hematocrit range. J Clin Invest 32:1309–1321, 1953
17. Donaldson GWK, MacArthur M, MacPherson AIS: Blood volume changes in splenomegaly. Br J Haematol 18:45–55, 1970
18. Dosik H, Prasad B: Coulter S hematocrit and microhematocrit in polycythemic patients. Am J Hematol 5:51–54, 1978
19. Ellis JT: Polycythemia Vera Study Group unpublished data, 1982
20. Ferrant A, Lewis SM, Szur L: The elution of ^{99m}Tc from red cells and its effect on red volume measurement. J Clin Pathol 27:983–985, 1974
21. Ferrant A, Rodhain J, Cauwe F, et al: Assessment of bone marrow and splenic erythropoiesis in myelofibrosis. Scand J Haematol 29:373–380, 1982
22. Finch CA, Deubelbeiss K, Cook JD, et al: Ferrokinetics in human. Medicine 49:17–53, 1970
23. Fouad FM, Tadena-Thome L, Bravo EL, Tarazi RC: Idiopathic hypovolemia. Ann Intern Med 104:298–303, 1986
24. Fudenberg H, Baldini M, Mahoney JP, Dameshek W: The body hematocrit/venous hematocrit ratio and the "splenic reservoir." Blood 17:71–82, 1961
25. Gelman RC, Tormey DC, Betensky R, et al: Actual versus ideal weight in the calculation of surface area. Cancer Treat Rep 71:907–911, 1987
26. Gilbert HS: Definition, clinical features and diagnosis of polycythemia vera. Clin Haematol 4:263–290, 1975
27. Glass HI, Brant A, Clark JC, et al: Measurement of blood volume using red cells labelled with radioactive carbon monoxide. J Nucl Med 9:571–575, 1968
28. Harker LA: Platelet kinetics in autonomous thrombocytosis. *In* Paulus JM (ed): Platelet Kinetics. Amsterdam, North Holland, 1971, pp 308–309
29. Heaton WAL, Keegan T, Hanbury CM, et al: Studies with non radio-isotopic sodium chromate. Transfusion 29:703–707, 1989
30. Hedge UM, Williams CD, Lewis SM, et al: Measurement of splenic cell volume and visualisation of the spleen with [99m]Tc. J Nucl Med 14:769–771, 1973
31. Hochweiss S, Fruchtman J, Hahn EG, et al: Increased serum procollagen III amino-terminal peptide in myelofibrosis. Am J Hematol 15:343–351, 1983
32. Hope A, Verel D: Observation on the distribution of red cells and plasma in disease: The low body haematocrit/venous haematocrit ratio. Clin Sci 14:501–508, 1955
33. Huber H, Lewis SM, Szur L: The influence of anaemia, polycythaemia and splenomegaly on

the relationship between venous haematocrit and red cell volume. Br J Haematol 10:567–573, 1964

34. Hume R, Goldberg A: Actual and predicted normal red cell and plasma volumes in primary and secondary polycythaemia. Clin Sci 20:449–508, 1964

35. Humphrey PRD, Michael J, Pearson TC: Management of relative polycythaemia: I. Studies of cerebral blood flow and viscosity. Br J Haematol 46:427–433, 1980

36. Hurley JP: Red cell and plasma volumes in normal adults. J Nucl Med 16:46–52, 1975

37. International Committee for Standardization in Haematology (ICSH): Standard techniques for the measurement of red cell and plasma volume. Br J Haematol 25:795–814, 1973

38. Jones J, Mollison PL: A simple and efficient method of labelling red cells with ^{99m}Tc for determination of red cell volume. Br J Haematol 38:141–148, 1978

39. Klerk G, Rosengarten PCJ, Vet RJW, Goudsmit R: Serum erythropoietin titers in polycythemia. Blood 58:1171–1174, 1981

40. Kulkarni V, Ritchey K, Howard D, Dainiak N: Heterogeneity of Epo-dependent erythrocytosis. Br J Haematol 60:751–758, 1985

41. Kurnick JE, Mahmood T, Napoli N, Block MA: Extension of myeloid tissue into the lower extremities in polycythemia. Am J Clin Pathol 71:427–431, 1980

42. Kutti J, Safai-Kutti S, Saroulis GC, Good RA: Plasma levels of beta-thromboglobulin and platelet factor 4 in relation to the venous platelet concentration. Acta Haematol 46:1–5, 1980

43. Lahtinen R, Lahtinen T, Hyodyumaa S: Increased bone marrow flow in polycythemia vera. Eur J Nucl Med 3:19–22, 1983

44. Linderkamp O, Betke K, Fendel H, et al: Tc-99m labeled red blood cells for the measurement of red cell mass in newborn infants. J Nucl Med 21:637–640, 1980

45. Locking JB, Wilson E: The whole body/venous haematocrit ratio in chronic non specific obstructive lung disease. Scand J Haematol 9:433–436, 1972

46. Ludlam CA: Evidence for the platelet specificity of beta-thromboglobulin and studies on its plasma concentration. Br J Haematol 41:271–278, 1979

47. Ludlam CA, Moore S, Bolton AE, et al: The release of a human platelet specific protein measured by a specific radioimmunoassay. Thromb Res 6:543–548, 1975

48. Marsh JCW, Hibben J, Marsh GW: Primary proliferative polycythaemia without splenomegaly: A diagnostic problem. Clin Lab Haematol 9:123–128, 1987

49. Marsh JCW, Liu Yin JA, Lewis SM: Blood volume measurement in pseudo-polycythaemia: When and why? Clin Lab Haematol 9:115–122, 1987

50. Milner GR, Geary CG, Wadsworth LD, Doss A: Erythrokinetic studies as a guide to the value of splenectomy in primary myeloid metaplasia. Br J Haematol 25:467–484, 1973

51. Modan B: Interrelationship between polycythemia vera leukemia and myeloid metaplasia. Clin Haematol 4:427–439, 1975

52. Nadler SB, Hidalgo JU, Bloch T: Prediction of blood volume in normal human adults. Surgery 51:224–232, 1962

53. Najean Y, Ardaillou N, Dresch C: Utilisation des techniques isotopiques en hématologie. Paris, Baillière, 1969, p 188

54. Najean Y, Arrago JP, Rain JD, Dresch C: The "spent" phase of polycythemia vera: Hypersplenism in the absence of amplifibrosis. Br J Haematol 56:163–170, 1984

55. Najean Y, Cacchione R: Blood volume in health and disease. Clin Haematol 6:543–566, 1977

56. Najean Y, Cacchione R, Castro-Malespina H, Dresch C: Erythrokinetic studies in myelofibrosis their significance for prognosis. Br J Haematol 40:205–217, 1978

57. Najean Y, Cacchione R, Dresch C, Rain JD: Intérêt pratique de la mesure du volume globulaire dans les polyglobulies. Nouv Presse Med 4:1633–1636, 1975

57a. Najean Y, Deschamps A, Dresch C, et al: Acute leukemia and myelodysplasia in polycythemia vera. Cancer 11:89–95, 1988

58. Najean Y, Deschryver F: The body-venous haematocrit ratio and its use for calculating total blood volume from fractional volumes. Eur J Nucl Med 9:558–560, 1984

58a. Najean Y, Legrand M, Poirier O, et al: The clinical significance of serum procollagen III in chronic myeloproliferative disorders. Eur J Haematol 45:239–243, 1990

59. Najean Y, Poirier O, Lokiec F: The clinical significance of beta thromboglobulin and platelet factor 4 in polycythaemic patients. Scand J Haematol 31:298–304, 1983

60. Najean Y, Triebel F, Dresch C: Pure erythrocytosis: Reappraisal of a study of 51 cases. Am J Hematol 10:129–136, 1981

61. Nielsen S, Rodbro P: Validity of rapid estimation of erythrocyte volume in the diagnosis of polycythemia vera. Eur J Nucl Med 15:32–37, 1989

62. Payne RW: Predictor of red cell mass from weight and height: A normogram. J Clin Pathol 31:1003–1008, 1978

63. Pearson TC, Glass UH, Wetherley-Mein G: Interpretation of measured red cell mass in the diagnosis of polycythaemia. Scand J Haematol 21:153–162, 1978

64. Pearson TC, Wetherley-Mein G: The course and complications of idiopathic erythrocytosis. Clin Lab Haematol 1:189–196, 1979

65. Penn D, Williams PR, Durcher TF, Adair RM: Comparison of hematocrit determination by micro-hematocrit and electronic particle counter. Am J Clin Pathol 72:71–74, 1979

66. Pernot C: Accidents cérébraux des cardiopathies congénitales. Presse Med 12:1009–1013, 1983

67. Peters AM, Klonizakis I, Lavender JP, Lewis SM: Use of indium 111-labelled platelets to measure spleen function. Br J Haematol 46:587–592, 1980

68. Pettit JE, Lewis SM, Goolden AWG: Polycythemia vera: Transformation to myelofibrosis and subsequent reversal. Scand J Haematol 20:43–69, 1978

69. Pettit JE, Lewis SM, Williams ED, et al: Quantitative studies of splenic erythropoiesis in polycythemia vera and myelofibrosis. Br J Haematol 34:465–475, 1976

70. Pettit JE, Lewis SM, Nicholas AW: Transitional myeloproliferative disorder. Br J Haematol 43:167–184, 1979

71. Phillips MJ, Harkness J: Plasma and whole blood viscosity. Br J Haematol 43:167–184, 19XX

72. Pollycove M, Winchell HS, Lawrence JH: Classification of patterns of erythropoiesis in polycythemia vera as studied by iron kinetics. Blood 28:807–829, 1966

73. Rain JD, Dresch C, Said A, Najean Y: Les éléments du choix thérapeutique dans les polyglobulies vraies: 2. Évolutions à long terme de 286 malades traités par le ^{32}P. Nouv Presse Med 2:1499–1503, 1973

73a. Rain JD, Najean Y: Bone marrow scintigraphy in myelofibrosis. Nouv Rev Fr Hematol 35:101–105, 1993

74. Rocker L, Laniado M, Kirsch K: The effect of physical exercise on plasma volume and red blood cell mass. In: Dunn CDR (ed): Current Concepts in Erythropoiesis. New York, Wiley, 1983, pp 246–276

75. Rothschild MA, Bauman A, Yalow RS, Berson SA: Effect of splenomegaly on blood volume. J Appl Physiol 6:701–706, 1954

75a. Schlageter MH, Toubert ME, Podgorniak MP, Najean Y: Radioimmunoassay of erythropoietin: Analytical performance and clinical use in hematology. Clin Chem 36:1731–1735, 1990

76. Silverstein MN: The evolution into and the treatment of late stage polycythemia vera. Semin Hematol 13:79–84, 1976

77. Silverstein MN, Brown AL, Linhon JW: Idiopathic myeloid metaplasia: Its evolution into acute leukemia. Ann Intern Med 132:709–713, 1973

78. Smith JR, Landaw SA: Smoker's polycythemia. N Engl J Med 298:6–10, 1978

79. Stenstrom G, Kutti J: The blood volume in pheochromocytoma patients. Acta Med Scand 218:381–387, 1985

80. Sterling K: Turnover rate of serum albumin using ^{131}I. J Clin Invest 30:1128–1139, 1951

81. Szur L: The nonleukaemic myeloproliferative disorders. In Hoffbrand AV, Lewis SM (eds): Tutorials in Postgraduate Medicine: Haematology. London, Heinemann, 1972, p. 257

82. Szur L, Lewis SM: Iron kinetics. Clin Haematol 4:407–425, 1975

83. Takacsi-Nagy L, Graj F: Definition, clinical features and diagnosis of myelofibrosis. Clin Haematol 4:291–308, 1975

84. Thomas DH, Boulay GH, Marshall J, et al: Cerebral blood flow in polycythaemia. Lancet 2:161–163, 1977

85. Toghill PJ, Green S: The influence of spleen size on the distribution of red cells and plasma. J Clin Pathol 25:570–573, 1972

86. Tubiana M, Flamant R, Attie E, Nayat M: A study of hematological complications occurring in patients with polycythemia vera treated with ^{32}P. Blood 32:536–548, 1968

87. Turitto VT: Blood viscosity, mass transport and thrombogenesis. Prog Hemost Thromb 6:139–177, 1982

88. Vellenga E, Mulder NH, Van Zanten AK, et al: The significance of the amino-terminal propeptide of type III procollagen in paroxysmal nocturnal haemoglobinuria and myelofibrosis. Eur J Nucl Med 8:499–501, 1983

89. Villalta IA, Pramanik AK, Diaz Blanco J, Herbest JJ: Diagnostic errors in neonatal polycythemia based on method of hematocrit determination. J Pediatr 115:460–462, 1989

90. Waddel CC, Brocon JA: Abnormal platelet function in myeloproliferative disorders. Arch Pathol Lab Med 105:432–435, 1981

91. Walsh PN, Murphy S, Barry WE: The role of platelets in the pathogenesis of thrombosis and hemorrhage in patients with thrombocytosis. Thromb Haemost 4:1085–1096, 1977

92. Ward HP, Block MH: The natural history of agnogenic myeloid metaplasia (AMM) and a critical evaluation of its relation-ship with the myeloproliferative syndrome. Medicine 50:357–420, 1971

93. Wasserman LR: Polycythemia vera: Its course and treatment. Relation to myeloid metaplasia and leukemia. Bull NY Acad Med 30:343–375, 1954

94. Wasserman LR: The treatment of polycythemia vera. Semin Hematol 13:57–78, 1976

95. Wawern F, Lewis SM: Blood volume, erythrokinetics and spleen function in thrombocythaemia. Acta Haematol 73:219–223, 1985

96. Weinreb NJ, Shih CF: Spurious polycythemia. Semin Hematol 12:397–407, 1975

97. Wood GA, Levitt SH: Simultaneous red cell mass and plasma volume determination using ^{51}Cr tagged red cells and ^{125}I-labelled albumin. J Nucl Med 6:433–440, 1965

98. Wright RP, Tono M, Pollycove M: Blood volume. Semin Nucl Med 5:63–78, 1975

99. Whohat M, Merlob P, Reisner SH: Neonatal polycythemia. Pediatrics 73:7–13, 1984

100. Wennersland R, Brown E, Hopper J, et al: Red cell, plasma and blood volume in healthy men measured by ratio-chromium bagging and haematocrit. J Clin Invest 36:1065–1077, 1959

101. Wehneier A, Scharf RE, Fricke S, Schneider W: Bleeding and thrombosis in chronic myeloproliferative disorders: Relation of platelet disorders to clinical aspects of the disease. Haemostasis 19:251–259, 1989

8

Cytogenetics

ROBERT V. PIERRE *and* JACQUELINE WHANG-PENG

Polycythemia vera (PV) is included conceptually in the group of chronic myeloproliferative disorders. There is clear evidence, based on both cytogenetic and isoenzyme studies, that PV represents a monoclonal stem-cell disorder.[1-10] Although PV is viewed predominately as a proliferative disorder of erythroid cells, it is usually accompanied by less prominent proliferation of the granulocytes and megakaryocytes. The neoplastic clone coexists in the bone marrow with the normal pluripotent and committed stem-cell populations. Unlike the normal erythroid stem cells, which are under humoral regulatory control, the neoplastic clone behaves in a nearly autonomous fashion.

The initiating events leading to the formation of the neoplastic clone are as yet unknown. Because of the possible role of chromosome abnormalities involving rearrangements of oncogenes and other structural genes in the causation of PV or in conferring proliferative advantages to the neoplastic clone, a study of cytogenetic abnormalities was initiated by the Polycythemia Vera Study Group (PVSG).[11-13] Cytogenetic studies were included in the design of the original protocol 01 of the PVSG. Cytogenetic studies were to be performed on all patients prior to randomization for therapy, and follow-up studies also were planned to document possible evolutionary changes.

The cytogenetic studies had the following objectives:

1. To describe the frequency and types of cytogenetic abnormalities observed in PV.
2. To determine whether the presence or absence of cytogenetic abnormalities was predictive of response to therapy, survival, or progression to acute leukemia.
3. To determine whether therapy would alter the cytogenetic status of the patient.

A review of the available literature data from other sources that address these same questions is also included in this chapter.

MATERIALS AND METHODS

The criteria for patient eligibility for protocol 01 are given in other chapters of this book. All patients included in the study have satisfied these criteria and had an unequivocal diagnosis of PV. All patients gave informed consent to participate in a randomized treatment trial. The investigators were requested to perform direct bone marrow cytogenetic studies prior to initiation of therapy and to repeat the studies at 2-year intervals during the course of therapy. The direct bone marrow chromosome preparation method of Tjio and Whang[14] was used. The interval between marrow aspiration and exposure to colchicine and subsequent hypotonic treatment was 2 hours in most instances. Institutions without cytogenetic laboratories were instructed how to prepare the direct slides or to prepare suspensions of fixed cells and mail them to reference cytogenetic laboratories staffed by certain members of the PVSG. If clonal chromosomal abnormalities were found in the bone marrow, particularly if they appeared to be balanced translocations or other abnormalities that might represent a constitutional abnormality, a PHA-stimulated peripheral blood leukocyte culture was suggested to eliminate the possibility of a constitutional abnormality. Direct bone marrow preparations were suggested at the initiation of the study because they were thought not to suffer from abnormalities induced by in vitro culture. It was not known at that time that short-term cultures of bone marrow without mitogens could give an improved fraction of successful studies, as has been shown by more recent studies.[15] In later stages of the study, banded chromosome studies utilizing Q bands, G bands, or R bands were done by the participating laboratories or the reference laboratories. Banding studies were not carried out on the majority of the specimens because the sample collections in many cases antedated the introduction of banding methods. The 01 protocol had 431 evaluable patients entered.

The scoring criteria for adequacy of the cytogenetic specimen is shown in Table 8–1. In order for a cytogenetic analysis to be adequate, chromosome spreads from 30 cells had to be counted and at least 5 metaphases karyotyped. In a number of patients insufficient material was present to constitute an adequate study, yet some information was available. If less than 30 but more than 10 metaphases were counted and less than 5 metaphases were karyotyped, the study was called "possibly adequate." If less than 10 metaphases were counted, the specimen was considered "inadequate," unless there was definite evidence of abnormalities, in which case it was accepted as "adequate." If no metaphases were examined, the study was called "unsuccessful." Successful pretreatment cytogenetic studies were completed on 208 of the 431 evaluable patients of the 01 protocol.

TABLE 8–1. SCORING CRITERIA USED IN CYTOGENETIC STUDIES

Adequate
  30 metaphases counted
  5 metaphases karyotyped (after 1972, G-banding or Q-banding analysis requested)
Possibly adequate
  Less than 30 metaphases counted
  Less than 5 metaphases karyotyped
Inadequate
  Less than 10 metaphases counted; if definite evidence of abnormalities existed, the scoring was accepted as adequate
Unsuccessful
  No metaphases could be examined

The data from each patient submitted by the participants and representative karyotypes from each case were reviewed by the Cytogenetic Committee of the PVSG, and the information from such reviews was coded for computer entry and analysis. In the initial cytogenetic report of the PVSG, the criteria for determining whether a study was normal or abnormal were based on studies of 50 subjects who were bone marrow donors and 55 patients who had cytogenetic studies performed for evaluation of anemic disorders and did not have evidence of any bone marrow malignancy. Subsequently, studies carried out by three of the PVSG reference laboratories demonstrated that there were consistent differences in the frequency of reported random hypodiploidy among the three laboratories. These differences appeared to be due to criteria for selection of metaphases for karyotype examination. For this reason, a more restrictive definition of abnormality was adopted and used for subsequent reports of the Cytogenetics Committee. The criteria used for definition of definitely or possibly abnormal are shown in Table 8–2.

TABLE 8–2. DEFINITIONS USED IN THIS STUDY

1. Definitely abnormal
   a. Two or more cells with pseudodiploidy or consistent whole or partial autosome gain in any one study, unless evidence for a constitutional defect is present
   b. Two or more cells, comprising at least 10 percent of spreads examined, which show consistent whole autosome loss, unless evidence for a constitutional defect is present
   c. Two cells with major structural abnormalities (ring, dicentrics, isochromosome, deletion, chromatid exchange, extensive fragmentation, or pulverization)
   d. Three percent or more polyploid cells
2. Possibly abnormal
   a. One cell with pseudodiploidy or hyperdiploidy
   b. Any study in which more than 20 percent of the cells show random chromosome loss
   c. One cell with structural abnormalities (ring, dicentrics, fragmentation, or pulverization)
   d. Any study with two or more cells showing breaks or fragments
   e. Ten percent, and at least two or more cells, with consistent loss of whole or partial chromosomes from the same group (unbanded)
3. Loss of the Y chromosome in two or more cells
4. Normal—none of the above

The chromosome nomenclature employed in this chapter is that of the Denver, Chicago, and Paris Conferences.[16-18] The Cytogenetics Committee reviewed the cytogenetic studies to determine how many patients had abnormal pretreatment findings. Correlation of successful pretreatment results with other clinical and laboratory parameters was carried out. Correlation of chromosomal abnormalities with death from acute leukemia or other causes was determined.

RESULTS

Pretreatment cytogenetic studies were completed successfully in only 208 of the 431 evaluable patients entered on protocol 01. There were several reasons for the low success rate. The principal reason was inexperience with bone marrow cytogenetic techniques in many of the participating institutions. An educational program was held by the PVSG which led to better compliance with the techniques. In some institutions, insufficient amounts of marrow were obtained and inadequate numbers of metaphases were available for study. Another factor was the selection of the direct bone marrow technique as the sole method.

In order to determine whether patients with unsuccessful cytogenetic studies had different clinical characteristics or bone marrow abnormalities, such as lower mitotic index or myelofibrosis, which might have been responsible for their unsuccessful studies, 223 patients with unsuccessful studies were compared with the 208 patients with successful studies. There were no differences in the following mean and range parameters: age in years, 60.8 (19 to 83) versus 60.4 (20 to 88); hematocrit, 61.7 percent (40 to 77) versus 60.3 percent (42 to 86); RBC $\times 10^6$, 7.1 (4.8 to 16.0) versus 7.1 (4.6 to 10.0); platelets $\times 10^3$, 611 (461 to 782) versus 614 (461 to 808); and WBC $\times 10^3$, 2.5 (0.18 to 4.16) versus 2.53 (1.50 to 3.85), respectively. The degree of bone marrow cellularity and reticulin fibrosis did not differ between the two groups. Furthermore, 22.5 percent of the successful studies showed marrow fibrosis.

The frequency of abnormal cytogenetic studies was determined by placing patients into three categories, as shown in Table 8–3: *definitely abnormal* (A), *possibly abnormal* (PA), and *normal* (N). The results of the 17 (8.2 percent) *definitely abnormal* patients are shown in Table 8–4. Seven (41.2 percent) of the *definitely abnormal* patients had polyploidy without evidence of structural chromosomal abnormalities. One patient had both hypodiploid and hyperdiploid cells. One patient was missing the Y chromosome in 85 percent of the metaphases in a study performed 2 years after randomization. Five of the 8 *definitely abnormal* patients were studied by nonbanded techniques, and only 3 had banding studies. Structural abnormalities were demonstrated in all 3 banded studies. A del(13)(q21) was found in 1 patient. A t(lq;15), int del(13q), and a missing chromosome 18 were found in the second case, and a 2q+ was found in the third case. Fifty-one (24.5 percent) of patients had *possibly abnormal* studies, and 140 (67.3 percent) were cytogenetically *normal*.

Long-term follow-up data were available in only 38 patients. The results of the cytogenetic analyses are shown in Tables 8–5 and 8–6. There were 16 patients with *normal* initial karyotypes who developed *definitely abnormal* status on follow-up. Their results are listed in Table 8–5. One patient had 6 percent polyploidy. Other patients had extra

TABLE 8-3. NUMBER OF PATIENTS IN EACH CATEGORY AND THE INCIDENCE OF LEUKEMIA IN 208 PATIENTS WITH SUCCESSFUL CYTOGENETIC STUDIES

	INITIAL STUDY (PERCENT)	FOLLOW-UP 2 TO 5 TIMES	LEUKEMIA
Definitely abnormal (A)	16 (7.7%)		0
Missing Y	1 (0.5%)		1
Possibly abnormal (PA)	51 (24.5%)		3
Normal (N)	140 (67.3%)		12
----------------------- A		16	6
-----------------------PA		14	1
------- PA-------------- N		8	0
TOTAL	208	38	16

TABLE 8–4. SEVENTEEN PATIENTS WITH INITIAL DEFINITELY ABNORMAL KARYOTYPES AND THEIR STATUS

PLOIDY	SPECIFIC ABNORMALITY	STATUS
Hypodiploidy		
24005	t(1q;15),del(13)(q21),−18	Died, colon cancer
27139*	−Y (85%)	Died, leukemia
29011	45,−E	Died, aspiration pneumonia
Pseudodiploidy		
6010	t(B;B)	Died, myocardial infarction
13008	46,+C,−D,−F,+cent fr.	Alive, well
14003	46,del(13)(q21)	Died, pulmonary embolus
18004	46,2q+ (25%)	Died, myelofibrosis, CHF
Hyperdiploidy		
0601	47,+C	Adenocarcinoma of colon
6007	Two cells with extra G	Alive, well
Hypo-, hyperdiploidy		
24006	Hypo (75%), hyper (18%)	Metastatic cancer
Polyploidy		
9002	10%	Alive, well
31003	15%	Died, aortic aneurysm
13004	15%	Alive, well
26028	20%	Alive, well
8029	43%	Alive, well
27167	57%	Alive, myocardial infarction
31002	100%	Alive, myocardial infarction

*First marrow sample was obtained 2 years after diagnosis.

TABLE 8–5. SIXTEEN PATIENTS WITH INITIALLY NORMAL KARYOTYPES (N) WHO LATER DEVELOPED AN ABNORMAL KARYOTYPE (A)

NUMBER	TREATMENT	STATUS	OUTCOME
08022	^{32}P	N→31 ms→A(+G,+C)→120 ms	Died, leukemia
26002	Chlor	N→14 ms→N→24 ms→leukemia→ 2 ms→del(20q)(60%)	Died, leukemia
27023	Chlor	N→3 ms→N→108 ms→del(11q),?+16(66%)→2 ms	Died, leukemia
37001	Phleb/chlor	N→31 ms→46,XY,−20,del(4q),rcp(4;20)/47, XY,+9,−20,+del(4q),rcp(4;20)(100%)→ 21 ms→A(100%)→16 ms→A(100%)→55 ms	Alive, leukemia
28009	^{32}P	N→34 ms→N→25 ms→N→4 ms→ring(50%)	Died, leukemia
32003	Chlor	NH→91 ms→leukemia→1 ms→47, XX,+C→chloroma	Died, non-Hodgkin's lymphoma
18016	^{32}P	N→27 ms→+8(15%)→30 ms→+8(90%)	Died, myelofibrosis (spent)
24002	Phleb	N→45 ms→N→21 ms→N→36 ms →N→ 24 ms−18,−21,−3C,−E,del(6q),2-4 markers (15%)	Alive, prostate cancer
26003	^{32}P	N→39 ms→N→37 ms→N→22 ms→del(13q)(84%)	Died, myelofibrosis
26007	Chlor	N→37 ms→PA→35 ms→t(1;5)(p36;q31)(90%)→13 ms→t(1;5)(95%)→1 ms→N→37 ms	Died, metastatic melanoma
26009	Chlor	N→55 ms→del(12P)(55%)→10 ms→del(12p)(95%),del(20q)(5%)→17 ms→del(12q)(100%)	Alive
26029	Phleb	N→36 ms→polyploidy(6%)	Died, CVA
27088	^{32}P	N→56 ms→N→24 ms→+marker(8%)	Alive
27120	Phleb	N→62 ms→del(2p)(10%)	Alive
27133	^{32}P	N→60 ms→N→22 ms→t(1p;1q)(67%)	Died, CHF
32007	Chlor	N→45 ms→N→37 ms→t(8;12)(q12;q24),18p+	Died, subdural hemorrhage

Abbreviations: N = normal; PA = possible abnormal; Chlor = chlorambucil; Phleb = phlebotomy; ms = months.

TABLE 8-6. FOURTEEN PATIENTS WITH INITIALLY NORMAL KARYOTYPES WHO DEVELOPED POSSIBLY ABNORMAL KARYOTYPES (PA)

NUMBER	TREATMENT	STATUS
35003	Chlor	N→12 ms→<45 chromosomes (50%)→13 ms (died, leukemia)
08019	Chlor	N→45 ms→N→40 ms→<45 chromosomes (30%)
20011	Chlor	N→25 ms→N→16 ms→<45 chromosomes (20%)
29010	Chlor	N→70 ms→N→49 ms→<45 chromosomes (28%)
29413	Chlor	N→63 ms→1 cell with 47 chromosomes
27117	^{32}P	N→26 ms→<45 chromosomes (60%)
28013	^{32}P	N→28 ms→<45 chromosomes (40%)
29008	^{32}P	N→33 ms→<45 chromosomes (25%)
11005	Phleb	N→81 ms→<45 chromosomes (32%)
03007	Phleb	N→24 ms→<45 chromosomes (20%)
23409	Phleb	N→33 ms→N→37 ms→<45 chromosomes (20%)
27021	Phleb	N→32 ms→1 cell with del(Gq)
08003	Phleb	N→12 ms→1 cell with +C,−D,+fragment
28003	Phleb	N→27 ms→N→39 ms→1 cell with +A

chromosomes; one had extra chromosomes in the G and C groups, one had a marker of unknown origin, and the third had an extra C-sized chromosome. One patient had a ring chromosome in 50 percent of the cells; the origin of the ring could not be determined because no banding studies were performed. One patient had an extra chromosome 8, one had multiple chromosome abnormalities[−18, −21, del(6q), −3C, −E, and 2−4 markers], one had del(13q), one had t(l;5)(p36;q31), one had del(12p), one had del(20q), one had del(11q) and ?+16, one had del(2p), one had t(8;12)(q12;q24) and 18p+, and one had 47,XY,+9,−20,+del(4q),rcp(4;20)/46,XY, del(4q),rcp(4;20).

Fourteen patients with an initially *normal* karyotype developed *possibly abnormal* karyotypes on follow-up (see Table 8–6). Ten of them had more than 20 percent hypodiploid cells as the only abnormality. Three other patients all had an extra chromosome, and one patient had deletion of a G-group chromosome; none of these patients had banded chromosome studies.

Eight patients who were initially *normal* progressed to *possibly abnormal* status but later returned to *normal*, suggesting that the *possibly abnormal* status was transient or due to artifact. Treatment of these 8 patients consisted of ^{32}P (4 patients), chlorambucil (3 patients), and phlebotomy (1 patient).

Study of the correlation of cytogenetic abnormalities and the development of acute leukemia were carried out. Of the 17 patients with initial *definitely abnormal* karyotypes, only 1 progressed to acute leukemia. This patient had a missing Y chromosome in 85 percent of the marrow cells. The studies do not permit us to determine whether the Y loss in this case was age-related or leukemia-related.[19,20]

Of the 16 patients who initially had *normal* karyotypes and later developed definite numerical or structural chromosome abnormalities (Table 8–5), 5 developed acute leukemia and 1 developed leukemia and chloroma and eventually died of non-Hodgkin's malignant lymphoma.

One patient who had a *normal* initial karyotype and later developed a *possibly abnormal* karyotype with 50 percent of the cells showing hypodiploidy of less than 45 chromosomes died of acute leukemia (Table 8–6). None of the 8 patients who developed transient possible abnormalities developed leukemia.

Comparison of the *definitely abnormal* cytogenetic changes in patients who developed leukemia and those who died of other causes without leukemia are shown in Tables 8–7 and 8–8. Thirty patients developed acute leukemia; 16 were among the 208 patients with cytogenetic studies, and 14 had no cytogenetic studies. Only 13 of the 16 patients with leukemia had *definitely abnormal* chromosomes (Table 8–7). Ten patients with *definitely abnormal* cytogenetic studies died of causes other than leukemia (Table 8–8). Chromosome 20 was involved in 3 (possibly 4) of the leukemic group and in only 1 of the nonleukemic group. Abnormalities of chromosomes 8, 9, 21, and 22 were seen in the leukemic group, whereas 3 patients in the nonleukemic group had translocations involving chromosome 1. The status and out-

TABLE 8-7. DEFINITELY ABNORMAL PATIENTS WHO DIED WITH LEUKEMIA (ANLL)

PATIENT*	%A	CYTOGENETIC FINDINGS
PVSG		
26015	85%	48–50,XX,+8,+marker,+acro
26002	85%	del(20q)
27005	ND	del(20q)
27007	60%	48,XX,+9,+21
27023	55%	46,XY,del(11q)/47,XY,+16,del(11q)
27139	85%	45,X,−Y
28005	35%	del(20q)
28009	50%	ring
12801	ND	+2,−C,−18
32003	50%	47,XX,+C (leukemia→chloroma→non-Hodgkin's lymphoma)
35003	50%	Hypodiploid
08022	5%	+C,+22
37001	100%	47,XY,+9,−20,+del(4q),rcp(4;20)/46,XY,−20,+del(4q),rcp(4;20)
Zech et al.		
81F	18%	+9, multiple aberrations including a ring chromosome
Rege-Cambrin et al		
53/M	100%	47,XX,+8 (M2)
41/F	100%	47,XX,+9
73/F	100%	46,XX,del(7)(p14) (M5b)
42/F	100%	48,XX,+8,+mar
57/F	100%	46,XX,del(11)(q14),del(12q),8p+, (M4)
58/M	100%	43,XY,−5,−7,−11,−17,+mar/44, XX, del(5) (q12q23), −12, −13, −17, +M
Berger		
62/M	70%	47,XY,+9
67/M	96%	54,X,−Y
59/M	56%	46,XY,del(20q)/45,XY,−20,del(20q)
Testa et al.		
Case 32	100%	48,XX, −5,−5,+8,−17,−19,+21, del(5)(q13q31)?, +der(11), t(11;?)(p14;?), +2mar, +0-2 DMs
Case 33	100%	47,XY, −13, del(3)(q12?), del(5)(q12?), der(6), t(6;?)(q11?;?), +markers/51-52,XY, −13,−17,+21, del(5)(q12?), +markers.
Case 34	100%	47-49,XY, −7,−13,−16,−22, del(5)(q15?), i(8q), +2-13markers/48,XY, −7,−8,−13,−16,−22, del(5)(q15?), +dic(9), +4-7 markers/48,XY, −5,−7,−8,−13,−16,−22, del(q15?), dic(9), +6-9markers

*Patients from the PVSG and other published studies (listed by reference).

come of 208 patients in the randomized treatment programs are listed in Table 8–9.

Chromosome 13 deletion was found in 2 patients in the nonleukemic group but was not observed in the leukemic group. None of the leukemic patients had polyploidy as the sole abnormality. One patient in the leukemic group had 50 percent hypodiploid cells; the possibility of a structural or definite abnormality could not be ruled out because banding studies had not been done.

DISCUSSION

Adamson et al.[1] in 1976 proposed that PV was a clonal disorder as a result of studies of two black females with double heterozygosity for X-linked glucose-6-phosphate dehydrogenase loci. Each patient exhibited a single enzyme in her hemic cells. Additional evidence of the clonality of the disease has been derived from cytogenetic studies. Numerous reports of clonal chromosomal abnormalities in patients with PV have been published since 1966.[2–10] Studies of Ruutu et al.[19] helped to demonstrate that the disorder involves a pluripotent stem cell; they found the same clonal abnormality in erythroid and granulocytic-monocytic colonies grown from the marrow of three patients with PV. Price et al.[20] utilized FISH/APAAP (combined fluorescent in situ hybridization for trisomy 8 and alkaline phosphatase–antialkaline phosphatase immunostaining of cells) to determine that there was selective involvement of

TABLE 8–8. DEFINITELY ABNORMAL PATIENTS WHO DIED OF CAUSES OTHER THAN LEUKEMIA

PATIENT*	%A†	CYTOGENETIC FINDINGS	CAUSE OF DEATH
PVSG			
14003	100%	del(13)(q21)	Herpes zoster
08004	25%	2q+	CHF, myelofibrosis
06010	96%	t(B;B)	Myocardial infarction
24006	96%	Hypo- and hyperdiploidy	Metastatic adenocarcinoma, colon
24005	ND	t(1;15)	Metastatic adenocarcinoma, colon
29011	ND	45, − E	Aspiration pneumonia
30012	100%	polyploidy	Myocardial infarction
26007	ND	t(1;5)(p36;q31)	Disseminated melanoma
26003	ND	del(13q)	Spent phase of PV
27002	ND	t(1;3), + del(20q)	Heart failure, thrombosis
Berger			
73/F	17%	47,XX,+21	Esophageal carcinoma
72/M	33%	46,XY,del(16q)	Peritonitis
72/F	13%	46,XX,del(3p)	Heart failure
48/F	22%	46,t(13q;15q)/46, + 12, − 21	Myeloid metaplasia
78/M	6%	46, − B, + marker	Parathyroid carcinoma

* Patients from the PVSG and other published studies (listed by reference).
† Percent abnormal; ND, not done.

granulocytes and nucleated red cells in two cases of PV.

The chromosome abnormalities frequently seen in PV include trisomy 8, trisomy 9, and deletion of the long arm of chromosome 20 [del(20)(q12)] (see Tables 8–7 and 8–8). Mitelman[21] reviewed 86 cases of PV from different geographic locations: Illinois (USA), Israel (Asia), and Sweden, West Germany, and France (Europe). The incidence of trisomy 8 was similar in all five locations, whereas the incidence of trisomy 9 was quite variable: 47 percent in Sweden, 27 percent in Illinois and Israel, and very low percentages in West Germany and France. The incidence of the del(20q) marker showed similar variability: 32, 27, 20, 0, and 0 percent in Sweden, Illinois, France, West Germany, and Israel, respectively.

A review of chromosomal abnormalities in initial samples in the published literature[2, 4, 5, 8, 10, 22–25] revealed an incidence of 12.2 percent (51 of 417 patients) in untreated PV patients, 40 percent (126 of 287 patients) in treated patients, and 92.1 percent (35 of 38 patients) in treated patients who developed acute leukemia (Tables 8–10 and 8–11). It is apparent that clonal cytogenetic abnormalities do occur in untreated PV, but the incidence is quite low.

TABLE 8–9. STATUS AND OUTCOME OF 208 PATIENTS IN RANDOMIZED TREATMENTS

TREATMENT (TOTAL NO.)	INITIAL STATUS	TOTAL	PROGRESSION OF DISEASE TO:				
			Leukemia	Cancer	Thrombosis	Death	Well
Phlebotomy	A	4	0	0	2	0	2
(66)	PA	12	0	0	5	5	2
	N	50	1	3	16	13	17
Chlorambucil	A	6	0	1	2	2	1
(73)	PA	18	2	1	3	4	8
	N	49	9	6	11	23	0
^{32}P (69)	A	6	0	1	3	2	0
	PA	21	1	3	9	7	1
	N	41	2	8	10	12	9
Missing Y		1	1	0	0	0	0
TOTAL		208	16	23	61	68	40

TABLE 8-10. CYTOGENETIC RESULTS OF PUBLISHED DATA IN 417 UNTREATED PV PATIENTS

STUDY*	TOTAL NO. OF PATIENTS	NO. OF PATIENTS WITH ANEUPLOIDY	ABNORMAL CHROMOSOME†
Lawler et al.	33	5	+1 or +2 C (4X), −Y (1X)
Visfeldt et al.	8	0	
Shiraishi et al.	3	0	
Zech et al.	4	2	+9(1X), −Y,20q−(1X)
Westin et al.	50	7	+8, +9(3X), +9(1X),del (1)(p21)(1X) t(1;9) (q22;q13)(1X), del(20)(q11)(1X)
Testa et al.	13	4	+8, +9(1X), −Y(1X), −Y or −G(1X), t(12;17) (q13;p11),t(Y;1)(q12;q21), +1(1X)
Berger	30‡	7	+8(1X), del(11q)(2X), +9(2X) del(3)(p11p14) (1X), t(4;4)(p16;q21)(1X)
Rege-Chambrin et al.	68	9	del(20q)(1X), del(13q)(2X), +8 and/or +9(6X) t(7;19)(q21;q12)
PVSG	208	17	+G(1X), t(8;8)(1X), +C, −D, −F(1X), del(13) (q21)(1X), t(1q;15), del(13q), −18(1X), −Y(1x), 2q+(1X) −E(1X), Polyploidy (10-100% 7X), Hypo-Hyper(1X)
TOTAL	417	5(12.2%)	

* Listed by reference.
† In parentheses, the number of times a particular abnormality was observed.
‡ 22 patients treated by phlebotomy.

The current study revealed a definite chromosome abnormality in the initial bone marrow sample in 17 (8.2 percent) of the 208 patients with adequate studies. Detailed serial follow-up studies of 38 patients showed that 16 (42 percent) of them developed an abnormality after treatment with ^{32}P, chlorambucil, or phlebotomy. In this group, 6 cases of leukemia and 1 case of malignant lymphoma developed; 6 had *definitely abnormal* chromosome status and 1 was *possibly abnormal*.

Swolin et al.[26] have reported 12 patients with PV who have complete or partial trisomy 1q. Eight of their 12 patients had developed leukemia or a dysmyelopoietic syndrome. Only 3 of their patients had the trisomy 1q at the time of diagnosis; the remainder developed later in the course. Swolin et al.[27] subsequently reported long-term follow-up of 64 untreated PV patients (31 of whom are included in the PVSG protocol 01). Thirty-three patients were cytogenetically normal on initial study and remained normal. Twenty patients developed cytogenetic abnormalities after an initial normal study, and 11 patients had abnormal initial studies. Of the 11 patients with initial abnormal studies, trisomies of both chromosome 8 and 9 were seen in 3 patients and trisomy 1q in another 3 patients, 2 of whom

were trisomic for 9p as well. Thus complete or partial trisomy of chromosome 9 (9p) was the most common abnormality.

In the current PVSG study, chromosome 1 translocations were found in 3 patients, none of whom died of leukemia. One patient with t(−1;15) died of metastatic carcinoma of the colon, one with t(1;5) died of disseminated melanoma, and one with t(1;3) and +20q− died of heart failure and thrombosis. It is possible that the chromosome 1 abnormalities observed in the 2 patients with metastatic carcinoma may represent metastatic malignant cells, since chromosome 1 involvement in solid tumors is common.

Deletion of the long arm of chromosome 20 has been reported in a wide spectrum of hematologic malignancies. It is also seen commonly in patients with PV; the overall incidence in published cases is shown in Table 8−11. This marker accounted for 5 percent of aneuploidy seen in untreated patients and increased to 28 percent of aneuploidy in treated patients. In one study of PV, Millard et al.[28] stated that the deleted F chromosome probably arose during the course of the disease. In the PVSG series, no cases of del(20q) were seen on initial studies of untreated patients, but of the 13 patients with leukemia, 3 (possibly 4) patients had the deletion; 1 patient in the nonleukemic treated group

TABLE 8–11. CYTOGENETIC RESULTS OF PUBLISHED DATA IN 287 TREATED PV PATIENTS

STUDY*	NO. OF PATIENTS	A	DEL(20Q)	LEUKEMIA	CHROMOSOME ABNORMALITIES†
Lawler et al.	46	16	7	9/9	No banding available
Visfeldt et al.	42	21	8	5/8	No banding available
Shiraishi et al.	9	5	3	0/0	−Y(1X), del(11)(q11)(1X), del(13q)(1X)
Zech et al.	6	5	2	1/1	+9(3X),+8(1X),−Y(1X)
Testa et al.	21	16(?)	4(?)	3/3	+8(3X), i(8q)(1X), +9(2X), +8,+9(1X) −Y(2X), del(5q)(4X), 1X:del(7)(q22, del(11)(q21?), t(2;11) (p13;q21), t(1;15) (p1?;q1?), del(16)(q12), del(3)(q12?), t(6;?)(q11?;?), dic 9, −5, −7, 8, −9, −13, −15, −16, −17, −19, +12
Berger	105	28	5	3/3	+8(4X), +9(2X), del(1p)(3X), −Y(2X), 17p+(2X), del(11q)(2X), 1X: +12, +21, −7, 1p+, t(1;1)(q13;p36), t(4;4)(p16;q21), t(13q15q), del(16q), del(3p), del(3)(p11p14), del(10q)
Rege-Cambrin et al.	20	19	5	7/7	del(13)(q13q13 or q13q21)(5X), +8(X2), +9(3X), +8, +9(3X), 18p+(2X),1X: del(5)(q14q32), +21, −18, del(5)(q13q32), inv(12) (p13q23), del(12) (p13q23), del(12) (q14q21), t(7;19) (q21;q12), del(7) (q31qter), ins(4;11) (q26q35;q14), del(11)(q22), del(11p), t(16;18) (q11;q12)
PVSG	38	16	2	7/7	1X: +8, +9, +16, −18, −20, −21, del(2p), del(6q), del(12p), del(13q) t(1p;1q), t(8;12) (q12;q24), 18p+, del(4q), t(1;5) (p36;q31), del(11q), rcp(4;20),ring
TOTAL	287	126(40%)	35(28%)	35/38(92.1%)	

*Listed by reference.
†In parentheses, the number of times a particular abnormality was observed.

also had the deletion. In one published PV series,[22] this marker was the most frequent sole chromosomal abnormality (6 of 108 patients), but it was present in only 1 initial untreated bone marrow sample.

Trisomies of chromosomes 8 and 9 are among the most common abnormalities observed in PV, especially in initial untreated bone marrows; 3 cases of +8,+9 or combined were found in the PVSG study, and 6 cases were found among 108 patients studied by Rege-Cambrin et al.[22]

One patient, whose initial cytogenetic study (2 years after randomization) showed a missing Y chromosome in 85 percent of his bone marrow cells, developed leukemia with no additional abnormalities seen. In this par-

ticular patient, it is impossible to discern whether the Y loss was disease-related or age-related.[29,30] In this combined series, 4 patients (possibly 5) had a missing Y chromosome in the pretreatment marrow and 6 patients had a missing Y in the treated marrow. Although loss of the Y chromosome is age-related, it also appears to have a specific association with acute nonlymphocytic leukemia, particularly the FAB-M2 subtype associated with a t(8;21) chromosome abnormality[31] and with chronic granulocytic leukemia.[32] One patient with a normal initial study developed a ring chromosome in 50 percent of metaphases and leukemia after 53 months of ^{32}P treatment. The development of a chromosome abnormality during the course of the disease appears to carry a higher risk of transformation to acute leukemia or to a dysmyelopoietic syndrome.

In 1979, Van Den Berghe et al.[33] reported a characteristic interstitial deletion, del(5)(q14q32), that occurred late in the disease course in 3 patients with PV accompanying the transformation to myelofibrosis and the appearance of a preleukemic disorder. Another nonrandom abnormality seen in a variety of hematologic disorders is del(13)(q21). Two patients in the present series had this deletion; one patient, who died of a pulmonary embolus, had it in the initial marrow, and the other patient, who was initially normal, was found to have the del(13q) in 84 percent of marrow cells at the 98-month follow-up and died of myelofibrosis.

Miller et al.[34] have compared the patterns of karyotypic abnormalities in idiopathic myelofibrosis (MF) and in postpolycythemic myelofibrosis (PPMF). In MF, the abnormalities appeared to be unrelated to therapy, except possibly for an association with partial or complete loss of chromosomes 5 and 7. Trisomy 8 was the only chromosomal abnormality that was more common in MF than in PPMF. Other abnormalities were more common in PPMF, particularly del(20q), loss of chromosome 7, del(7q), trisomy 9, and, to a lesser extent, trisomy 1q and del(5q). The author concluded that cytogenetic studies are not useful in distinguishing between MF and PPMF and that karyotypic evolution has serious prognostic implications in the leukemic transformation of PPMF.

Diez-Martin et al.[35] reported a series of 104 patients with various stages of PV studied at the Mayo Clinic. Fifty-four had PV, 28 had post-PV with myeloid metaplasia (PPVMM), 12 had PV with myelofibrosis, and 10 had leukemia-myelodysplasia syndrome. Cytogenetic studies were successful in 86 (83 percent) of the 104 patients, and abnormalities were found in 37 (43 percent). Of untreated patients studied at diagnosis, 4 of 28 (14 percent) had an abnormal clone, whereas 78 percent of PPVMM patients and 100 percent of leukemia-myelodysplasia patients had abnormal clones. This study suggested that patients with chromosomal abnormalities at the time of diagnosis had a poorer survival than patients with only normal metaphases.

In reviewing the published cytogenetic data[5, 8, 10, 22, 23] on 26 PV patients who died with leukemia (ANLL) (see Table 8–7), del(20q), +8, +9, and del(5q) were found to be the most frequent abnormalities, but no chromosomal markers were found to be specific to this group of patients.

No identifiable pattern of chromosomal abnormalities was seen in the PV patients who died of causes other than leukemia (see Table 8–8). Chromosome segment 13q abnormalities were seen in 3 instances, but no specific breakpoint was observed. More such cases would have to be studied to determine whether 13q abnormalities are of any significance in this disease. The presence of a definite chromosome abnormality at the time of initial study does not appear to play any important role in progression to leukemia, cancer, thrombosis, or death (see Tables 8–10 and 8–11).

CONCLUSIONS

The presence of chromosome abnormalities in pretreatment bone marrow of patients with PV does not correlate with a subsequent diagnosis of leukemia or cancer, nor does it predict survival. Studies have shown, however, that the incidence of chromosomal abnormalities does increase after treatment (12.2 percent in initial untreated samples versus 40 percent in treated patients) and that an even higher percentage (92.1 percent) is seen in patients who develop leukemia. Polyploidy in the bone marrow has no significance and should not be regarded as an abnormality in PV patients. Random hypodiploidy also has no prognostic significance.

The PVSG data confirm the reports of others that numerical gain of chromosomes 8, 9, or both and a structural abnormality of chromosome 20 are common in PV. In addition, rearrangements of chromosome 5, 5q–, rearrangement of chromosome 12, and trisomy 1 are common in treated PV patients or in the transitional or leukemic phases of the disease. Serial follow-up of 38 previously karyotypically normal patients suggests that the development of a definite abnormality may be of prognostic significance for progression to leukemia or survival.

The cytogenetic data obtained by the PVSG in the 01 protocol suffered from poor compliance (approximately half the patients were actually studied prior to therapy), and many of the chromosome studies were of poor quality and nonbanded. A prospective study in which more complete data were obtained and modern banding methods were used might provide us with a more precise relationship between cytogenetic abnormalities and the clinical features of the disease and the emergence of acute leukemia.

REFERENCES

1. Adamson JW, Fialkow PJ, Murphy S, et al: Polycythemia vera: Stem cell and probable clonal origin of the disease. N Engl J Med 295:913–916, 1976
2. Shiraishi Y, Hayata I, Sakurai M, et al: Chromosomes and causation of human cancer and leukemia: XII. Banding analysis of abnormal chromosomes in polycythemia vera. Cancer 36: 199–202, 1975
3. Wurster-Hill D, Whang-Peng J, McIntyre OR, et al: Cytogenetic studies in polycythemia vera. Semin Hematol 13:13–32, 1976
4. Westin J, Wahlstrom J, Swolin B: Chromosome studies in untreated polycythemia vera. Scand J Haematol 17:183–196, 1976
5. Zech L, Gahrton C, Killander D, et al: Specific chromosomal aberrations in polycythemia vera. Blood 48:687–696, 1976
6. Nowell PC, Finan JB: Chromosome studies in preleukemic states: IV. Myeloproliferative versus cytopenic disorders. Cancer 42:2254–2261, 1978
7. Lawler SD: Cytogenetic studies in Philadelphia chromosome–negative myeloproliferative disorders, particularly polycythemia rubra vera. Clin Haematol 9:159–174, 1980
8. Testa JR, Kanofsky JR, Rowley JD, et al: Karyotypic patterns and their clinical significance in polycythemia vera. Am J Hematol 11:29–45, 1981
9. Wurster-Hill DH, McIntyre OR: Chromosome studies in polycythemia vera. Virchows Arch [B] 29:39–44, 1978
10. Berger R, Bernheim A, Le Coniat M, et al: Chromosome studies in polycythemia vera patients. Cancer Genet Cytogenet 3:217–223, 1984
11. Croce CM, Isobe M, Palumbo A, et al: Gene for alpha-chain of human T-cell receptor: Location on chromosome 14 region involved in T-cell neoplasms. Science 227:1044–1047, 1985
12. Davis MP, Dewald GW, Pierre RV, et al: Hematologic manifestations associated with deletions of the long arm of chromosome 20. Cancer Genet Cytogenet 12:63–71, 1984
13. Yunis JJ: The chromosomal basis of human neoplasia. Science 221:227–236, 1983
14. Tjio JH, Whang J: Chromosome preparations of bone marrow cells without prior in vitro culture or in vivo colchicine administration. Stain Technol 37:17–20, 1962
15. Knuutilas S, Vuopio P, Elonen E: Culture of bone marrow reveals more cells with chromosome abnormalities than the direct method in patients with hematologic disorders. Blood 58:369–375, 1981
16. Denver Conference: A proposed standard system of nomenclature of human mitotic chromosomes. Lancet 1:1063–1065, 1960
17. Bergsma D (ed): Chicago Conference: Standardization in human cytogenetics. New York, The National Foundation–March of Dimes, 1966
18. Paris Conference (1971): Standardization in human cytogenetics. Birth Defects 8:7, 1972
19. Ruutu T, Partanen SL, Knuutila S: Clonal karyotype abnormalities in erythroid and granulocyte-monocyte precursors in polycythemia vera and myelofibrosis. Scand J Haematol 31:253–256, 1983
20. Price CM, Kanfer EJ, Colman SM, et al: Simultaneous genotypic and immunophenotypic analysis of interphase cells using dual-color fluorescence: A demonstration of lineage involvement in polycythemia vera. Blood 80:1033–1038, 1993
21. Mitelman F: Geographic heterogeneity of chromosome aberrations in hematologic disorders. Cancer Genet Cytogenet 20:203–208, 1986
22. Whang-Peng J, McIntyre OR, Pierre RV, et al: Cytogenetic findings in the polycythemia vera: Long-term follow-up in patients randomized to treatment by the Polycythemia Vera Study Group. In Zanjani ED, Tavassoli M, Ascensao JL (eds): Regulation of Erythropoiesis. New York: Pergamon Press, 1987
23. Rege-Cambrin G, Mecucci C, Tricot G, et al: A chromosomal profile of polycythemia vera. Cancer Genet Cytogenet 25:233–245, 1987
24. Lawler SD, Millard RE, Kay HEW: Further cytogenetical investigations in polycythemia vera. Eur J Cancer 6:223–233, 1970
25. Visfeldt J: Primary polycythemia: 2. Types of chromosome aberration in 21 clones found in bone marrow samples from 50 patients. Acta Pathol Microbiol Scand [A] 79:513–523, 1971
26. Swolin B, Weinfeld A, Westin J: Trisomy 1q in polycythemia vera and its relationship to disease transition. Am J Hematol 22:155–167, 1986
27. Swolin B, Weinfeld A, Westin J: A prospective long-term cytogenetic study in polycythemia vera in relation to treatment and clinical course. Blood 72:386–395, 1988
28. Millard RE, Lawler SD, Kay HEW, et al: Further observations on patients with a chromosomal abnormality associated with polycythemia vera. Br J Haematol 14:363–374, 1968
29. Sandberg AA, Sakurai M: The missing Y chromosome and human leukemia. Lancet 1:375, 1973
30. Pierre RV, Hoagland HC: 45,X cell lines in adult men: Loss of Y chromosome, a normal aging phenomenon? Mayo Clin Proc 46:52–55, 1971
31. Fourth International Workshop on Chromosomes in Leukemia, 1982: Translocation (8;21) (q22;q22) in acute nonlymphocytic leukemia. Cancer Genet Cytogenet 11:284–287, 1984
32. Sandberg A: The Y chromosome in human neoplasia. In Sandberg AA (ed): The Y Chromosome, Part B: Clinical Aspects of Y Chromosome Abnormalities. New York, Alan R. Liss, 1985, pp 377–393
33. Van Den Berghe H, Broeckaert-van Orshoven A, Louwagie A, et al: Transformation of polycythemia vera to myelofibrosis and late appearance of a 5q chromosome anomaly. Cancer Genet Cytogenet 1:157–167, 1979
34. Miller JB, Testa JR, Lindgren V, et al: The pattern and clinical significance of karyotypic abnormalities in patients with idiopathic and postpolycythemic myelofibrosis. Cancer 55:582–591, 1985
35. Diez-Martin JL, Graham DL, Petitt RM, Dewald GW. Chromosome studies in 104 patients with polycythemia vera. Mayo Clinic Proc 66:287–299, 1991

9

Megakaryocytes, Platelets, and Coagulation in the Myeloproliferative Diseases

SCOTT MURPHY

Under the umbrella of the myeloproliferative diseases (MPDs), four specific entities are generally recognized: polycythemia vera (PV), essential thrombocythemia (ET), chronic myelocytic leukemia (CML), and the agnogenic myeloid metaplasia-myelofibrosis syndrome.[1] European workers have used the term *chronic megakaryocytic-granulocytic myelosis* to refer to the stage of the agnogenic myeloid metaplasia-myelofibrosis syndrome when the bone marrow is hyperplastic.[2] The Polycythemia Vera Study Group (PVSG) has used the term *undifferentiated myeloproliferative disease* in situations where classification is difficult and marrow fibrosis is not prominent.[1] These difficulties in terminology cannot be resolved at present, but in this chapter I will use the term *agnogenic myeloid metaplasia-myelofibrosis* (AMM-MF) to refer to this heterogeneous group that undoubtedly overlaps with the better-defined entities PV and ET. *Chronic myelocytic leukemia* (CML) refers to the disease in which the Philadelphia chromosome is present in the bone marrow karyotype and/or the *bcr.abl* gene rearrangement can be demonstrated in studies of marrow DNA or RNA.[3,4] In the past, hematologists have identified some patients as having Philadelphia chromosome–negative CML, but recent work has suggested that many are better classified with the dysmyelopoietic syndromes[5,6] unless the *bcr.abl* rearrangement is present.

In all these patients with MPDs, hemorrhage and thrombosis are major contributors to morbidity and mortality. There is no doubt that these clinical manifestations result from the interplay of a variety of pathologic forces. This chapter will review our knowledge of megakaryocytes, platelets, and coagulation in MPD. By necessity, in some circumstances this will involve a rather encyclopedic listing of abnormalities that have been described. However, I will attempt to place these abnormalities in perspective.

BONE MARROW AND MEGAKARYOCYTES

It is not possible to discuss megakaryocytes without discussing other features of the bone marrow. It must be stressed that the distribution of the bone marrow within the skeleton is abnormal in MPD. In normal adults, the marrow is confined to the central skeleton, and the cavities of the long bones are fatty. In MPD, there is extension of marrow into the long bones. This is most striking in AMM-MF, where the central marrow may be fibrotic while the long bones are cellular.[7] This is stressed because our picture of the bone marrow and, therefore, of megakaryocytes in MPD is derived predominantly from biopsy of the posterior iliac crest, which may or may not be representative of the total marrow organ.

102

With these reservations, the bone marrow is typically hypercellular in patients with PV[8] and ET,[9] while the iliac crest marrow may be hypercellular or show progressive hypocellularity due to replacement with fibrosis and osteosclerosis in AMM-MF.[10] In cellular areas, the number of megakaryocytes is increased. In one large series,[2] the respective increases in CML, PV, and AMM-MF were 1.5-fold, 2.5-fold, and 5.1-fold. In CML, dwarf or micro megakaryocytes predominate, whereas in PV, ET, and AMM-MF, giant forms are frequently seen.[2, 10–12] This information is presented graphically in Fig. 9–1. Furthermore, in normal marrow and in CML, megakaryocytes are distributed diffusely and are separated from each other by other cells. On the other hand, in ET and PV, clusters characterized by five or more megakaryocytes in proximity are common.[13, 14] In AMM-MF, these clusters may coalesce to form large sheets. The morphology of megakaryocytes in such sheets may be quite abnormal and atypical. Finally, Rabellino et al.[15] have used immunofluorescence of platelet protein markers to identify megakaryocytes in MPD marrow which are not recognizable using standard morphologic techniques. Thus standard microscopy may underestimate the degree of pathology. These abnormalities of distribution and morphology undoubtedly reflect cellular pathology, which would be expected to be reflected in abnormalities of the platelets derived from them.

We presume that these morphologic abnormalities in the bone marrow reflect the fact that the MPDs arise from the proliferation of a single, abnormal, pluripotent hematopoietic stem cell that gains a growth advantage over its normal counterparts. Analysis of glucose-6-phosphate dehydrogenase (G-6-PD) isoenzyme types in selected black females with ET, PV, CML, and AMM-MF have demonstrated that circulating erythrocytes, granulocytes, and platelets all arise from a single cell.[16–18] This experimental approach is based on the fact that one X chromosome in each female somatic cell is randomly inactivated early in embryogenesis. All the progeny of that cell have the same single active X chromosome. Since the locus for G-6-PD is on the X chromosome, a female heterozygous for the usual Gd^B gene and the Gd^A variant will have a population of cells synthesizing type B and a population of cells synthesizing type A. When females with MPD and heterozygous for G-6-PD were examined, erythrocytes, granulocytes, and platelets contained only one enzyme type, confirming the unicellular origin of the disease. Involvement of all three cell lines suggested that the cell of origin was an abnormal hematopoietic stem cell. Therefore, the megakaryocytes described above are all the progeny of an abnormal hematopoietic stem cell, and we assume that the abnormalities that they display reflect this origin. More recent studies with molecular techniques have essentially confirmed these findings, although occasional patients have been described with lack of involvement of one or more cell lines.[19]

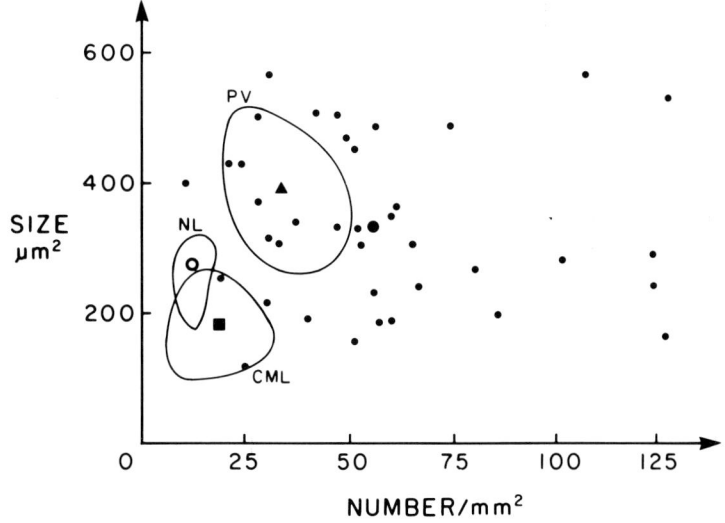

FIGURE 9–1. *Megakaryocyte size and number in MPD. Mean size and number per surface area of marrow biopsy are shown for a series of patients. The regions labeled NL, PV, and CML refer to data for normal individuals, PV patients, and CML patients (individual patient points not shown). The small solid circles represent individual AMM-MF patients. The large symbols represent means for normal individuals, ○; CML, ■; PV, ▲; and AMM-MF, ●. (Redrawn with permission from Thiele J, et al: Scand J Haematol 31:329–341, 1983.)*

In ET (always, by definition) and in PV (commonly), the platelet count is elevated at the time of diagnosis. Many studies have shown that this reflects an increase in the rate of platelet production, sometimes to as much as 15 times the normal rate.[11, 12, 20] In PV, the increased rate of erythrocyte production occurs despite the fact that circulating erythropoietin levels are unmeasurably low.[21] Knowledge of the control mechanisms for platelet production is still evolving but has not reached the state we have for control of red cell production. However, it has been proposed that megakaryocyte colony-stimulating activity (M-CSA) may play an analogous role to erythropoietin.[22] Gewirtz et al.[22] have shown that serum M-CSA levels are not elevated in patients with thrombocytosis and MPD. This would appear to be analogous to the low levels of erythropoietin in PV.

Furthermore, in PV, erythroid colonies grow in in vitro marrow cultures without the addition of exogenous erythropoietin (so-called endogenous colonies). Erythropoietin is required for growth from normal marrow. When such studies were performed in females with PV who were heterozygous for G-6-PD, endogenous colonies were all of one enzyme type.[23] However, addition of exogenous erythropoietin resulted in the formation of colonies of the other enzyme type, showing that residual normal erythroid stem cells were present but not proliferating and differentiating. At any concentration of erythropoietin, the number of colonies formed from PV marrow was greater than the number formed from normal marrow. Several groups have presented data suggesting that similar events are occurring for megakaryocytes.[22, 24, 25] Gewirtz et al.[22] grew megakaryocyte colonies from peripheral blood in plasma clots and showed that the number of colonies formed by MPD patients with thrombocytosis was increased 19-fold relative to normal individuals without the addition of M-CSA. Furthermore, there was a 3-fold increase in the number of megakaryocytes per colony in MPD. Conversely, in reactive thrombocytosis, the number and size of megakaryocyte colonies formed with or without M-CSA was identical to normal. Thus, in MPD with erythrocytosis and thrombocytosis, there is an increase in the number of both red cell and platelet precursors which will proliferate at low or absent levels of stimulatory hormone.

These studies strongly suggest that in MPD, red cell precursors and megakaryocytes proliferate either autonomously or in response to extremely low levels of poietic hormones. For megakaryocytes, this concept is supported by measurements of cell volume. As mentioned earlier, the mean volume of individual megakaryocytes is increased approximately 1.5 to 2 times normal in both ET and PV.[11, 12, 26] On the other hand, in experimental animals hypertransfused with platelets, there is a reduction in megakaryocyte volume associated with the increased number of platelets in the circulation.[27] The maintenance of increased megakaryocytic volume in the presence of thrombocytosis in MPD is consistent with relative autonomy from physiologic control mechanisms. Megakaryocytes are polyploid cells, and there is evidence that there is a correlation between megakaryocyte size and DNA content. Normal megakaryocytes display a 16n ploidy class in two-thirds of the population. In PV and ET there is a characteristic shift of the megakaryocyte ploidy distribution to higher levels, whereas in CML there is a shift to lower levels.[28–32] This provides a correlation with the observations of megakaryocyte size.

THROMBOKINETICS

Several studies have indicated that platelet survival time in PV and ET is normal or nearly normal.[11, 12, 20] One can calculate the rate of platelet production from such survival measurements. Furthermore, there are techniques for estimating the total-body megakaryocyte volume. When these two measurements have been compared in PV and ET, the rate of platelet production and total-body megakaryocyte volume increased in parallel, suggesting that platelet production is effective, with an appropriate number of platelets being released into circulation for the amount of megakaryocyte cytoplasm present.[33] However, erythrokinetic studies using radioactive iron have provided clear demonstration that red cell production becomes increasingly ineffective in the AMM-MF syndrome.[34] One can view the bone marrow abnormalities seen in AMM-MF and in the similar syndrome that arises as a late event in the course of PV as reflecting advancing degeneration of the abnormal clone of cells responsible for the disease. Although direct evidence is lacking, it seems likely that the megakaryocytes in AMM-MF which are increased in number but abnormal in morphology and location do not produce an equivalently increased number of platelets. Therefore, platelet production may be ineffective as well as red cell production. Normally, megakaryocytes lie adjacent to marrow sinusoids and shed their cytoplasm into them. Alternatively, they may enter the sinusoids intact and shed their cytoplasm in the lungs. Burkhardt et al.[13] have proposed that there is interstitial deposition of megakaryocyte cytoplasm when the megakaryocytes are clustered as they are in advanced forms of MPD. This would be the histologic counterpart of ineffective platelet production. Since megakaryocytopoiesis is more abnormal in AMM-MF than it is in PV and ET, one would expect that the circulating platelets in AMM-MF would be more abnormal as well. This indeed has been found to be the case and will be discussed in the section on platelets.

The hypothesized release of megakaryocyte cytoplasm into the interstitium may play a role in the etiology of the fibrosis seen in AMM-MF. Several lines of evidence indicate that the proliferating fibroblasts are reacting to some stimulus and are not progeny of the abnormal hematopoietic clone. This inference is based on G-6-PD and karyotypic data,[18] as well as on the similarity in in vitro behavior of fibroblasts from normal and MPD marrow.[35] Within specific granules called *alpha granules*, platelets contain a growth factor, platelet-derived growth factor (PDGF), that can bind to bone marrow fibroblasts and induce their proliferation in vitro.[36] It has been shown that PDGF is synthesized in the megakaryocyte. It can be hypothesized that release of cytoplasm from abnormal megakaryocytes into the interstitium allows release of PDGF, which then may elicit bone marrow fibrosis.[37] While this is an attractive hypothesis to explain myelofibrosis in MPD, there is no direct evidence for it. Circumstantial evidence is derived from the hereditary gray platelet syndrome, in which there is myelofibrosis and apparently premature release of alpha granules from megakaryocytes in the bone marrow.[38]

Two other platelet-specific proteins are also localized in alpha granules, beta-thromboglobulin (βTG) and platelet factor 4 (PF4).

Reliable radioimmunoassays are available for βTG and PF4. Many investigators have measured serum, plasma, and urine concentrations of βTG and PF4 with the hope that light can be shed on platelet kinetics and the tendency to thrombosis in MPD. It has been reasoned that elevated levels in plasma would reflect in vivo release of platelet granules and thrombosis. In addition, βTG and PF4 have been proposed as surrogates for PDGF in an attempt to understand the etiology of marrow fibrosis. Most investigators have found that plasma levels of βTG and PF4 are elevated in many patients with MPD, but there has always been concern that these elevated levels may be due to in vitro release after phlebotomy and not reflect in vivo release.[39] Furthermore, it is uncertain how to correct elevated levels in plasma for the elevated blood platelet count in patients, since an increased rate of platelet production would be expected to increase "physiologic" release.[40] From a practical point of view, a large study by Najean et al.[41] in 192 cases of PV and ET found no statistical difference in the levels of these markers in patients who did and did not experience subsequent vascular accidents. Thus, at this time, there are no established guidelines to allow interpretation of plasma βTG or PF4 levels as reflections of platelet kinetics or in vivo thrombosis. On the other hand, Burstein et al.[42] studied 24-hour urinary PF4 excretion and found it to be normal in patients with ET and PV who did not have marrow fibrosis. Conversely, it was elevated in 9 of 12 patients with AMM-MF. They interpreted their data as consistent with the possibility that release of PDGF from platelet or megakaryocyte alpha granules played an etiologic role in the development of marrow fibrosis in some patients with MPD. It is quite clear that there is more important work to be done in this interesting area.

PLATELETS IN MYELOPROLIFERATIVE DISEASE

Table 9–1 lists abnormalities that have been described for platelets in MPD. Abnormalities of morphology, the surface membrane, arachidonic acid and energy metabolism, granule content and structure, and function have all been described. A detailed review was published recently.[43] The table

TABLE 9-1. PLATELET ABNORMALITIES IN MYELOPROLIFERATIVE DISEASE

I. Platelet morphology
   a. Size—normal mean cell volume with increased dispersion of size distribution by Coulter counter. Increased cell area on peripheral smear perhaps reflecting increased spreading on glass.[44,45]
   b. Shape—normal disk configuration.[44]
   c. Density—decreased mean cell density correlating with decreased concentration of cytoplasmic constituents.[47]
   d. Cytoplasm—hypertrophy of dense tubular and open cannilicular systems by electron microscopy.[60]

II. Surface membrane
   a. Glycoproteins—decreased glycoprotein Ib,[48–50] IIb, IIIa.[99]
   b. Receptors—decreased alpha-adrenergic,[52] prostaglandin D_2[53] receptors. Increased expression of Fc receptors.[54] Not necessarily concurrently.
   c. Coagulant activity—increase or decrease in collagen-induced coagulant activity, intrinsic factor Xa–forming activity, contact product–forming activity, reduction in factor X–activating activity.[88–89]
   d. Membrane function—decreased serotonin transport.[90] Abnormal fatty acid composition.[51]

III. Arachidonic acid metabolism
   a. Normal production of malondialdehyde (MDA) and cyclooxygenase pathway products[57,91] (one report[92] of reduced MDA production).
   b. Reduced lipoxygenase activity.[55,56]

IV. Granules
   a. Decreased alpha granules by light and electron microscopy.[60,93]
   b. Decreased dense granules with decreased content of nucleotides and serotonin.[64,94]
   c. Decreased beta-thromboglobulin content[95] with abnormal thrombospondin molecule.[96]

V. Metabolism
   a. Increased glyoxalase I activity.[97]
   b. Overproduction of lactate.[98]

VI. Function
   a. Bleeding time—generally normal, although increased in myeloid metaplasia.[58,62]
   b. Aggregation—in vitro spontaneous aggregation[57] in some cases. Reduced response to epinephrine most prominent with lesser abnormalities with collagen in ADP.[58,59]

and the review can be summarized by saying that the mean platelet size is normal, although the size distribution is widened, reflecting an increase in both small and large platelets.[44,45] The abnormality in size is associated with a uniform reduction in the density distribution of the platelets,[46] reflecting primarily a decrease in the density of the cytoplasm as well as a decrease in the number of granules.[47] A variety of abnormalities in membrane glycoproteins have been described, most consistently a decreased content of glycoprotein Ib.[48–50] Membrane fatty acid content has been found to be abnormal,[51] as well as alpha-adrenergic,[52] prostaglandin D_2,[53] and Fc[54] receptor function. The cyclooxygenase pathway has been found to be intact, but there is deficient lipoxygenase activity.[55,56] When platelets are studied in vitro in an aggregometer, spontaneous aggregation is sometimes seen,[57] generally in the proliferative phases of PV and ET, while a lack of response to epinephrine is very common with lesser degrees of reduced response to collagen and ADP.[58,59] It is characteristic for there to be a complete absence of primary wave aggregation in response to epinephrine. All these abnormalities are generally not present in patients with reactive thrombocytosis.

There are important unanswered questions about this host of abnormalities which seem to involve almost every aspect of cell structure, metabolism, and function. It would be attractive to find a basic underlying abnormality or at least a few underlying abnormalities from which all the recorded defects would flow. Such a fundamental defect has not been discovered. Furthermore, although there are exceptions, most reports have not been able to establish a clear relationship between any of the abnormalities described and clinical events, particularly the occurrence of thrombosis and hemorrhage. This will be discussed further in the clinical section.

Finally, there is debate as to the cause of these abnormalities. Two major hypotheses have been proposed. The first is that the abnormalities originate at the time of platelet production by abnormal megakaryocytes derived from an abnormal stem cell. An alternative view is that the abnormalities reflect damage to platelets in the circulation, presumably as they function in thrombotic events that characterize these illnesses. A great deal of evidence supports origin at the megakaryocyte level, at least for the morphologic and functional abnormalities. The morphologic abnormalities are relatively minimal during the proliferative phase of PV and ET, whereas they are much more prominent in patients with the AMM-MF syndrome. This generalization can be supported with objective techniques measuring size and density distribution,[47] and it correlates with the clinical observation that platelet morphology on peripheral blood smear is most strikingly abnormal during the advanced stages of AMM-MF.[60] These changes in platelets correlate with the spectrum of morphologic abnormalities of megakaryocytes described above. Abnormalities of megakaryocytic size, morphology, and distribution are much more striking in AMM-MF than in PV and ET.[2, 13] Furthermore, the bleeding time is often prolonged in AMM-MF[58, 61] but rarely prolonged in early PV or ET even when the patient has clinical hemorrhage.[62] This suggests that the advanced morphologic changes characteristic of AMM-MF correlate with an advanced stage of platelet dysfunction leading to a prolonged bleeding time. These observations argue against an origin for platelet abnormalities in MPD in thrombotic events in the microcirculation. Thrombotic complications are most common in PV and ET and less common in AMM-MF. One can infer from these clinical observations that the tendency to small-vessel thrombosis and therefore to damage to platelets in the circulation would be more likely to occur in the proliferative phase of PV and ET and less likely to occur in AMM-MF. Yet the morphologic and functional abnormalities are actually more severe in AMM-MF.

Further support for this point of view comes from the observations of Malpass et al.[63] They labeled platelets from patients with MPD with both ^{51}Cr and [^{14}C]serotonin and reinfused them. They found that the disappearance of serotonin was more rapid than the disappearance of chromium, suggesting that there was accelerated release of serotonin during circulation. It could be argued that this was due to hemostatic encounters. However, they, as well as most other investigators,[64] have found that the decrease in the contents of dense granules (serotonin, ADP, and ATP) of platelets from patients with MPD is far greater than the decrease in alpha-granule contents (βTG and PF4). They called on data from other systems[39] which indicated that with stimulation the platelet typically releases alpha-granular contents earlier and more readily than dense granular contents. If accelerated serotonin release in vivo were due to stimulation by hemostatic encounters, they should have observed decreased platelet βTG and PF4 levels as well, since βTG and PF4 would have been released and the platelet cannot resynthesize protein. They interpreted all their data to suggest that the accelerated loss of serotonin from MPD platelets in the circulation was due to membrane or granular defects with which the platelet was endowed at the time of release from megakaryocytes. Of course, these arguments do not exclude the possibility that some of the many abnormalities of platelets in MPD have their origin in thrombotic encounters in the circulation.

This alternate view has been sponsored predominantly by Boughton and colleagues.[65] Certainly, there is strong evidence that the turnover of clotting factors, specifically fibrinogen, is increased in patients with uncontrolled polycythemia[66] and thrombocytosis.[67] This is consistent with ongoing thrombosis in vivo. The accelerated turnover of fibrinogen tends to return toward normal with therapy either by phlebotomy[66] or myelosuppressive chemotherapy.[67] Since such treatment reduces the risk of thrombosis clinically, it is reasonable to hypothesize that platelets would be less likely to be damaged during thrombotic encounters after therapy. Boughton and colleagues have been impressed that platelet functional[68] and morphologic[69] abnormalities improve with therapy with phlebotomy or aspirin. Therefore, they propose that platelet abnormalities in MDP develop in the circulation. Until more definitive data become available, it is probably safest to assume that platelets are released with abnormalities from the megakaryocytes and that these abnormalities are aggravated as the platelets circulate.

THROMBOSIS IN MYELOPROLIFERATIVE DISEASE

Thrombotic complications are common in MPD, particularly PV. Of 431 patients randomized to the major PVSG protocol, a total of 119 thrombotic events had been reported after the patients had been on study for an average of 12 years.[70] Of these, the most common were cerebrovascular accidents, which accounted for one-third, followed by myocardial infarction, peripheral arterial occlusion, pulmonary infarction, and deep vein thrombosis in descending order of frequency. Clinicians agree that the incidence of thrombosis will be very high in PV when the hematocrit is not reduced to near the normal range. It must be emphasized that the patients on the PVSG protocol had their thrombotic complication when the hematocrit was reasonably well controlled by phlebotomy or myelosuppression. Despite the large number of laboratory studies of platelet and coagulation function in patients with MPD, we do not understand the cause of this increased thrombotic risk. Much of the insight that we do have is derived from clinical observations, some from prospective studies, but unfortunately, many from retrospective, anecdotal analysis.

First of all, the thrombotic risk appears to vary greatly from patient to patient. In the major PVSG study, thrombosis was most frequent in patients treated with phlebotomy alone without myelosuppression.[70] However, these excess thrombotic events in patients treated with phlebotomy alone occurred within the first 3 years on study. Thereafter, the risk for the group treated with phlebotomy alone was no greater than for patients treated with myelosuppression. This suggests that the thrombotic risk is particularly great in a subgroup of patients. In fact, complication-free survival is extraordinarily good for the subgroup of patients treated with phlebotomy alone who survive the first 7 years on study. Similarly, large numbers of untreated patients with ET do well for many years without complications.[71,72]

There are no convincing data that one can predict the thrombotic risk from a laboratory test. It is widely believed that the thrombotic tendency in MPD is related to thrombocytosis and that the excess incidence of thrombosis in PV treated with phlebotomy alone is related to the lack of control of thrombocytosis by that therapy. Yet there is little evidence that thrombocytosis per se causes thrombosis. In the major PVSG protocol, a matched-pair study was conducted in which each patient who suffered a thrombosis was matched with a thrombosis-free control of similar age, sex, treatment group, and duration on study.[70] Platelet counts at the nearest times before the thrombotic events of the index cases were not significantly different from those of the matched controls, suggesting that the level of the platelet count itself is not responsible for thrombosis. Furthermore, in the subsequent PVSG protocol 05 study,[73] 83 patients were treated with phlebotomy and "antiaggregating platelet therapy" consisting of aspirin, 300 mg three times daily, and dipyridamole, 75 mg three times daily. Analysis of this study in comparison with the PVSG protocol 01 as a historical control suggested no benefit in preventing thrombotic complications for such "antiplatelet therapy." In fact, there was an excess incidence of hemorrhage, particularly gastrointestinal, in patients treated with aspirin and dipyridamole. Since that study was started in 1977, there have been suggestions that a lower dose of aspirin might have been more appropriate[74] and that dipyridamole is a weak antithrombotic agent.[75] Nonetheless, the study is at least suggestive that thrombocytosis is at best only one of several factors leading to thrombosis in PV patients. Further evidence that thrombocytosis per se is not a major risk factor for thrombosis comes from observations in patients with reactive thrombocytosis, since thrombotic complications are rare in this setting. Even in the dramatic situation of reactive postsplenectomy thrombocytosis, several large studies have not shown an excess incidence of thrombosis in comparison with other postoperative groups.[76-78] Finally, several investigators have commented that thrombosis is not common in patients with thrombocytosis secondary to CML in chronic phase.[79]

Yet many clinicians have felt that lowering of the platelet count in patients with MPD leads to a reduction in thrombotic complications. This appeared to have been prospectively confirmed in the major PVSG study, in which myelosuppressive therapy was associated with fewer thrombotic complications than therapy with phlebotomy alone.[70] As mentioned earlier, Martinez et al.[67] reported that prothrombin and fibrinogen turnover rates were increased in patients with thrombocytosis and MPD. In that study, treatment with myelosuppressive therapy resulted in a return of fibrinogen and prothrombin kinetics toward normal. They ascribed the favorable effect of therapy to reduction of the platelet count. One must ask whether myelosuppressive therapy reduces the incidence of thrombosis because of reduction of the platelet count or whether thrombosis results from some other aspect of MPD which is as yet undefined but which is altered by myelosuppressive therapy. The unique observations of Valla et al.[80] support the latter point of view. Patients with MPD and particularly PV develop thrombosis at unusual anatomic sites, particularly involving the hepatic, portal, and mesenteric venous beds. In a literature review,[80] 42 percent of patients with hepatic vein thrombosis (Budd-Chiari syndrome) had PV. Valla et al. found that the majority of patients with hepatic vein thrombosis who did not have MPD by the usual clinical criteria did have autonomous erythroid colony growth when bone marrow was cultured in the absence of erythropoietin. They hypothesized that these patients had occult MPD and that almost all patients with hepatic vein thrombosis have underlying MPD. The corollary to this hypothesis is that the predisposition to thrombosis in MPD and particularly PV may be present in the absence of sufficient degrees of erythrocytosis, leukocytosis, and thrombocytosis to allow the diagnosis of MPD to be made.

In patients treated with phlebotomy alone in the major PVSG protocol, there was an increased risk of thrombosis as the rate of phlebotomy increased.[70] It may be that the high rate of phlebotomy itself increases the risk of thrombosis, but it seems at least equally likely that a high phlebotomy rate is merely a manifestation of increased disease activity which predisposes to thrombosis in a way that is not yet identified. Review of the current literature suggests that studies of megakaryocytes, platelets, and coagulation in MPD have not identified the crucial factors related to thrombosis so that we may estimate risk for it. One can only say that myelosuppressive therapy reduces risk.

Having said that thrombocytosis cannot be identified as a major risk factor for the thrombosis of major vessels seen in PV, there is a specific syndrome associated with thrombocytosis in ET and PV that has been termed *erythromelalgia*. The symptoms are burning pain in the feet, hands, and digits, sometimes associated with pallor, erythema, or cyanosis, occasionally progressing to frank gangrene. Peripheral pulses commonly remained palpable. Patients often discover for themselves that aspirin (300 to 600 mg daily) controls these symptoms. Michiels et al.[81] showed that this syndrome was associated with hyperthermia in affected areas and that biopsies of local arterioles showed inflammation and fibromuscular intimal proliferation. Narrowing of the arteriolar lumen appeared to result from proliferation of smooth-muscle cells associated with thrombus formation. This syndrome is not seen in reactive thrombocytosis, again confirming that the myeloproliferative process itself has unique features. Easy control of the clinical manifestations with aspirin suggests that platelet release of prostaglandins and thromboxanes plays some role in vessel damage. Anecdotal reports and the studies of Michiels et al.[81] suggest that suppression of the myeloproliferative process with myelosuppressive therapy reduces symptoms and vascular damage as well as aspirin does. Since both aspirin and myelosuppression are effective, it is hard to escape the conclusion that myelosuppression is affective in this particular situation by lowering the platelet count.

Patients with thrombocytosis and MPD frequently have neurologic symptoms, particularly transient ischemic attacks, which also respond to myelosuppressive therapy.[82] On the other hand, many patients with thrombocytosis and MPD are asymptomatic. All one can say is that in some patients uncontrolled thrombocytosis and MPD result in vascular symptomatology due to as yet undefined components of the MPD process. Laboratory studies have not yet clarified the differences between the symptomatic and the asymptomatic patient.

HEMORRHAGE IN MYELOPROLIFERATIVE DISEASE

In addition to thrombosis, patients with MPD also have an excessive incidence of pathologic hemorrhage. The type of bleeding is characteristic of platelet disorders: easy bruising, epistaxis, and mucosal hemorrhage. Hemorrhages more typical of clotting factor deficiencies such as hemarthroses are much less common. There are no unique types of hemorrhage seen almost exclusively in MPD, in contrast with hepatic and mesenteric vein thrombosis, which so commonly has MPD as its cause. The most straightforward type of hemorrhage is that seen in advanced AMM-MF. In these patients, the platelet count is often reduced, and the advanced morphologic abnormalities described above are associated with an intrinsic defect in platelet function and a prolongation of the bleeding time out of proportion to the reduction in the platelet count. When the platelet count is reduced to the 20,000 to 50,000/mm^3 range, pathologic hemorrhage typical for patients with thrombocytopenia and/or platelet function defects is common.

More difficult to explain is the bleeding that is seen when the platelet count is normal or elevated. In this situation, platelet morphology is only minimally abnormal, and most studies have indicated that the bleeding time will be normal.[58,62] First, one must separate the effects of an increased hematocrit, which in itself predisposes to hemorrhage. The mechanism is not clear, but presumably, increased blood viscosity interferes with normal hemostasis. In addition, hemorrhage is seen in ET and in PV when the hematocrit has been controlled by phlebotomy but the platelet count is elevated. As a generalization, hemorrhage has not correlated with the abnormalities listed in Table 9–1, but the literature is rather consistent, if anecdotal, in observing that reduction of the platelet count with myelosuppressive therapy reduces the incidence of hemorrhage.[83,84] If bleeding were due to an intrinsic platelet defect, it would be difficult to understand how lowering the number of defective platelets would improve the situation. Thus thrombocytosis per se appears to have a causative role. However, the situation is further complicated by the fact that pathologic hemorrhage appears not to be characteristic of the thrombocytosis in reactive thrombocytosis or CML.[79] Thus, although thrombocytosis per se appears to have a role, this must be combined with some as yet undefined abnormality present in PV and ET.

Two hypotheses have been raised. Martinez et al.[67] showed that thrombocytosis in

MPD was accompanied by a marked increase in the rate of catabolism of prothrombin and fibrinogen. These measurements returned to normal after myelosuppressive therapy. It might be proposed that, prior to therapy, there was accelerated intravascular coagulation and thrombosis in small blood vessels that could lead to infarction with hemorrhage from distal tissue as a result. The second hypothesis has been developed based on recently recognized abnormalities of vonWillebrand factor in MPD.[85–87] vonWillebrand factor circulates as a series of multimers, with the largest multimers reaching a molecular weight of 20,000,000.[85] vonWillebrand's disease may result from a simple decrease of circulating vonWillebrand factor protein or from a selective decrease of the larger vonWillebrand factor multimers. These high-molecular-weight multimers are believed to be required for platelet adhesion to subendothelial tissue during the initial phases of hemostasis. Budde et al.[85] and Fabris et al.[86] demonstrated a decrease in these large multimers and prolonged bleeding times in patients with MPD, the majority of whom had thrombocytosis. In some cases, myelosuppression resulted in improvement. Many explanations for these findings are possible. Budde et al.[87] have identified increased protease activity in the blood of patients with MPD. Also, one may speculate that high-molecular-weight vonWillebrand factor multimers may be absorbed from plasma during the active, proliferative phase of MPD. Further work in this interesting area is clearly indicated.

REFERENCES

1. Laszlo J: Myeloproliferative disorders (MPD): Myelofibrosis, myelosclerosis, extramedullary hematopoiesis, undifferentiated MPD, and hemorrhagic thrombocythemia. Semin Hematol 12:409–430, 1975
2. Thiele J, Holgado S, Choritz H, et al: Density distribution and size of megakaryocytes in inflammatory reactions of the bone marrow (myelitis) and chronic myeloproliferative diseases. Scand J Haematol 31:329–341, 1983
3. Blennerhassett GT, Forth ME, Anderson A, et al: Clinical evaluation of a DNA probe assay for the Philadelphia (Ph¹) translocation in chronic myelogenous leukemia. Leukemia 2:648–657, 1988
4. Kawasaki ES, Clark SS, Coyne MY, et al: Diagnosis of chronic myeloid and acute lymphocytic leukemias by detection of leukemia-specific mRNA sequences amphified in vitro. Proc Natl Acad Sci USA 85:5698–5702, 1988

5. Pugh WC, Pearson M, Vardiman JW, et al: Philadelphia chromosome–negative chronic myelogenous leukaemia: A morphological reassessment. Br J Haematol 60:457–467, 1985
6. Travis LB, Pierre RV, DeWald GW: Ph¹-negative chronic granulocytic leukemia: A nonentity. Am J Clin Pathol 85:186–193, 1986
7. Gilbert HS, Hanna MM, Goldsmith SJ, et al: Evidence that bone marrow density determination by computed tomography is a reliable indicator of peripheral expansion and fibrosis. Blood 66:174a, 1985
8. Ellis JT, Peterson P, Geller SA: Studies of the bone marrow in polycythemia vera and the evolution of myelofibrosis and second hematologic malignancies. Semin Hematol 23:144–155, 1986
9. Murphy S, Iland H, Rosenthal D, et al: Essential thrombocythemia: An interim report from the polycythemia vera study group. Semin Hematol 23:177–182, 1986
10. Ward HP, Block MH: The natural history of agnogenic myeloid metaplasia (AMM) and a critical evaluation of its relationship with the myeloproliferative syndrome. Medicine 50:357–413, 1971
11. Branehog I, Ridell B, Swolin B, et al: Megakaryocyte quantifications in relation to thrombokinetics in primary thrombocythaemia and allied diseases. Scand J Haematol 15:321–332, 1975
12. Harker LA, Finch CA: Thrombokinetics in man. J Clin Invest 48:963–974, 1969
13. Burkhardt R, Bartl R, Jager K, et al: Working classification of chronic myeloproliferative disorders based on histological, haematological, and clinical findings. J Clin Pathol 39:237–252, 1986
14. Thiele J, Funke S, Holgado S, et al: Megakaryopoiesis in chronic myeloproliferative diseases: A morphometric evaluation with special emphasis on primary thrombocythemia. Anal Quant Cytol 6:155–167, 1984
15. Rabellino EM, Levene RB, Nachman RL, et al: Human megakaryocytes: III. Characterization in myeloproliferative disorders. Blood 63:615–622, 1984
16. Fialkow PJ, Faguet GB, Jacobson RJ, et al: Evidence that essential thrombocythemia is a clonal disorder with origin in a multipotent stem cell. Blood 58:916–919, 1981
17. Adamson JW, Fialkow PJ, Murphy S, et al: Polycythemia vera: Stem-cell and probable clonal origin of the disease. N Engl J Med 295:913–916, 1976
18. Jacobson RJ, Salo A, Fialkow PJ, et al: Agnogenic myeloid metaplasia: A clonal proliferation of hematopoietic stem cells with secondary myelofibrosis. Blood 51:189–194, 1978
19. Gilliland DG, Blanchard KL, Bunn HF: Clonality in acquired hematologic disorders. Annu Rev Med 42:491–506, 1991
20. Kutti J, Ridell B, Weinfeld A, et al: The relation of thrombokinetics to bone marrow megakaryocytes and to the size of the spleen in polycythaemia vera. Scand J Haematol 10:88–95, 1973
21. Erslev AJ, Caro J, Kansu E, et al: Plasma erythropoietin in polycythemia. Am J Med 66:243–247, 1979
22. Gewirtz AM, Bruno E, Elwell J, et al: In vitro studies of megakaryocytopoiesis in thrombocytotic disorders of man. Blood 61:384–389, 1983
23. Prchal JF, Adamson JW, Murphy S, et al: Polycythemia vera: The in vitro response of normal and abnormal stem cell lines to erythropoietin. J Clin Invest 61:1044–1047, 1978
24. Komatsu N, Suda T, Sakata Y, et al: Megakaryocytopoiesis in vitro of patients with essential thrombocythaemia: Effect of plasma and serum on megakaryocytic colony formation. Br J Haematol 64:241–252, 1986
25. Deschamps JF, Bodevin E, Caen JP: Increased spontaneous number of megakaryocyte colonies in essential thrombocythemia (ET). Thromb Haemost 58:201, 1987
26. Franzen S, Strenger G, Zajicek J, et al: Microplanimetric studies on megakaryocytes in chronic granulocytic leukaemia and polycythaemia vera. Acta Haematol 26:182–193, 1961
27. Harker LA: Kinetics of thrombopoiesis. J Clin Invest 47:458–465, 1968
28. Woodruff RK, Bell WR, Castaldi PA, et al: Essential thrombocythaemia. Haemostasis 9:105–125, 1980
29. Penington DG, Weste SM: Megakaryocyte ploidy measurements in thrombocytosis. In Paulus JM (ed): Platelet Kinetics. Amsterdam, North-Holland, 1971, pp 311–313.
30. Queisser W, Weidenhauer G, Queisser U, et al: Megakaryocyte polyploidization in myeloproliferative disorders. Blut 32:13–20, 1976
31. Lagerlof B: Cytophotometric study of megakaryocyte ploidy in polycythemia vera and chronic granulocytic leukemia. Acta Cytol 16:240–244, 1972
32. Ridell B, Kutti J, Revesz P, et al: DNA content and nuclear size of megakaryocytes in thrombocythaemia. Acta Pathol Microbiol Immunol Scand 98:845–850, 1990
33. Murphy S: Thrombocytosis and thrombocythaemia. Clin Haematol 12:89–106, 1983
34. Pollycove M, Winchell HS, Lawrence JH: Classification and evolution of patterns of erythropoiesis in polycythemia vera as studied by iron kinetics. Blood 28:807–829, 1966
35. Castro-Malaspina H, Gay RE, Jhanwar SC, et al: Characteristics of bone marrow fibroblast colony-forming cells (CFU-F) and their progeny in patients with myeloproliferative disorders. Blood 59:1046–1054, 1982
36. Bryckaert MC, Wasteson A, Lindroth M, et al: Platelet derived growth factor (PDGF) binds to human bone marrow fibroblasts and stimulate their proliferation. Thromb Haemost 58:188, 1987
37. Castro-Malaspina H, Rabellino EM, Yen A, et al: Human megakaryocyte stimulation of proliferation of bone marrow fibroblasts. Blood 57:781–787, 1981
38. Breton-Gorius J, Vainchenker W, Nurden A, et al: Defective α-granule production in megakaryocytes from gray platelet syndrome: Ultrastructural studies of bone marrow cells and megakaryocytes growing in culture from blood precursors. Am J Pathol 102:10–19, 1981
39. Files JC, Malpass TW, Yee EK, et al: Studies of human platelet alpha-granule release in vivo. Blood 58:607–618, 1981
40. Ireland H, Lane DA, Wolff S, et al: In vivo platelet release in myeloproliferative disorders. Thromb Haemost 48:41–45, 1982

41. Najean Y, Porier O, Lokiec F: The clinical significance of beta-thromboglobulin and platelet factor-4 in polycythaemia patients. Scand J Haematol 31:298–304, 1983

42. Burstein SA, Malpass TW, Yee E, et al: Platelet factor-4 excretion in myeloproliferative disease: Implications for the aetiology of myelofibrosis. Br J Haematol 57:383–392, 1984

43. Holme S, Murphy S: Platelet abnormalities in myeloproliferative disorders. Clin Lab Med 4: 873–888, 1990

44. Holme S, Simmonds M, Ballek R, et al: Comparative measurements of platelet size by Coulter counter, microscopy of blood smears, and light-transmission studies. J Lab Clin Med 97:610–622, 1981

45. Small BM, Bettigole RE: Diagnosis of myeloproliferative disease by analysis of the platelet volume distribution. Am J Soc Clin Pathol 76:685–691, 1981

46. Boneu B, Nouvel C, Sie P, et al: Platelets in myeloproliferative disorders: I. A comparative evaluation with certain platelet function test. Scand J Haematol 25:214–220, 1980

47. Holme S, Murphy S: Studies of the platelet density abnormality in myeloproliferative disease. J Lab Clin Med 103:373–383, 1984

48. Bolin RB, Okumura T, Jamieson GA, et al: Changes in distribution of platelet membrane glycoproteins in patients with myeloproliferative disorders. Am J Hematol 3:63–71, 1977

49. Clezardin P, McGregor JL, Dechavanne M: Platelet membrane glycoprotein abnormalities in patients with myeloproliferative disorders and secondary thrombocytosis. Br J Haematol 60: 331–344, 1985

50. Eche N, Sie P, Caranobe C, et al: Platelets in myeloproliferative disorders: III. Glycoprotein profile in relation to platelet function and platelet density. Scand J Haematol 26:123–129, 1981

51. Leoncini G, Maresca M, Balestrero F, et al: Platelet membrane fatty acids in thrombocytosis due to myeloproliferative disorders. Cell Biochem Funct 2:23–25, 1984

52. Kaywin P, McDonough M, Insel PA, et al: Platelet function in essential thrombocythemia. N Engl J Med 299:505–509, 1978

53. Cooper B, Ahern D: Characterization of the platelet prostaglandin D_2 receptor. J Clin Invest 64:586–590, 1979

54. Moore A, Nachman RL, et al: Platelet Fc receptor: Increased expression in myeloproliferative disease. J Clin Invest 67:1064–1071, 1981

55. Okuma M, Uchino H: Altered arachidonate metabolism by platelets in patients with myeloproliferative disorders. Blood 54:1258–1271, 1979

56. Schafer AI: Deficiency of platelet lipoxygenase activity in myeloproliferative disorders. N Engl J Med 306:381–386, 1982

57. Wu KK: Platelet hyperaggregability and thrombosis in patients with thrombocythemia. Ann Intern Med 88:7–11, 1978

58. Murphy S, Davis JL, Walsh PN, et al: Template bleeding time and clinical hemorrhage in myeloproliferative disease. Arch Intern Med 138: 1251–1253, 1978

59. Zucker S, Mielke CH: Classification of thrombocytosis based on platelet function tests: Correlation with hemorrhagic and thrombotic complications. J Lab Clin Med 80:385–394, 1972

60. Maldonaldo JE, Pintado T, Pierre RV: Dysplastic platelets and circulating megakaryocytes in chronic myeloproliferative diseases: I. The platelets: Ultrastructure and peroxidase reaction. Blood 43:797–809, 1974

61. Didisheim P, Bunting D: Abnormal platelet function in myelofibrosis. Am J Clin Pathol 45: 566–573, 1966

62. Berger S, Aledort, LM, Gilbert HS, et al: Abnormalities of platelet function in patient with polycythemia vera. Cancer Res 33:2683–2687, 1973

63. Malpass TW, Savage B, Hanson SR, et al: Correlation between prolonged bleeding time and depletion of platelet dense granule ADP in patients with myelodysplastic and myeloproliferative disorders. J Lab Clin Med 103:894–904, 1984

64. Pareti FI, Gugliotta L, Mannucci L, et al: Biochemical and metabolic aspects of platelet dysfunction in chronic myeloproliferative disorders. Thromb Haemost 47:84–89, 1982

65. Boughton BJ, Corbett WEN, Ginsburg AD: Myeloproliferative disorders: A paradox of in-vivo and in-vitro platelet function. J Clin Pathol 30:228–234, 1977

66. Boughton BJ, Dallinger KJC: [125]I fibrinogen turnover in polycythaemia: The effect of phlebotomy. Br J Haematol 53:97–102, 1983

67. Martinez J, Shapiro SS, Holburn R, et al: Metabolism of human prothrombin and fibrinogen in patients with thrombocytosis secondary to myeloproliferative states. Blood 42:35–46, 1973

68. Boughton BJ: Chronic myeloproliferative disorders: Improved platelet aggregation following venesection. Br J Haematol 39:589–598, 1978

69. Boughton BJ, Jerrome DW, Rychetnik M: Chronic myeloproliferative disorders: A quantitative assessment of platelet ultrastructure. Acta Haematol 64:319–323, 1980

70. Berk PD, Goldberg JD, Donovan PB, et al: Therapeutic recommendations in polycythemia vera based on polycythemia vera study group protocols. Semin Hematol 23:132–143, 1986

71. Kessler CM, Klein HG, Havlik RJ, et al: Uncontrolled thrombocytosis in chronic myeloproliferative disorders. Br J Haematol 50:157–167, 1982

72. Hoagland HC, Silverstein MN: Primary thrombocytopenia in the young patient. Mayo Clin Proc 53:578–580, 1978

73. Tartaglia AP, Goldberg JD, Berk PD, et al: Adverse effects of antiaggregating platelet therapy in the treatment of polycythemia vera. Semin Hematol 23:172–176, 1986

74. Herschel R, Harter MD, Burch JW, et al: Prevention of thrombosis in patients on hemodialysis by low-dose aspirin. N Engl J Med 301:577–579, 1979

75. Fitzgerald GA: Dipyridamole. N Engl J Med 316: 1247–1257, 1987

76. Boxer MA, Braun J, Ellman L, et al: Thromboembolic risk of postsplenectomy thrombocytosis. Arch Surg 113:808–809, 1978

77. Coon WW, Penner J, Clagett GP, et al: Deep venous thrombosis and postsplenectomy thrombocytosis. Arch Surg 113:429–431, 1978

78. Starksen NF, Day AT, Gazzaniga AB: Does splenectomy result in a higher incidence of limb deep venous thrombosis? Am J Surg 135:202–206, 1978

79. Mason JE, DeVita VT, Canellos GP: Thrombocytosis in chronic granulocytic leukemia: Incidence and clinical significance. Blood 44: 483–487, 1974

80. Valla D, Casadevall N, Lacombe C, et al: Primary myeloproliferative disorder and hepatic vein thrombosis: A prospective study of erythroid colony formation in vitro in 20 patients with Budd-Chiari syndrome. Ann Intern Med 103: 329–334, 1985

81. Michiels JJ, Abels J, Steketee, J, et al: Erythromelalgia caused by platelet-mediated arteriolar inflammation and thrombosis in thrombocythemia. Ann Intern Med 102:466–471, 1985

82. Jabaily J, Iland HJ, Laszlo J, et al: Neurologic manifestations of essential thrombocythemia. Ann Intern Med 99:513–518, 1983

83. Gunz FW: Hemorrhagic thrombocythemia: A critical review. Blood 15:706–723, 1960

84. Bensinger TA, Logue GL, Rundles RW: Hemorrhagic thrombocythemia: Control of postsplenectomy thrombocytosis with melphalan. Blood 36:61–69, 1970.

85. Budde U, Schaefer G, Mueller N, et al: Acquired von Willebrand's disease in the myeloproliferative syndrome. Blood 64:981–985, 1984

86. Fabris F, Casonato A, Del Ben MG, et al: Abnormalities of von Willebrand factor in myeloproliferative disease: A relationship with bleeding diathesis. Br J Haematol 63:75–83, 1986

87. Budde J, Dent JA, Berkowitz SD, et al: Subunit composition of plasma von Willebrand factor in patients with the myeloproliferative syndrome. Blood 68:1213–1217, 1986

88. Walsh PN, Murphy S, Barry WE: The role of platelets in the pathogenesis of thrombosis and haemorrhage in patients with thrombocytosis. Thromb Haemost 38:1085–1096, 1977

89. Semeraro N, Cortellazzo S, Colucci M, et al: A hitherto undescribed defect of platelet coagulant activity in polycythaemia vera and essential thrombocythaemia. Thromb Res 16:795–802, 1979

90. Caranobe C, Sie P, Fernandez F, et al: Abnormal platelet serotonin uptake and binding sites in myeloproliferative disorders. Thromb Haemost 51:349–353, 1984

91. Cunietti E, Gandini R, Mascaro G, et al: Defective platelet aggregation and increased platelet turnover in patients with myelofibrosis and other myeloproliferative diseases. Scand J Haematol 26:339–344, 1981

92. Keenan JP, Wharton J, Shepherd AJN, et al: Defective platelet lipid peroxidation in myeloproliferative disorders: A possible defect of prostaglandin synthesis. Br J Haematol 35: 275–283, 1977

93. Zeigler Z, Murphy S, Gardner FH: Microscopic platelet size and morphology in various hematologic disorders. Blood 51:479–486, 1978

94. Caranobe C, Sie P, Nouvel C, et al: Platelets in myeloproliferative disorders. Scand J Haematol 25:289–295, 1980

95. Boughton BJ, Allington MJ, King A: Platelet and plasma thromboglobulin in myeloproliferative syndromes and secondary thrombocytosis. Br J Haematol 40:125–132, 1978

96. Booth WJ, Berndt MC, Castaldi PA: An altered platelet granule glycoprotein in patients with essential thrombocythemia. J Clin Invest 73: 291–297, 1984

97. Leoncini G, Maresca M, Balestrero F, et al: Platelet glyoxalases in thrombocytosis. Scand J Haematol 33:91–94, 1984

98. Leoncini G, Maresca M, Armani U, et al: Lactate overproduction in platelets of subjects affected with myeloproliferative disorders. Scand J Haematol 35:229–232, 1985

99. Mazzucato M, Del Ben MG, Casonato A, et al: Platelet membrane glycoproteins abnormalities in myeloproliferative disorders: Structure/function relationship. Thromb Haemost 58:192, 1987

ACKNOWLEDGMENTS: I wish to thank Drs. Allan Erslev, Andrew Schafer, and Allan Gewirtz for their critical review of this chapter.

10

Rheology in Normal Individuals and Polycythemia Vera

SHU CHIEN *and* STEPHEN GALLIK

The hematocrit is a major determinant of blood viscosity, which, in turn, affects resistance to flow and circulatory transport.[1] Hence knowledge of blood rheology in polycythemia vera (PV) serves to elucidate the pathophysiologic mechanisms of hemodynamic derangements and to provide a rational basis for guiding the clinical management of this condition.[2] In this chapter we shall first review the factors determining the rheologic behavior of normal blood as measured in vitro, and then we shall examine the changes in these factors and their contributions to blood hyperviscosity in PV. These will be followed by a discussion of the role of blood rheology in affecting circulatory transport in vivo under normal conditions and in PV.

FACTORS DETERMINING BLOOD VISCOSITY

Some Basic Definitions Related to Viscosity

The definitions of some rheologic terms can be illustrated by considering the flow of a fluid between two parallel plates (Fig. 10–1). If the lower plate is stationary and the upper plate is moved horizontally by the application of a tangential force, the fluid in the gap will move as laminar layers with a velocity v (in cm/s) that decreases in the direction y (in cm) from a maximum at the top to zero velocity at the bottom. This velocity gradient is referred to as the *shear rate* γ (in s^{-1}):

$$\gamma = dv/dy \qquad (10.1)$$

The unit for force F is the newton (N) in the standard system and the dyne (dyn = 0.1 N) in the centimeter-gram-second (cgs) system. The tangential force applied per unit plate area A (in m^2 or cm^2) is defined as the *shear stress* τ (in N/m^2 or dyn/cm^2, with $1 N/m^2 = 10$ dyn/cm^2):

$$\tau = F/A \qquad (10.2)$$

For a given fluid, the shear rate varies with the shear stress, and the relation between these two parameters depends on the flow property of the fluid, i.e., the viscosity η. *Viscosity* is defined as the ratio of shear stress τ to shear rate γ:

$$\eta = \tau/\gamma \qquad (10.3)$$

The unit of viscosity is pascal-second (Pa = $N \cdot s/m^2$) in the standard system and poise (P = $dyn \cdot s/cm^2$) in the cgs system, with $1 Pa = 10 P$. The normal values of blood viscosity are such that the unit usually used is millipascal (1 mPa = 0.001 Pa) or centipoise (1 cP = 0.01 P), with 1 mPa = 1 cP.

Fluids (e.g., water) with a constant η under varying conditions of shear are called *Newtonian fluids*. A plot of shear stress versus shear rate for Newtonian fluids shows a straight line going through the origin (Fig. 10–2). Plasma is a Newtonian fluid with a viscosity η_P of approximately 1.2 cP at 37°C. Blood, being a suspension of blood cells in plasma, is a nonNewtonian fluid. A plot of shear stress versus shear rate for blood shows a nonlinear relationship, with blood viscosity decreasing

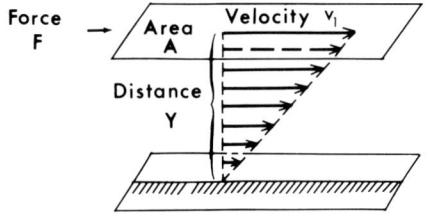

Shear stress = F/A   Shear rate = dv/dy = v_1/Y

$$\text{Viscosity} = \frac{\text{Shear stress}}{\text{Shear rate}}$$

FIGURE 10–1. The relation between shear stress and shear rate when a fluid is sheared between two parallel plates. *(Used with permission from Chien S, in Messmer K, Schmid-Schönbein H (eds): Hemodilution: Theoretical Basis and Clinical Application. Basal, Karger, 1972, pp 1–45.)*

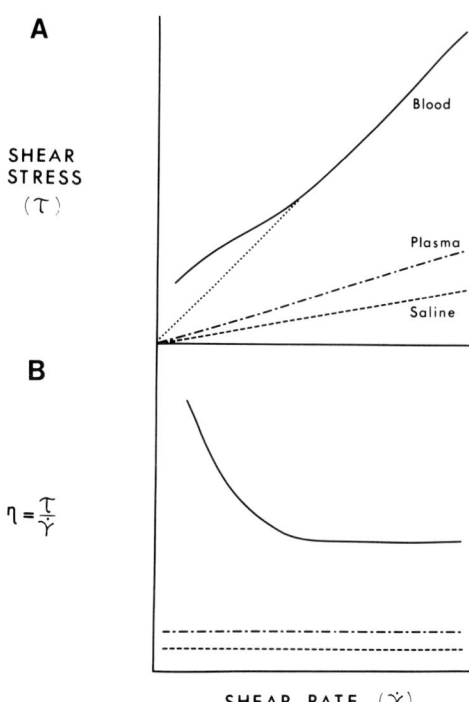

FIGURE 10–2. Plots of shear stress versus shear rate for saline, plasma, and blood (A) and viscosity versus shear rate for the same fluids (B). *(Used with permission of Chien S, in Surgenor DMN (ed): The Red Blood Cell, vol 2, 2d ed. New York, Academic Press, 1975, pp 1031–1133.)*

as the shear stress or shear rate is increased; i.e., blood exhibits a shear thinning behavior (see Fig. 10–2).

Factors Determining Blood Viscosity in Bulk Flow

The viscosity of blood η_B, like that of other liquids, varies inversely with temperature. At a given temperature, blood viscosity is primarily a function of cell concentration, plasma viscosity, cell aggregation, and cell deformation.[1]

Red Cell Concentration (Hematocrit). Because the red blood cells (RBCs) occupy the largest volume fraction of blood cells, hematocrit (Hct) is a major determinant of blood viscosity. White blood cells (WBCs) and platelets are much lower in their volume concentrations (sum < 1 percent), and they normally have no significant influence on the flow behavior of blood during bulk flow in large vessels. The role of WBCs in affecting blood flow through very narrow vessels is discussed below. When the Hct of normal blood is altered experimentally in vitro, the η_B-Hct relationship obtained is strongly nonlinear (Fig. 10–3); the rise in blood viscosity becomes increasingly more pronounced when the Hct level is raised above 50 to 60 percent.

Plasma Viscosity. The viscosity of normal human plasma at 37°C is approximately 1.2 cP.[3] Plasma viscosity is a function of the concentration of plasma proteins, especially

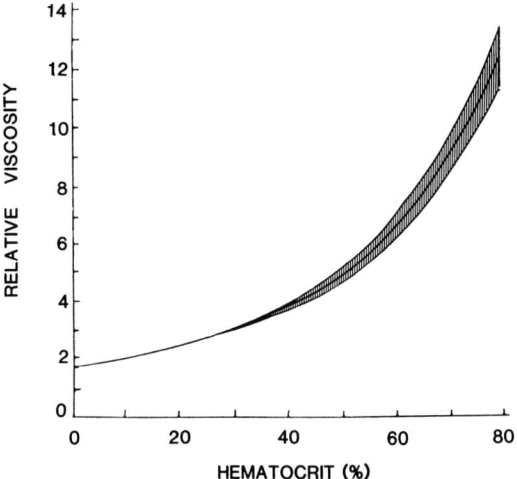

FIGURE 10–3. Blood viscosity relative to water viscosity at high shear rates (>1000 s^{-1}). *(Used with permission from Chien et al, in Renkin EM, Michel C (eds): Handbook of Physiology, Circulation: Section on Microcirculation. Bethesda, Md, American Physiological Society, 1984, pp 217–249.)*

those with molecular asymmetry, i.e., fibrinogen and some globulin fractions. In a variety of normal and pathologic conditions, plasma viscosity can be correlated with the sum of the plasma concentrations of fibrinogen and globulins.[4,5] The ratio η_B/η_P is referred to as the *relative blood viscosity*. The relative viscosity of a blood sample with Hct adjusted to a constant level, e.g., 45 percent, serves to normalize variations in Hct and plasma viscosity among samples, and it reflects primarily variations in RBC aggregation and RBC deformability, which are the two factors outlined below.

Red Cell Deformability. Normal human RBCs are remarkably deformable, and the degree of RBC deformation depends on the level of shear stress acting on the cell surface. With an increase in either shear rate or the plasma viscosity surrounding the cells, the deforming stress becomes greater and the RBCs become elongated. Under these conditions, the deforming stress can cause the RBC membrane to undergo rotational motion and transmit the stress to the internal fluid for the latter to participate in flow.[6-8] This allows the RBC to maintain a stable, deformed shape with its long axis aligned with flow and reduces the viscous resistance of the cell. This effect of mechanical shearing on RBC deformation is another microrheologic mechanism, in addition to the shear-dependent aggregation-disaggregation, for the macrorheologic finding of the shear-thinning behavior of blood viscosity.

RBC deformability serves to lower blood viscosity under physiologic high flow conditions and makes possible the passage of RBCs through narrow capillaries. The remarkable deformability of RBCs results from (1) the fluidity of internal hemoglobin-rich fluid, (2) the favorable geometric relationship between membrane surface area and cell volume, and (3) the viscoelastic properties of the cell membrane.

The internal fluid viscosity of normal human RBCs is approximately 7 cP at 37°C[9,10]; it increases with hemoglobin concentration, and the rise becomes very steep when the hemoglobin concentration approaches 40 g/dl or higher.[10] The relationship between viscosity and hemoglobin concentration may change in the presence of abnormal hemoglobins. Thus the viscosity curve is markedly elevated for deoxygenated hemoglobin S,

constituting the main rheologic basis for abnormal RBC deformability in sickle cell disease.

The normal discoid RBC has a surface area (≈ 140 μm^2) in excess of that required to enclose a sphere with the same volume (≈ 90 μm^2). Therefore, the normal RBC can deform into a variety of shapes without changing its surface area or volume.

The rheologic behavior of RBC membrane has been the subject of many reviews (see, for example, refs. 11 and 12). RBC deformation under most physiologic conditions, e.g., during transit through a narrow capillary, involves primarily deformation at a constant surface area. The elastic modulus for such shear deformation can be determined by the use of micropipette aspiration, and the normal value is approximately 5×10^{-3} dyn/cm.[13-15] When RBC deformation involves membrane area expansion, e.g., during RBC swelling in a hypotonic medium, the elastic modulus is more than 4 orders of magnitude higher.[11] RBC membrane exhibits time-dependent behavior during deformation[14] and recovery,[13] with time constants on the order of 10^{-1} s. From the time constant and the shear elastic modulus, one can calculate the membrane viscosity. The viscoelastic behavior of the RBC membrane is primarily governed by the cytoskeletal protein network on its endoface formed by spectrin, actin, band 4.1, and other proteins and is connected to glycoprotein molecules (e.g., band 3 and glycophorin) spanning the thickness of the membrane.[16] The membrane lipids do not play a significant role in the elastic behavior, but they may contribute to membrane viscosity in micro domains.

Red Cell Aggregation. Red blood cells aggregate to form rouleaux as a result of the bridging of cell surfaces by fibrinogen and some globulin fractions, e.g., α_2-globulin.[17,18] The degree of red cell aggregation reflects an energy balance in which the adhesive energy between the bridging macromolecules and the red cell surface is counteracted by several sources of disaggregating energies.[19,20] The disaggregating energy under resting conditions is mainly the electrostatic repulsive energy existing between the negatively charged cell surfaces[21] due to the presence of sialic acid;[22] in the presence of flow, disaggregating energy is also provided by the work done by the mechanical shear stress.[23]

The difference between the aggregating energy and the disaggregating energies is the *net aggregation energy*. A positive net aggregation energy leads to the close apposition of adjacent RBCs linked by the bridging macromolecules, and the resulting change in strain energy stored in the cell membrane is manifested by shape alteration of aggregated cells.[24]

Consideration of the energy balance indicates that RBC aggregation is enhanced when there is an increase in the plasma concentrations of fibrinogen and some globulins, a lowering of red cell surface charge density, and/or a decrease in shear stress under low-flow conditions. Under physiologic flow conditions, the shear stresses in most parts of the circulatory system are sufficiently high to prevent RBC aggregation; the only possible exception is the postcapillary venules, where the shear stress is the lowest.[25] An increase in shear stress causes a progressive disaggregation of rouleaux and a decrease in blood viscosity (Fig. 10–4). This effect of mechanical shearing on RBC aggregation is an important microrheologic mechanism for the macrorheologic finding of the shear-thinning behavior of blood viscosity.

Rheology of Blood in Flow Through Narrow Tubes

In blood flow through narrow tubes, its particulate or cellular nature becomes more important than in bulk flow through large tubes.[26] In tubes with diameters smaller than approximately 300 μm, the Hct of blood flowing in the tube is lower than the Hct in the discharge (outflow) blood.[17,27] This lowering in tube Hct becomes increasingly pronounced as tube diameter is reduced, to reach a minimum value in 15- to 20-μm tubes. Further decreases in tube diameter then causes the ratio of tube Hct to discharge Hct to rise toward unity (Fig. 10–5). The low Hct in narrow tubes is accompanied by a reduction in blood viscosity,[28] thus serving to partially compensate for the high resistance due to the small radii. In tubes with very narrow diameters (e.g., less than 4 to 5 μm), however, the blood viscosity would rise because of the need of RBCs to undergo marked deformation in passing through these narrow vessels.[1] When the tube diameter is reduced to less than 3 μm, the limit for RBC passage is reached, and blood viscosity increases sharply toward infinity.

While the white blood cells normally do not play a significant role in affecting the flow properties of blood during bulk flow through large tubes, they become increasingly important in blood flow through narrow tubes. Because of their larger volume and lower deformability, each WBC offers nearly 1000-fold the resistance of a RBC during flow into a 5-μm cylindrical channel. Therefore, although the concentration of WBCs is normally only ¹/₇₀₀ that of RBCs, the small proportion of WBCs present in a given volume of blood is as important as all the RBCs there in affecting the flow resistance through such a narrow channel. In vivo, WBCs may cause microvascular plugging due to their rigidity,[29–32] thus becoming a significant rheologic factor, especially in some pathologic conditions.

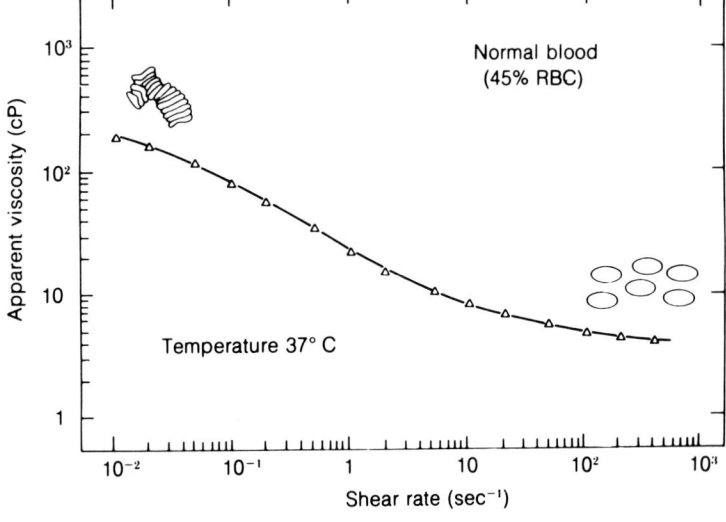

FIGURE 10–4. Logarithmic relation between blood viscosity and shear rate in normal human blood containing 45 percent RBCs by volume. Insets show RBC aggregation at low shear rates and RBC diaggregation and deformation at high shear rates. (*Used with permission from Chien et al, in Renkin EM, Michel C (eds): Handbook of Physiology, Circulation: Section on Microcirculation. Bethesda, Md, American Physiological Society, 1984, pp 217–249.*)

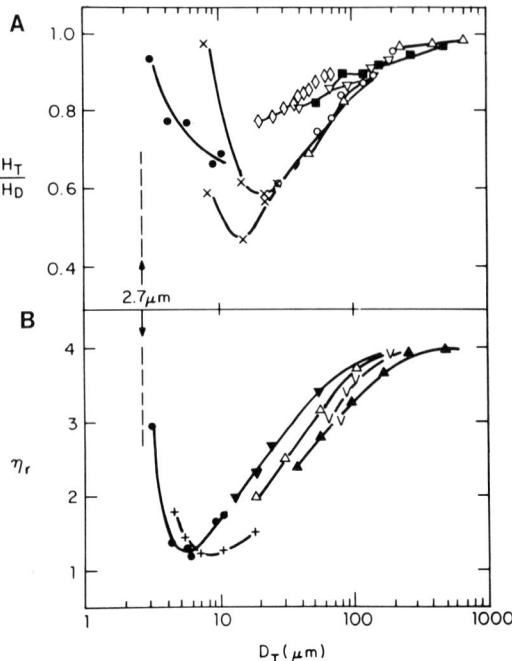

FIGURE 10-5. Variations of the ratio of tube Hct to discharge Hct (H_T/H_D) (A) and the viscosity ratio of the cell suspension to the suspending medium (η_r) (B) as a function of the diameter d of capillary tubes. Different symbols refer to data obtained by various investigators. *(Modified with permission from Chien et al, in Renkin EM, Michel C (eds): Handbook of Physiology, Circulation: Section on Microcirculation. Bethesda, Md, American Physiological Society, 1984, pp 217–249.)*

BLOOD VISCOSITY AND ITS COMPONENTS IN POLYCYTHEMIA VERA

The preceding discussions indicate that the rheologic behavior of blood is determined not only by hematocrit but also by other factors. Therefore, an understanding of alterations in blood viscosity in PV requires an analysis of these components determining blood viscosity.

Whole-Blood Viscosity

The principal hemorheologic abnormality in PV is an elevated whole-blood viscosity. The blood viscosity of PV patients is higher than that of normal controls at all shear rates (Fig. 10–6). Viscosity measurements of PV blood with the use of a coaxial cylinder viscometer demonstrated a 70 percent increase at a high shear rate of 208 s^{-1} and a 115 percent increase at a low shear rate of 0.5

s^{-1}.[33] Similar results were found using a Brookfield cone-plate viscometer.[34]

Hematocrit

PV is characterized by elevations in total red cell volume and hematocrit.[35-37] When comparisons are made at matched Hct values, the viscosity of PV blood becomes rather close to that of normal blood (see Fig. 10–6). Hence the high Hct is the main contributor to the elevation in whole-blood viscosity in PV. Thomas et al.[38] and Wade[39] showed that when PV patients were venesected to a Hct of approximately 45 percent, their blood viscosity values decreased to within the normal range. However, Procidano et al.[40] and Pearson et al.[41] found that some PV patients maintained a higher than normal whole-blood viscosity despite the normalization of Hct. Hence, in such patients, the increase in Hct may not be the only factor responsible for the increased blood viscosity in PV.

Plasma Viscosity

The plasma viscosity of PV patients is not significantly different from that of normal

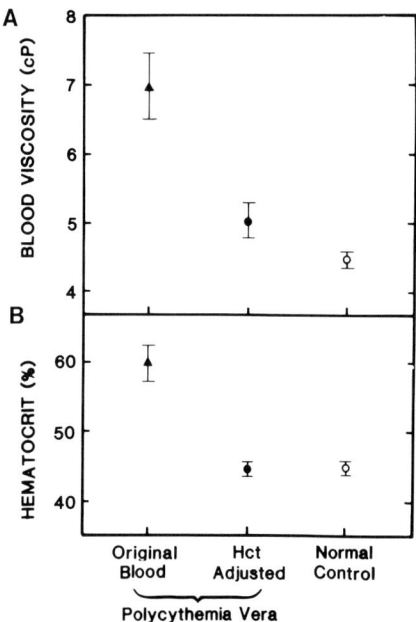

FIGURE 10-6. (A) Logarithmic relation between viscosity of blood samples obtained from PV patients and shear rate compared with that of normal blood. (B) Also shown are the data on PV blood adjusted to a normal hematocrit of 45 percent.

individuals.[33,34] Pearson et al.,[41] however, found a wider range of plasma viscosity values for PV patients than for normal individuals; i.e., some patients had a hyperviscous plasma.

The plasma protein profile is generally normal in PV. Dintenfass[42] and Procidano et al.[40] have reported that some PV patients display an increased plasma fibrinogen concentration.

Red Cell Deformability

The viscosity of suspensions of PV RBCs in a Ringer-albumin solution at an adjusted Hct of 45 percent is significantly higher than that of control RBCs.[33] Since variations in Hct, plasma viscosity, and RBC aggregation are eliminated in this system, the results suggest a decrease in RBC deformability in PV. The filtration time of RBC suspensions in autologous plasma (Hct = 40 percent) through 5-μm-pore polycarbonate sieves was 2.4-fold longer in PV over control.[43] The results have been interpreted to mean a decreased RBC deformability, but possible differences in RBC aggregation could not be ruled out in this system. Procidano et al.[40] found no increase in mean corpuscular hemoglobin concentration (MCHC), which is a major determinant of the internal viscosity of the RBC, in PV. Hougland and Luethke[44] demonstrated 34 percent fewer sulfhydral groups on the RBCs of PV patients and suggested that this alteration in membrane organization may contribute to a decrease in RBC deformability and an increase in blood viscosity in PV. There are needs for further studies on RBC deformability in PV, including micropipette tests, and on the mechanisms underlying the altered deformability.

It has been suggested that the hypochromic microcytosis in PV treated by venesection contributes to the blood hyperviscosity.[45-47] Hutton[45] demonstrated a linear correlation between the natural logarithms of mean corpuscular hemoglobin (MCH) and the viscosity of blood from iron-deficient PV and anemic patients at a standard hemoglobin concentration of 20 g/dl. On this basis, he concluded that iron deficiency and the associated decrease in the MCH contributes significantly to increased blood viscosity. Milligan et al.,[46] through the statistical analysis of viscosity measurements on PV whole blood, also arrived at the conclusion that in addition to the high Hct, reductions in MCH or mean corpuscular volume (MCV) also contribute significantly to the elevation in blood viscos-

ity, especially at low shear rates. In venesected PV patients, Pearson et al.[48] also found an inverse relationship between blood viscosity and MCH at a standard hemoglobin concentration but found no relationship when Hct was adjusted to a standard value of 45 percent. This has been confirmed by the findings of Birgegard et al.[49] that at a fixed Hct there is no significant relationship between blood viscosity and MCV in PV; these authors concluded that the iron deficiency in treated PV does not cause an increased blood viscosity. Lane[50] reported that when the whole blood is corrected to a standard RBC count of $5 \times 10^{12}/\mu l$, a linear correlation between blood viscosity and MCV is found. Under this experimental condition, Hct varies with MCV, and the results actually reflect the major influence of Hct on blood viscosity in microcytic PV. Therefore, the question of whether hypochromic microcytosis in treated cases of PV leads to an elevated blood viscosity remains unresolved. Part of the difficulty arises from the interdependence of the various hematologic indices (i.e., MCH = MCHC × MCV and MCV = Hct/[RBC]), and the correlation between blood viscosity and any one of these parameters depends on the conditions of the others. Mechanistically, it is easier to visualize a reduction in RBC deformability and a consequent rise in bulk blood viscosity with an increase in MCHC or an increase in flow resistance through narrow channels with an increase in MCV (see above). There does not appear to be a direct rheologic mechanism by which a decrease in MCH or MCV would raise blood viscosity. If an inverse correlation does exist between these parameters, the rheologic effects probably are exerted by other concurrent changes, e.g., a stiffening of the RBC membrane and/or an enhancement of RBC aggregation, rather than by decreases in MCH or MCV per se.

Red Cell Aggregation

The viscometric aggregation index, which is derived from low-shear viscosity measurements of PV blood adjusted to a Hct of 45 percent,[33] is not significantly different between the PV and normal blood. By stereologic evaluation of light photomicrographs of aggregating RBCs in vitro, Dintenfass et al.[51] found that the rates of aggregation of PV and normal RBCs (Hct = 30 percent) upon flow cessation were not significantly different, but the initial aggregate diameter was significantly larger in PV RBCs. Measuring the dynamics of RBC aggregation of PV blood by the use of a transient flow viscometric method, Joly et al.[52] found that while its steady-state aggregation behavior is normal, the PV blood had slower rates of rouleaux disaggregation; this increased rouleau stability is reduced by adjusting the Hct to 45 percent. It is known that a high Hct would enhance RBC aggregation by facilitating cell-cell encounters.[18]

It has been shown that the electrophoretic mobility and the sialic acid content of PV RBCs were significantly increased compared with normal controls.[53] This should lead to an increase in the electrostatic repulsive forces between RBC surfaces[22] in PV, thus reducing the probability of aggregation. Since fibrinogen promotes red cell aggregation, probably through the intercellular bridging of RBC surfaces,[19] those PV patients with an increased fibrinogen concentration[40,42] would have an increase in RBC aggregation. Red cell aggregation is enhanced in low flow states when there is insufficient shear force to displace the rouleaux. The whole-blood hyperviscosity in PV would lead to a low-flow condition, thus favoring RBC aggregation and causing a further increase in blood viscosity to constitute a vicious cycle.

In summary, the available evidence seems to suggest that in some PV patients there is an increase in the intrinsic aggregability of the blood (due to plasma and/or RBC factors) and that the high Hct and low flow may facilitate RBC aggregation in all cases of PV. Figure 10–7 presents a summary diagram that dissects the contributions of the various rheologic components to the changes in blood viscosity in PV.[2]

Leukocytes and Platelets

Among the 325 patients in the Polycythemia Vera Study Group (PVSG),[54] 50 to 60 percent had a WBC count greater than 12,000/μl, with a maximum count of approximately 52,000/μl. In view of the dominant resistance effects of WBCs during flow through narrow vessels (see above), this high WBC count may exert significant rheologic effects in narrow vessels. The high concentration of WBCs may exert detrimental rheologic effects in the microcirculation due

not only to their low deformability but also to the increased likelihood of their adhesion to the vascular endothelium, especially in the presence of the low-flow state and enhanced RBC-WBC interactions.[55]

The platelet count is also elevated in PV. Approximately 63 percent of the patients in the PVSG had a platelet count greater than 400,000/μl, with a maximum count of 3 million/μl.[54] The enhanced collisions between RBCs and platelets due to their increased concentrations in blood would increase the frequency at which platelets are brought to vessel surfaces,[56] thus enhancing the probability of platelet-endothelial interactions.

When there is an increase in RBC aggregation, which may occur in PV due to the high Hct and low-flow state (see above), the leukocytes and platelets are excluded from the rouleaux in the core and displaced toward the vessel wall.[26] This microrheologic effect of RBC aggregation may further enhance the interactions of WBCs and platelets with the vessel wall in PV.

IN VIVO RELEVANCE OF BLOOD RHEOLOGY IN NORMAL AND POLYCYTHEMIC STATES

Apparent Blood Viscosity and Shear Rate in Vivo

Because of the complexity of vascular geometry in vivo and the non-Newtonian behavior of blood, it is difficult to determine shear rate in the circulation in vivo. A rough estimate of wall shear rate in a blood vessel can be obtained as 4 × mean velocity/vessel radius ($4v/r$), which is wall shear rate for a Newtonian fluid in Poiseuille flow. The values for $4v/r$ in various parts of the circulation are plotted in Fig. 10–8.[25]

Shear rates in the arteries are sufficiently high to cause RBC deformation and disaggregation, resulting in a low blood viscosity. The highest shear rate is normally found in the capillaries; the high values of shear rate and shear stress in the capillaries serve to ensure the stress deformation of RBCs where it is needed. The postcapillary venules and small veins have the lowest shear rate in the circulation (see Fig. 10–8), and they represent the most likely sites of RBC aggregation.

Similar to the findings in narrow tubes in vitro (see above), Hct and blood viscosity are

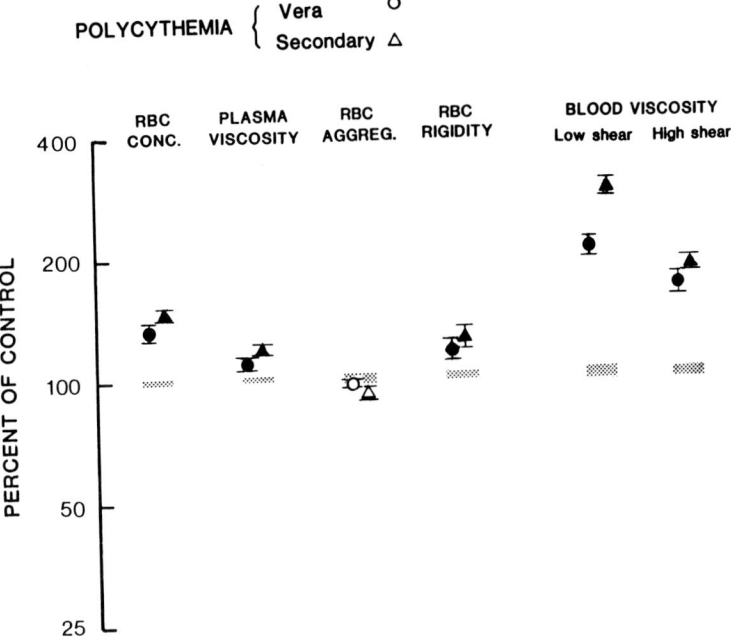

FIGURE 10-7. Diagram showing the blood viscosity at two shear rates and the four major determinants of blood viscosity of 7 patients with PV (*circles*) and 22 patients with secondary polycythemia (*triangles*) compared with the results on 30 normal human subjects. Red cell rigidity (reciprocal of deformability) was estimated by determining the viscosity (shear rate = 0.5 s^{-1}) of RBC suspension at 45 percent hematocrit in a Ringer-albumin solution. RBC aggregation was estimated by determining the viscosity (shear rate = 0.5 s^{-1}) of a blood sample adjusted to 45 percent hematocrit in the patient's own plasma and dividing it by the plasma viscosity to yield a relative viscosity; this relative viscosity value is further divided by the relative viscosity of the suspension of 45 percent RBC in Ringer-albumin solution to give an index for RBC aggregation after correcting for any alteration in the other three determinants of blood viscosity. The mean values for the normal data are taken as 100 percent, and the ordinate is in logarithmic scale. The values given are means ± SEM, with symbols and bars for the PV patients and shaded areas for normal controls. Whenever the data on PV patients are significantly different from controls ($p < 0.05$), closed symbols are used instead of open ones. The control values are hematocrit: 42.6 ± 0.6 percent; plasma viscosity: 1.24 ± 0.01 cP; RBC aggregation index: 2.86 ± 0.08; RBC rigidity index: 6.32 ± 0.11 cP; and the values of blood viscosity at the low shear rate of 0.5 s^{-1}: 29.4 ± 1.1 cP, at the high shear rate of 200 s^{-1}: 4.03 ± 0.08 cP.

lower in microvessels than in large vessels. It has been shown in the cat mesentery that the microvessel Hct is reduced to approximately three-quarters the large vessel Hct in 70-μm vessels, to half in 40-μm vessels, and to nearly one-quarter in 20-μm vessels.[30] Similar trends of decreases in microvessel Hct with diameter have been found in the hamster cheek pouch,[57] rat mesentery,[58] and rat cremaster muscle.[59] From simultaneous measurements of pressure drop, blood flow velocity, and vessel geometry in single arterioles of cat mesentery, Lipowsky et al.[30] have demonstrated that apparent blood viscosity decreases in parallel with microvessel Hct; i.e., the viscosity-Hct relationship is the same as that determined in viscometers during bulk flow in vitro.

The effect of acute normovolemic hemoconcentration on microvessel Hct has been investigated in the arterioles of the cat mesentery.[60] The results indicate that as the large-vessel Hct was doubled from a mean control value of 36 to 71 percent, the mean Hct in 35-μm arterioles also was doubled from 17 to 34 percent. Thus the arteriolar Hct increased in parallel with the large-vessel Hct under the condition of experimental hemoconcentration, and this would lead to a corresponding rise in arteriolar blood viscosity. Intravital measurements of RBC velocity showed that the volumetric flow in these arterioles decreased in experimental hemoconcentration.

The effect of experimental hemoconcentration on capillary hematocrit has not been

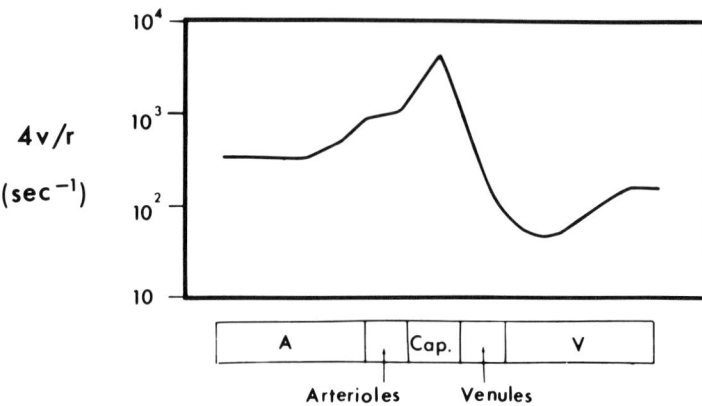

4v/r

(sec⁻¹)

Arterioles   Venules

FIGURE 10–8. Variation in $4v/r$, where v is mean velocity and r is vessel radius, in various parts of the circulation (A = arteries; Cap. = capillaries; V = venules). The parameter $4v/r$ gives a rough estimate of the shear rate in these vessels. (*Used with permission from Chien et al, in Renkin EM, Michel C (eds): Handbook of Physiology, Circulation: Section on Microcirculation. Bethesda, Md, American Physiological Society, 1984, pp 217–249.*)

reported. If, like the arteriolar Hct, the capillary Hct also rises in parallel with the large-vessel Hct during hemoconcentration (i.e., if the 1 : 4 ratio[30] is maintained), the capillary Hct would rise to only 20 percent when the large-vessel Hct is raised to 80 percent. It appears that the narrow capillaries are protected from a large rise in Hct even in severe cases of PV.

The existence of lower shear rates in the postcapillary than in the precapillary segments (see Fig. 10–8) may affect transcapillary fluid exchange in low-flow states.[25] In the normal circulation, the shear rate is high in both the pre- and postcapillary segments, and the discrepancy in shear rate may not be associated with a significant difference in blood viscosity. With a reduction in shear rate down to the shear-dependent portion of the

η_B—γ curve, however, the lower shear rate in postcapillary segments would lead to a high blood viscosity (Fig. 10–9). This preferential elevation of postcapillary blood viscosity would cause an increase in the postcapillary/precapillary resistance ratio and an elevation in capillary pressure. Under conditions of normovolemic hemoconcentration, the η_B—γ curve is steepened by the increase in Hct; consequently, the low-flow and hyperviscosity conditions in the postcapillary venules are exaggerated. The low shear condition in the postcapillary venules would enhance not only RBC aggregation but also WBC–endothelial cell interaction (see above). These rheologic changes would further worsen the elevation of capillary pressure and transcapillary fluid loss. Such a vicious cycle involving rheologically induced fluid loss may

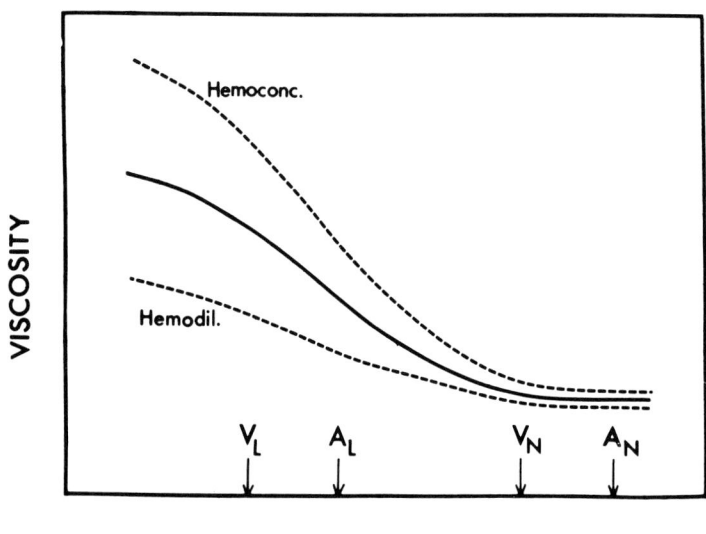

VISCOSITY

Hemoconc.

Hemodil.

V_L A_L V_N A_N

SHEAR RATE

FIGURE 10–9. Showing the disproportionate influence of flow rate on viscosity of postcapillary (V) and precapillary (A) segments of the circulation. Solid line indicates the relation between viscosity and shear rate for normal blood. According to Fig. 10–11, the normal shear rate in the postcapillary segment (V_N) is lower than that in the precapillary segment (A_N). In low-flow states, the shear rates in these segments are reduced to V_L and A_L, respectively. The broken lines above and below the solid curve indicate the relations obtained when the shear dependence of blood viscosity is altered by hemoconcentration and hemodilution, respectively. (*Used with permission from Chien S: Adv. Microcirc 2:89–103, 1969.*)

play a significant role in affecting micro-vascular hemodynamics and plasma volume balance in PV. The hypervolemia in PV, however, would serve to increase the systemic and microcirculatory blood flow (see below) and alleviate some of the rheologic consequences due to the high-viscosity, low-flow condition in hemoconcentration.

Theoretical computations[61,62] and experimental measurements[56,63] have shown that a rise in Hct causes a blunting of the parabolic velocity profile of blood flow in tubes. Thus the velocity gradient is flattened near the center of the lumen, while it is steepened near the wall of the tube. These changes lead to an expansion of the central cell-rich, low-shear region and a narrowing of the peripheral cell-poor, high-shear layer, with enhancements of shear rate and shear stress at the wall. Such microrheologic alterations not only would alter the apparent blood viscosity in the vessel but also may exert biophysical and biochemical effects on the vascular endothelium via the changes in wall shear stress.[64]

Correlation Between Blood Viscosity and Flow Resistance

The arterial blood pressure decreases along the vascular tree as energy is dissipated due to the resistance R to flow. The resistance can be defined as the ratio of pressure drop P to flow Q:

$$R = P/Q \qquad (10.4)$$

The large arteries and veins contribute little to the overall flow resistance, and the major sites of resistance are in small vessels, especially small arteries, arterioles and capillaries.[65,66] In these small blood vessels, the flow characteristics are laminar, and the energy dissipation is entirely viscous in nature. According to the Poiseuille-Hagen law for laminar flow, the resistance is governed by blood viscosity and vascular geometry, which includes the radius r, the length L, and the parallel number N of vessels:

$$R = 8\eta_B L/N\pi r^4 \qquad (10.5)$$

The contribution by the vascular geometry to resistance may be called *vascular hindrance Z*, which in Eq. (10.2) is represented by $8L/N\pi r^4$.[67] Thus resistance is a product of vascular hindrance and blood viscosity:

$$R = Z \times \eta_B \qquad (10.6)$$

The Poiseuille-Hagen law applies quantitatively to the steady, laminar flow of a simple fluid through a straight, rigid tube with a uniform radius. The blood vessels, however, are distensible and have complicated geometry, with their radii varying in space and time; Eq. (10.5) would not hold quantitatively for the complex flow conditions in the circulation in vivo. Nevertheless, the relative roles of the various geometric factors and blood viscosity in affecting flow resistance, as formulated in Eq. (10.5), are still valid; e.g., in vivo measurements on single microvessels have shown that the vascular hindrance is strongly dependent on vessel radius, with an exponent close to being 4.[68]

According to Eq. (10.6), the simultaneous measurements of in vivo flow resistance and blood viscosity would allow the estimation of vascular hindrance. In several experimental and clinical conditions, this approach has been used to dissect the relative contributions of blood viscosity and vascular hindrance to the total peripheral resistance, which can be calculated from the ratio of arterial pressure and cardiac output determined in vivo.[2,4,69] Similar analysis has been applied to hemodynamic and rheologic studies on experimental animals subject to hematocrit variations and on patients with PV, as discussed below.

Systemic Hemodynamics in PV. Experimental and clinical investigations on the effect of hemoconcentration on systemic blood flow have led to the conclusion that in addition to Hct, blood volume is another important parameter in determining systemic blood flow in PV. Richardson and Guyton[70] demonstrated that the cardiac output (or systemic blood flow) is inversely proportional to Hct following isovolemic exchange transformation in dogs. Murray et al.[71] later showed that this inverse relationship is a function of the blood volume; at a given Hct, the cardiac output is directly related to blood volume. Thus cardiac output may be increased in the presence of an expanded blood volume, despite the elevated Hct. Similar results have been found in PV patients. In 10 PV patients with a mean Hct of 60 percent, Cobb[72] found a 32 percent increase in the cardiac index as compared with 6 normovolemic, normocythemic individuals; in these patients, the red cell volume increased by 116 percent, and the total-blood volume increased by 58 percent above normal. Examining 27 PV patients, Segel and Bishop[73] also found increased cardiac output and total blood volume and suggested that the increase in cardiac output was due to the expanded blood volume. Likewise, in a study of 24 patients with PV, Weber et al.[74] found a direct relationship between cardiac output and blood volume and an inverse relationship between cardiac output and Hct (Fig. 10–10). The increase in cardiac output in PV is due primarily to an increase in the stroke volume, with the heart rate being nearly normal. The results of these investigations indicate that in normovolemic PV, systemic blood flow is reduced due to the elevated blood viscosity, whereas in hypervolemic PV, the expansion of blood volume facilitates venous return and thus increases stroke volume and cardiac output despite the elevated blood viscosity.

In PV, the arterial pressure is usually not markedly altered. Hence, as a corollary to the findings on cardiac output, the total peripheral resistance varies directly with Hct at a given blood volume and inversely with blood volume at a given Hct. The relative roles of blood viscosity and vascular hindrance to the observed changes in total peripheral resis-

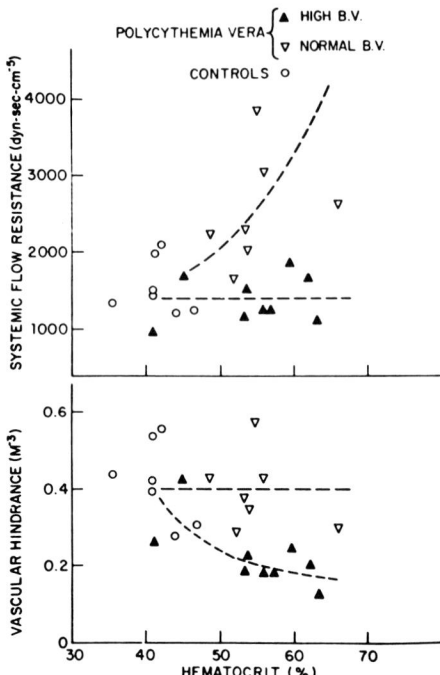

FIGURE 10–11. Systemic flow resistance (= mean arterial pressure/cardiac output, from ref. 74 and vascular hindrance in PV patients with a high blood volume and those with normal blood volume. (Reprinted from Chien S: Clin Hemorheol 1:319–342, 1981 with kind permission from Elsevier Science Ltd, The Boulevard, Langford Lane, Kidlington 0X5 1GB, UK.)

tance can be analyzed by calculating the vascular hindrance from the data on total peripheral resistance and blood viscosity (Eq. 10.6). As shown in Fig. 10–11, the vascular hindrance of normovolemic PV patients is essentially the same as that of normal controls, while in hypervolemic PV patients it decreases as Hct is raised.[2] In the 27 PV patients studied by Segel and Bishop,[73] the systemic vascular hindrance was estimated to be 74 percent less than normal. These findings have led to the hypothesis that the expanded blood volume in PV patients makes possible the compensatory reduction in vascular hindrance, resulting in an increase in blood flow through the microcirculation in PV.[2] This also would increase the cardiac preload by facilitating venous return and decrease the afterload by reducing peripheral impedance, thus increasing stroke volume and cardiac output under hypervolemic/polycythemic conditions.

Regional Blood Flow in PV. The elevation of Hct in PV leads to a decrease in cerebral blood flow. Thomas et al.[38] showed a 45

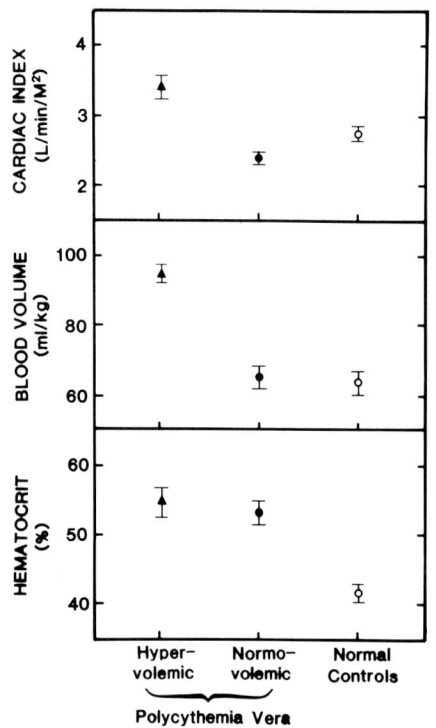

FIGURE 10–10. Relationships between cardiac output and blood volume and hematocrit in PV patients.

percent decrease in cerebral blood flow in PV patients (Hct = 53 percent) compared with normal individuals (Hct = 41 percent). Treatment by venesection reduced the Hct and increased the cerebral blood flow to near-normal levels. Wade[39] also showed in 6 PV patients that when the Hct was reduced by venesection from 56 to 45 percent, the cerebral blood flow rose by 36 percent, and the rate of oxygen delivery (= flow x arterial O_2 content) increased by 7.2 percent. A decrease in Hct lowers the blood viscosity as well as the oxygen-carrying capacity. There is a lack of agreement as to the relative roles of blood viscosity and oxygen-carrying capacity in the Hct dependency of cerebral blood flow. The data of Thomas[38] suggest that the viscosity, not the oxygen-carrying capacity, of the blood is the important factor determining cerebral blood flow in PV. Brown et al.,[75] using a stepwise inclusion multiple regression to statistically analyze their data from PV patients, concluded that blood viscosity had no significant effect on cerebral blood flow after the arterial O_2 content had been considered. It is to be noted that arterial O_2 content and blood viscosity are not completely independent variables. In young lambs, Hudak et al.[76] maintained the arterial O_2 content at a constant level while increasing the Hct by isovolemic exchange with RBCs containing methemoglobin. Under these conditions, cerebral blood flow decreased and fractional O_2 extraction increased, suggesting that cerebral blood flow is dependent on blood viscosity when arterial O_2 content has been eliminated as a variable. On the other hand, there is also ample evidence that when the Hct and blood viscosity are kept constant, decreases in arterial O_2 saturation and O_2 content would increase cerebral blood flow.[77] It appears that both blood viscosity and arterial O_2 content should be taken into account when interpreting the Hct dependence of cerebral blood flow.

There are a limited number of studies of regional blood flow in other tissues in PV. Bollinger and Luthy[78] showed that the resting arm blood flow in PV patients is not significantly different from that in control subjects. Milligan et al.[79] found that the calf blood flow in PV patients is not significantly altered by a reduction in Hct through venesection. Since the arterial blood pressure was found to be normal in PV,[78] the normal blood flow in these regions indicates that the regional resistance also must be normal. A normal resistance in the face of a significant increase in blood viscosity indicates the occurrence of a compensatory decrease in vascular hindrance. Using the pressure-flow data of Bollinger and Luthy[78] and the Hct-viscosity relationship found in vitro, we calculate the forearm vascular hindrance in these PV patients to be approximately 45 percent lower than in control subjects. This is in agreement with the conclusion reached from analysis of the systemic hemodynamic and rheologic data, as discussed above.

Optimal Hematocrit for Oxygen Transport

The rate of oxygen delivery (I_{O_2}) to tissues is equal to the product of blood flow and the arterial O_2 content (A_{O_2}).

$$J_{O_2} = Q \times A_{O_2} \qquad (10.7)$$

From Eqs. (10.4) and (10.6), blood flow can be expressed as

$$Q = P/\eta_B Z \qquad (10.8)$$

The arterial O_2 content is mainly that carried with the hemoglobin, and this is

$$A_{O_2} = k \times O_2 \text{ sat.} \times MCHC \times Hct \quad (10.9)$$

where k is a constant, and O_2 sat. is the percent O_2 saturation of the hemoglobin.

Hence, if P, O_2 sat., and MCHC are normal, the rate of O_2 delivery is

$$J_{O_2} = k' Hct/\eta_B Z \qquad (10.10)$$

where k' is a constant. If Z is also unchanged, then the rate of O_2 delivery varies with the ratio Hct/η_B. This O_2 delivery parameter (Hct/η_B) is small at very low Hct levels because of the insufficient arterial O_2 content, and it is also small at very high Hct levels because of the high blood viscosity and reduced blood flow. Therefore, there exists a range of optimal Hct values over which the O_2 delivery is at a maximum (Fig. 10–12). Under normal conditions, when Hct is the only variable, the optimal Hct range encompasses the normal Hct levels.

Experimental studies on dogs subjected to Hct variations by isovolemic exchange have provided evidence that the optimal Hct for maximum O_2 delivery to the systemic and coronary circulations is near the normal Hct levels and that the rates of O_2 consumption were essentially constant over a Hct range of

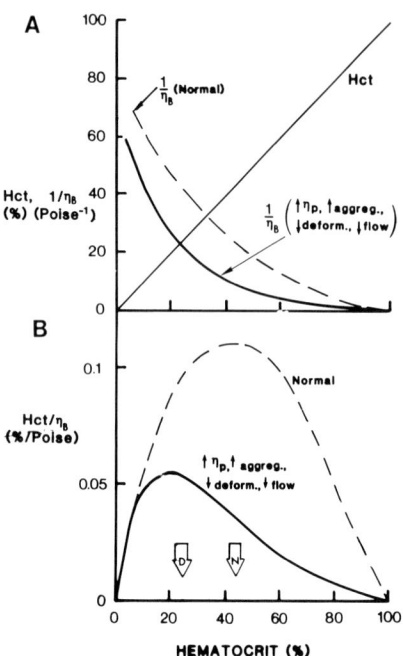

FIGURE 10–12. (A) The variations in Hct and $1/\eta_B$ with Hct. (B) Effects of variations in hematocrit (Hct) on O_2 transport as reflected by the calculated parameter Hct/η_B. Dashed lines indicate results obtained when Hct is the only variable, with other rheologic parameters remaining normal. Solid lines indicate results obtained when there are increases in plasma viscosity (η_P) or RBC aggregation or decreases in RBC deformability or flow rate. Arrow marked N shows normal Hct level and that marked D shows Hct level found in patients with abnormal plasma viscosity, RBC deformability, RBC aggregation, and/or low-flow states.

20 to 60 percent.[80, 81] The optimal hematocrit range for maximum O_2 delivery is narrower in some other organs.[81] Low-flow states lead to an increase in blood viscosity at a given Hct (see Fig. 10–4). Under these conditions, O_2 delivery is better maintained at lower Hct levels (see Fig. 10–12). This has been verified by investigations on the effects of Hct variations in dogs subjected to hemorrhagic hypotension at an arterial pressure of 50 mmHg.[82] The range of optimal Hct for myocardial O_2 transport and consumption shifted from 20 to 60 percent in the control state to 20 to 25 percent in the low-flow state.

The preceding discussions are based on an unchanged vascular hindrance, and O_2 delivery is considered only in terms of the ratio Hct/η_B. When PV is accompanied by a decrease in vascular hindrance, Eq. (10.10) indicates that O_2 delivery would be improved. Therefore, the decrease in vascular hindrance in hypervolemic PV serves an impor-

tant function by counteracting the increase in blood viscosity and minimizing the decrease in O_2 delivery.

SUMMARY

Blood viscosity at a given temperature is dependent on hematocrit, plasma viscosity, red cell deformability, and red cell aggregation. Red cell deformation and aggregation are flow-dependent phenomena; low-flow states are accompanied by a reduction in shear stresses for the deformation and disaggregation of red blood cells, thus raising the blood viscosity. In blood flow through narrow tubes, the larger and less deformable leukocytes may play a significant role in increasing the resistance to flow. The basic knowledge derived from studies on normal blood can be used to analyze the blood rheology in PV.

In PV, whole-blood viscosity is elevated. This blood hyperviscosity is primarily due to the high hematocrit, but other rheologic factors also may play contributory roles. The plasma viscosity is elevated in some PV patients. There is some evidence suggesting that red cell deformability is decreased in PV. In addition to a slight increase in intrinsic aggregability in some PV patients, the facilitation of red cell aggregation by high hematocrit may contribute to abnormal blood rheologic properties at low shear rates in PV. The rheologic behavior of PV blood in narrow vessels also may be affected by the high WBC count.

In the circulation in vivo, blood viscosity and vascular geometry together determine the resistance to blood flow. In major resistance vessels (arterioles and capillaries), the Hct and blood viscosity are lower than the corresponding values in large conduit vessels, and this serves to reduce the high resistance in such narrow vessels. Under experimental conditions of acute normovolemic hemoconcentration, the increases in Hct and blood viscosity are proportionately translated to the arterioles, and microcirculatory blood flow is often significantly reduced. Under conditions of hypervolemic hemoconcentration, however, this hyperviscosity effect due to high Hct may be compensated by a reduction in vascular hindrance due to increases in the size and/or number of resistance vessels, thus resulting in a normal blood flow despite the elevated blood viscosity.

Measurements on the systemic circulation in PV have demonstrated that blood volume and Hct are both important determinants of hemodynamic functions. For normal blood volume levels, the peripheral resistance is directly proportional to blood viscosity as Hct is elevated, with the vascular hindrance remaining essentially unchanged. At a given high Hct level, the vascular hindrance is inversely related to blood volume. In the presence of hypervolemia, the peripheral resistance remains normal despite the elevation of Hct, since the increase in blood viscosity is counterbalanced by the compensatory decrease in vascular hindrance. The data suggest that the hypervolemia due to an increased red cell mass in PV leads not only to an improvement in venous return and increase in stroke volume but also to a decrease in systemic vascular hindrance and maintenance of peripheral blood flow. The cerebral blood flow is diminished in PV, and it can be raised to normal levels following the normalization of Hct by venesection. Unlike cerebral blood flow, the resting arm and calf blood flows are normal in PV; these findings reflect a compensatory decrease in vascular hindrance in the extremities.

In postcapillary vessels, a detrimental low-flow condition could develop which is characterized by increased red cell aggregation and enhanced interactions of leukocytes and platelets with the vascular endothelium. These detrimental low-flow conditions may be ameliorated by a concomitant hypervolemia.

The optimal hematocrit for maximum O_2 delivery and consumption normally has a fairly wide range encompassing and extending beyond the normal values. An elevation of Hct above 60 percent leads to a decrease in O_2 availability and utilization. The effect of high Hct on O_2 utilization has regional variations and depends on flow conditions; high Hct is particularly detrimental for the coronary circulation under low-flow state.

REFERENCES

1. Chien S: Biophysical behavior of red cells in suspensions. *In* Surgenor DMN (ed): The Red Blood Cell, vol. 2, 2d ed. New York, Academic Press, 1975, pp 1031–1133
2. Chien S: Hemorheology in disease, pathophysiological significance and therapeutic implications. Clin Hemorheol 1:319–342, 1981
3. Harkness J: The viscosity of human blood plasma: Its measurement in health and disease. Biorheology 8:171–193, 1971
4. Scholz PM, Kinney JM, Chien S: Effects of major abdominal operations on human blood rheology. Surgery 77:351–359, 1975
5. Letcher RL, Chien S, Pickering TG, et al: Direct relationship between blood pressure and blood viscosity in normal and hypertensive subjects: Role of fibrinogen and concentration. Am J Med 70:1195–1202, 1981
6. Schmid-Schönbein H, Wells R: Fluid drop like transition of erythrocytes under shear. Science 165:288–291, 1969
7. Fischer TM, Stoher-Liesen M, Schmid-Schönbein H: The red cell as a fluid droplet: Tank tread-like motion of the human erythrocyte membrane in shear flow. Science 202:894–896, 1978
8. Keller SR, Skalak R: Motion of a tank-treading ellipsoidal particle in a shear flow. J Fluid Mech 120:27–47, 1982
9. Cokelet GR, Meiselman HJ: Rheological comparison of hemoglobin solutions and erythrocyte suspension. Science 162:275–277, 1968
10. Chien S, Usami W, Bertles JF: Abnormal rheology of oxygenated blood in sickle cell anemia. J Clin Invest 49:623–634, 1970b
11. Evans EA, Skalak R: Mechanics and Thermodynamics of Biomembranes. Cleveland, Chemical Rubber Company, 1980
12. Lux SE, Shohet SB: The erythrocyte membrane: Biochemistry. Hosp Pract 19:77–83, 1984
13. Evans, EA, Hochmuth RM: Membrane viscoelasticity. Biophys J 16:1–11, 1976
14. Chien S, Sung KLP, Skalak R, et al: Theoretical and experimental studies on viscoelastic properties of red cell membrane. Biophys J 24:463–487, 1978
15. Waugh R, Evans EA: Viscoelastic properties of erythrocyte membranes of different vertebrate animals. Microvasc Res 12:291–304, 1976.
16. Palek J, Lux SE: Red cell membrane skeletal defects in hereditary and acquired hemolytic anemias. Semin Hematol 20:189–224, 1983
17. Fåhraeus R: The suspension stability of blood. Physiol Rev 9:241–274, 1929
18. Chien S, Usami S, Dellenback RJ, Gregersen MI: Shear-dependent interaction of plasma proteins with erythrocytes in blood rheology. Am J Physiol 219:143–153, 1970
19. Chien S, Jan KM: Red cell aggregation by macromolecules: Roles of surface absorption and electrostatic repulsion. J Supramol Struct 1:385–409, 1973
20. Chien S: Aggregation of red blood cells: An electrochemical and colloid chemical problem. *In* Bioelectrochemistry: Ions, Surfaces, Membranes. Advances in Chemistry Series. Washington, American Chemical Society, 1980, pp. 1–32
21. Jan K-M, Chien S: Role of surface electric charge in red blood cell interactions. J Gen Physiol 61:638–654, 1973
22. Seaman GVF: Electrokinetic behavior of red cells. *In* Surgenor DMN (ed): The Red Blood Cell, vol. 2, 2d ed. New York, Academic Press, 1975, pp. 1135–1229
23. Chien S, Sung AL, Kim S, et al: Determination of aggregation force in rouleaux by fluid mechanical technique. Microvasc Res 13:327–333, 1977

24. Skalak R, Zarda PR, Jan KM, Chien S: Mechanics of rouleau formation. Biophys J 35:771–781, 1981

25. Chien S: Blood rheology and its relation to flow resistance and transcapillary exchange, with special reference to shock. Adv Microcirc 2:89–103, 1969

26. Chien S, Usami S, Skalak R: Blood flow in small tubes. In Renkin EM, Michel C (eds): Handbook of Physiology, Circulation: Section on Microcirculation. Bethesda, Md, American Physiological Society, 1984, pp 217–249

27. Cokelet GR: Blood rheology interpreted through the flow properties of the red cell. In Grayson J, Zingg W (eds): Microcirculation, vol 1. New York, Plenum Press, 1976, pp 9–32

28. Fåhraeus R, Lindqvist T: The viscosity of the blood in narrow capillary tubes. Am J Physiol 96:562–568, 1931

29. Lichtman MA: Rheology of leukocytes, leukocyte suspensions and blood in leukemia. J Clin Invest 52:350–358, 1973

30. Lipowsky HH, Usami S, Chien S: In vivo measurements of "apparent viscosity" and microvessel hematocrit in the mesentery of the cat. Microvasc. Res 19:297–319, 1980

31. Bagge U, Amundson B, Louritzen C: White blood cell deformability and plugging of skeletal muscle capillaries in hemorrhagic shock. Acta Physiol Scand 108:159–163, 1980

32. Engler RL, Schmid-Schönbein GW, Pavelec RS: Leukocyte capillary plugging in myocardial ischemia and reperfusion in the dog. Am J Pathol 111:98–111, 1983

33. Chien S: Blood rheology in hypertension and cardiovascular diseases. Cardiovasc Med 2:356–360, 1977

34. Girolami A, Martino R, Procidano M, Saltarin P: Integral viscosity: A useful parameter in evaluating whole blood and plasma viscosities in health and disease. Folia Hematol 109:488–494, 1982

35. Berlin NI, Lawrence JH, Gartland J: Blood volume in polycythemia as determined by ^{32}P-labeled red blood cells. Am J Med 9:747–751, 1950

36. Modan B: The Polycythemic Disorders. Springfield, Ill, Charles C Thomas, 1971

37. Wetherley-Mein G, Pearson TC: The myeloproliferative disorders. In Hardisty RM, Weatherall DJ (eds): Blood and Its Disorders, 2d ed. Oxford, Blackwell Scientific Publications, 1982, pp 1269–1316

38. Thomas DJ, Du Boulay GH, Marshall J, et al: Cerebral blood-flow in polycythaemia. Lancet 2(8030):161–163, 1977

39. Wade JPH: Transport of oxygen to the brain in patients with elevated haematocrit values before and after venesection. Brain 106:513–523, 1983

40. Procidano M, Zanolli FA, Fornasiero L, Girolami A: Blood viscosity in native and reconstituted polycythemic blood. Folia Haematol 111:671–680, 1984

41. Pearson TC, Ring CP, Wetherley-Mein G: Plasma and whole-blood viscosity in treated primary polycythemia. Clin Lab Haematol 2:73–82, 1980

42. Dintenfass L: Rheology of Blood in Diagnostic and Preventive Medicine. London, Butterworths, 1976

43. Rewald E, Rosasco MG: Delay in red cell filtration in polycythemic patients (letter). Br J Haematol 47:485, 1981

44. Hougland MW, Luethke JM: Quantitation of sulfhydral groups on erythrocytes in polycythemia vera. Histochemistry 76:57–60, 1982

45. Hutton, RD: The effect of iron deficiency on whole blood viscosity in polycythemic patients. Br J Haematol 43:191–199, 1979.

46. Milligan DW, MacNamee R, Roberts BE, Davies JA: The influence of iron-deficiency indices on whole blood viscosity in polycythemia. Br J Haematol 50:467–473, 1982

47. Milligan DW, Roberts BE, Davies JA: Iron deficiency and whole blood viscosity in polycythemia (letter). Br J Haematol 51:501–503, 1982

48. Pearson TC, Grimes AJ, Slater NGP, Wetherley-Mein G: Viscosity and iron deficiency in treated polycythemia. Br J Haematol 49:123–127, 1981.

49. Birgegard G, Carlsson M, Sandhagen B, Mannting F: Does iron deficiency in treated polycythemia vera affect whole blood viscosity? Acta Med Scand 216:165–269, 1984

50. Lane DW: The influence of iron deficiency indices on whole blood viscosity in polycythemia (letter). Br J Haematol 51:503–504, 1982

51. Dintenfass L, Jedrzejczyk H, Willard A: Photographic, stereological, and statistical methods in evaluation of aggregation of red cells in disease: I. Kinetics of aggregation. Biorheology 19:567–577, 1982

52. Joly M, Lacombe C, Quemada D: Application of the transient flow rheology to the study of abnormal human bloods. Biorheology 18:445–452, 1981

53. Streichman S, Segal E, Tatarsky I, Marmur A: ¹²Moving boundary electrophoresis and sialic acid content of normal and polycythaemic red blood cells. J Haematol 48:273–279, 1981

54. Berlin NI: Diagnosis and classification of the polycythemias. Semin Hematol 12:339–351, 1975

55. Schmid-Schönbein GW, Usami S, Skalak R, Chien S: The interaction of leukocytes and erythrocytes in capillary and postcapillary vessels. Microvasc Res 19:45–70, 1980

56. Goldsmith HL: Deformation of human red cells in tube flow. Biorheology 7:235–242, 1971

57. Sarelius IH, Duling BR: Direct measurement of microvessel hematocrit, red cell flux, velocity, and transit time. Am J Physiol 243:H1018–1026, 1982

58. Kanzow G, Pries AR, Gaehtgens P: Analysis of the hematocrit distribution in the mesenteric microcirculation. Int J Microcirc Clin Exp 1:67–79, 1982

59. House S, Lipowsky HH: Distribution of microvessel hematocrit and blood flow in cremaster muscle. Microvasc Res 29:225–226, 1985

60. Lipowsky HH, Firrell JC: Microvascular hemodynamics during systemic hemoconcentration and dilution. Am J Physiol (in press)

61. McDonald DA: Blood Flow in Arteries. London, Edward Arnold, 1960

62. Oka S: Theoretical considerations of the flow of blood through a capillary. In Copley AL (ed): Proc. 4th Int. Congr. Rheol., Providence, Rhode Island, 1963 (Pt.4: Symp. Biorheology). New York, Interscience, 1965, pp 89–102

63. Goldsmith HL, Karino T: Physical and mathematical models of blood flow: experimental studies. *In* Cokelet GR, Meiselman HJ, Brooks DE (eds): Erythrocyte Mechanics and Blood Flow. New York, Liss, 1980, pp 165–194

64. Chien S: Transport across arterial endothelium. *In* Spaet TH (ed): Progress in Hemostasis and Thrombosis, vol 4. New York, Grune and Stratten, 1978, pp 1–36

65. Caro CG, Pedley TJ, Schroter RC, Seed WA: The Mechanics of the Circulation. Oxford, Oxford University Press, 1978

66. Fung YC: Biodynamics Circulation. New York, Springer-Verlag, 1984

67. Lamport H: Hemodynamics. *In* Fulton JF (ed): Texbook of Physiology, 17th ed. Philadelphia, Saunders, 1955, p 595

68. Lipowsky HH, Zweifach BW: Methods for the simultaneous measurement of pressure differentials and flow in single unbranched vessels of the microcirculation for rheological studies. Microvasc Res 14:345–361, 1977

69. Chien S, Dellenback RJ, Usami S, et al: Blood volume, hemodynamic and metabolic changes in hemorrhagic shock in normal and splenectomized dogs. Am J. Physiol 225:866–879, 1973

70. Richardson TQ, Guyton AC: Effects of polycythemia and anemia on cardiac output and the circulatory factors. Am J Physiol 197:1167–1170, 1959

71. Murray JF, Gold P, Johnson BL Jr: The circulatory effects of hematocrit variation in normovolemic and hypervolemic dogs. J Clin Invest 42:1150–1159, 1963

72. Cobb LA, Kramer RJ, Finch CA: Circulatory effects of chronic hypervolemia in polycythemia vera. J Clin Invest 39:1722–1728, 1960

73. Segel N, Bishop JM: Circulatory studies in polycythemia vera at rest and during exercise. Clin Sci 32:527–549, 1967

74. Weber PM, Pollycove M, Bacaner MB, Lawrence JH: Cardiac output in polycythemia vera. J Lab Clin Med 73:753–762, 1969

75. Brown MM, Wade JPH, Marshall J: Fundamental importance of arterial oxygen content in the regulation of cerebral blood flow in man. Brain 108:81–93, 1985

76. Hudak ML, Koehler RC, Rosenberg AA, et al: The effect of hematocrit on cerebral blood flow: differentiation of viscosity and oxygen content effects. Microvasc Res 29:226, 1985

77. Kety SS, Schmidt CF: The effects of altered arterial tensions of carbon dioxide and oxygen on cerebral blood flow and cerebral oxygen consumption of normal young men. J Clin Invest 27:484–499, 1948.

78. Bollinger A, Luthy E: Blood viscosity and blood flow in the human forearm. Helv Med Acta 34:255–264, 1967

79. Milligan DW, Tooke JE, Davies JA: Effect of venesection on calf blood flow in polycythemia. Br Med J 284:619–620, 1982

80. Jan KM, Chien S: Effect of hematocrit variations on coronary hemodynamics and oxygen utilization. Am J Physiol 233:H106–H133, 1977

81. Fan F-C, Schuessler GB, Chen RYZ, Chien S: Effect of hematocrit alteration on the regional hemodynamics and oxygen transport. Am J Physiol 238:H545–H552, 1980

82. Jan K-M, Heldman J, Chien S: Coronary hemodynamics and oxygen utilization after hematocrit variations in hemorrhage. Am J Physiol 239:H326–H332, 1980

83. Chien S: Present state of blood rheology. *In* Messmer K, Schmid-Schönbein H (eds): Hemodilution: Theoretical Basis and Clinical Application. Basel, Karger, 1972, pp 1–45

ACKNOWLEDGMENTS: We wish to acknowledge the support of NIH Grants P01 HL-43026 and R01 HL 44147 from the National Heart, Lung and Blood Institute.

11

Urate Metabolism in the Polycythemias

TS'AI-FAN YU

Excessive hematopoiesis in polycythemia vera (PV) results in varying degrees of overproduction of granulocytes, thrombocytes, and erythrocytes. The bone marrow and circulating cells appear morphologically normal but display chromosomal and functional characteristics suggesting that PV ultimately is caused by proliferation of abnormal hematopoietic clones.[1] The excessive cellular proliferation in PV results in increased synthesis and degradation of nucleoprotein and the production of increased amounts of uric acid. Serum uric acid greater than 7.0 mg/dl is present in 30 to 50 percent of patients. Hyperuricosuria is prevalent unless renal function is impaired. Both hyperuricemia and hyperuricosuria tend to increase in frequency and severity as PV progresses to the spent phase and eventually to the myeloid metaplasia stage with marked hepatosplenomegaly related to extramedullary hematopoiesis. Symptomatic gout may develop in 5 to 10 percent of these patients.[2]

Gout associated with PV may present a quite different clinical picture from what one sees in primary gout. The incidence of females with primary gout is usually 5 percent, but in PV it is more than 10 percent. Mean age of onset for primary gout is 44 years, with a very wide range from 13 to 81 years of age. The mean age of onset of gout in PV is usually more than a decade older, and the interval between the onset of PV and of gout is usually about 10 years. The range of age of onset is not very wide, apparently related to the limited life span in those with

this blood disorder. The incidence of positive family history of gout is approximately 30 percent in primary gout, but it is much lower in gout with PV (Fig. 11–1). The higher incidence of females, later age of onset, and positive family history of gout become more pronounced in spent-phase PV and myeloid metaplasia.

SERUM URATE CONCENTRATION AND URINARY URIC ACID

Mean serum urate concentrations in healthy nongouty men vary between 5.0 and 7.0 mg/dl, and the value is approximately 1 mg/dl less for females. In primary gout, the mean serum urate level is approximately 9.0 mg/dl. Serum urate above 11 mg/dl occurs in about 14 percent of patients, and normouricemia less than 7.0 mg/dl occurs in 3 percent only. Hyperuricemia in PV may be seen in as many as 30 to 50 percent of patients. In those with secondary gout, the mean serum urate level is even higher, more than 11 mg/dl in 60 percent, reflecting a distinct increase in uric acid biosynthesis (Fig. 11–2A).

In normal men, the 24-hour urinary uric acid level is usually between 400 and 600 mg, and the uric acid nitrogen to total nitrogen ratio is 1.5 ± 0.3 percent if intake of dietary protein is 75 to 100 g/d. Approximately 20 percent of patients with primary gout may have a significantly increased daily excretion of uric acid to more than 800 mg, with the

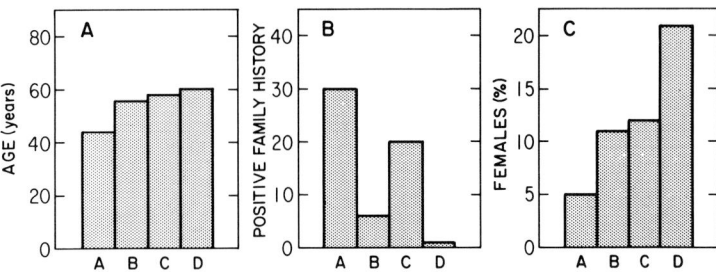

FIGURE 11-1. Clinical history: (A) age of onset, (B) family history, and (C) incidence of females (1 = primary gout, 2 = gout in polycythemia vera, 3 = gout in spent polycythemia, 4 = gout in myeloid metaplasia).

uric acid nitrogen to total nitrogen ratio exceeding 1.5 percent on similar protein intake, indicative of an increased endogenous uric acid metabolism. In PV with gout, urinary excretion of uric acid of more than 800 mg/d occurs in almost 40 percent, indicative of an even more active urate biosynthesis and excretion (Fig. 11-2B).

With spent-phase PV and myeloid metaplasia, hyperuricemia and hyperuricosuria become even more striking (Fig. 11-3). However, when kidney function is impaired, the excessive excretion disappears regardless of the stages of the blood dyscrasia.

MISCIBLE POOL AND TURNOVER RATE OF URIC ACID

A more precise way to know the amount of uric acid within the body is to assess the size of the miscible pool of uric acid. Following a single intravenous injection of uric acid-1,3-^{15}N or uric acid-2-^{14}C of known isotope abundance, the pool size can be calculated from the rate of decline in the isotope abundance in daily urine of the succeeding days.[3-9] In a normal steady state, the miscible pool of uric acid is constant in size, and its rate of replacement should balance the rate of removal. Studies have shown that the quantity of uric

acid turnover each day exceeds the quantity appearing in urine. The difference in amount is indicative of uric acid disposed of by routes other than the kidney.

In the nongouty man, the uric acid pool approximates 1100 mg, with a range of about 800 to 1300 mg. The turnover rate of uric acid is approximately 60 percent of the total pool size. The size of the pool is generally increased in gout, and so is the turnover rate. In nontophaceous gout or gout with minimal tophi, the pool size may be increased two to three times. In patients with severe tophaceous involvement, the uric acid pool may show a 10- to 20-fold increase.[10,11] Following the use of uricosuric agents, uric acid pool size is usually diminished.[11,12] In one report, the pool size was dramatically reduced from 31,000 to 2000 mg after salicylate administration. This clearly indicates a dynamic equilibrium between body fluid and the tophus. In estimating the isotope abundance in a tophus, it has been shown that the superficial surface is miscible with the uric acid pool, but the deeper layers are not.

In PV, the size of the miscible pool of uric acid depends likewise on the presence or absence of tophi. In nontophaceous cases, the pool size may be normal or slightly elevated. In tophaceous cases, the pool size is usually much more enlarged. As shown in Table

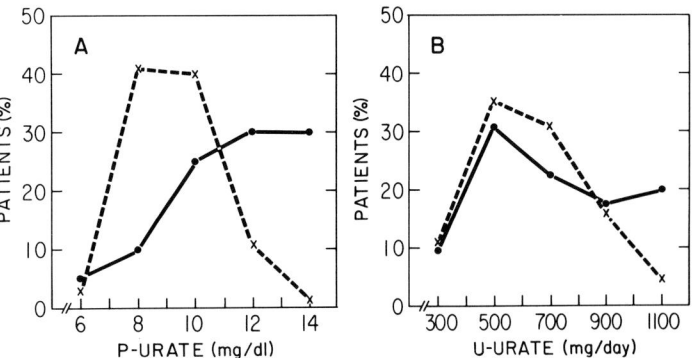

FIGURE 11-2. Distribution of (A) plasma urate (mg/dl) and (B) urinary urate (mg/d) (broken line = primary gout; solid line = gout secondary to polycythemia vera).

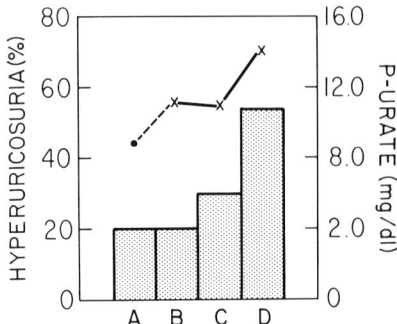

FIGURE 11-3. Hyperuricemia and hyperuricosuria in (A) primary gout, (B) polycythemia vera, (C) spent polycythemia, and (D) myeloid metaplasia.

11-1, case 1 had a slightly enlarged uric acid pool size of 1555 mg, a turnover rate of 935 mg/d, and renal excretion of 570 mg/d. Thus about 60 percent of the daily uric acid production was excreted by the kidneys, and 40 percent was eliminated by extrarenal routes. In case 2, the miscible pool size was further increased. The turnover rate was greatly augmented to 1463 mg/d, and urinary excretion was 664 mg/d, not much increased, and the extrarenal excretion was up to 799 mg/d. It is conceivable that only a part of this quan-

tity of uric acid was excreted by way of the intestinal tract, with some retained to form tophi. This is even more striking in the last patient, in whom the miscible pool was 3180 mg, the turnover rate was markedly increased to 2200 mg/d, and yet the renal excretion was 813 mg/d. Extrarenal disposal amounted to almost 1.4 g/d. A large part of this amount presumably was diverted to subcutaneus tissues and joints to form the tophi.

BIOSYNTHESIS OF URIC ACID FROM [15N]GLYCINE

Glycine is a specific precursor of carbon atoms 4 and 5 and nitrogen atom 7 of uric acid (Fig. 11–4). In studying the biosynthesis of uric acid using labeled glycine, each subject is given 15N-glycine (60 atom percent excess 15N) in a single oral dose of 100 mg/kg of body weight. Daily 24-hour urine collection is made for a varying number of days. After 15N-glycine feeding, there is a relatively rapid incorporation of the isotope into urinary uric acid. In nongouty subjects, the peak isotope abundance of uric acid is approximately 0.1 atom percent excess within 2

TABLE 11-1. MISCIBLE POOL OF URIC ACID IN GOUT SECONDARY TO POLYCYTHEMIA VERA

CASE	TOPHI	MISCIBLE POOL (mg)	TURNOVER RATE (mg/d)	URINARY URIC ACID (mg/d)	EXTRARENAL EXCRETION (mg/d)
1*	0	1555	935	570	365
2	+ +	3070	1463	664	799
3	+ + +	3180	2200	813	1387

* Patient subsequently developed gout, but not at time of the study.

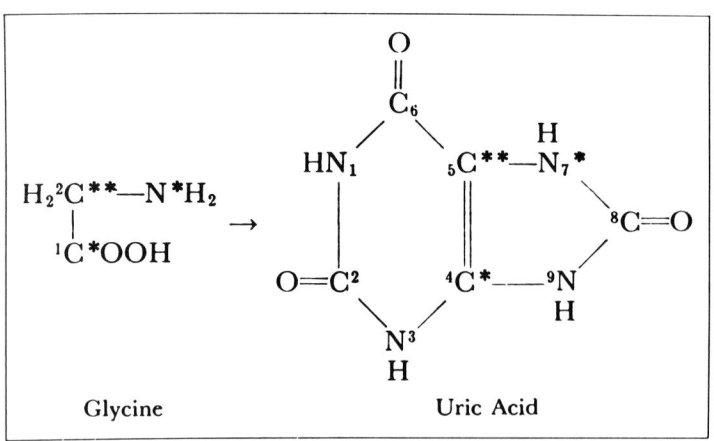

FIGURE 11-4. Glycine as specific precursor of uric acid for carbon atoms 4 and 5 and nitrogen atom 7 of uric acid. (Reproduced with permission from Gutman et al: Am J Med 25:917, 1958.)

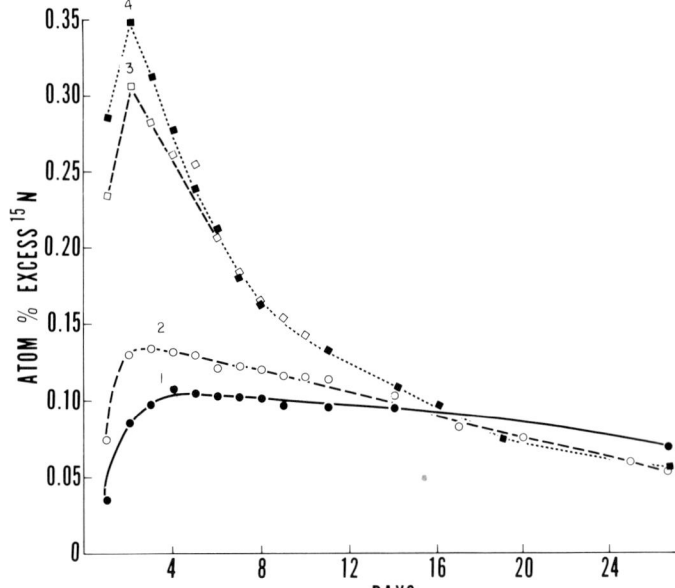

FIGURE 11-5. Rate of ^{15}N incorporation into uric acid after ^{15}Nglycine (1,2 = normal; 3,4 = primary gout).

to 4 days, followed by a very slow rate of decline in excretion of urinary uric acid ^{15}N for weeks thereafter. The incorporation of ^{15}N from labeled glycine into urinary uric acid in some gouty patients, notably in those who habitually excrete excess uric acid, reaches its maximum during the first and second days, indicative of a direct overproduction of uric acid via a shunt pathway. The excessive incorporation of uric acid is approximately three times normal (Fig. 11-5). A number of gouty subjects without excess urinary uric acid excretion frequently show no indication of overincorporation of uric acid. The ^{15}N

incorporation into uric acid in such patients nevertheless is significantly increased at the N-9 and N-3 positions (Fig. 11-6). Similar results showing excessive biosynthesis of uric acid are also demonstrable using ^{14}C or ^{13}C precursors of uric acid.[9,15]

In PV, there is some diversion of glycine into the metabolic pathways leading to synthesis of hemoglobin and nucleic acid in order to meet the increased requirements of excessive hematopoiesis. Studies of ^{15}N-glycine incorporation into hemin in PV reveal a more than two-fold increase in the rate of red cell and hemoglobin production.

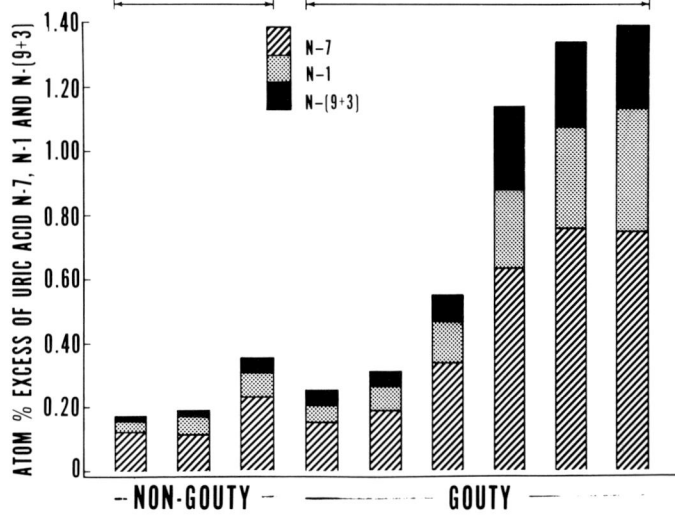

FIGURE 11-6. Intramolecular distribution of atom percent excess in uric acid ^{15}N after ^{15}Nglycine in three nongouty and six gouty subjects.

Augmented hematopoiesis in the polycythemias is reflected also in the rate and magnitude of ^{15}N-glycine incorporation into uric acid. Different patterns of isotopic incorporation into uric acid are seen in patients with PV (Fig. 11–7). After oral ^{15}N-glycine administration in PV, there is a less than normal incorporation into uric acid ^{15}N in the first few days, and then there is a slow steady enrichment of ^{15}N in urinary uric acid. A peak abundance is not reached until about the fifteenth day, and then there is a very slow decline over a period of weeks, as seen in the normal subject. The low initial concentration of the isotope in urinary uric acid is not accounted for solely by dilution with slowly formed unlabeled uric acid. It is probably due to some diversion of glycine from the rapid shunt pathways of uric acid biosynthesis to the slower metabolic routes involving incorporation into intracellular nucleic acids, a redistribution consistent with the exaggerated hematopoietic requirements of this disorder. A high percentage of ingested ^{15}N-glycine also may be diverted to urea formation instead of uric acid. The cumulative incorporation of ^{15}N-glycine into urinary uric acid is high. This demonstrates unequivocally that uric acid overproduction is sometimes comparable with that seen in overproducers with primary gout. It is of interest to note that there is no difference in the rate and magnitude of ^{15}N-glycine incorporation into uric acid in patients with PV with or without gout (see Fig. 11–7).

In secondary polycythemia, the rate of incorporation of ^{15}N-glycine into urinary uric acid may differ from case to case. The rate curve in one of the two subjects studied is comparable with that seen in PV. The slope of the curve of isotope incorporation is slightly less than normal during the first 4 days; then there is a slow progression to reach a peak abundance of 0.12 atom percent excess on or about the tenth day and thereafter a gradual decline after the thirtieth day. In another patient, the rate of incorporation is not unlike that in a normal subject without polycythemia or gout. Such differences in the rate of incorporation may be due to the varying rates of erythrogenesis. It may also be related to the differences in metabolic pathways of hematopoiesis and the enhanced production of myeloid cells characteristic of the late phases of the myeloproliferative disorders play a part.[16]

URINARY EXCRETION OF PURINE BASES

Enzymatic hydrolysis of polynucleotide chains of nucleic acids to form oligonucleotides occurs through the action of various nucleases. Oligonucleotides are cleaved to form mononucleotides and then nucleosides by various nucleotidases and phosphatases. The nucleosides may be absorbed intact or may be broken down further to form purine bases by respective enzymes. Whereas adenine, hypoxanthine, and guanine are formed exclusively from the corresponding nucleosides, xanthine may be formed from xanthosine, hypoxanthine, and guanine. These

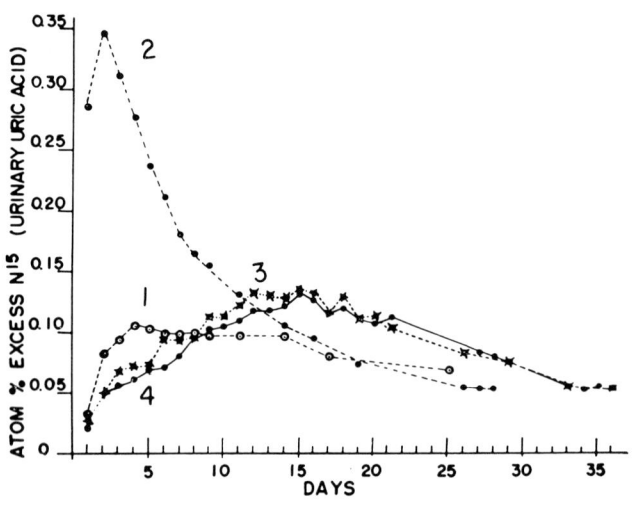

FIGURE 11–7. Rate of ^{15}N incorporation into uric acid after ^{15}Nglycine (1 = normal; 2 = primary gout; 3 = polycythemia vera with gout; 4 = polycythemia vera with no gout).

purine bases, except adenine, are readily converted to form uric acid. Small amounts of purine bases, some methylated, are excreted in urine.

In normal humans, the daily urinary excretion of hypoxanthine is approximately 10 mg, and that of xanthine and 7-methylguanine is 6 mg each. Excretion of other purine bases ranges between 0.5 and 1.5 mg daily (Table 11–2). The excretion of individual purine base may vary 50 to 100 percent within a group of normal subjects and may vary over a 50 percent range in the same individual over an extended time interval.[16]

Hypoxanthine and xanthine excretion in primary gout is significantly less. A twofold increase in 8-OH,7-methylguanine may be observed during an attack of acute gouty arthritis. A decreased excretion of hypoxanthine and xanthine is likewise observed in PV. This decrease is exaggerated in patients with advanced disease, such as myelofibrosis in the terminal stage. There is also a two- to threefold elevation of 8-OH,7-methylguanine excretion. On the other hand, hypoxanthine and xanthine excretion is not strikingly low, nor is there any abnormal increase in 8-OH,7-methylguanine in a patient with mild secondary polycythemia. The less than normal excretion in hypoxanthine and xanthine may be related to the overactivity of xanthine oxidase, which converts hypoxanthine and xanthine to uric acid. The mechanism of high 8-OH,7-methylguanine excretion is not understood.

ACUTE GOUTY ARTHRITIS

Patients with primary gout may go to bed without symptoms or any premonitory warning. The pain may start suddenly in sleep, reaching to intolerable distress in a few hours, with all the cardinal signs of acute inflammation. With appropriate therapeutic measures, such patients may become perfectly asymptomatic in a day or two or even in a briefer period of time.

Acute gouty arthritis in PV can be quite atypical. The onset of an attack may be insiduous. Instead of the classical podagra, frequently other joints are attacked. The attack is usually polyarticular instead of monarticular. The clinical course may be quite irregular despite the use of various potent antigout measures.[17] Whereas satisfactory response to treatment for acute attack in primary gout usually occurs within several days in more than 90 percent, in gout secondary to active PV, it is about 70 percent only. The efficacy is further reduced to less than 40 to 50 percent in spent-phase PV and myeloid metaplasia (Fig. 11–8A).

In primary gout, the most apparent precipitating cause of an acute attack is attributable to emotional stress or overindulgence in food and drink. In gout secondary to PV, acute attacks may follow phlebotomy, blood transfusion, or chemotherapy. In other words, attacks are more likely due to stress related to the underlying blood dyscrasia.

NEPHROLITHIASIS[18]

It is well known that many patients suffering from gout also may have kidney stones. The suggestion of a causal relationship between gout and urinary tract stones dates back to the time of Galen in the second century A.D. As many as 25 percent of patients with primary gout may have kidney stones.

TABLE 11–2. URINARY EXCRETION OF PURINE BASES (mg/dl) IN NORMAL, POLYCYTHEMIA VERA, MYELOFIBROSIS IN THE TERMINAL PHASE, AND SECONDARY POLYCYTHEMIA

	NORMAL		POLYCYTHEMIA VERA, RANGE	MYELOFIBROSIS, RANGE	POLYCYTHEMIA SECONDARY
	Mean	Range			
Hypoxanthine	9.7	5.9–13.2	2.5–7.5	1.6–3.1	7.5
Xanthine	6.1	5.1–8.6	2.7–4.7	1.1–2.6	3.1
1-Methyl and 7-methyl-guanine	6.5	5.5–7.8	2.6–7.3	3.2–7.7	4.2
Adenine	1.4	1.1–1.7	1.4–1.5	1.7–1.7	1.1
Guanine	0.4	0.2–0.6	0.2–0.7	0.3–0.3	0.5
8-OH, 7-Methyl-guanine	1.6	1.1–2.0	3.3–4.3	2.2–3.7	1.1

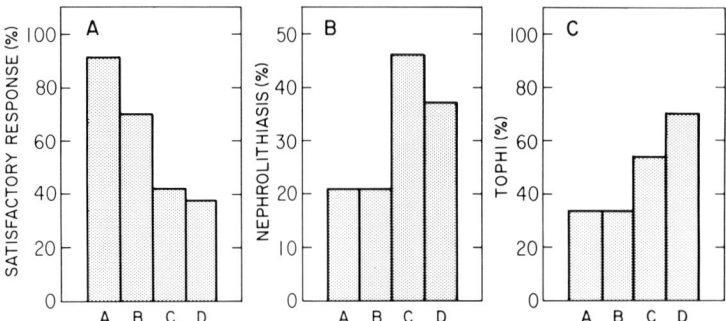

FIGURE 11-8. Clinical features: (A) response to treatment in acute gouty arthritis, (B) prevalence of nephrolithiasis, (C) prevalence of tophi (1 = primary gout, 2 = gout in polycythemia vera, 3 = gout in spent polycythemia, 4 = gout in myeloid metaplasia).

Chemical composition of the stones is uric acid and/or urate in 80 percent of cases.

Under normal circumstances, urine pH is subject to wide diurnal fluctuations, being more acid at night and in the early morning and less acid after meals. In primary gout, the circadian rhythm is not apparent, and urine is usually unduly acidic. Urine collected in the morning after an overnight fast has a pH of 5.0 or less in more than 40 percent of patients and a pH of 5.7 or more in less than 10 percent. Under similar conditions, barely 15 percent of normal subjects may have a pH of 5.0 or less, and nearly 30 percent have a pH of 5.7 or more (Table 11-3).

Daily urinary uric acid in primary gout is more or less within a similar range to that of normal subjects if serum uric acid is less than 9 mg/dl. When serum urate gets above 11 mg/dl, excess urinary uric acid occurs much more frequently. The chance of uric acid lithiasis is 40 to 50 percent if urinary uric acid exceeds 1 g/d (Table 11-4). About half those patients with stones may have recurrent renal lithiasis. On very rare occasions, obstructive uropathy, anuria, and pyelonephritis may result.

In PV, excessive uric acid production and augmented turnover of nucleic acids lead to very high serum uric acid and urinary uric

TABLE 11-4. PREVALENCE OF RENAL CALCULI IN PRIMARY GOUT: CORRELATION WITH PLASMA URATE AND URINARY URATE EXCRETION

PLASMA URATE (P) URINARY URATE (U)	RENAL CALCULI
P: <9 mg/dl U: <600 mg/d	<30%
P: 9–11 mg/dl U: 600-799 mg/d	30–40%
P: >11 mg/dl U: 800–1000 mg/d	40–50%

acid excretion levels, which in turn cause precipitation of uric acid in the urinary tract. This hazard is further increased with acceleration of uric acid degradation after radio- or chemotherapy. Prevalence of lithiasis is double that in primary gout (Fig. 11-8B), particularly during the spent stage and the myeloid metaplasia stage.

Urinary obstruction by aggregates of uric acid crystals at the ureteropelvic junction may result in hydronephrosis, which on rare occasions may require surgical intervention. With repeated obstruction and surgical maneuvers, urinary tract infection may result. With infection by urea-splitting organisms, staghorn stones composed of magnesium ammonium phosphate (struvite), may form, occupying the entire ureteropelvic junction, with dilatation of renal pelvis and calyces and thinning of the renal cortex (Fig. 11-9). Aggregates of uric acid crystals at times may cause cavitation in the renal parenchyma. The kidney may reveal urate deposits or microcalculi in the collecting tubules. There may be evidence of acute or chronic pyelonephritis. Struvite stones are friable and tend to recur. With recurrent stones and persistent infection, nephrectomy may become

TABLE 11-3. URINE PH IN PRIMARY GOUT AND NORMAL SUBJECTS

URINE	PRIMARY GOUT		NORMAL SUBJECTS	
	No.	Percent	No.	Percent
<4.8–5.0	133	41	12	15
5.1–5.6	166	51	47	59
5.7–6.5	26	8	21	26
TOTAL	325		80	

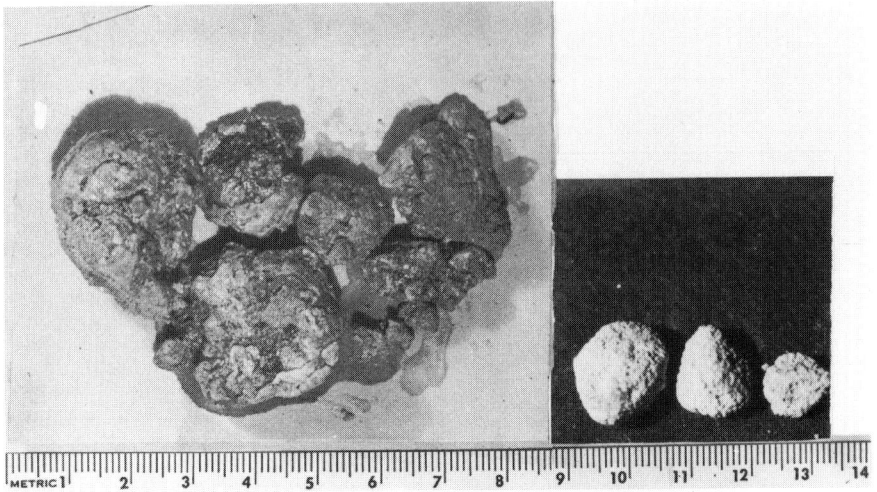

FIGURE 11-9. Renal calculi: (A) staghorn calculus, (B) uric acid calculi.

necessary. In some cases, renal function deteriorates, and renal insufficiency follows.

Prevention of nephrolithiasis is largely accomplished by the use of allopurinol, which reduces the rate of uric acid production. Better control of the primary condition likewise lessens urate production and excretion rate. Thus one has less frequently encountered poorly controlled nephrolithiasis and its various complications in the last two decades.

TOPHI

Formation of tophi depends on the degree of hyperuricemia and its duration. In primary gout, about 40 percent of patients may become tophaceous, mostly minimal at 5 years after the first attack. At 10 years, its incidence increases to 50 percent, and some tophi may become quite extensive.[19]

Tophi rarely occur before the first attack of acute gouty arthritis and seldom appear if the serum urate level remains less than 9 mg/dl. In PV, prevalence of tophi is 33 percent in its active stage, increased to 53 percent in the spent stage, and to 70 percent in the myeloid metaplasia stage (Fig. 11–8C). Tophi may be detectable shortly after or even before the first attack of acute gouty arthritis in about a third of patients. Tophi in some patients may develop very rapidly and cause disability in a short time. In some, discharging sinuses develop, resulting in sepsis and

gangrene, at times requiring amputation. As shown in a patient with gout secondary to PV, the tophi of both hands and one foot were extensive, and the other foot had been amputated for extremely extensive tophi with gangrene (Fig. 11–10). In a rare patient, urate deposits were found in the mitral ring of the left side of the heart in addition to extensive tophi in various organs, including the kidneys and subcutaneous tissues. By correcting the abnormal urate metabolism with allopurinol, such formidable consequences of urate deposits are prevented.

THERAPEUTIC MEASURES

Since secondary gout in PV can be quite atypical, it is important to use prophylactic colchicine daily. Colchicine, 0.6 mg daily, is advisable, particularly if the treatment for the blood dyscrasia is not under control.

The hyperuricemia in PV is often associated with excessive excretion of uric acid and nephrolithiasis. Thus uricosuric agents, such as probenecid or sulfinpyrazone, should not be used. Allopurinol is the drug of choice, since its main action is reduction of uric acid production.

A satisfactory uric acid level in blood and urine is frequently reached with a daily dose of 200 to 300 mg allopurinol. Adequate hydration is always important. Slow and steady weight reduction is preferable. Weight fluc-

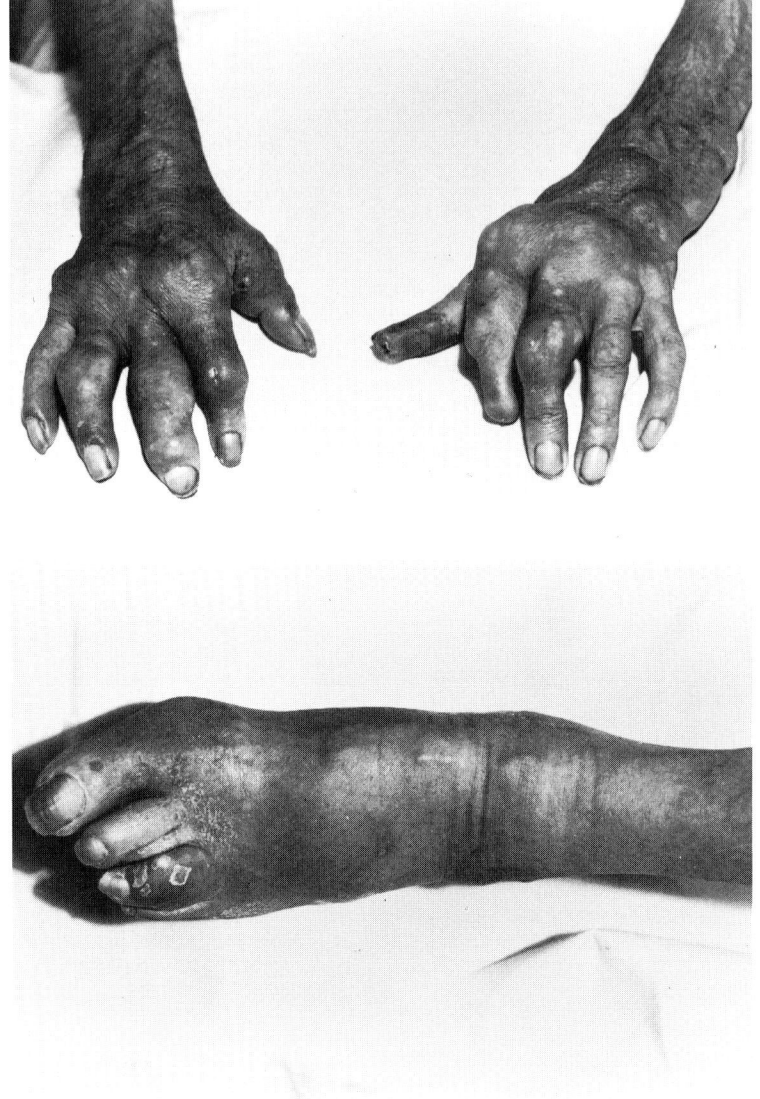

FIGURE 11-10. Tophi in gout secondary to polycythemia vera: (A) both hands, (B) left foot.

tuation by frequent change in dietary habits should be avoided. In those with renal function impairment, dietary fat and proteins should be reduced, and the degree of hydration should be carefully observed. Unsatisfactory response is usually related to poor control of hematologic conditions and severe damage to renal function. And lastly, too many drugs administered concurrently may cause unfavorable drug interactions. Most important is that the patient's physician know what medications, particularly homeopathic drugs, the patient is taking. Periodic blood

examination, including liver and kidney functions, are necessary. Medications may be changed periodically according to one's clinical conditions and laboratory findings.

SUMMARY

Increased hematopoiesis in PV is characterized by increased turnover of nucleic acid, which is associated with marked hyperuricemia, excessive hyperusicosuria, an augmented uric acid pool, and an accelerated rate of its biosythesis, particularly in spent-phase PV and myeloid metaplasia. Acute gouty arthritis in PV is frequently atypical in its clinical presentation. Colchicine prophylaxis is therefore indicated. Extensive tophaceous deposits and recurrent nephrolithiasis frequently complicate the clinical course. With better control of the blood picture in PV and the use of allopurinol in more recent years, urate biosynthesis tends to be normalized and the clinical sequelae modified or entirely prevented.

REFERENCES

1. Adamson JW, Fialkow PJ, Murphy S, et al: Polycythemia vera: Stem cell and probably clonal origin of the disease. N Engl J Med 295:913–916, 1976
2. Yu TF: Secondary gout associated with myeloproliferative diseases. Arthritis Rheum 8:765–771, 1965
3. Benedict JD, Forsham PH, Stetten D Jr: The metabolism of uric acid in the normal and gouty human studied with the aid of isotopic uric acid. J Biol Chem 181:183–193, 1949
4. Geren W, Bendich A, Bodansky O, Brown GB: The fate of uric acid in man. J Biol Chem 183:21–31, 1950
5. Bishop C, Garner W, Talbott JH: Pool size turnover rate and rapidity of equilibration of injected isotopic uric acid in normal and pathological subjects. J Clin Invest 30:879–888, 1951
6. Buzard J, Bishop C, Talbott JH: Recovery in humans of intravenously injected isotopic uric acid. J Biol Chem 196:179–184, 1952
7. Wyngaarden JB, Stetten D Jr: Uricolysis in normal man. J Biol Chem 203:9–21, 1953
8. Wyngaarden JB: Overproduction of uric acid as the cause of hyperuricemia in primary gout. J Clin Invest 36:1508–1515, 1957
9. Sorensen LB: Elimination of uric acid studied by means of ^{14}C-labeled uric acid. Scand J Clin Lab Invest Suppl 54:90–111, 1960
10. Seegmiller JE, Grayzel AI, Laster L, Liddle L: Uric acid production in gout. J Clin Invest 40:1304–1314, 1961
11. Benedict JD, Forsham PH, Roche M, et al: The effect of salicylate and adrenocortical hormone upon the miscible pool of uric acid in gout. J Clin Invest 29:1104–1111, 1950
12. Bishop C, Rand R, Talbott JH: The effect of benemid p-(di-n-propylsulfamyl) benzoic acid in uric acid metabolism in one normal and one gouty subject. J Clin Invest 30:889–895, 1951
13. Benedict JD, Roche M, Yu TF, et al: Incorporation of glycine nitrogen into uric acid in normal and gouty man. Metabolism 1:3–12, 1952
14. Gutman AB, Yu TF, Adler J, Javitt NB: Intramolecular distribution of uric acid-^{15}N after administration of glycine-^{15}N and ammonium-^{15}N chloride to gouty and nongouty subjects. J Clin Invest 41:623–636, 1962
15. Gutman AB, Yu TF, Black H, et al: Incorporation of glycine-1-^{14}C, glycine-2-^{14}C and glycine-^{15}N into uric acid in normal and gouty subjects. Am J Med 25:917–932, 1958
16. Yu TF, Weissman B, Sharney L, et al: On the biosynthesis of uric acid from glycine-^{15}N in primary and secondary polycythemia. Am J Med 21:901–917, 1956
17. Yu TF, Weinreb N, Wittman R, Wasserman LR: Secondary gout associated with chronic myeloproliferative disorders. Semin Arthritis Rheum 5:247–256, 1976
18. Yu TF: Nephrolithiasis. In Yu TF, Berger L (eds): The Kidney in Gout and Hyperuricemia. Mount Kisco, NY, Futura, 1982, Chap 6, pp 195–232
19. Yu TF, Gutman AB: Principles of current management of primary gout. Am J Med Sci 254:893–904, 1967

12

The Epidemiology of Polycythemia Vera

BARUCH MODAN

Once almost strictly limited to the study of infectious diseases, epidemiologic methods have now become an indisputable component in the assessment of any condition leading to health impairment. Establishment of the epidemiologic features of a specific disease may shed light on its etiology and be indicative of potential preventive measures.

The epidemiologic approach to causality infers three major phases: (1) descriptive characteristics or mapping, (2) analytic design or risk-factor determination, and (3) prognostic assessment or health care evaluation. Of these, only the former has been more than sparsely undertaken in the study of polycythemia vera (PV). In this framework, fairly adequate information has been accumulated on the incidence of PV and on its relationship to certain other clinical syndromes. Evidence on the role of environmental factors in the disease etiology is still lacking.

MAGNITUDE

Because of the relatively benign nature of PV, efforts to assess its population occurrence from mortality records would be futile, while analysis of morbidity data necessitates a thorough search of hospital records, outpatient specialty clinics, and files of hematologists practicing in the community. Estimates of the incidence of PV are therefore weighted by hospital admissions and confounded by the significant proportion of patients treated at home by general practitioners and those referred to ambulatory clinics, where only little registration exists.

In recent years, PV has been added to the neoplastic categories of the U.S. National Cancer Institute SEER Program, the IARC publications, and the International Classification of Diseases (ICD). Although this administrative decision may be questioned on nosologic grounds, it has contributed valuable knowledge and will doubtless enable a more comprehensive assessment in the future.

On the basis of worldwide information collated from those cancer registries which have followed the new classification routine,[1] the modal annual incidence of PV in Western countries in the 1970s ranged between 5 and 15 cases per 1 million population, while in developing countries it was barely noticeable. It must be emphasized that these figures depend strongly on the quality of medical care and on the completeness of registration in each individual country.

Estimates based on more refined evaluation of cancer registry data range from an annual incidence of 9.1 per 1 million in England and Wales[2] for the 1968–1982 period up to 14.6 per 1 million in western Australia[3] during 1960–1969. These rates reflect varying degrees of flexibility with regard to the diagnostic criteria. An annual mortality rate of 2.7 estimated for England and Wales[2] is an obvious underestimate, since PV is only infrequently marked on death certificates.

More finite information can be deduced from several population studies undertaken over the past 20 years. The first community-wide study of PV, conducted in Baltimore, Maryland, was based on all hospital admissions in the area during the 1951–1969 time period.[4] An estimate of 4.9 new cases per 1 million residents per year and a mean annual prevalence of 6.3 per 1 million were observed. This estimate is compatible with the results obtained in the course of a subsequent nationwide study conducted in Israel for the 1955–1966 period,[5] where a mean annual incidence of 6.6 cases per 1 million was found, and with the incidence rate of 3.5 million observed in Oklahoma City[6] during 1965–1971.

Data obtained in three smaller communities differ markedly. An annual incidence of 16 per 1 million was observed in Rochester, Minnesota,[7] during 1935–1969, while an extreme rate of 35 per 1 million was noted in Elyria, Ohio, in 1977–1979.[8] The latter figures may reflect, however, an exceedingly high awareness in the vicinity of the Mayo Clinic and an a priori selection of one town, Elyria, on the basis of its high PV prevalence. More recently, an incidence rate of 26 per 1 million was obtained in Malmo, Sweden,[9] on the basis of hospital records. Again, this may reflect better awareness in recent years.

HOST FACTORS

The disease usually appears during middle age and is slightly more prevalent in males.[10] Community studies yielded an age at diagnosis ranging between 57.5 and 61.5 years and a sex ratio ranging from 1.1 to 2.7. Data derived from series of patients seen in several major medical centers[11] showed a median age at diagnosis of 56.9 years (mean of 55.0 years) in both sexes, and a male-to-female ratio of 1.4 : 1. Both figures are almost identical with those obtained in the course of the long-term clinical trial[12] conducted by the Polycythemia Vera Study Group (PVSG), based on approximately 40 institutions in the United States and abroad (mean age at diagnosis 60.6 ± 0.6 years and a sex ratio of 1.3 : 1). Since a considerable number of patients included in the selected hospital series were treated by radioactive phosphorus, they could reflect, to a certain extent, the reluctance to subject a woman of child-bearing age to ionizing radiation.

Only a small number of PV cases have been reported in childhood, and barely a few of these[13-15] would meet the currently accepted strict diagnostic criteria for the disease. Others would be categorized today as familial polycythemia, a separate nosologic entity[16,17] that is referred to in more detail further on. The scattered reports of polycythemia of the newborn[18-21] probably represent physiologic variants and maternal-fetal or sibling transfusion.

On the other hand, there is practically no upper age limit to the development of PV. Gunale and Zelkowitz[23] reported a case in a 96-year-old woman, and Devesa et al.[24] pointed out two 97-year-old individuals observed in the course of the third U.S. National Cancer Survey and 17 additional subjects aged 85 to 89 years. These yielded a combined annual incidence rate of 43 per 1 million in 1969–1971 and an estimated total of 65 PV cases in the United States as a whole for the 85 years and above age category. In the 80- to 84-year age group, the incidence was 52 per 1 million, or roughly 120 cases for the whole country.

HIGH- AND LOW-RISK POPULATIONS

As in other chronic diseases, an assessment of a differential incidence of PV in distinct ethnic or racial groups may provide clues to etiologic risk factors,[25] although, as has already been noted, a wide spectrum of incidence rates could reflect variations in the level of medical care administered. Nevertheless, at least some of the discrepancies observed in the distribution of PV in distinct populations seem genuine.

More specifically, it is generally accepted that Jews have an increased risk of PV and blacks a lower one. Reznikoff et al.,[26,27] who examined the ethnic background of PV patients in six hospital clinics in New York City over 50 years ago, noted that almost 50 percent were Jews of eastern European extraction, as compared with less than 10 percent of total admissions to those hospitals. Subsequently, Damon and Holub[28] found that 33 percent of PV patients in a large New York Medical Center were Jewish, as compared with 16.1 percent of those receiving blood transfusions at the same institution. Among white patients, the respective frequencies were 34.2 and 19.7 percent.

These clinically based data could be biased by a higher tendency of Jews to obtain medical care for an essentially benign condition,[29] but they are compatible with findings obtained on a population basis in Baltimore, a city that contains a large Jewish population, and the results of a nationwide study in Israel. In the Baltimore study,[2] the rate of PV in Jewish patients was about fourfold higher than in Protestants and sixfold higher as compared with Catholics. In Israel,[3] the incidence in European-born Jews was found to be in the same range of magnitude as among Baltimore Jews, who are mostly of European origin (8.4 per 6 million and 10.4 per 6 million, respectively), but significantly higher than in Asian- and African-born Israelis. It seems, therefore, that PV is not necessarily "a Jewish disease" but is more frequently encountered in Jews of European parentage. The gradient has been confirmed recently by Chaiter et al.[30]

The apparently lower incidence of PV in blacks is more difficult to assess due to the lower referral of this population segment to specialty clinics in the past. Damon and Holub[28] observed 3.6 percent of blacks in their group of PV patients, as compared with 16.4 percent among controls. Similarly, in the Baltimore community study,[2] only 8 percent of blacks were accrued, while blacks comprised about 35 percent of the city inhabitants during the study period. The white/black ratio declined to 2:1 following age adjustment.

The practical absence of PV in African countries' cancer registries[1] also may be seen in the context of a lesser recognition of an essentially nonmalignant disease, combined with a genuine low risk to develop PV.

GENETIC PREDISPOSITION

A familial tendency of PV patients is more strongly substantiated. A number of investigators, starting already with Nikhamin[31] in 1907, reported multiple cases of PV in a single family. Spodaro and Forkner,[32] who reviewed the literature up to 1933, accepted a familial nature in the presence of a well-established PV in only six instances. They noted that such cases tend to have a more benign course, usually with splenomegaly but no leukocytosis, and suggested that these

should be considered as a separate entity—coined as *benign familial polycythemia*. This definition also has been referred to subsequently as *primary erythrocytosis*[14] or *familial erythrocytosis*.[33] Nevertheless, a familial tendency has definitely been noted in undisputed PV as well.[34-37]

Recently, the issue of genetic predisposition to PV was reassessed by Brubaker et al.[38] on the basis of the substantial material accumulated in the course of the PVSG multicenter study. Out of a total of 652 PV cases registered over close to 20 years—478 on the main protocol and 174 on various associated ones—there were 5 documented cases of PV that met the strict diagnostic criteria of the PVSG group among parents of PV patients: two fathers and two mothers of male patients and one mother of a female patient. Twenty additional patients had a suggestive family history, but only three of these had a nonparental relative with PV that met the PVSG criteria. Assuming a life span of up to 75 years and comparing the data with the Connecticut Tumor Registry, a tenfold excess was estimated.

An association of PV with specific blood groups showed a slight excess of blood group O in one study,[39] but no deviation from the expected distribution was found in three others.[28,40,41] All four studies were hampered by small samples.

Familial aggregation does not necessarily imply a genetic predisposition, since the possibility of a common exposure to an environmental substance shared by family members must always be explored. At least two families have been encountered where both husband and wife had PV.[41,42] More recently, Ratnoff and Gress[43] described the occurrence of PV in a father and son, both of whom had an intermittent exposure to organic solvents. The father, a Jewish executive, was diagnosed in 1955 at the age of 53, while his son, a chemical salesman who worked for years in his father's chemical supply firm, was diagnosed 22 years later at the age of 44. This family illustrates the difficulty of delineating genetic factors from a possible exposure to environmental bone marrow stimulants that could have led to a proliferation of a pluripotential hematopoietic stem cell or, for that matter, from a purely chance association.

POTENTIAL RISK FACTORS

There have been practically no attempts to assess the role of environmental factors in PV etiology in a controlled manner, although the literature abounds with sporadic reports of polycythemia developing in patients or in animals exposed to supposedly toxic substances. Most of such observations were confined to the period preceding World War II, and one may suspect that the lesser impact in the scientific literature subsequently is related to more effective preventive measures, more rigorous diagnostic criteria, or abandonment of the old practice of drawing conclusions from individual case histories.

Lawrence et al.[44] mentioned that 6 percent of their patients gave a history of exposure to fumes from oil, gas, or paint, but this observation was nullified by Tubiana et al.,[45] who found similar frequencies of positive history in their control patients as well. Mondon and Andre[46] reported two cases of PV in men occupationally exposed to benzene. This is supported by several other clinical observations[47,48] suggesting that this substance, in small experimental doses, is capable of producing polycythemia. Bernard[49,50] found that injection of tar into the rat bone marrow resulted in increased red and white blood cell counts, a bone marrow reaction that was considered by him to be similar to the one found in human PV, and the appearance of young white blood cells in the peripheral blood.

Several other chemical substances have at one time or another been suspected of producing polycythemia.[51-54] Of these, cobalt received most attention, first in animals and then in human subjects.[55,56] Polycythemia also was observed in 11 of 24 chronic alcoholics and attributed to the toxicity of cobalt added to the beer in the brewery.[57] Today it is well established that cobalt polycythemia is not a manifestation of PV, and with the possible exception of benzene derivates, the same is probably true for the other chemicals sporadically incriminated in PV etiology. As in many other neoplastic conditions, smoking also may play an etiologic role.[58]

The only attempt for a systematic exploration of a causal environmental factor for PV in a concrete study population was made by Caldwell et al.[59] in the course of a follow-up of approximately 3200 participants of the detonation of the "Smoky" nuclear device in August of 1957 who were traced through 1981. Two definite and two suspected cases of PV were found, while on the basis of previously described community studies, only 0.2 cases were expected to occur during 25 years in a population of this size. It is of interest to quote a single case report that detailed sequential development of PV and chronic myelocytic leukemia in a patient following radiation exposure from nuclear weapons tests.[60]

These findings may be construed as consistent with the relatively high incidence rate of PV reported in the Nagasaki Cancer Registry, a rate that stands out in comparison with other Japanese prefectures and with other Far Eastern populations. However, intriguing as they are, it is hard to accept these data as indicating a causal association with prior ionizing radiation exposure, in view of the extremely minute radiation dose involved, and the lack of supporting data from other cohorts of individuals exposed to x-radiation. It seems therefore much more likely that this is just one other example of a better detection of a rare and essentially nonmalignant disease in a cohort of healthy individuals subjected to a careful and regular follow-up procedure.

ASSOCIATION WITH OTHER DISEASES

The association of PV with other disease entities is reviewed here primarily in the context of possible common etiology. The relationship of PV with cancer, and particularly leukemia, has always stood out as a major element in understanding the nature of PV. The possible relationship of PV to leukemia was first raised in 1905 by Blumental,[61,62] who described a patient with leukocytosis and immature white cells in the peripheral blood. Myeloid leukemia was supposedly confirmed by autopsy. Numerous similar reports followed.[63-65]

With better understanding of the leukemogenic effect of ionizing radiation,[66] doubts were expressed as to whether leukemia is part of the basic process in PV or results from massive x-ray and/or ^{32}P treatment. The issue was further confounded by the argument that patients treated radioactively allegedly survive longer than those treated otherwise[67] and reach a later, supposedly natural stage of the disease that could not have been reached by a patient treated otherwise.

This led to the establishment of two schools of thought:

1.   PV is a neoplastic disorder in which an early benign course accelerates toward a fulminant neoplastic development as part and parcel of its natural course.

2. The disease is essentially benign with a subsequent induction of leukemia by radiation therapy.

Today it is quite evident[11,68,69] that although acute leukemia may occur in about 1 percent of patients naturally, its frequency is increased by tenfold or more following ^{32}P or radiomimetic therapy.[70] This issue is discussed more elaborately in Chaps. 14 and 15.

As expected, most of the leukemias are of the acute variety, only occasionally chronic myeloid. The rare association with chronic lymphocytic leukemia[71,72] must be construed as a chance association. By the same token, the occurrence of PV in association with multiple myeloma and/or gammopathy,[73-76] which has been described in the context of a possible interrelationship within the group of myeloproliferative disorders,[77,78] also may be seen as an illustration of a higher probability to detect a second blood dyscrasia in patients regularly followed by a hematologist.

The prolonged contemplation of the potentially neoplastic nature of polycythemia has raised questions about a possible association with other neoplastic disorders as well.[79,80] This issue also has been resolved recently in the course of the long-term follow-up studies mentioned above.[10,81] Since radiation carcinogenesis is by no means limited to leukemia,[82] the findings are not surprising. It is of interest, though, that the excess of non-leukemia cancer in PV patients treated by radiation or by radiomimetic agents is smaller than the respective excess of leukemia. This difference could perhaps be due to the inherent difference in the critical dose needed for the induction of distinct tumors or a variation in latency periods.

It should be mentioned that a large number of *benign* tumors have been related to polycythemia,[6,83-87] which disappeared following the tumor's extirpation, but except for a chance association, these must be considered as manifestations of secondary polycythemia.

In contrast, the thrombotic and hemorrhagic events that are frequently observed in the course of PV,[88-90] and often are singled out as leading causes of death, constitute part of the natural course of the disease even though occasionally they are related to the treatment administered.

PROSPECT

In conclusion, although PV has probably been more extensively studied than most other chronic diseases of the same magnitude for almost a full century, our knowledge regarding its epidemiology is still in the budding stage and diluted by information inferred from series of cases in which rigid diagnostic criteria have not been applied.

The disease has a late onset, peaking in the second part of the sixth decade of life, with a male-to-female ratio of about 1.3 : 1, which is similar to the one observed in most neoplastic syndromes. The annual incidence is on the order of 0.5 to 1 per 100,000 population and is strongly affected by the availability of medical care and the degree of referral of patients with benign chronic disorders to specialists. Nevertheless, a higher incidence noted among Jews of European extraction and a somewhat lower one in blacks seem to be most probably genuine.

Despite occasional suggestions of underlying environmental factors such as radiation or chemical substances, none has been demonstrated definitely in PV etiology. On the other hand, a familial tendency has been well substantiated, though it is still premature to differentiate between genetic predisposition and a familial aggregation on the basis of a commonly shared environment.[91,92]

A better understanding of the disease etiology is mandatory for the implementation of preventive measures. Modern diagnostic techniques, e.g. one based on the recently identified IGF-1 hypersensitivity[93] would be helpful to achieve this goal. More massive accumulation of descriptive data regarding the disease distribution in distinct communities could pave the way toward analytic case-control studies that might delineate much needed etiologic clues.

REFERENCES

1. Waterhouse J, Muir C, Shanmugaratnam K, Powell J: Cancer Incidence in Five Continents, vol 4. Lyon, IARC, 1982
2. Prochazka AV, Markowe HLJ: The epidemiology of polycythaemia rubra vera in England and Wales, 1968–1982. Br J Cancer 53:59–64, 1986
3. Dougan LE, Matthews MLV, Armstrong BK: The effect of diagnostic review on the estimated incidence of lymphatic and hematopoietic neoplasms in Western Australia. Cancer 48: 866–872, 1981
4. Modan B: An epidemiological study of polycythemia vera. Blood 26:657–666, 1965
5. Modan B, Kallner H, Zemer D, Yoran C: A note on the increased risk of polycythemia vera in Jews. Blood 37:172–176, 1971
6. Goin JE: Polycythemia vera in Oklahoma hospitals. J Oklahoma State Med Assoc 66:71–75, 1973

7. Silverstein MN, Lanier AP: Polycythemia vera, 1935–1969: An epidemiologic survey in Rochester, Minnesota. Mayo Clin Proc 46:751–753, 1971

8. Bender GP, Young D, Balcerzak SP: Polycythemia vera in a small Ohio town. Ohio State Med J 82:631–635, 1986

9. Berglund S, Zettervall O: Incidence of polycythemia vera in a defined population. Eur J Haematol 48:20–26, 1992

10. Modan B. The Polycythemic Disorders. Springfield, Ill, Charles C Thomas, 1971

11. Modan B, Lilienfeld AM: Polycythemia vera and leukemia: The role of radiation treatment. Medicine 44:305–344, 1965

12. Wasserman LR: Polycythemia vera study group: A historical perspective. Semin Hematol 23:183–187, 1986

13. Marlow AA, Fairbanks VF: Polycythemia vera in an eleven-year-old girl. N Engl J Med 263:950–952, 1960

14. Cap J: Prava polycytemia u 11-rocneho diatata drenovy utlm po liecbe draprimon. Cesk Pediatr 16:49–53, 1961

15. Aggeler PM, Pollycove M, Hoag S, et al: Polycythemia vera in childhood: Studies of iron kinetics with Fe^{59} and blood clotting factors. Blood 17:345–350, 1961

16. Auerback ML, Wolff JA, Mettier SR: Benign familial polycythemia in childhood. Pediatrics 21:54–58, 1958

17. Knock HL, Githens JH: Primary erythrocytosis of childhood. Am J Dis Child 100:189–195, 1960

18. Sacks MO: Occurrence of anemia and polycythemia in phenotypically dissimilar single-ovum human twins. Pediatrics 24:604–608, 1959

19. Michael AF, Jr., Mauer AM: Maternal-fetal transfusion as a cause of plethora in the neonatal period. Pediatrics 28:456–461, 1961

20. O'Connor JF, Shapiro JH, Ingall D: Erythrocythemia as a cause of respiratory distress in the newborn: Radiologic findings. Radiology 90:333–335, 1968

21. Salvesen DR, Brudenell MJ, Nicolaides KH: Fetal polycythemia and thrombocytopenia in pregnancies complicated by maternal diabetes mellitus. Am J Obstet Gynecol 166:1287–1292, 1992

22. Kurlat I, Sola A: Neonatal polycythemia in appropriately grown infants of hypertensive mothers. Acta Paediatr 81:662–664, 1992.

23. Gunale SR, Zelkowitz L: Polycythemia vera in nonagenarian. JAMA 228:1148, 1974

24. Devesa SS, Young JL, Williams RR: Polycythemia vera among the elderly. JAMA 232:706–707, 1975

25. Modan B: Role of migrant studies in understanding the etiology of cancer. Am J Epidemiol 112:289–295, 1980

26. Reznikoff P, Foot NC, Bethea JM: Etiologic and pathologic factors in polycythemia vera. Am J Med Sci 189:753–759, 1935

27. Reznikoff P, Foot NC, Bethea JM, Du Bois EF: Racial and geographic origin of patients suffering from polycythemia vera and pathological findings in blood vessels of bone marrow. Trans Assoc Am Physicians 49:273–276, 1934

28. Damon A, Holub DA: Host factors in polycythemia vera. Ann Intern Med 49:43–60, 1958

29. MacMahon B, Koller EK: Ethnic differences in the incidence of leukemia. Blood 12:1–10, 1957

30. Chaiter Y, Brenner B, Aghai E, Tatarsky I: High incidence of myeloproliferative disorders in Ashkenazi Jews in northern Israel. Leuk Lymphoma 7:251–255, 1992

31. Nikhamin SB. Ein Fall von Erythraemia (Polyglobulia Splenomegalica) (abstract). Folia Haematol 6:301, 1908

32. Spodaro A, Forkner CE: Benign familial polycythemia. Arch Intern Med 52:593–602, 1933

33. Greenberg BR, Golde DW: Erythropoiesis in familial erythrocytosis. N Engl J Med 296:1080–1084, 1977

34. Levin WC, Houston EW, Ritzmann SE: Polycythemia vera with Ph^1 chromosomes in two brothers. Blood 30:503–512, 1967

35. Lawrence JH, Goetsch AT: Familial occurrence of polycythemia and leukemia. Calif Med 73:361–364, 1950

36. Erf LA: Radioactive phosphorus in the treatment of primary polycythemia (vera). Progr Hematol 1:153–165, 1956

37. Manohanar A, Garson OM: Familial polycythaemia vera: A study of 3 sisters. Scand J Haematol 17:10–16, 1976

38. Brubaker LH, Wasserman LR, Goldberg JD, et al: Increased prevalence of polycythemia vera in parents of patients on polycythemia vera study group protocols. Am J Hematol 16:367–373, 1984

39. Sievers ML, Calabresi P: Gastric pepsin secretion and ABO blood groups in polycythemia vera. Am J Dig Dis 4:515–521, 1959

40. Perkins J, Israels MCG, Wilkinson JF: Polycythemia vera: Clinical studies on a series of 127 patients managed without radiation therapy. Q J Med 33:499–518, 1964

41. Modan B: Unpublished data, 1994

42. Miller RL, Purvis JD, Weick JK: Familial polycythemia vera. Cleve Clin J Med 56:813–818, 1989

43. Ratnof WD, Gress RE: The familial occurrence of polycythemia vera: Report of a father and son, with consideration of the possible etiologic role of exposure to organic solvents, including tetrachloroethylene. Blood 56:233–236, 1980

44. Lawrence JH, Berlin NI, Huff RL: The nature and treatment of polycythemia. Medicine 32:323–388, 1953

45. Tubiana M, Vallee G, Boiron M, Perez R: Le devenir des polyglobulies essentielles traitees par le phosphore radioactif: A propos d'une serie de 310 cas. Nouv Rev Fr Hematol 1:445–459, 1961

46. Mondon H, Andre JJL: Maladie de Vaquez et intoxication benzolique. Presse Med 49:989–991, 1941

47. Nissen NI, Soeborg-Ohlsen A: Erythromyelosis: Review and report of a case in a benzene (benzol) worker. Acta Med Scand 145:56–71, 1953

48. Mallory TB, Gall EA, Brickley WJ: Chronic exposure to benzene (benzol): III. The pathologic results. J Indust Hyg 21:355–393, 1939

49. Bernard J: L'erythro-leucemie experimentale provoquee par le goudron. Sangre (Barc) 8:28–38, 1934

50. Bernard J: Polyglobulies et leucemies provoquees par les injection intramedullaries de goudron. Ann Med 40:373, 1936

51. Harrop GA Jr: Polycythemia. Medicine 7:291–344, 1928

52. Kleinberg W: The hemopoietic effects of cobalt and cobalt-manganese compounds in rabbits. Am J Physiol 108:545–549, 1934

53. Myerson A, Loman J, Dameshek W: Physiologic effects of benzedrine and its relationship to other drugs affecting the autonomic nervous system. Am J Med Sci 192:560–574, 1936

54. Davis JE: The production of experimental polycythemia in dogs, rabbits and man by daily administration of ephedrine and by amphetamine in dogs. Am J Physiol 134:219–224, 1941

55. Cartwright GE: The relationship of copper, cobalt and other trace elements to hemopoiesis. Am J Clin Nutr 3:11–19, 1955

56. Davis JE, Fields JP: Experimental production of polycythaemia in humans by administration of cobalt chloride. Proc Soc Exp Biol Med 99:491–493, 1958

57. Kesteloot H, Roelander J, Willems J, et al: An inquiry into the role of cobalt in the heart disease of chronic beer drinkers. Circulation 37:854–864, 1968

58. Aitchison R, Russell N: Smoking, a major cause of polycythaemia. J R Soc Med 81:89–91, 1988

59. Caldwell GG, Kelley DB, Health CW Jr, Zack M: Polycythemia vera among participants of a nuclear weapons test. JAMA 252:662–664, 1984

60. Weinberg JB: Sequential development of polycythemia vera and chronic myelocytic leukemia in a patient following radiation exposure from nuclear weapons tests. Am J Med 87:121–123, 1989

61. Blumenthal R: Un cas de polycythemie myelogene. J Med Bruxelles 10:545–554, 1905

62. Blumenthal R: Sur l'origine myelogene de la polycythemie vraie. Arch Med Exp Anar Pathol 19:697, 1907

63. Schwartz E: Erythraemia und Myelose. Folia Haematol 62:261–335, 1939

64. Merskey C: The relationship between polycythemia vera and myeloid leukemia. Clin Proc 8:150–162, 1949

65. Schwartz SO, Ehrlich L: The relationship of polycythemia vera to leukemia: A critical review. Acta Haematol (Basel) 4:129–147, 1950

66. Modan B: Cancer and leukemia risks after low level radiation controversy, facts and future. Med Oncol Tumor Pharmacother, 4:151–161, 1987

67. Modan B: Computing the length of survival in long term disease. JAMA 192:609–612, 1965

68. Landaw SA: Acute leukemia in polycythemia vera. Semin Hematol 23:156–165, 1986

69. Berk PD, Goldberg JD, Silverstein MN, et al: Increased incidence of acute leukemia in polycythemia vera associated with chlorambucil therapy. N Engl J Med 304;441–447, 1981

70. Nand S, Messmore H, Fisher SG, et al: Leukemia transformation in polycythemia vera: Analysis of risk factors. Am J Hematol 34:32–36, 1990

71. Wang G, Ahn YS, Whitcomb CC, Harrington WJ: Development of polycythemia vera and chronic lymphocytic leukemia during the course of refractory idiopathic thrombocytopenic purpura. Cancer 53:1770–1776, 1984

72. Polkowska KE, Matusewicz W, Golebiowska A, et al: The coexistence of chronic lymphocytic leukaemia and polycythaemia vera terminating in acute myeloid leukaemia. Folia Haematol (Leipz) 115:647–652, 1988

73. Lawrence JH, Rosenthal RL: Multiple myeloma associated with polycythemia: Report of four cases. Am J Med Sci 218:149–154, 1949

74. Brody JI, Beizer LH, Schwartz S: Multiple myeloma and myeloproliferative syndromes. Am J Med 36:315–319, 1964

75. Franzen S, Johansson B, Kaifas M: Primary polycythemia associated with multiple myeloma. Acta Med Scand 179(suppl 445):336–343, 1966

76. Dittmar K, Kochwa S, Zucker-Franklin D, Wasserman LR: Coexistence of polycythemia vera and biclonal gammopathy (GK and AL) with two Bence-Jones proteins (BJK and BJL). Blood 31:81–92, 1968

77. Spickard A: Multiple myeloma with myelofibrosis and with polycythemia vera: Further evidence for relationship between myeloproliferative disorders. Bull Johns Hopkins Hosp 107:234–240, 1960

78. Reed RE: Polycythemia vera and agnogenic myeloid metaplasia. Med Clin North Am 64:667–681, 1980

79. Videbaek A: Polycythemia vera co-existing with malignant tumors (particularly hypernephroma). Acta Med Scand 138:239–245, 1950

80. Bernard J, Tubiana M, Boiron M, Perez R: Etude de l'association polyglobulie-cancer. Nouv Rev Fr Hematol 1:473–478, 1961

81. Berk P: Personal communication, 1993

82. Sinclair WK: Risk, research, and radiation protection. Failla Memorial Lecture. Radiat Res 112:191–216, 1987

83. Golde DW, Hocking WG, Koeffler HP, et al: Polycythemia: mechanisms and management. Ann Intern Med 95:71–87, 1981

84. Da Silva J-L, Lacombe C, Bruneval P, et al: Tumor cells are the site of erythropoietin synthesis in human renal cancers associated with polycythemia. Blood 75:577–582, 1990

85. Reman O, Reznik Y, Casadevall N, et al: Polycythemia and steroid overproduction in a gonadotropin-secreting seminoma of the testis. Cancer 68:2224–2229, 1991

86. Trimble M, Caro J, Talalla A, Brain M: Secondary erythrocytosis due to a cerebellar hemangioblastoma: Demonstration of erythropoietin mRNA in the tumor. Blood 78:599–601, 1991

87. Tachibana I, Yamashima T, Yamashita J: Immunohistochemical study of erythropoietin in cerebellar hemangioblastomas associated with secondary polycythemia. Neurosurgery 28:24–26, 1991

88. Wasserman LR, Gilbert HS: Surgical bleeding in polycythemia vera. Ann NY Acad Sci 115:122, 1964

89. Orlowitz HL, Brodsky I: Busulphan treatment of polycythemia vera. Br J Haematol 52:1–6, 1982

90. Randi ML, Casonato A, Fabris F, et al: The significance of thrombocytosis in old age. Acta Haematol (Basel) 78:41–44, 1987

91. Shpitberg O, Modan M, Modan B, et al. Familial aggregation of haematological neoplasms—a controlled study. Br J Haematol (in press)

92. Prchal JT, Prchal JF. Evolving understanding of the cellular defect in polycythemia vera: implications for its clinical diagnosis and molecular pathophysiology. Blood 83:1–4, 1994

93. Correa PN, Eskinazi D, Axelrad AA. Circulating erythroid progenitors in polycythemia vera are hypersensitive to insulin-like growth factor-1 *in vitro*: Studies in an improved serum-free medium. Blood 83:99–112, 1994

13

Early Approaches in the Treatment of Polycythemia Vera

FRANK H. GARDNER

Polycythemia vera (PV) is a disease entity first described accurately in the present century. When one realizes that the marked skin color changes would be evident to the clinician, it is surprising that there were no definitive comments until those of 1892 by Vasquez. By 1908, Osler[1] had reviewed 18 cases. The increased clinical recognition was documented rapidly, and by 1912, Harrop had noted that 179 cases were in the literature. The disease had enough recognition to enable Parkes-Weber in 1921 to classify PV as a separate entity from secondary (anoxic) polycythemia.[2]

A number of therapies were used in the first 50 years to reduce plethora, and it is difficult to find a particular program that was more helpful than others. To evaluate the therapies that were used in this interval, I reviewed the records from 1928 until 1965, when the Polycythemia Vera Study Group (PVSG) was started, at the Peter Bent Brigham Hospital (now Brigham & Women's Hospital) in Boston. Over this 38-year span, 158 cases were found in the record files of this 300-bed hospital that appeared to satisfy a diagnosis of PV. Some cases were rejected if they were considered by current criteria to be a diagnosis of myeloid metaplasia. While numerous cases of presumably spurious polycythemia could be found, the absence of other peripheral blood abnormalities or splenomegaly allowed their exclusion. After 1950, most cases had confirmatory red cell mass studies done. When the PVSG was begun, it was intended that all patients would be

enrolled in its protocols; therefore, the use of different random therapies was discontinued at the Brigham in 1965. I believed that the therapies used in a teaching hospital would reflect the types of therapies that were available in the United States before the advent of a prospective protocol.

As one might anticipate, the largest percentage of patients had their initial therapy with a phlebotomy program, although the hematocrit levels were maintained nearer to 50 percent than to the currently recommended level of 45 percent (Table 13–1). A review of the hospital charts indicated that the majority of patients had phlebotomies to a normal hematocrit before other therapies were added. Until the initial reports by Lawrence and associates[3] of the use of radiophosphorus, phlebotomy was used primarily to maintain the lower hematocrit for years despite some discomfort from the symptoms of iron deficiency. Long bone irradiation to suppress erythropoiesis had only a limited appeal (18 cases) in the 1930s, in part related to poor calibration of dosage. A few patients continued to have an overlap with radiophosphorus therapy and skeletal irradiation, but in the mid-1940s the hospital staff began to use only radioactive phosphorus. Radioactive phosphorus also was used in conjunction with busulfan in the 1950s.[4] From the tabulation and hospital charts, the combined protocol of long bone irradiation and phenylhydrazine had minimal use because of difficulties in achieving a satisfactory hemoglobin level. A few patients received liver ex-

TABLE 13-1. TREATMENT OF POLYCYTHEMIA VERA (158 PATIENTS), 1928-1966, PETER BENT BRIGHAM HOSPITAL (300 BEDS)

Phlebotomy	55
Phlebotomy + ^{32}P*	50
Phlebotomy + ^{32}P + busulfan	14
Phlebotomy + radiation	7
Phlebotomy + ^{32}P + 6MP*	3
Phlebotomy + ^{32}P + radiation + busulfan	2
Phlebotomy + liver extract	1
Phlebotomy + phenylhydrazine + ^{32}P	1
Phlebotomy + radiation + phenylhydrazine + liver extract	1
Phlebotomy + busulfan	1
Phlebotomy + radiation + ^{32}P	1
Phlebotomy + radiation + phenylhydrazine	1
TOTAL phlebotomized patients	137
Radiation + liver extract	3
^{32}P	8
Radiation + Fowler's solution* + liver extract	1
Radiation + phenylhydrazine	1
Radiation + phenylhydrazine + liver extract	1
^{32}P + busulfan	1
^{32}P + radiation	1
Fowler's solution	1
Liver extract	1
Phenylhydrazine	1
6MP	1
Busulfan	1
TOTAL nonphlebotomized patients	21

*6MP = 6-mercaptopurine; ^{32}P = IV sodium phosphate; Fowler's solution = potassium arsenite.

tract injections when a satisfactory parenteral product was available, but there were no data to suggest that it was helpful. Despite some enthusiasm for Fowler's solution (potassium arsenite),[5] this treatment had little therapeutic application in this teaching hospital. Patients treated with long bone x-ray therapy had other marrow-suppressive therapies.

From this potpourri of therapies, no firm conclusion could be reached to say that any one marrow-suppressive therapy was more helpful than another. The hospital record review was of interest because it demonstrated that 85 percent of the patients had a prolonged phlebotomy program as the initial therapy. By the 1960s, radiophosphorus had become the predominate therapy to follow the initial phlebotomy program. However, the hospital division had no protocol of a specific program, and some of the staff used busulfan as the long-term intermittent therapy after the initial phlebotomy period (usually 2 to 4 months). One can appreciate that this medical school teaching hospital had no data collection and the staff was hopeful that

the PVSG protocol would demonstrate that radioactive phosphorus was the best therapy.

In the literature review of treatment programs historically, phlebotomy usually has been the initial therapy and continues to be part of all current protocols. A carefully controlled program of frequent bleedings can rapidly alleviate many of the symptoms described and often may be a major factor in the early rehabilitation of the patient. Usually, patients with hematocrits less than 70 percent may be bled twice weekly to reduce the hematocrit to the range of 40 percent. Patients with severe plethora who have altered mentation or associated vascular compromise can be bled more vigorously; indeed, 500 ml of blood can be removed daily. Older patients (> 60 years of age) should have the volume of the phlebotomy replaced with saline solution at each bleeding. Many years ago I replaced volume for volume with plasma or a plasma expander, but in recent years, electrolyte solutions have worked as well. There is always some risk of cerebral vascular complications if the patient has some congestive heart failure, and in such patients, plasma expanders may be more protective, along with a more cautious initial phlebotomy (250 ml of whole blood).[6] In the older patient, postural hypotension may develop after the beginning of phlebotomies. The use of oral fluorocortisone acetate (Florinef) tablets, 0.1 mg per day, prior to and for 2 days after the phlebotomy has been helpful in maintaining expanded plasma volume during an active phlebotomy program.[7] In all programs, the physician should continue reduction of the red cell mass until a hematocrit of 40 percent is achieved. With automated blood cell separators, hematocrits can be reduced to normal (45 percent) in a 1- to 2-hour interval.[8,9] In these procedures, blood is maintained temporarily by replacement with plasma protein fractions. I suspect that this equipment will allow more physiologic rheology, especially if the patient needs to have a normal red cell mass for surgical intervention.

In our geographic area of the world, blood letting has been intermittent, but we should recognize that induction of an artificial hookworm disease can be quite successful as a method to achieve slow blood loss, and this has been advocated as a therapeutic modality in third world countries.[10,11] Control of the infection can be related to the elevated hematocrit and the number of larvae applied to the skin. When the hematocrit has returned to normal, the infection can be eliminated.

What are the immediate benefits of phlebotomy to reduce the red cell mass?

1. *Central nervous system symptoms.* The lethargy and vague descriptions of inactivity and headache are improved rapidly as the hematocrit returns to a normal range. With plethora, the central blood flow is impaired. With the return of the hematocrit to the 45 percent range, cerebral blood flow will increase by 70 percent, related to a decrease of the blood viscosity by 30 percent.[13] It is important to recognize that the cerebral blood flow begins to be impaired as the hematocrit exceeds 50 percent.[14] This observation may explain the marked improvement in objective psychological testing and alertness that has been described when the hematocrit percentage was lowered to the forties, for the improved scores in this type of testing did correlate with the increased cerebral blood flow.[15] A variety of confusing diagnoses with different neurologic deficits has been noted with high hematocrits. Such patients should have the red cell mass reduced by phlebotomy before special neurologic studies are pursued, especially that group of patients with "stroke in evolution." In this latter group, I would urge the use of equal volume amounts of plasma expanders after phlebotomy, although there is no comparative study available. Even hearing loss can improve with reduction of red cell mass.[16]

2. *Peripheral vascular symptoms.* The number of patients who have the initial diagnosis made because of peripheral vascular symptoms vary with the physician's interest in the medical referral pattern. Many years ago I was impressed with the number of patients sent to the clinic at the Peter Bent Brigham Hospital by peripheral vascular surgeons. Indeed, two-thirds of a small group of 26 patients had entry for medical care because of red or cyanotic toes or burning pain in the hands or feet.[17] Such types of erythromelagia have dramatic improvement with phlebotomy. Early ischemic extremity ulceration may heal when the hematocrit returns to the low normal range.[18] In the event that the ischemia is irreversible, the hematocrit should be normalized before any surgical procedures.[19]

Can PV be treated only by phlebotomy? Certainly many patients can be supervised with only phlebotomy. In the review of these 158 cases at the Peter Bent Brigham Hospital, 55 had only phlebotomy for therapy over many years. Such therapy has been emphasized as satisfactory, recognizing that some patients may have symptoms of iron deficiency (pica, burning tongue, and cheilosis). If the patient has tolerance for these symptoms, phlebotomy can be continued indefinitely.[20] However, in my experience, the discomfort of cheilosis and the glossitis can be distressing, and accordingly, a myelosuppressive agent frequently was added for patient well-being. Certainly the observation of patients treated only with phlebotomy for 25 years at the Johns Hopkins Hospital would support the belief that there were no serious long-term complications from chronic iron deficiency. For safety, it may be the ideal therapy if vascular complications can be controlled. This issue is considered in greater detail in the two chapters that follow.

Three additional techniques utilizing red cell hemolysis to reduce the red cell mass have been applied, namely, administration of lead acetate,[21] phenylhydrazine,[22] and immune antisera.[24] As with many special therapies, they were successful in a few clinics that knew how to control these agents effectively. Although I find no published records, Dr. E. H. Falconer in San Francisco attempted to compare the efficacy of intravenous colloidal lead acetate with radioactive phosphorus in the 1940s with equivalent results in his clinic. In such short-term studies of a few years, the knowledge of how to use this agent allowed him to use lead safely for such a comparative study. Compared with the predictability of phlebotomy, these hemolytic techniques had little in their favor aside from conservation of iron stores. Indeed, the excess and often uncontrolled hemolysis with phenylhydrazine probably explains why it was tabulated only five times in the Brigham study and only once without other therapies. More recently, infusion of high-titer blood group antibodies has been used to reduce the hematocrit. This is a unique type of hemolysis that would need careful observation to prevent acute intravascular hemolysis, but it did emphasize again the conservation of iron stores.

Aside from the hemolytic effect from phenylhydrazine and lead acetate, the early efforts to suppress the hyperactive marrow were related to the use of irradiation. Although irradiation was proposed as early as 1907, by the 1920–1940 period, irradiation of the long bones and vertebral column had become an acceptable although capricious method to suppress marrow function.[25] While the calculations were not specific and dosage schedule varied, the normalization of blood values was the response used to define the amount of irradiation used. In later years, with further experience, whole-body irradiation was used successfully (usually 100 to 200 rad over a 3- or 4-week interval).[26, 27] However, the introduction of radioactive sodium phosphate in 1938 more or less eliminated the use of external irradiation, especially as the isotope became more available after 1945.[28] Casual comments in the literature have implied that radiophosphorus gained acceptance rapidly because the physician was not dependent on the radiologist for therapy and control of the patients. Thereafter, as more restrictions were placed on the use of isotopes, hematologists again embraced chemical myelosuppressive drugs to have more complete personal supervision of their patients.[29] A number of other isotopes have been used to suppress marrow prolif-

eration, but none has had widespread use in the past 40 years.[30, 31] Multiple series have been published to extoll the comfort and convenience of radioactive phosphorus.[32, 33] In the Brigham series, 79 of 158 patients received radioactive phosphorus alone or in combination with other myelosuppressive drugs after an initial phlebotomy program. By the mid-1950s, there were increasing reports of acute myeloblastic leukemia as a complication of external irradiation or radioactive phosphorus. If the patients could be observed for 10 years, the clinician could expect a 10 to 12 percent leukemic complication. These leukemic manifestations are documented in detail elsewhere in this book.

With the introduction of nitrogen mustard to treat malignant disease, it was apparent that PV also could respond to the same variety of drugs that suppressed cell proliferation for leukemias or lymphoma.[34] During the next 15 years (1948–1963), small series of patients were evaluated with different drugs, of which the most popular are listed in Table 13–2. Clinicians assumed that the patients would have no leukemogenic complications from these agents. It is apparent from review of their use that all these agents have had transient benefits in decreasing the trilineage proliferation of PV. From the large list, two agents, busulfan and melphalan, have had consistent popularity.[35, 36] Busulfan was used predominantly in the United States, since there was a general assumption that this alkylating agent was not leukemogenic and would decrease the risk of leukemia that was accumulating in the literature with the use of radiophosphorus. Certainly because of ease of oral administration and the opportunity

TABLE 13–2. DRUGS USED IN POLYCYTHEMIA VERA

Busulfan (Myleran) (35)
Chlorambucil (Leukeran) (36)
Cyclophosphamide (cytoxan) (49)
Cytosine arabinoside (40)
Hydroxyurea (41)
L-Phenyl alanine mustard (Melphalan) (36)
Myelobromol (42)
Nitrogen mustard (39)
Pipobroman (Vercyte) (43)
Procarbazine (44)
Pyrimethamine (Daraprim) (45)
6-Mercaptopurine (6MP) (46)
6-Thioguanine (47)
Thiotepa (51)
Triethylene melamine (48)
Uracil mustard (50)

for the clinician to use it without the need for an isotope license, it rapidly became popular in the United States and Europe. Despite the continued use of busulfan, all clinicians experienced the problem of sudden changes in the hemogram after months of stable values with small daily oral doses. Especially frustrating was the observation of sudden neutropenia or thrombocytopenia. In my personal experience, such variable hematologic responses prompted me to prefer radiophosphorus (Table 13–1).

In the Brigham clinic during the 1950s and 1960s, after the patient had obtained a normal hematocrit (50 percent) by phlebotomy, the patient received 3 to 5 mCi of IV radiophosphorus. Busulfan was used sparingly and for the most part only if the total dose of radioactive phosphorus was high, i.e., above 16 to 20 mCi. The complication of altered hydroxylation of cortisone by busulfan has made the incidence of abnormal skin pigmentation and pulmonary fibrosis a risk that must be explained to the patient. Although in my experience these complications have been limited largely to chronic myelocytic leukemia, these possible developments contributed to the exploration of other alkylating drugs in the 15 years prior to the PVSG protocol. Chlorambucil was chosen instead of busulfan as the alkylating agent in the initial PVSG protocol in anticipation that the patient would have fewer unpredictable swings in white count and platelet levels. More recently, a comparative study in the treatment of PV with radiophosphorus and busulfan has been published by the European Organization for Research and Treatment of Cancer.[37] They have reported on an 8-year follow-up period in which they imply that busulfan was the better choice. As noted in Chapter 15, a longer period may be needed to be certain that the mutagenic complications are less than those observed in the PVSG results. Nevertheless, these results do suggest that busulfan may be a relatively safe alkylating agent and may have fewer leukemogenic complications as used in their protocol. It may well be that busulfan now can be used more effectively with less intermittent thrombocytopenia and leukopenia than in the programs followed from 1955 to 1965.

With the frequent laboratory monitoring required of all oral myelosuppressive drugs, the patient must be educated to the need to accept this close medical supervision. In contrast, radiophosphorus can be used effectively while requiring probably only a third of the professional visits. In the older patient, I would use radiophosphorus for the patient's comfort and accept the risk of leukemia. Certainly, as noted in the phlebotomy arm of the PVSG protocol, there is a need to have some program to reduce the incidence of vascular complications in the initial 2 years of treatment. Finally, we have had, in the Brigham experience, combined therapies with radiophosphorus and busulfan. This approach probably should be discouraged in view of the increased risk noted in the treatment of Hodgkin's disease when chemotherapy has been added to irradiation.

Another unique type of marrow suppression has been proposed on the basis that a marrow inhibitor is present in plasma of the patient with PV.[38] In 37 of 41 patients, prolonged hematologic remissions have been reported following the reinfusion of autologous plasma. The initial improvement was maintained for varying intervals up to 2 years. These patients have maintained a lower hematocrit longer than one would expect from phlebotomy per se. Further clinical data will be needed to indicate whether this method may replace the current protocols.

This review of past therapies has focused on the program of one hospital over a period of approximately 40 years, when most current therapies were developed. Such retrospective data were of interest because phlebotomy remained the predominant therapy throughout four decades. The small number of patients who received hemolytic therapies or external irradiation reflects the unacceptable variability of response. By 1965, radiophosphorus and an alkylating agent (busulfan) were the major additions to phlebotomy, and this pattern followed the general practice in the United States in the 1950–1965 interval.

REFERENCES

1. Osler W: Erythremia (polycythemia with cyanosis, Maladie de Vaquez). Lancet 1:143–146, 1908
2. Parkes-Weber PF: Polycythemia, Erythrocytosis and Erythremia. London, HK Lewis, 1921
3. Lawrence JH: Polycythemia: Physiology, Diagnosis and Treatment Based on 303 Cases. Modern Medical Monographs. New York, Grune & Stratton, 1955, pp 13–136

4. Killman S, Cronkite EP: Treatment of polycythemia vera with myleran. Am J Med Sci 241: 124–130, 1961

5. Forkner CE, Scott TFM, Wu SC: Treatment of polycythemia vera (erythremia) with a solution of potassium arsenite. Arch Intern Med 51: 616–629, 1933

6. Kiraly JF III, Feldmann JE, Wheby MS: Hazards of phlebotomy in polycythemic patients with cardiovascular disease. JAMA 236:2080–2081, 1976

7. Hickler RB, Thompson GR, Fox LM, Hamlin JT: Successful treatment of orthostatic hypotension with 9-alpha fluorohydrocortisone. N Engl J Med 261:788–791, 1959

8. Klein HG, Winslow RM, Monge C, et al: Rapid isovolemic hemodilation in subjects with chronic high altitude polycythemia (abstract). Transfusion 22:423, 1982

9. Newland AC, Cotter FE, Wedzicha JA, Empey DW: Rapid isovolemic haemodilation in subjects with 1° and 2° polycythemia (abstract). Br J Haematol 55:177–178, 1983

10. Brumpt LC, Gujar BJ: The treatment of polycythemia by artificial infection with Ancylostoma duodenale. Ind Med Gaz 166–169, 1948

11. Myhre J, Wallace F: Hookworm treatment of polycythemia vera. Minn Med 39:99, 1956

12. Wasserman LR, Bassen F: Polycythemia. J Mt Sinai Hosp 26:1–49, 1959

13. Thomas DJ, Marshall J, Ross Russell RW, et al: Cerebral Blood-flow in polycythaemia. Lancet 12:161–163, 1977

14. Kremer M, Lambert CD, Lawton N: Progressive neurological deficits in primary polycythaemia. Br Med J 22:216–218, 1972

15. Willison JR, du Boulay GH, Paul EA, et al: Effect of high haematocrit on alertness. Lancet 846–848, 1980

16. Davis EC, Nilo ER: Hearing improvement induced by phlebotomy in polycythemia. Laryngsc 1847–1852, 1964

17. Edwards EA, Cooley MH: Peripheral vascular symptoms as the initial manifestation of polycythemia vera. JAMA 214:1463–1467, 1970

18. Pagrell B, Mellstedt H: Polycythemia vera as a cause of ischemic digital necrosis. Acta Chir Scand 144:129–132, 1978

19. Wasserman LR, Gilbert HS: Surgery in polycythemia vera. N Engl J Med 269:1226–1230, 1963

20. Rector WG Jr, Fortuin NJ, Conley CL: Non-hematologic effects of chronic iron deficiency: A study of patients with polycythemia vera treated soley with venesections. Medicine 61:382–389, 1982

21. Falconer EH: The treatment of polycythemia vera with lead compounds. Am J Med Sci 203: 856–857, 1942

22. Kennedy AM: Untoward effect of phenylhydrazine in polycythemia. Br Med J 1:659–661, 1934

23. Pengelly CDR: Reduction of excessive haematocrit levels in patients with polycythaemia due to hypoxic lung disease by phenylhydrazine hydrochloride and pyrimethamine. Postgrad Med J 45:583–590, 1969

24. Hrubiski M, Libusa F, Lipsic T: Therapeutische Beein flussung der polycythaemia vera durch ubertragene antierythrozytare antikorper. Haematologia 7:25–33, 1973

25. Pack TT, Craver LF: Radiation therapy of polycythemia vera. Am J Med Sci 180:609–617, 1930

26. Hunter FT: "Spray x-ray therapy" in polycythemia vera and in erythroblastic anemia. N Engl J Med 214:1123–1127, 1936

27. Richardson W, Robbins LL: The treatment of polycythemia vera by spray irradiation. N Engl J Med 238:78–82, 1948

28. Hall BE: Therapeutic use of radiophosphorus in polycythemia vera, leukemia, and allied diseases. *In* The Use of Isotopes in Biology and Medicine. Madison, Wisc, University of Wisconsin Press, 1948, p 353.

29. Najean Y, Dresch C: Myelosuppression in polycythemia vera: Chemotherapy or radiotherapy? Blut 44:1–5, 1982

30. Sailer J: Polycythemia treated with radium. Trans Assos Am Physicians 31:172–176, 1916

31. Greenbero J, Sawitsky A, Dudley HC, et al: Therapy of polycythemia vera with radioyttrium (Y-90). J Nucl Med 3:18–25, 1962

32. Erf LA, Jones HW: Primary polycythemia: Remission induced by therapy with radiophosphorus. Blood 1:202–208, 1946

33. Friedberg HD: The treatment of polycythaemia vera by irradiation: A follow-up study of 52 cases. J Facial Radiol 10:77–79, 1959

34. Shullenberger CC, Watkins CH: Effects of nitrogen mustard on the bone marrow in polycythemia vera. Ann Intern Med 33:841–853, 1950

35. Brodsky I: Annotation: Busulphan treatment of polycythaemia vera. Br J Haematol 52:1–6, 1982

36. Logue GL, Gutterman JU, McGinn TG, et al: Melphalan therapy of polycythemia vera. Blood 36:70–86, 1970

37. Leukemia and Hematosarcoma Cooperative Group, European Organization for Research on Treatment of Cancer (EORTC) Haanen C (Chair), Mathe G (Counc), Hayat M (Sec): Treatment of polycythaemia vera by radiophosphorus or busulphan: A randomized trial. Br J Cancer 44:75–80, 1981

38. Stefanovic S, Radotic M, Dukic M, et al: Treatment of polycythaemia vera with reinfusion of autologous blood plasma obtained by phlebotomy. Haematologia 8(1–4):473–476, 1974

39. Spurr CL, Smith TR, Block MH, Jacobson LO: Clinical study of the use of nitrogen mustard in polycythemia vera. J Lab Clin Med 35:252–264, 1950

40. Goldenberg DM: Cytosine arabinoside in the treatment of erythremia. Chemotherapy 14:133–139, 1969

41. West WO, Ruff JD, Yarbro JW: Response of polycythemia to treatment with a new agent: Hydroxyurea (abstract). Ann Intern Med 72:795, 1970

42. Szentklaray J: Treatment of polycythaemia vera with myelobromol. Ther Hung 14:143–148, 1966

43. Najman A, Stachowiak J, Parlier Y, et al: Pipobroman therapy of polycythemia vera. Blood 59: 890–894, 1982

44. Penttila O, Ikkala E: Procarbazine (Natulan) and busulfan in the treatment of polycythemia vera. Ann Med Int Fenn 57:99–101, 1968

45. Isaacs R: Treatment of polycythemia vera with daraprim. JAMA 156:1491–1493, 1954

46. Shullenberger CC: Long-range treatment of polycythemia vera with 6-mercaptopurine. Cancer Chemother Rep 16:251–252, 1962

47. Milligan DW, Thein SL, Roberts BE: Secondary treatment of polycythemia rubra vera with 6-thioquanine. Cancer 50:836–839, 1982

48. Rosenthal N, Rosenthal RL: Treatment of polycythemia vera with triethylene melamine: Summary of thirty cases. Arch Intern Med 90:379, 1952

49. Gilbert HS: Problems relating to control of polycythemia vera: The use of alkylating agents. Blood 32:500–505, 1968

50. Perkins J, Israels MCG, Wilkinson JF: Polycythaemia vera: Clinical studies on a series of 127 patients managed without radiation therapy. Q J Med 33:499–518, 1964

ACKNOWLEDGMENT: I am indebted to Miss Agnes Cochran, who collected and tabulated the patient data at the Peter Bent Brigham Hospital.

14

Acute Leukemia in Polycythemia Vera

STEPHEN A. LANDAW

In polycythemia vera (PV), the interrelationships among natural history, treatment, and complications are complex and controversial. The Polycythemia Vera Study Group (PVSG) was founded by Dr. Louis R. Wasserman in 1967, with a view toward standardizing the diagnosis of PV and determining long-term complications and survival by means of a randomized, prospective three-armed clinical trial. With regard to the occurrence of acute leukemia (AL) in PV, the following questions were asked: (1) What is the incidence of AL in PV treated with phlebotomy, ^{32}P, and chlorambucil? (2) Are there agents without leukemogenic potential that are able to control symptoms in PV? (3) Are there clinical and/or laboratory characteristics that predict for the development of AL? (4) Is the development of AL the result of prolongation of survival, thereby unmasking a potential for AL not realized because of short survival in the untreated disease? (5) Is the presence of myelofibrosis with myeloid metaplasia (MF-MM) a risk factor for the development of AL?

This chapter will review observations and conclusions relative to the preceding questions arising from the results of the various research protocols of the PVSG as well as some newer observations concerning the relationships between chromosomal abnormalities, treatment, and the development of myelodysplastic or preleukemic states in patients with PV.

BACKGROUND

Many reviews concerning the occurrence of AL in PV have been published over the past 35 years.[1-4] The review by Schwartz and Ehrlich[4] in 1950 provided working diagnostic criteria for both PV and AL to document whether the cases appearing in the literature have verifiable PV and/or AL. The review by Modan and Lilienfeld[3] in 1965 was a retrospective analysis of records from seven large medical centers, whereas that by Lawrence et al.[2] in 1969 was an analysis of the experience of the Donner Laboratory in Berkeley. A review[1] in 1976 presented anecdotal information from a questionnaire circulated to members of the American Society of Hematology concerning the occurrence of AL in PV patients treated with phlebotomy alone or with various alkylating agents and added additional cases from the literature. Difficulties with documentation of the diagnosis of PV and/or AL, as well as with widely differing conclusions based on the type of information available, were multiple and are best appreciated by a careful reading of these articles.

Lawrence[5] introduced ^{32}P as treatment for PV in the late 1930s, and the first recorded case of AL following ^{32}P treatment of PV was reported about 7 years later by Tinney et al.[6] The concept of the myeloproliferative disorders, and of MF-MM and AL as specific stages in the evolution of PV were developed in the early 1950s by Rosenthal,[7] Dameshek,[8] and Wasserman.[9] Between 1950 and 1965, more than 11 large series of PV patients were presented in which analysis of the complication of AL was a prominent part.[1] The review by Modan and Lilienfeld[3] in 1965 reported on 1222 patients with polycythemia and concluded that the incidence of AL in PV was chiefly the result of therapeutic ionizing radiation.

Between 1964 and 1968, three reports appeared in which PV patients were treated with various chemotherapeutic agents without the use of ionizing radiation (^{32}P, x-ray).[3, 10, 11] For these series of patients, the incidence of AL appeared to be less than 1 percent, leading to enthusiasm for the choice of an alkylating agent for one of the arms of the PVSG major protocol. Because of available experience with chlorambucil (Leukeran[10]), this agent was chosen for the chemotherapy arm. By the 1970s, other reports appeared concerning patients treated with radiation and chemotherapy in which the incidence of AL was as high as 21 to 57 percent when stated in terms of the percentage of deaths.[12–14] By 1975, the first cases of AL in the chemotherapy arm of the PVSG major protocol (protocol 01) were reported,[1] and by 1979, the incidence of AL in that arm was shown to be significantly higher statistically than that in the other two arms (phlebotomy, ^{32}P).[15, 16] After August of 1979, patients on the chlorambucil arm were treated with phlebotomy only. For those patients with symptomatic thrombocytosis requiring myelosuppression, hydroxyurea (Hydrea, E.R., Squibb & Sons, Princeton, N.J.) was to be used. These findings were reported in abstract form[16] in December of 1979 and published[5] in February of 1980.

When the PVSG protocol 01 stopped accruing new patients, attempts were made to start efficacy (phase II) trials of potentially nonleukemogenic agents. A trial of tri-acetyl-6-azauride (Azaribine), an agent approved by the FDA for use in psoriasis, was thwarted when it was reported that use of this agent was associated with a higher incidence of thrombosis in psoriasis patients.[17] Thereafter, attention was paid to hydroxyurea (Hydrea), a metabolic inhibitor of DNA synthesis with limited carcinogenic potential in experimental animal systems.[18] Additionally, a second randomized trial (PVSG protocol 05), comparing ^{32}P with phlebotomy-aspirin-dipyridamole (Persantine) was begun in the hope that the addition of aspirin and Persantine to the phlebotomy arm would yield an acceptable nonleukemogenic treatment unassociated with an increased incidence of thrombosis.[19] Addition of aspirin and Persantine in the doses chosen by that study did not reduce the incidence of thrombosis, and PVSG protocol 05 was terminated shortly thereafter.[20] Initial results of the PVSG protocol 08 phase II trial of hydroxyurea indicated that it was remarkably effective in controlling symptoms of PV. Approximately 51 patients with previously untreated PV were enrolled in this study; long-term follow-up of this group (see below) will allow us to make some conclusions concerning leukemogenicity of this agent.

Although ^{32}P and the alkylating agents are leukemogenic per se, the manner of giving these agents may influence the incidence of AL, and there may be better ways of delivering such treatment. In PVSG protocol 01, chlorambucil was given in alternating cycles (i.e., one month "on," one month "off"). In contrast, the European Organization for Research on Treatment of Cancer (EORTC) initiated a phase III comparative trial in previously untreated PV patients comparing ^{32}P (0.5 to 1.0 mCi per 10 kg of body weight IV) versus busulfan (Myleran) given in short-term courses (4 to 6 mg/d for 4 to 6 weeks and withheld for a platelet count of less than 120,000/μl). When used in this manner, remissions were noted to last for months to years before reinstitution of busulfan treatment. The EORTC trial was initiated in 1967, and by the time it was reported in the literature in 1981,[21] 50 percent of the patients had a follow-up of at least 8 years. Of the 140 patients randomized to ^{32}P, 2 developed AL, whereas in the 145 patients treated with busulfan, there were 3 with AL. Although these numbers are too small to make comparisons, clearly this manner of giving an alkylating agent did not result in a lower incidence of AL when compared with ^{32}P, although it should be noted that the overall incidence of AL in their series (<2 percent) was exceedingly low, perhaps because the follow-up period was too short.[52]

PVSG PROTOCOL 01 STUDY

Between 1967 and 1974, 478 patients were randomized to the three treatment arms of PVSG protocol 01 (phlebotomy, chlorambucil, ^{32}P). Of these, 431 were considered eligible and 47 ineligible. The physical examination and laboratory characteristics of patients from the three groups did not differ significantly, although there were some differences in sex distribution.[15] Follow-up of the 47 ineligible patients did not disclose any previously unreported cases of AL, removing this as a possible source of bias. As of January 1986, minimal and maximal follow-up times for surviving patients were 12 and 18 years, respectively. Table 14–1 indicates the status regarding occurrence of AL as of January 1986. The difference in leukemia-free survival between the chlorambucil- and ^{32}P-treated groups that was evident previously[15] and that was statistically significant ($p <$ 0.025) is no longer significant ($0.50 > p >$ 0.30). The incidence of AL in the phlebotomy arm (1.5 percent), now representing 2 cases, is significantly different from that of the two myelosuppressive arms ($p < 0.01$).

The time to develop AL from time of randomization was analyzed for the 47 cases reported to date; results are shown in Table 14–2. Both the cases seen in the phlebotomy arm occurred within the first 5 years after randomization. In the chlorambucil arm, one-half the cases occurred in the first 5 years, with the remainder equally split between the second and third 5-year periods. In contrast, over 60 percent of the AL cases in the ^{32}P arm occurred 6 to 10 years after randomization. These results suggest that for the phlebotomy arm, development of AL is not due to prolongation of survival, such as that resulting from improvement in general medical care. This is consistent with results obtained from the American Society of Hematology survey,[1] in which the cases of AL reported in patients treated with phlebotomy alone occurred an average of 4 to 5 years

TABLE 14–1. OCCURRENCE OF ACUTE LEUKEMIA IN PVSG PROTOCOL 01 (DATA AS OF JANUARY 1986)

TREATMENT	ELIGIBLE PATIENTS	ACUTE LEUKEMIA	
		Cases	Percent
Phlebotomy	134	2	1.5
Chlorambucil	141	19	13.5
^{32}P	156	15	9.6
TOTAL	431	36	8.4

TABLE 14–2. RELATIONSHIP BETWEEN YEARS OF TREATMENT AND DEVELOPMENT OF ACUTE LEUKEMIA

YEARS OF TREATMENT	PERCENT OF ACUTE LEUKEMIA CASES*		
	Phlebotomy	Chlorambucil	^{32}P
0–5	100	53	25
6–10	0	26	62
11–15	0	21	12

* For PVSG protocol 01 data as of January 1986.

earlier than those appearing after treatment with ^{32}P.

Although the retrospective data for development of AL after chemotherapy suggested that acute leukemias occurred in a time-dependent manner quite similar to that seen in phlebotomy-treated patients, this was not seen in the prospective data shown in Table 14–2. Since chlorambucil was stopped in 1979, no patient can have received this agent for more than 12 years. However, three cases of AL were reported after follow-up of 13, 14, and 15 years, respectively. Analysis of the hazard function, the instantaneous incidence of leukemia at the midpoint of each study year (given survival without AL at the beginning of that year), is virtually flat for the chlorambucil arm from 2 to 7 years after randomization[15] (Fig. 14–1). As noted for the development of AL in the phlebotomy arm, the large number of cases occurring very early after randomization suggests that this is not the result of prolongation of survival. More important, the function for chlorambucil becomes alarmingly high after 10 years on study, suggesting that the risk of developing AL increases with time, even after the drug has been stopped.

Both the retrospective and prospective data tend to agree for the time course of appearance of AL after ^{32}P, with the first cases appearing about 2 years after treatment and with most of the cases appearing more than 5 years after treatment[1] (see Table 14–2). Both sets of data also agree with the time course for development of AL in survivors of the atomic bombings in Hiroshima and Nagasaki,[22] with the first cases of AL appearing at 3 years and the maximal number appearing at about 7 years after exposure. The mean interval noted by Rosner and Grunwald between onset of Hodgkin's

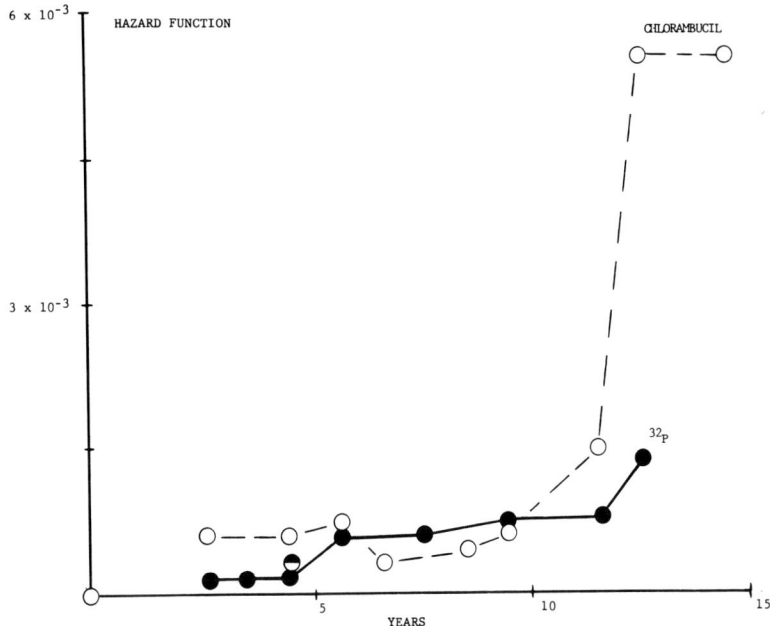

FIGURE 14–1. Hazard function for development of acute leukemia in PVSG protocol 01 (data as of January 1986). The function shown is the instantaneous rate of AL at the midpoint of the study year, given survival without AL at the start of that year. The open circles represent the chlorambucil-treated patients, closed circles represent the [23]P-treated patients, and the half-closed circle represents the phlebotomy-treated patients. *(Reproduced with permission from Berk PD, Goldberg JD, Silverstein MN et al: Increased evidence of acute leukemia in polycythemia vera associated with chlorambucil therapy. N Engl J Med 304:444–447, 1981.)*

disease and acute nonlymphocytic leukemia (ANLL) was 6.5 years, with all but three of the patients having received radiation therapy.[23] It appears that the time course for development of AL in these three separate groups of subjects is quite similar, despite differences in ethnic origin, average age, type of radiation received, and nature of underlying disorders.

RISK FACTORS FOR DEVELOPMENT OF AL

Myelofibrosis with Myeloid Metaplasia[24]

Nine cases of AL developed after there had been evidence for the development of myelofibrosis with myeloid metaplasia (MF-MM) based on the presence of increased reticulin and/or collagen in bone marrow biopsies, clinical evidence for increasing splenic size, worsening anemia, and the presence in the peripheral blood of teardrop poikilocytes, nucleated erythrocytes, and granulocytic precursors more immature than band forms.[9] The incidence of MF-MM was identi-

cal in the three arms, being 10 percent. Of the 43 PV patients developing MF-MM, 9 subsequently developed AL, for an incidence of 21 percent. On the other hand, for the 388 patients not developing MF-MM, there were 27 cases of AL, for an incidence of 7 percent. This statistically significant difference ($p <$ 0.001) for the entire group of patients also was seen within each of the three treatment arms (Table 14–3). If, in fact, AL and MF-MM are entirely independent endpoints, then the incidence of patients having both complications should be equal to the product of their relative frequencies. Table 14–4 indicates that this is not the case and that there are approximately two to three times as many patients as would be expected. For those patients in the myelosuppression arms who developed MF-MM, the incidence of AL was 28 percent, making this a particularly hazardous combination (see Table 14–3).

Silverstein and Brown[25] had noted that half of their patients with PV and AL developed MF-MM before their AL, and Lawrence et al.[2] had speculated that the usual progression in PV is for MF-MM to precede the development of AL. These findings of the PVSG also might be used to corroborate

TABLE 14-3. RELATIONSHIP BETWEEN TREATMENT, DEVELOPMENT OF MYELOFIBROSIS WITH MYELOID METAPLASIA, AND DEVELOPMENT OF ACUTE LEUKEMIA IN PVSG PROTOCOL 01 (DATA AS OF JANUARY 1986)

| | MF-MM ABSENT | | | MF-MM PRESENT | | |
| | | Acute Leukemia | | | Acute Leukemia | |
TREATMENT	Total Cases	Cases	Percent	Total Cases	Cases	Percent
Phlebotomy	120	1	0.8	14	1	7.1
Chlorambucil	127	14	11.0	14	5	36.0
[32]P	141	12	8.5	15	3	20.0
All chemotherapy	268	26	9.7	29	8	27.6

claims by other authors that splenic size,[26] presence of immature granulocytes in the circulation,[3] and higher leukocyte counts[26] might be predictors for the ultimate development of AL in PV patients. Najean et al.,[52] on the other hand, believe that the presence of MF-MM in PV is not a predictor for AL and is simply a function of the number of years of disease activity. While they did not give the number of patients in their series who had MF-MM and then went on to develop AL, 11 of the 33 patients (33 percent) in their series who developed AL had MF-MM before the diagnosis of AL was made. Similarly, Swolin et al.[39] noted that in their collected series of 13 patients with PV, MF-MM, and trisomy 1q, 5 (38 percent) went on to develop AL or myelodysplastic syndrome.[39] Based on this information, caution should be exercised in giving further chemotherapy to PV patients in whom evolution to MF-MM has occurred.[1, 27]

Chlorambucil (Leukeran)

In the 1981 PVSG publication the sole factor significantly associated with development of AL was randomization to one of the two myelosuppression arms (chlorambucil or ^{32}P). For patients taking chlorambucil, there was a fourfold increase in relative risk of developing AL if the dose was more than 4 mg/d (relative to a smaller dose; $p < 0.01$[15]) and a fivefold relative increase if this agent was given more than 50 percent of the available days (as opposed to 50 percent or less of available days; $p < 0.005$[15]). It has not been possible to determine the independent contributions of each of the two preceding variables to the development of AL.

Fully half the cases of AL reported to date in the chlorambucil arm occurred within 5 years of randomization (see Table 14-2) and are thus attributable to the effect of the drug alone rather than to prolongation of survival. Because this agent seemed to confer no sig-

TABLE 14-4. INCIDENCE OF THE COMBINATION OF MYELOFIBROSIS WITH MYELOID METAPLASIA AND ACUTE LEUKEMIA: OBSERVED VERSUS EXPECTED FOR PVSG PROTOCOL 01 (DATA AS OF JANUARY 1986)

| | TREATMENT ARM OF PVSG PROTOCOL 01 | | | |
CHARACTERISTIC	Phlebotomy	Chlorambucil	[32]P	ALL CASES
Incidence of AL (%)	1.5	13.5	9.6	8.4
Incidence of MF-MM (%)	10.4	9.9	9.6	10.0
Expected incidence of AL and MF-MM (%)*	0.156	1.34	0.922	0.833
Observed incidence of AL and MF-MM (%)	0.746	3.55	1.92	2.09
Observed/expected for the combination of AL and MF-MM	4.8	2.6	2.1	2.5

*Assumes that the complications are independent and that the probability of having both complications is equal to the product of the incidence of each taken separately.

nificant benefits over ^{32}P, use of this agent as one of the arms of PVSG protocol 01 was stopped in 1979. However, it was realized at that time that the future follow-up data might indicate an even higher incidence of AL, approximating the highest incidences reported for [32]P.[15] Indeed, despite the later onset for the majority of cases of AL following ^{32}P, the incidence of AL in the chlorambucil arm (13.5 percent) is higher (although not in a statistically significant amount) than that noted in the ^{32}P arm (9.6 percent) as of the 1986 data analysis.

Finally, it was noted that cases of AL have occurred on the chlorambucil arm 1 to 3 years after this drug was stopped. Moreover, the hazard function (Fig. 14–1) suggests that such patients are at an extremely high risk for development of AL more than 10 years after beginning treatment with this agent. Whether such late events (occurring with or without MF-MM) will continue to appear will require further follow-up of the surviving subjects in PVSG protocol 01.

Radioactive Phosphate (^{32}P)

As of the 1981 PVSG publication, the risk of developing AL was 2.3 times higher for patients in the chlorambucil arm than for those in the ^{32}P arm ($p < 0.025$). Although the risk of developing AL in the ^{32}P arm (6 percent) was much higher than that in the phlebotomy arm (1 percent), this difference was not statistically significant in 1979. At the latest available analysis (January 1986), this circumstance is changed, with the incidence of AL in the ^{32}P arm (9.6 percent) being significantly ($p < 0.01$) greater than that in the phlebotomy arm (1.5 percent) and not significantly different from that in the chlorambucil arm (13.5 percent; $0.50 > p > 0.30$). No analysis is yet available to determine whether, as in the case of the chlorambucil arm, there is any relationship between the total dose of ^{32}P and the relative risk of developing AL, as was suggested by Modan and Lilienfeld's data,[3] but that was not considered to be an important factor by Osgood[28] or by Lawrence et al.[2]

To a first approximation, survival is similar in the three arms, whereas the incidence of AL is significantly greater in the myelosuppression arms. One would therefore have to conclude that the high incidence of AL in the ^{32}P arm is due to the leukemogenic potential of this agent rather than to an effect of prolongation of survival. Retrospective data suggested that half the ^{32}P-associated cases of AL would occur more than 11 years after start of treatment and that they would continue to occur for at least 20 years. It is thus possible that future follow-up will establish a higher incidence of AL following ^{32}P treatment than that herein reported.

Phlebotomy

The presence of fully documented cases of AL in the phlebotomy arm firmly establishes AL as a part of the natural history of the "untreated" disease, with an incidence of 1.5 percent. Because the incidence of acute myelogenous leukemia (AML) in the U.S. population is about 10 cases per 100,000 per year for patients 55 to 75 years of age,[29] one would have expected about 0.07 cases in 1979 (1 observed) and 0.13 cases in 1984 (2 observed). Because both cases of AL occurred in patients prospectively randomized to phlebotomy and within 5 years of such randomization, this finding cannot be ascribed to bias in patient selection or prolongation of survival and establishes a low but significant incidence of AL when PV is treated with phlebotomy alone. Table 14–3 shows that for phlebotomy-treated patients, the incidence of AL was 0.8 percent when MF-MM was absent and 7 percent (1 case in 14) when it was present. Although based on a small subpopulation, this suggests that the presence of MF-MM might be an additional risk factor for development of AL in phlebotomy-treated PV patients.

Prolongation of Survival

Truly untreated patients with PV are rare in this era, but when reported in the past, they had a 50 percent survival time of about 18 months.[30] Because all reported treatments prolong survival well beyond 1 1/2 years,[31,32] it is unethical to withhold some sort of treatment. However, when the PVSG was organized, survival after phlebotomy was felt to be approximately 3 to 9 years and that for ^{32}P in the range of 10 to 15 years.[32] It was because of this prevailing belief in the superiority of survival of the ^{32}P treated patients that the issues of prolongation of survival and leukemogenicity of ^{32}P became critical. Thus, the following quotations:

The incidence of acute leukemia in our patients treated with ^{32}P may be primarily a result of prolonged survival rather than radiation dose.

Lawrence et al.[2]

Most persons would rather die at an advanced age with some risk of acute leukemia than at an earlier age from some other cause.

Osgood[33]

However, the latest analyses of PVSG protocol 01 data indicate that overall survival in the first 7 years after randomization is virtually identical in the phlebotomy, chlorambucil, and ^{32}P arms, although the complications suffered by patients in the three arms during this time are decidedly different.[19, 34] It is thus possible to conclude, in general, that the complications are the result of the treatment to which the patient was randomized rather than being due to longer survival with the uncovering of complications obscured by early deaths. Thus phlebotomy treatment is associated with thrombotic events, especially in the first 4 years after randomization, chemotherapy with leukemia and other malignancies, mostly occurring within 3 to 5 years of institution of therapy, and ^{32}P with AL and other malignancies having the more delayed onset typical of radiation carcinogenesis.

Hydroxyurea

The number of patients originally enrolled in PVSG protocol 08 and treated with hydroxyurea as the sole myelosuppressive agent is 51. Maximum follow-up is now more than 8 years. Thus far, with the addition of the case reported by Holcombe et al.,[53] the incidence of AL in the hydroxyurea-treated patients (4 cases of AL out of 51, 7.8 percent) is now significantly higher than that of the historical controls (PVSG protocol 01, phlebotomy arm: 2 cases of AL out of 134, 1.5 percent; $p < 0.03$.[35, 53] One additional patient was noted by the author (S.A.L.) to have developed and died of myelodysplastic syndrome (RAEB/T by the FAB classification). Further follow-up of this group of patients is eagerly awaited to determine whether this agent will prove to be significantly less leukemogenic than other effective myelosuppressive agents.

Nand et al.[54] reported the development of AL in 28 percent of their 18 patients treated with hydroxyurea. Of the 8 PV patients treated with hydroxyurea as the sole myelosuppressive agent, 12 percent developed AL, while this complication developed in 4 of 10 patients (40 percent) in whom hydroxyurea was used in combination with other myelosuppressive agents. Recently, Murphy et al. noted 1 case of AL in a series of 23 patients (4 percent) with essential thrombocythemia treated with hydroxyurea alone but in 5 of 6 patients (83 percent) initially treated with hydroxyurea and later switched to therapy with an alkylating agent (Murphy, Peterson, Iland, and Fruchtman, submitted to 14th Congress of the International Society on Thrombosis and Hemostasis). Such results as those reported above indicate that hydroxyurea may be leukemogenic when used in this setting as a single agent and suggest that the risk of treatment-associated AL may be quite high when hydroxyurea is one of multiple myelosuppressive agents used in a single patient.[54]

Other Chemotherapeutic Agents

The retrospective and anecdotal review[1] of 1976 indicated that fully 50 percent of collected cases of AL in chemotherapy-treated PV patients were associated with busulfan (Myleran) therapy. Average time from onset of PV to death from AL after busulfan was 7 years, and average age at the time of death was 58 years. These data suggested that busulfan would not be an effective alternative to chlorambucil in terms of reducing the incidence of AL. The EORTC phase III trial comparing ^{32}P with short-term courses of busulfan showed a similar incidence of AL in the two arms at a mean follow-up time of 8 years.[21]

Brusamolino et al.[36] have reported their experience with 100 consecutive PV patients treated with Pipobroman, a piperazine derivative alkylating agent. Seventy-three of these patients were previously untreated, and median follow-up for all patients was 5 years (range 1 to 12 years). Median actuarial survival for all patients was 11.7 years, and the cumulative risk of developing AL was 6 percent at 5 years and 9 percent at 7 years. The first leukemias were seen at 2 years after institution of therapy, and none has been seen more than 7 years after treatment. For those patients treated only with this agent and followed a mean of 5.2 years, the cumulative risk of developing AL was 6.8 percent.[36] It thus appears that this agent is comparable in leukemogenicity to ^{32}P and less leukemogenic than chlorambucil when compared with the PVSG protocol 01 data.

Toh et al.[55] reported on the use of uracil mustard in 11 PV patients and noted 2 cases of AL after 6 to 7 years of treatment with this agent (18 percent). Those patients who developed AL had been treated for longer periods of time and at higher doses than those patients not developing this complication.

Chromosomal Abnormalities

Chromosomal abnormalities in PV are discussed elsewhere in this book (Chapter 8). Although the incidence of structural and/or numerical clones was appreciable in the PV patients entered in the PVSG protocol 01 study, none was found to predict for the development of AL.[37] Similarly, Testa et al.[38] concluded that chromosomal abnormalities do not necessarily predict for the eventual occurrence of leukemia, although evolutionary changes during the course of treatment may be important prognostically.

Swollin et al.[39] reported on 12 of their patients with complete or partial trisomy of the long arm of chromosome 1 (trisomy 1q). Myelofibrosis with myeloid metaplasia (MF-MM) was present in 5 cases, and 5 developed AL. In an additional 19 cases taken from the literature, 12 of which had clinical details, there was evidence for AL in 3, and 7 to 9 may have had MF-MM. Thus, for this collected group of 24 cases, the incidence of MF-MM was approximately 50 to 58 percent and that of AL 33 percent—many times higher than that noted for patients randomized to the chemotherapeutic arms of PVSG protocol 01. The authors pointed out, however, that there was no consistent relationship between the occurrence of trisomy 1q and the development of MF-MM and/or AL. Although virtually all the 24 patients received some sort of chemotherapy, 3 did not, and none of these developed frank AL, while 2 did develop MF-MM. It is thus possible that trisomy 1q may be a marker for development of MF-MM and that those who are *also* treated with myelosuppressive drugs are the ones at further risk for development of AL. Indeed, the incidence of AL in the 24 patients (33 percent) is very close to that found in our cases of PV with MF-MM treated with ^{32}P or Leukeran (28 percent; see Table 14–3).

Pisciotta et al.[40] reported on the presence of leukemia associated with antigens (LAAs) in patients with PV. Although these were generally negative in patients with PV but without evidence for AL, three nonleukemic patients with PV were found to have a positive reaction that became progressively stronger with time. All three patients subsequently developed AL. The authors suggested that, in some cases, the presence of reactivity to LAAs may be predictive for the development of AL, although they could not rule out the possibility that such patients may already have had AL at a cellular burden too low for making a clinical diagnosis.[40]

CHARACTERISTICS OF ACUTE LEUKEMIA SEEN IN PV PATIENTS (INCLUDING DEVELOPMENT OF THE PRELEUKEMIC STATE)

There were significant improvements in our ability to diagnose and treat acute leukemia and the preleukemic (myelodysplastic) states occurring simultaneously with the PVSG protocols, including availability of cell markers and the increasing use of the more aggressive chemotherapeutic regimens. Because these were not made part of the protocols, it is not possible to comment, for example, on the breakdown of AL into the various subtypes of the modern FAB classification. However, some general observations concerning the nature of survival of such patients can be made at this time, and more complete analyses will be the subject of future PVSG publications.

Morphology

Classically, the AL occurring in PV has been of the nonlymphoblastic type, or ANLL. There are reports of eight cases of coexisting PV and chronic lymphocytic leukemia (CLL),[41] well-documented cases of acute lymphoblastic leukemia (ALL) occurring in PV,[42] and one case of basophilic leukemia.[43] In two series comprising a total of 16 patients,[44,45] 5 were described as myeloblastic, 5 as myelomonocytic, 4 as erythroleukemic, and 1 each as promyelocytic and undifferentiated. In a series of 13 patients with PV and AL taken from members of the PVSG (PVSG protocol 06[46]), all 13 were classified as ANLL. Although no formal attempt was made to classify these patients further, one was described as undifferentiated. One additional patient was found to have cells positive for terminal transferase, although these same cells contained Auer rods and had other morphologic characteristics of ANLL. This patient failed to respond to initial treatment with vincristine and prednisone and obtained complete remission after conventional anti-ANLL treatment with cytosine arabinoside and an anthracycline.

Clinical Characteristics

The earlier literature[1] suggested that AL was more common in male patients with PV. However, in the three series noted in the preceding paragraph[44-46] containing 29 patients, there were 15 males and 14 females. Additionally, analysis for risk factors for the first 26 cases of AL occurring in PVSG protocol 01 did not indicate that "maleness" was a statistically significant risk factor for the development of AL in PV.

Initial clinical experience with PV also suggested that the development of AL was abrupt, with few patients exhibiting a distinct "preleukemic" phase. However, starting in about 1986, reports appeared indicating that a distinct myelodysplastic disorder has preceded the development of AL in about 1 to 6 percent of PV patients[39,52,53,56-60] after a median interval of about 10 years. In the 24 cases reviewed by Shandas et al.[56] of RAEB and PV, 9 had structural or numerical abnormalities in either chromosome 5 or 7. Two patients had been treated with phlebotomy alone, and 18 were treated with ^{32}P alone or in combination with other myelosuppressive agents. Najean et al.[52] noted that fully 50 percent of their patients with AL and PV developed a myelodysplastic disorder (RAEB) before the diagnosis of AL. Other investigators have noted that many of the patients developing myelodysplasia in PV have shown chromosomal abnormalities such as trisomy 11,[57] deletions of chromosomes 5 and 7,[59-61] and translocations such as t(3;21) and t(1;7)[62,63] which are often seen in treatment-related AL occurring in the course of other malignancies, infrequently seen in stable-phase PV, and uncommon in patients treated with phlebotomy alone.

Treatment of the AL occurring in PV has generally been disappointing, although cases exhibiting complete remission and prolonged disease-free survival have been reported.[47] Three cases have been reported

with PV and AL who reverted back to a phase of active PV after induction, requiring institution of phlebotomy or myelosuppressive (cyclophosphamide, Cytoxan, Bristol Laboratories, Syracuse, N.Y.) therapy.[47,48,53] Because the average age of onset of PV is 60 years[15] and AL ensues some years after that (see Table 14–2), the patients definitely fall into a poor-risk category due to age alone.[49] Because the majority of cases (over 94 percent; see Table 14–1) in our series occurred in patients treated with chemotherapy, there is also the problem of underlying marrow damage, as reflected in the chromosomal abnormalities and/or accompanying myelodysplastic states (see above). Generally, it is the experience that secondary leukemias occurring in both malignant and nonmalignant conditions treated with chemotherapy (such as multiple myeloma and Hodgkin's disease) are especially refractory to therapy.[23,50,51] However, as noted by Bloomfield and Brunning,[51] few such patients have been treated with the effective combination chemotherapy now available.

Based on evidence that patients with chronic myelogenous leukemia (CML) may develop an ALL-like picture with terminal transferase positivity and response to vincristine-prednisone combinations, 13 consecutive patients with PV and AL were entered into a protocol (PVSG protocol 06) that involved initial treatment for 2 weeks with vincristine (1.3 mg/m^2 IV on days 1 and 8) and prednisone (60 mg/m^2 per day orally for 14 days). All 13 patients failed to respond to this treatment,[46] and 4 died during the initial 2 weeks. The 9 remaining patients were treated with anthracycline (Adriamycin, Adria Laboratories, Columbus, Ohio), 30 mg/m$_2$ IV on days 1, 2, and 3) and cytosine arabinoside (100 mg/m^2 by continuous IV infusion for 7 days, starting on day 1). Of these 9 patients, 5 died during the first 30 days of treatment due either to bleeding or infection. One patient obtained a partial response but refused further treatment and died at 33 weeks. One patient did not respond, did not receive further treatment, and survived a total of 52 weeks despite having a bone marrow containing about 50 percent blast cells. One patient obtained complete remission status lasting 38 weeks. Reinduction therapy in this patient was unsuccessful. Finally, a single patient not responding to the first course of therapy was treated with 2 consecutive days of Adriamycin and 5 days of cytosine arabinoside, failed to respond, and died shortly thereafter. Median survival for this group of 13 patients was only 32 days from the start of vincristine-prednisone, and only 1 of the 9 patients treated with Adriamycin–cytosine arabinoside achieved complete remission status (11 percent). It was clear from this study that not only was the vincristine-prednisone therapy ineffective, but it also was harmful, in that it represented 14 days during which the patient was not receiving effective therapy, while the prednisone was predisposing that patient to be at increased risk for infection.

Two final comments may be in order. There is some likelihood of response to combination chemotherapy schedules for AL in PV, which can be attempted in younger patients with good performance status. For the others, as in the patient who lived 52 weeks in continuous relapse status, supportive therapy with transfusions and antibiotics often can be associated with appreciable survival and an acceptable quality of life.

CONCLUSIONS

Acute leukemia is part of the natural history of PV, occurring at a frequency of 1 to 2 percent in phlebotomy-treated patients. When PV patients are treated with chemotherapy, ^{32}P, or x-ray, the incidence of AL approaches 10 to 15 percent. The AL is usually of the ANLL variety, may be preceded by MF-MM, and/or a myelodysplastic state, and is less responsive to therapy than is de novo ANLL. There appears to be no generally applicable way to predict which PV patient requiring chemotherapy is likely to develop AL. Patients with PV and transformation into MF-MM are at a higher risk of developing AL, and it would be prudent to limit further chemotherapy in these patients if at all possible.

REFERENCES

1. Landaw SA: Acute leukemia in polycythemia vera. Semin Hematol 13:33–48, 1976
2. Lawrence JH, Winchell HS, Donald WG: Leukemia in polycythemia vera: Relationship to splenic myeloid metaplasia and therapeutic radiation dose. Ann Intern Med 70:763–771, 1969
3. Modan B, Lilienfeld AM: Polycythemia vera and leukemia: The role of radiation treatment. A study of 1222 patients. Medicine 44:305–344, 1965
4. Schwartz SO, Ehrlich L: The relationship of polycythemia vera to leukemia: A critical review. Acta Haematol 4:129–147, 1950
5. Lawrence JH: Polycythemia: Physiology, Diagnosis, and Treatment. Orlando, Fla, Grune & Stratton, 1955
6. Tinney WS, Hall BE, Giffin HZ: Hematologic complications of P. vera. Proc Staff Meet Mayo Clin 18:227–230, 1943
7. Rosenthal MC: Extramedullary hematopoiesis, myeloid metaplasia. Bull N Engl Med Center 12:154, 1950
8. Dameshek W: Some speculations on the myeloproliferative syndromes. Blood 6:372–375, 1951
9. Wasserman LR: Polycythemia vera: Its course and treatment. Relation to myeloid metaplasia and leukemia. Bull NY Acad Med 3:343–375, 1954
10. Gilbert HS: Problems relating to control of polycythemia vera: The use of alkylating agents. Blood 32:500–505, 1968
11. Perkins J, Israels MCG, Wilkinson JF: Polycythaemia vera: Clinical studies on a series of 127 patients managed without radiation therapy. J Med 33:499–518, 1964
12. Logue GL, Gutterman JV, McGinn TG, et al: Melphalan therapy of polycythemia vera. Blood 36:70–86, 1970
13. Najean Y, Dresch C, Rain JD, et al: Les elements du choix therapeutique dans les polyglobulies vraies: 1. L'efficacite de la chimiotherapie. Nouv Presse Med 2:1431–1435, 1973
14. Rain JD, Dresch C, Said A, et al: Les elements du choix therapeutique dans les polyglobulies vraies: II. Evolution a long terme de 286 malades traites par ^{32}P. Nouv Presse Med 2:1499–1503, 1973
15. Berk PD, Goldberg JD, Silverstein MN, et al: Increased incidence of acute leukemia in polycythemia vera associated with chlorambucil therapy. N Engl J Med 304:441–447, 1981
16. Silverstein MN, Goldberg JD, Balcerzak SP, et al: The incidence of acute leukemia in a randomized clinical trial for polycythemia vera. Blood 54(suppl):209A, 1979
17. Shubin S: Triazure and public drug policies. Perspect Biol Med 22:185–204, 1979
18. United States Public Health Service: Survey of compounds which have been tested for carcinogenic activity. Public Health Service Publication No. 149. Washington, US Government Printing Office, 1951 (supplements through 1971)
19. Wasserman LR, Balcerzak SP, Berk PD, et al: Influence of therapy on causes of death in polycythemia vera. Trans Assoc Am Physicians 94:30–38, 1981
20. Tartaglia AP, Goldberg JD, Berk PD, Wasserman LR: Adverse effects of antiaggregating platelet therapy in the treatment of polycythemia vera. Semin Hematol 23:172–176, 1986
21. Haanen C, Mathe G, Hayat M: Treatment of polycythaemia vera by radiophosphorus or busulphan: A randomized trial. Br J Cancer 44:75–80, 1981

22. Bizzozero OJ, Johnson KG, Ciocco A: Radiation-related leukemia in Hiroshima and Nagasaki, 1946–1964. N Engl J Med 274:1095–1101, 1966

23. Rosner F, Grunwald H: Hodgkin's disease and acute leukemia: Report of 8 cases and review of the literature. Am J Med 58:339–353, 1975

24. Ellis JT, Peterson P, Geller SA, Rappaport H: Studies of the bone marrow in polycythemia vera and the evolution of myelofibrosis and second hematologic malignancies. Semin Hematol 23:144–155, 1986

25. Silverstein MN, Brown AL: Idiopathic myeloid metaplasia. Arch Intern Med 132:709–712, 1973

26. Tubiana M, Flamant R, Attie E, et al: A study of hematological complications occurring in patients with polycythemia vera treated with ^{32}P. Blood 32:536–548, 1968

27. Silverstein MN: Post-polycythemia myeloid metaplasia. Arch Intern Med 134:113–120, 1974

28. Osgood EE: Contrasting evidence of acute monocytic and granulocytic leukemia in ^{32}P-treated patients with polycythemia vera and chronic lymphocytic leukemia. J Lab Clin Med 64:560–573, 1964

29. Cutler SJ, Young JL (eds): Third National Cancer Survey: Incidence Data. National Cancer Institute Monograph No. 41. Washington, US Government Printing Office, 1975, p 102

30. Chievitz E, Thiede T: Complications and causes of death in polycythemia vera. Acta Med Scand 172:513–523, 1962

31. Videbaek A: Polycythemia vera: Course and prognosis. Acta Med Scand 138:179–187, 1950

32. Wasserman LR: The treatment of polycythemia vera. Semin Hematol 13:57–78, 1976

33. Osgood EE: Polycythemia vera: Age relationships and survival. Blood 26:243–256, 1965

34. Berk PD, Goldberg JD, Donovan PB, et al: Therapeutic recommendations in polycythemia vera based on Polycythemia Vera Study Group Protocols. Semin Hematol 23:132–143, 1986

35. Kaplan ME, Mack K, Goldberg JD, et al: Long-term management of polycythemia vera with hydroxyurea: A progress report. Semin Hematol 23:167–171, 1986

36. Brusamolino E, Salvaneschi L, Canevari A, et al: Efficacy trial of pipobroman in polycythemia vera and incidence of acute leukemia. J Clin Oncol 2:558–561, 1984

37. Berk PD, Wasserman LR: Acute leukemia in polycythemia vera (letter). N Engl J Med 305:342–343, 1981

38. Testa JRM, Kanofsky JR, Rowley JD, et al: Karyotypic patterns and their clinical significance in polycythemia vera. Am J Hematol 11:29–45, 1981

39. Swolin B, Weinfeld A, Westin J: Trisomy 1q in polycythemia vera and its relation to disease transition. Am J Hematol 22:155–167, 1986

40. Pisciotta AV, Cronkite C, Hanson GA, et al: Leukemia-associated antigens in leukemic transformation of polycythemia vera. J Lab Clin Med 101:432–440, 1983

41. Jacobsen N, Theilade K, Videbaek A: Two additional cases of coexisting polycythemia vera and chronic lymphocytic leukemia. Scand J Haematol 29:405–410, 1982

42. Hoffman R, Estren S, Kopel S, et al: Lymphoblastic-like leukemic transformation of polycythemia vera. Ann Intern Med 89:71, 1978

43. Eagan JW, Kaughman KL, Miller S, et al: Systemic mastocytosis in a patient with polycythemia vera treated with radioactive phosphorus. Blood 49:563–571, 1977

44. Rosenthal DS, Moloney WC: Occurrence of acute leukemia in myeloproliferative disorders. Br J Haematol 36:373–382, 1977

45. Weinfeld A, Westin J, Ridell B, et al: Polycythaemia vera terminating in acute leukaemia. Scand J Haematol 19:255–272, 1977

46. Donovan PB, Landaw SA, Dresch C, et al: Resistance to therapy of acute leukemia developing in the course of polycythemia vera. Nouv Rev Fr Hematol 23:187–192, 1981

47. Hazani A, Tatarsky I, Barzilai D: Prolonged remission of leukemia associated with polycythemia vera. Cancer 40:1297–1299, 1977

48. Daly HM, Scott GL: Acute monocytic leukaemia complicating polcythaemia rubra vera: Successful response to chemotherapy with recurrence of polycythaemia. Clin Lab Haematol 5:319–321, 1983

49. Henderson ES: Acute myelogenous leukemia. In Williams WJ, Beutler E, Erslev AJ, et al (eds): Hematology, 3d ed. New York, McGraw-Hill, 1983, p 239

50. Preisler HD, Lyman GH: Acute myelocytic leukemia subsequent to therapy for a different neoplasm: Clinical features and response to therapy. Am J Hematol 3:209–218, 1977

51. Bloomfield CD, Brunning RD: Acute leukemia as a terminal event in nonleukemic hematopoietic disorders. Semin Oncol 3:297–317, 1976

52. Najean Y, Deschamps A, Dresch C, et al: Acute leukemia and myelodysplasia in polycythemia vera: A clinical study with long-term follow-up. Cancer 61:89–95, 1988

53. Holcombe RF, Treseler PA, Rosenthal DS: Chronic myelomonocytic leukemia transformation in polycythemia vera. Leukemia 5:606–610, 1991

54. Nand S, Messmore H, Fisher SG, et al: Leukemic transformation in polycythemia vera: Analysis of risk factors. Am J Hematol 34:32–36, 1990

55. Toh BT, Gregory SA, Knospe WH: Acute leukemia following treatment of polycythemia vera and essential thrombocythemia with uracil mustard. Am J Hematol 28:58–60, 1988

56. Shamdas GJ, Spier CM, List AF: Myelodysplastic transformation of polycythemia vera: Case report and review of the literature. Am J Hematol 37:45–48, 1991

57. Ohyashiki K, Nagasu M, Hojo H, et al: Myelodysplastic syndrome with trisomy 11 associated with polycythemia vera. Am J Hematol 31:122–125, 1989

58. Heim S, Sorensen AG, Christensen BE, et al: Reemergence in remission of primary clone in acute myelogenous leukemias with multiple chromosomal aberrations at diagnosis. Br J Haematol 82:332–336, 1992

59. Diez-Martin JL, Graham DL, Petitt RM, et al: Chromosome studies in 104 patients with polycythemia vera. Mayo Clin Proc 66:287–299, 1991

60. Testa JR, Kanofsky JR, Rawley JD, et al: Karyo-typic patterns and their clinical significance in polycythemia vera. Am J Hematol 11:29, 1981

61. Mertens F, Johannson B, Heim S, et al: Karyotypic patterns in chronic myeloproliferative disorders: Report on 74 cases and review of the literature. Leukemia 5:214–220, 1991

62. Rubin CM, Larson RA, Anastasi J, et al: t(3;21) (q26;q22): A recurring chromosomal abnormality in therapy-related myelodysplastic syndrome and acute myeloid leukemia. Blood 76: 2594–2598, 1990

63. Morrison-DeLap SJ, Kuffel DG, Dewald GW, et al: Unbalanced 1;7 translocation and therapy-induced hematologic disorders: A possible relationship. Am J Hematol 21:39–47, 1986

15

Treatment of Polycythemia Vera: A Summary of Clinical Trials Conducted by the Polycythemia Vera Study Group

PAUL D. BERK, LOUIS R. WASSERMAN,
STEVEN M. FRUCHTMAN, *and* JUDITH D. GOLDBERG

The Polycythemia Vera Study Group (PVSG) was founded in 1967 to conduct clinical studies in polycythemia with three explicit goals: (1) to develop a set of diagnostic criteria that could then become the basis for defining patient populations for future studies (Chapt. 3), (2) to gather information about the epidemiology, natural history, and pathophysiology of the disorder (Chaps. 4-6, 8-11, 13 and 22), and (3) to determine the optimal treatment for polycythemia vera (PV). Since its creation in 1967, the group has conducted a total of 14 separate studies addressing various questions concerning PV and the other myeloproliferative diseases. Some of these protocols were principally natural history studies, and others dealt with myeloproliferative disorders other than PV, including entities such as essential thrombocythemia (ET) and myelofibrosis with myeloid metaplasia. Seven protocols dealt specifically with treatment issues related to PV, and it is the three major PV treatment protocols that form the focus of this chapter. These studies, which in the aggregate involved almost 10,000 patient-years of follow-up, permit the PVSG to make a series of therapeutic recommendations in this disorder which are based on extensive, systematic, and well-designed clinical trials.

The organization of the PVSG followed by 2 years the landmark publication[1] in which Modan and Lilienfeld, following a massive review of the literature, claimed that the frequent occurrence of acute leukemia in patients with PV was directly linked to the use of radioactive phosphorus (^{32}P) as a treatment modality. These conclusions argued strongly against the continued use of ^{32}P therapy. In fact, acute leukemia as a complication of the treatment of PV with ^{32}P had first been reported in 1943 by Tinney et al.[2] After World War II, with the increased availability of ^{32}P, there were numerous anecdotal comments and discussion about its safety and efficacy compared with phlebotomy. Some argued that phlebotomy was the treatment of choice because it was not associated with acute leukemia; others held that ^{32}P was preferable because only for that treatment modality were there substantial data indicating a life expectancy approaching that of a normal control population. There were no acceptable data permitting a direct comparison of results in patients treated with ^{32}P compared with phlebotomy alone. The data of Chievitz and Thiede[3] and others (reviewed in ref. 4) were at best of limited value. While Modan and Lilienfeld summarized data from seven institutions indicating a median life expectancy of approximately 10 years in patients treated with ^{32}P, there were no comparable data for phlebotomy-treated patients or patients treated with other myelosuppressive agents.

Because radioactive phosphorus had been so widely employed in this disorder and provided by far the most trouble-free management of the disease for long periods of time in many patients, many clinicians were reluctant to accept the conclusions of the Modan and Lilienfeld study without the confirmation of a prospective, randomized, controlled trial. The first study undertaken by the PVSG, designated PVSG protocol 01, was therefore precisely such a prospective, randomized trial that compared the efficacy of phlebotomy alone with that of two different myelosuppressive regimens supplemented by phlebotomy. The myelosuppressive regimens studied were radioactive phosphorus and chemotherapy with the alkylating agent chlorambucil. While the use of alkylating agents for the control of PV was a growing practice in the 1960s, the specific choice of chlorambucil was based on a relatively limited experience, predominantly at the Mount Sinai Hospital in New York City, suggesting that this agent was effective in the control of PV with a minimum of short-term side effects. Subsequent PVSG studies have, among other issues, investigated the use of platelet antiaggregating agents for the prevention of thrombotic complications in PV (PVSG protocol 05), the treatment of acute leukemia which develops during the course of PV (PVSG protocol 06), the effectiveness of hydroxyurea as a nonalkylating myelosuppressive agent in the control of PV (PVSG protocol 08), the use of androgen therapy for the treatment of the spent phase of PV (PVSG

protocols 04 and 11), and the use of H_1 (PVSG protocol 14) and combined $H_1 + H_2$ (PVSG protocol 15) histamine receptor antagonists for the control of intractable pruritus in PV. The design of the PVSG protocol 01, 05, and 08 studies and essential results derived from them will be discussed in detail below.

DIAGNOSIS OF POLYCYTHEMIA VERA

A pathophysiologic approach to the diagnosis of PV, involving the exclusion of other secondary causes of erythrocytosis and the demonstration of such diagnostic features as the presence of "endogenous colonies" in blood and bone marrow, was described in Chap. 3. This approach has been incorporated into a useful and effective diagnostic algorithm. However, completion of the entire algorithm is both time-consuming and expensive. To rapidly identify patients with PV, facilitating their enrollment in clinical studies, the PVSG devised a set of formal criteria that facilitated establishing the diagnosis within two visits in an ambulatory setting. These criteria are summarized in Table 15–1. The PVSG has established by detailed follow-up that patients who meet these simple criteria are highly likely to have PV; the false-positive rate is approximately 0.5 percent. Accordingly, the criteria listed in Table 15–1 were used as standard entry criteria for the PVSG protocols described below.

In applying these criteria, false-positive results are most likely to be found in patients who are excessive users of both alcohol and tobacco. In this context, excessive compensatory erythroid activity associated with carboxy-

TABLE 15–1. PVSG CRITERIA FOR THE DIAGNOSIS OF POLYCYTHEMIA VERA

A1.	Increased RBC mass Male: ≥36 ml/kg Female: ≥32 ml/kg	B1.	Thrombocytosis: Platelet count >400,000/μl	
A2.	Normal arterial O_2 saturation (≥92%)	B2.	Leukocytosis: >12,000/μl (no fever or infection)	
A3.	Splenomegaly	B3.	Increased leukocyte alkaline phosphatase (LAP > 100)	
		B4.	Increased serum B_{12}/binders B_{12}: >900 pg/ml Unbound B_{12} binding capacity: >2200 pg/ml	

Note: Diagnosis of PV virtually certain in the presence of A1 + A2 + A3 or A1 + A2 + any two from category B.

hemoglobinemia from smoking ("smoker's polycythemia"), in combination with the splenomegaly, leukocytosis, and increased serum B_{12} and leukocyte alkaline phosphatase activities associated with alcoholic liver disease, may confound the diagnosis. In addition, patients with early disease who do not yet meet the PVSG criteria may prove to have PV discernible only through special studies such as bone marrow colony assays.

POLYCYTHEMIA VERA STUDY GROUP PROTOCOL 01

Description of the Protocol

The basic features of PVSG protocol 01 are outlined in Fig. 15–1. Patients with PV who satisfied the required PVSG diagnostic criteria (see Table 15–1) and in whom the diagnosis of PV had been made within 4 years were initially registered for the study. They were then phlebotomized to a normal hematocrit and observed. If the hematocrit rose by 10 percent within the subsequent 3 months or rose to a level greater than 55 percent within 1 year, the patient was then randomized to one of the three treatment arms of the study. This prerandomization component to the protocol was incorporated in order to ensure that only patients in the active, proliferative stage of the disease were entered into the study.

Between 1967 and 1974, a total of 431

patients were found to be fully eligible and were randomized to one of the three treatment arms of the study. Thus the initial patient was entered more than 25 years ago, and the minimum period of follow-up in surviving patients exceeds 19 years as this review is written.

In patients randomized to receive phlebotomy treatment, the procedure was performed as often as necessary to maintain a normal hematocrit value. This was defined early in the study as a hematocrit of 52 percent or less. Subsequently, our experience and that of others[5–7] led to a modification of the protocol to require maintenance of a hematocrit of 45 percent or less. Patients randomized to receive ^{32}P therapy were initially phlebotomized to achieve a normal hematocrit, as defined above. Subsequently, ^{32}P, 2.3 mCi/m^2 of body surface area (maximum dose limit 5 mCi), was administered intravenously. Patients were classified as complete responders, partial responders, or nonresponders based on their hematocrit and platelet and white cell counts, according to previously reported criteria.[8] Radioactive phosphorus administration could be repeated as often as every 12 weeks, according to the clinical response. In patients in whom there was no response to the initial dose, subsequent doses were increased by 25 percent. Phlebotomy was used as often as necessary to maintain a hematocrit equal to or less than the current limit established by the phlebotomy regimen during the interval be-

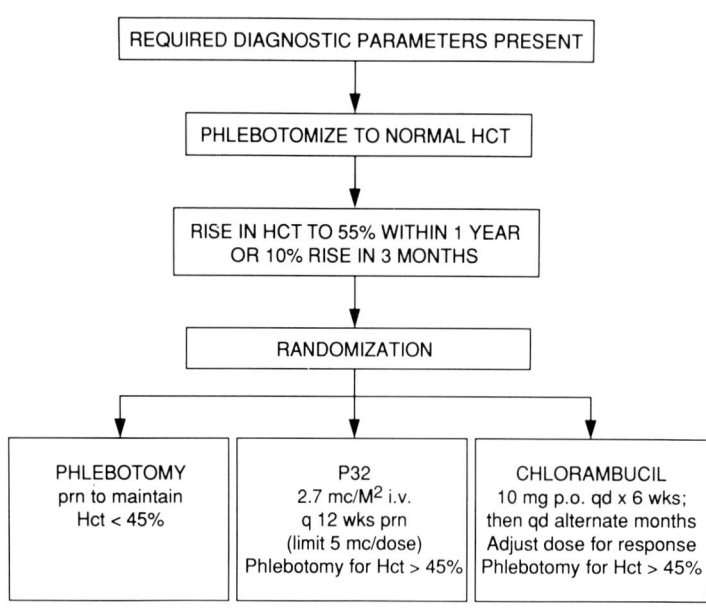

FIGURE 15–1. Schematic outline of Polycythemia Vera Study Group protocol 01.

tween ^{32}P doses. Patients initially randomized to chlorambucil treatment also were initially phlebotomized to achieve a normal hematocrit. Subsequently, chlorambucil, 10 mg PO, was administered daily for 6 weeks. Administration was followed by a 30-day rest period. The patient was then placed on a maintenance regimen that consisted of 30 days of treatment alternating with 30 days of rest. The daily dose during each treatment period was adjusted to avoid either thrombocytopenia or leukopenia.

Patients entered into the study were seen as often as necessary for appropriate clinical management, but at least every 12 weeks. Reports of physical examinations, detailed laboratory data, functional status reports, and information concerning a variety of specific endpoints were submitted to the central office on each patient at specified intervals. Major developments, complications of treatment, and deaths were reported as soon as they occurred. A quality control committee reviewed each patient's initial data in order to confirm his or her eligibility. This committee also reviewed all follow-up data semiannually in order to ensure appropriate adherence to the protocol and to confirm diagnosed causes of death and other reported complications. This review was performed concurrently with reviews performed by the cytogenetics and histopathology committees, which examined all submitted specimens in order to ensure uniformity of interpretation and diagnosis. Those patients whose treatment resulted in minor protocol violations were maintained in the study, and their treatment was adjusted appropriately to conform with the protocol. In a few instances, as a result of major protocol violations, the quality control committee required that patients be removed from the study. Data on such patients were handled as described below in the section on statistical procedures. Every effort was expended to continue to obtain follow-up data on all patients initially entered into the study until death, including those patients who were subsequently excluded because of protocol violations.

The clinical courses of patients were examined for the first occurrence of the following major endpoints: a major thrombotic event, the development of acute leukemia or lymphoma, the development of a nonhematologic neoplasm, or death. Transformation of PV from the active proliferative stage to the "spent" phase and the occurrence of major hemorrhagic events also were recorded but were not considered endpoints for analysis. The criteria for the diagnosis of acute leukemia included the clinical status, the presence of blast cells in the peripheral blood, and the presence of 25 percent or more blasts in a bone marrow specimen of at least normal cellularity.[9]

Through 1978, reports of physical examinations, detailed laboratory data, functional status reports, and information concerning a variety of specific endpoints were submitted to the central office quarterly on each patient. From 1978 through 1981, such reports were submitted semiannually. Because of the infrequency of significant changes in many of the parameters under study and the stability of many long-term trends, annual follow-up is now required for surviving patients only for the occurrence of major endpoints, as defined above. Through 1981, an extensive update of the entire data file was conducted semiannually. Data bases are now updated as new data are accessioned, principally for monitoring purposes. Periodically, major efforts are made to retrieve delinquent data; these are followed by a major update of the entire data base. The most recently completed major update and analysis were conducted in 1987, for all events reported as of January 1, 1987. Collection of data for a new major update was initiated during the summer of 1993 and is in process as this is written. Although, for the sake of uniformity, this analysis is based principally on the results of the 1987 data base update and analysis, preliminary analyses of all data received through the early spring of 1993 indicate that the more recent data do not alter any of the conclusions presented below.

At the time of the 1987 data base update and analysis, 16.3 percent of the initial randomized patient population was alive and on active study, and 50.8 percent had died while on study. An additional 29.0 percent of the initial patient population had been removed from active participation in the study for a variety of reasons, most commonly for a major protocol violation. For the most part, the data presented in this chapter are based on analyses only of events that occurred while patients were still actively on study. However, parallel statistical analyses also have been carried out including events reported to the central office subsequent to the removal from study. To date, inclusion of events reported after removal from study has not changed any of the major findings to be reported. As of 1987, only 3.9 percent of the initial total study population of 431 patients had been irretrievably lost to follow-up after major efforts to obtain relevant information.

Statistical Methods

The primary aim of this report is to compare the rates of occurrence of the specified endpoints of the study among the three treatment groups. Therefore, Kaplan-Meier curves for the incidence of these endpoints were compared with the use of Breslow's extension of generalized Wilcoxon and Kruskal-Wallis tests,[10, 11] as well as the log-rank chi-squared procedure.[12, 13] These significance testing procedures differ in that the Breslow method gives more weight to earlier events and the log-rank procedure gives more weight to later events.

To ensure that the balance sought by the randomization procedure was achieved, methods of descriptive statistics were used to compare the characteristics of patients randomized to the three treatment groups at entry. These exploratory analyses of entry characteristics also were used to identify imbalances among the treatment groups that would suggest possible covariates for adjustment in the multivariate analyses described below.

Analysis of the incidence of each of the specified endpoints or disease complications also used Cox regression models for censored data[14-16] to assess whether the observed treatment effects might be explained by other factors. These models permit simultaneous adjustment for variables that may influence prognosis. With these models, each variable thought to be related to prognosis was examined individually or jointly for its contribution to the likelihood function. Reduced models were then developed that included only factors that appeared important on statistical or clinical grounds through procedures similar to those described by Byar and Corle.[17] With the simplified coding of dichotomous variables employed (0 = low level, 1 = high level), relative risks are readily estimated from the coefficients calculated from the Cox model and the approximate significance of coefficients assessed by referencing the appropriate distribution.

Possible sources of bias introduced by assumptions in the analytical procedures, patient exclusion, patient management, and data reporting have been examined. As noted earlier, patients who were lost to follow-up, had never been treated according to protocol, or had been withdrawn because of violations of protocol were classified in these analyses as censored at the time of loss, termination, or violation. Events or endpoints that occurred in these patients after withdrawal from the study were excluded from the primary analysis; however, the data also were reanalyzed including events reported later among patients withdrawn from the study while still alive. These additional analyses have in no instance resulted in an alteration of a major conclusion of the study. All secondary analyses confirm that the results described below were not influenced by identifiable biases; these include analyses based on all reported events in all patients ever randomized.

Results

Overall Survival and Causes of Death. Cumulative survival curves for the three treatment arms of PVSG protocol 01 are presented in Fig. 15–2. As of January 1, 1987, 219 patients, or 50.8 percent of the initial randomized cohort, had died while on study. Median survival from entry into the study until death was 9.1 years for patients treated with chlorambucil, 10.9 years for those treated with ^{32}P, and 12.6 years for patients in the phlebotomy group. As indicated in the figure, long-term survival from randomization is significantly poorer for patients treated with chlorambucil than for those treated with either radioactive phosphorus supplemented by phlebotomy or with phlebotomy alone. Survival in these latter two groups is comparable. This conclusion is essentially unchanged since the analysis of March 1983, even though 56 additional deaths have occurred in the intervening 4 years. Maximum follow-up as of January 1, 1987 was 17.5 years in the ^{32}P group, 18.5 in the phlebotomy group, and 19.1 years in the chlorambucil group.

Of the causes of death reported to the central office as of January 1, 1987, the most common, accounting for 29.2 percent of on-study fatalities, was thrombosis, followed in descending order by leukemia, lymphoma,

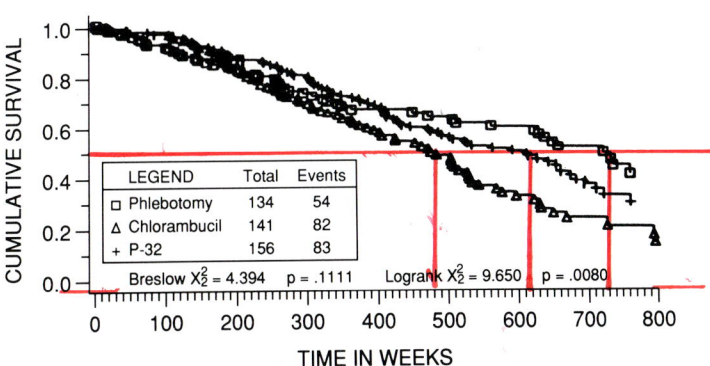

FIGURE 15–2. Cumulative survival curves for patients randomized to each of the three treatment arms of PVSG protocol 01. Curves reflect on-study events reported to the statistical office from the initiation of the study in 1967 through January 1, 1987. See text for details.

and other hematologic malignancies, which accounted for 23.3 percent; nonhematologic malignancies, 16.0 percent; hemorrhage, 6.8 percent; and the development of spent phase with myelofibrosis and/or myeloid metaplasia, 3.2 percent. Thus only five entities accounted for more than three-quarters of all deaths reported. The relative frequency of these five principal causes of death did not change appreciably if deaths occurring off study were included in the analysis. The remaining 21.5 percent of deaths were distributed over a wide variety of other causes.

As suggested by a comparison of the results of the log-rank procedure, which emphasizes later events, and the Breslow procedure, which emphasizes earlier events, current differences in overall survival among the three treatment arms are principally the result of difference in the incidence of fatalities late in the study (Fig. 15–2). Indeed, over the first 7 years after randomization, overall survival was equivalent in the three treat-

ment groups, although the causes of death varied as a function of treatment.[18] Thrombosis occurred appreciably more frequently among phlebotomy-treated patients during the first 3 years of the study, while leukemia and cancer have occurred predominantly in the myelosuppressive-group patients, particularly after the fifth year. If attention is restricted to survival in patients who have remained alive and on study for at least 7 years, the progressive disadvantage of patients treated with myelosuppressive therapy, resulting from an inexorable increase in both hematologic and nonhematologic malignancies, is apparent (Fig. 15–3).

The distribution of thrombotic, leukemic, and other malignant deaths among the three treatment arms of the study will be described in the sections that follow.

Thrombosis

As of January 1, 1987, 146 patients had had a thrombotic event as a primary end-

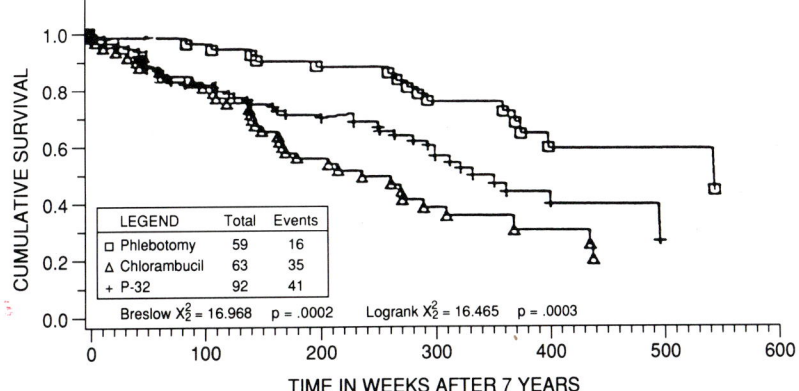

FIGURE 15–3. Cumulative survival after 7 years on study for patients in each of the treatment arms of PVSG protocol 01. Compared with Fig. 13–2, this analysis emphasizes the progressive disadvantage of patients treated with either of the two myelosuppressive regimens (chlorambucil or ^{32}P). See text for discussion.

point while on study. An additional 17 thrombotic events occurred in patients who had been removed from the study for the reasons enumerated above. These off-study events were evenly distributed among the three treatment arms of the study.

The nature of the initial thrombotic events occurring on this study is summarized in Table 15-2. The most common were cerebral vascular accidents, which accounted for approximately 35 percent of the reported initial thrombotic episodes. In descending order of frequency, myocardial infarction, peripheral arterial occlusion, pulmonary infarcts, and venous thromboses other than thrombophlebitis accounted for an additional 31 percent. The venous thromboses included catastrophic situations such as mesenteric vein thrombosis, axillary vein thrombosis, and two instances of hepatic vein thrombosis. Twenty-two percent of the initial thrombotic events occurring in this study represented uncomplicated deep vein thrombosis, while the remaining 12 percent represented a miscellaneous group of conditions. Recent reports attributing numerous episodes of apparently idiopathic portal or hepatic vein thrombosis[19, 20] to "latent" myeloproliferative disease, diagnosed solely from the presence of apparently erythropoietin-independent ("endogenous") erythroid colony growth in vitro, are in striking contrast to the occurrence of only three cases of Budd-Chiari syndrome (one of which occurred off study) in the almost 5000 patient-years of follow-up in this study of patients with overt myeloproliferative disease.

TABLE 15-2. PVSG PROTOCOL 01: INITIAL THROMBOTIC EVENTS (ON-STUDY EVENTS)

TYPE OF EVENT	NUMBER	PERCENT OF EVENTS
Cerebral vascular accident	51	35
Myocardial infarct	18	12
Peripheral arterial occlusion	13	9
Pulmonary infarct	8	6
Venous thrombosis (other than thrombophlebitis)	6	4
Deep vein thrombophlebitis	32	22
Miscellaneous	18	12
TOTAL	146	100

It is important to emphasize that the thrombotic events that occur during the course of PV include both arterial and venous occlusive phenomena. If uncomplicated deep vein thrombophlebitis and the various miscellaneous conditions are excluded, one-quarter of the initial thrombotic events were fatal. To date, approximately one-third of individuals who survived an initial thrombosis have had a second or subsequent thrombotic episode. The case-fatality rate in these subsequent thrombotic episodes has been approximately 35 percent.

The thrombosis-free cumulative survival curves are illustrated in Fig. 15-4. With regard to thrombotic events, phlebotomy-treated patients did significantly less well statistically than those of the two groups treated with myelosuppression during the first 3 years of the study. Subsequently, however, curves of thrombosis-free survival in the three treatment arms have been essentially parallel, and the incidence of late thrombotic events in the [32]P- and chlorambucil-treated patients has gradually caught up with the earlier incidence observed in phlebotomy-treated patients. Indeed, the high incidence of thrombotic events early in the study in patients treated with phlebotomy posed appreciable ethical difficulties for the investigators. Since thrombosis-free cumulative survival in the phlebotomy treatment group was significantly poorer than in the other two treatment arms (Fig. 15-4A: Breslow $\chi^2_2 = 8.4, p = 0.015$), a number of the investigators in the group argued that the study should be terminated at that point because patients in the phlebotomy arm were being exposed to an undue risk of thrombosis. Other investigators, with the support of the group's biostatistical office, argued that this decision would be premature, and the study was permitted to continue while being monitored frequently with respect to the trend toward excess thrombosis in the phlebotomy-treated patients. The decision to continue the study proved to be a highly appropriate one. Among patients who remained on study 3 years or longer, there have been no differences among the three treatment arms with respect to the incidence of thrombotic complications (Fig. 15-4B: logrank $\chi^2_2 = 0.508$, $p = 0.78$), and as noted above, phlebotomy-treated patients over the long run have proved to have the best overall survival.

Thrombosis-Related Risk Factors. In an effort to define the factors associated with an

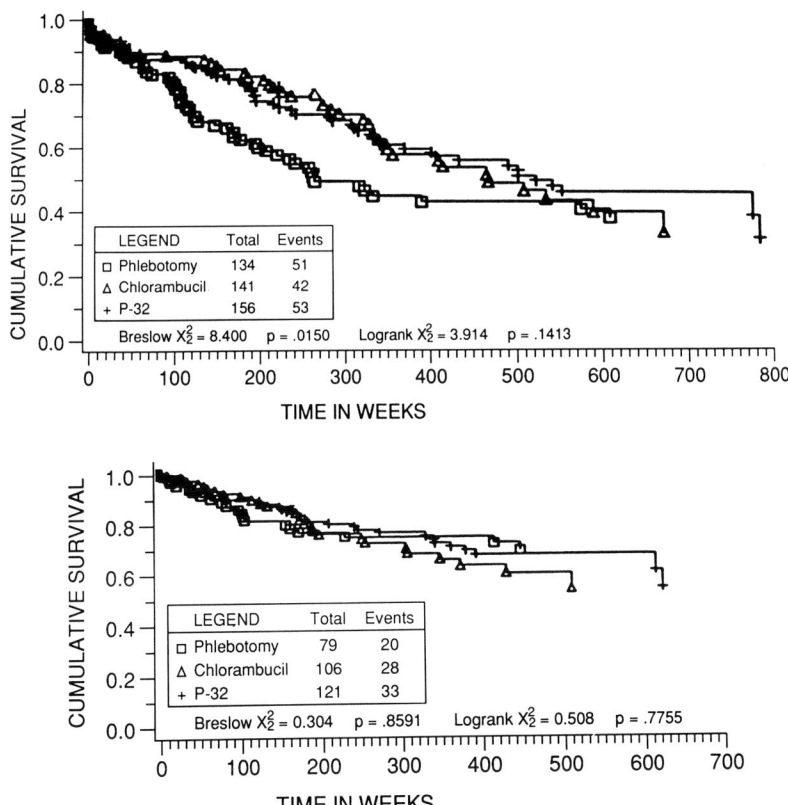

FIGURE 15-4. (A) Thrombosis-free cumulative survival in PVSG protocol 01. Note that during the early years of the study there were significantly more thrombotic events among phlebotomy-treated patients than among those treated with either of the myelosuppressive regimens. This difference disappeared as the study continued. (B) Thrombosis-free cumulative survival in PVSG protocol 01 after 3 years among patients who remained on study longer than 3 years. Comparison with part (A) emphasizes that the excess of thrombotic events in phlebotomy-treated patients was largely limited to the initial 3 years of treatment.

increased risk of early thrombosis, data from the entire cohort of 431 patients were examined in 1983 using a variety of multivariate methods including Cox models. Of all the variables examined, treatment with phlebotomy, in and of itself, was found to be associated with a statistically significant increased risk of early thrombosis. History of prior thrombosis and advanced age were the two other risk factors that contributed significantly to the overall risk of thrombosis. The addition of other variables to the Cox model, including such parameters as sex, history of hemorrhage, and pretreatment hematologic indices (e.g., hematocrit, white count, platelet count, and red cell indices), individually or collectively, did not contribute significantly to the explanation of the observed data. Among patients treated with phlebotomy alone, one additional variable, the phlebotomy rate, also was found to contribute

significantly to the incidence of thrombosis; i.e., there was an increased risk of thrombosis as the phlebotomy rate increased. We have been unable to determine whether the combination of a high phlebotomy rate and an increased risk of thrombosis are causally related or if the two are simply manifestations of increased disease activity. Results of a preliminary analysis were published in 1981.[18]

Role of Hematocrit and Platelet Count.
At the start of the study, there was a preexisting bias among the investigators that an elevated platelet count was a risk factor for thrombotic complications. However, attempts to demonstrate an association between the platelet count and risk of thrombosis within the entire data set of 431 patients were confounded by the wide scatter of values reported not only between treatment groups but also in the courses of individual patients. To obviate some of these problems,

a retrospective study was conducted. In this matched-pair design, for each patient who suffered a thrombosis, a thrombosis-free control patient of similar age, sex, treatment group, and duration on study was selected. Hematologic parameters measured at the closest observation prior to the thrombotic event of the index case were then compared with those in the matched control patient at the corresponding time on study. Within this retrospective study, neither elevations in platelet count nor in hematocrit were associated with increased risk of a thrombotic event.[18] In this analysis, the number of patients with platelets greater than 1,500,000/μl or with hematocrits above 52 percent was small; therefore, these conclusions cannot be extrapolated to patients whose hematologic parameters exceeded these limits. Nevertheless, these analyses strongly suggest that (1) treatment with phlebotomy alone, particularly among patients with a high phlebotomy requirement, (2) advanced age, and (3) a history of prior thrombosis, appear per se to be major factors contributing to the increased risk of early thrombotic events in patients treated by this modality. As described below, attempts to ameliorate the high incidence of early thrombosis in phlebotomy-treated patients by the addition of aspirin and Persantine to the phlebotomy regimen (PVSG protocol 05) were unsuccessful.[21] In PVSG protocol 05, there was no beneficial reduction in the incidence of thrombosis in patients receiving these platelet antiaggregating agents, but there was, by contrast, a significant increase in the incidence of serious gastrointestinal hemorrhages. Hence the combination of aspirin and Persantine, at least at the doses used in PVSG protocol 05, cannot be recommended in patients with PV.

Hematologic Malignancies

Acute Leukemia. In 1981, the PVSG reported that treatment with chlorambucil was associated with a statistically significantly increased risk of developing acute leukemia.[22] At the time of that report, 18 cases of acute leukemia had been reported on the chlorambucil arm of the study, 1 on the phlebotomy arm, and 9 among patients receiving radioactive phosphorus. The role of chlorambucil as a leukemogen was further documented by the observed association among chlorambu-

cil-treated patients between the incidence of leukemia and the average daily dose of the drug employed to achieve control of the disease, as well as between the incidence of leukemia and proportion of time on study that the drug was employed. No other potential risk factor of the many examined was found to explain the observation. Therefore, the group recommended that treatment with chlorambucil be stopped and that patients who had been treated with chlorambucil on the protocol 01 study continue to be followed.

Although the incidence of acute leukemia among ^{32}P-treated patients was greater than that observed in the phlebotomy arm in 1981, this difference was not statistically significant at the time of that original report.[22] Nevertheless, analyses of earlier noncontrolled trials suggested that the peak incidence of leukemia on ^{32}P-treated patients tended to occur later than among patients treated with alkylating agents.[4] Hence the group anticipated that further follow-up might confirm that ^{32}P also was a leukemogenic agent.

Since 1981, 5 of the chlorambucil-treated patients originally diagnosed as having acute leukemia were reclassified as having a lymphocytic lymphoma (see below). However, 7 additional cases of documented acute leukemia have occurred in chlorambucil-treated patients. In the same interval, there has been 1 additional reported case of acute leukemia in the phlebotomy-treated group and 6 additional cases among patients treated with [32]P. Hence, as of January 1, 1987, 37 cases of acute leukemia, thoroughly documented by our histopathology committee, had occurred among patients on study. An additional 7 cases of probable acute leukemia, diagnosed locally, have not been confirmed by our histopathology committee, most often because submitted specimens were not considered adequate. This brings the total number of leukemias reported to 44.

As indicated in the leukemia-free cumulative survival curves (Fig. 15–5), the incidence of acute leukemia in both the chlorambucil and ^{32}P treatment arms of the study is now statistically significantly greater than among phlebotomy-treated patients. It is noteworthy that although the use of chlorambucil was abandoned in 1981, approximately one-third of the total cases of acute leukemia observed on the chlorambucil arm of the study were reported following cessation of use of the drug. The most recent case of acute leu-

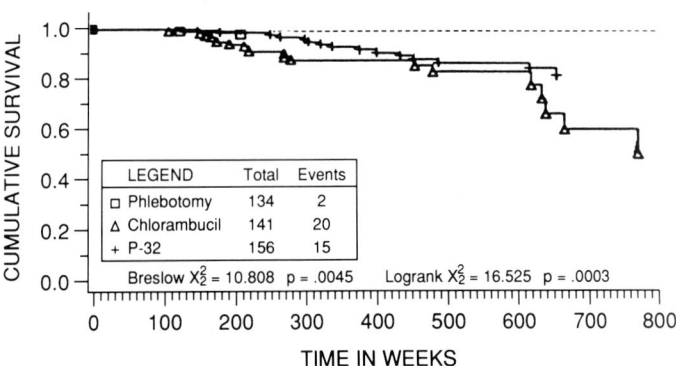

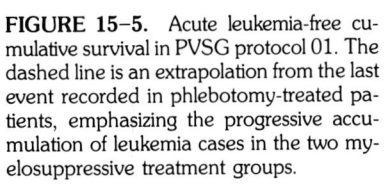

FIGURE 15-5. Acute leukemia-free cumulative survival in PVSG protocol 01. The dashed line is an extrapolation from the last event recorded in phlebotomy-treated patients, emphasizing the progressive accumulation of leukemia cases in the two myelosuppressive treatment groups.

kemia in the chlorambucil-treated population reported to the PVSG was diagnosed in 1985, 6 years after exposure to this agent was terminated. However, since a comprehensive data update and analysis have not been completed since 1987, it is possible that additional cases of chlorambucil-associated acute leukemia have occurred even longer after cessation of treatment with this drug.

The experience of the PVSG with postpolycythemic leukemia has been reported in detail elsewhere.[9] Since there have been no new findings since that earlier report, the topic will be given only brief mention here. Of particular note is the finding that the incidence of biphenotypic leukemias is greater in this population than in a population in which acute leukemia develops de novo and does not follow a prior hematologic malignancy (Fig. 15–6). The group's experience is similar in this regard to that observed in a variety of other settings in which acute leukemia develops secondarily following ei-

ther a preexisting hematologic disorder or develops in the postpolycythemic state is particularly aggressive and poorly responsive to chemotherapy. In PVSG protocol 06, which will not be described in further detail here, 13 patients with postpolycythemic acute leukemia were treated initially with 2 weeks of vincristine and prednisone, followed by a combination of cytosine arabinoside and Adriamycin. Based on the anecdotal experience of PVSG group members,[23, 24] the vincristine and prednisone treatment was initiated while terminal transferase studies, then not widely available, were conducted at a reference laboratory in the hope that occasional postpolycythemic leukemias, like occasional blast transformation in chronic myelogenous leukemia, would be lymphoblastic and responsive to these agents.[25] The choice of Adriamycin rather than daunorubicin in the second portion of the protocol resulted from the unavailability of daunorubicin at that time at a number of the international centers

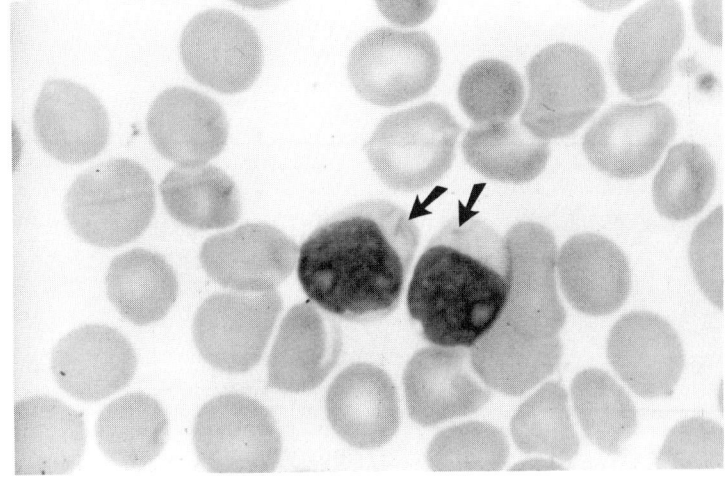

FIGURE 15-6. Peripheral blood smear from a patient with postpolycythemic acute leukemia. Although the patient was TdT-positive, many of the blasts in the peripheral blood contained Auer rods (*arrows*).

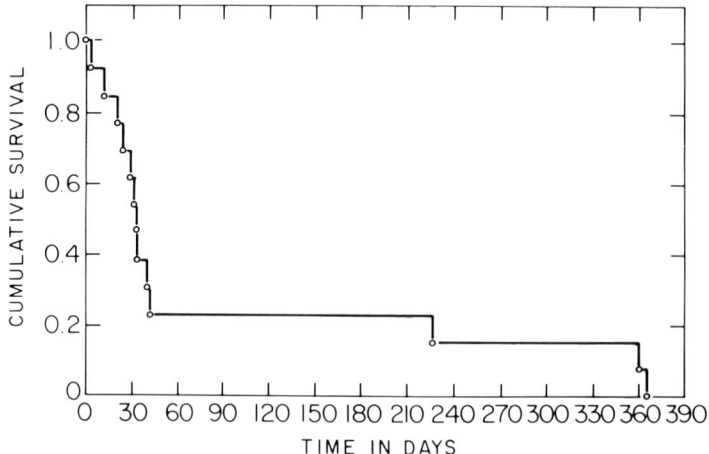

FIGURE 15–7. Cumulative survival in patients with postpolycythemic acute leukemia treated with combination chemotherapy on PVSG protocol 06.

participating in the study. There were considerable data to support this alternative therapy as being effective in conventional de novo leukemias.[26] In PVSG protocol 06, only 1 complete and 1 partial remission was achieved among 13 patients, in whom median survival was 32 days (Fig. 15–7). By contrast, expected remission rates at participating institutions ranged from 60 to 80 percent in adult patients with de novo acute myelogenous leukemia, with median survivals in excess of 1 year being the rule. Subsequent to the completion of PVSG protocol 06, there have been several anecdotal reports suggesting a higher success rate of achieving complete remissions in postpolycythemic acute leukemia using the high-dose cytosine arabinoside (ARA-C) regimen of Capizzi et al.[27] The authors' experience is that these remis-

sions, however, are usually very short-lived and that the development of acute leukemia in the setting of PV is an extremely grave prognostic feature.

Lymphomas. At the time of autopsy, two chlorambucil-treated patients initially diagnosed as having acute lymphoblastic leukemia were found to have significant bulk tissue disease in the abdomen and were reclassified as having large-cell lymphocytic lymphoma (Fig. 15–8). Three other patients with a similar clinical and pathologic picture have subsequently been reported to the PVSG central office. Of the five patients with this unusual constellation of large-cell lymphocytic lymphoma with a predominantly abdominal presentation, all had been treated with chlorambucil. This group of patients has been the subject of a separate report.[28]

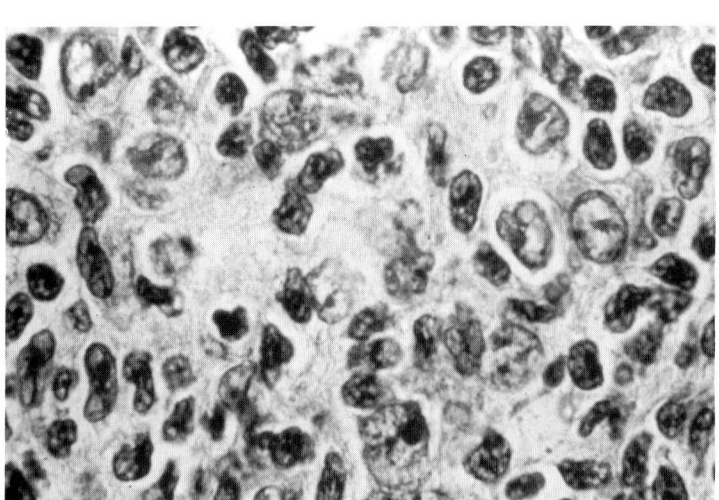

FIGURE 15–8. Large-cell lymphocytic lymphoma with bulk tissue disease within the abdomen in a patient treated with chlorambucil in PVSG protocol 01 (original magnification × 250).

No cases of non-Hodgkin's lymphoma have been reported to the study group among patients treated with either phlebotomy or radioactive phosphorus. Kaplan-Meier plots illustrating leukemia and lymphoma-free cumulative survival for the three treatment arms of PVSG protocol 01 are presented in Fig. 15–9; they indicate a highly significant increase in the risk of developing a hematologic malignancy in patients treated with either chlorambucil or ^{32}P compared with those treated with phlebotomy alone.

Spent Polycythemia

Although the development of the spent phase of PV was not a formal endpoint of the study, both the histopathology and quality control committees of the PVSG have recently examined with particular interest the evolution of this late stage of the disease. The diagnosis of the spent phase was based on the presence of increased reticulin and/or collagen in bone marrow biopsy specimens, clinical evidence for increasing spleen size, the development and subsequent worsening of

anemia, and the presence in the peripheral blood of the characteristic leukoerythroblastic picture, including teardrop poikilocytes, nucleated erythrocytes, and granulocytic precursors more immature than bands.[29, 30]

The incidence and the time to development of the spent phase of PV, with myelofibrosis and myeloid metaplasia, were virtually identical in the three arms of study; the incidence averaged approximately 9 percent overall by 650 weeks into the study. These data differ somewhat from results reported by Silverstein[31] some 10 years earlier. In the earlier data, there appeared to be an increased incidence of bone marrow fibrosis and the spent phase in patients treated with radioactive phosphorus.

Prior investigators, and in particular Silverstein and Brown[32] and Lawrence et al.,[33] had noticed an increase in acute leukemia among patients who had developed post-polycythemic myelofibrosis with myeloid metaplasia and had in fact speculated that the usual progression in PV was for myelofibrosis with myeloid metaplasia to precede the development of leukemia. These

FIGURE 15–9. Leukemia and lymphoma-free cumulative survival in PVSG protocol 01. The only three events among phlebotomy-treated patients occurred within the first 200 weeks. Since that time, there has been a progressive and highly significant accumulation of hematologic malignancies in patients treated with either ^{32}P or chlorambucil.

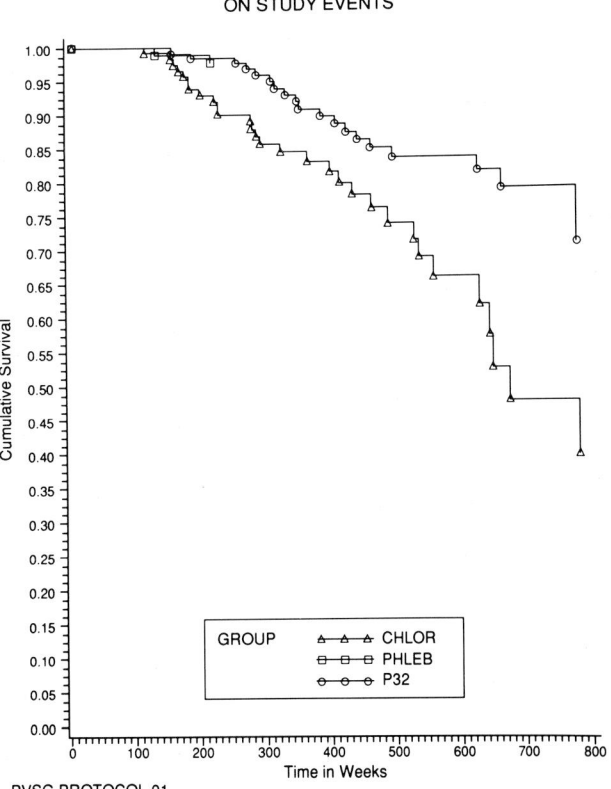

ALL LEUKEMIA/LYMPHOMA
ON STUDY EVENTS

PVSG PROTOCOL 01

TABLE 15–3. PVSG PROTOCOL 01: OCCURRENCE
OF ACUTE LEUKEMIA IN POLYCYTHEMIA VERA
BY THERAPY AND SPENT PHASE

	TREATMENT			
	Phleb*	Chlor*	^{32}P	Total
Spent PV*	15	11	12	38
With AL*	1 (6.7%)	5 (45.5%)	3 (25%)	9 (23.7%)
Not spent PV	119	130	144	393
With AL	1 (1.7%)	14 (10.8%)	12 (8.3%)	28 (7.1%)

* Phleb: phlebotomy; Chlor: chlorambucil; PV: polycythemia vera; AL: acute leukemia.

observations were confirmed in PVSG protocol 01.[34] In this study, among the 38 patients who had developed spent-phase PV with biopsy-proven myelofibrosis by 650 weeks, the incidence of acute leukemia was 23.7 percent. By contrast, among the 393 patients in whom myelofibrosis and myeloid metaplasia were not diagnosed within the same time interval, the incidence of acute leukemia was only 7.1 percent (Table 15–3). The increased incidence of acute leukemia in patients with spent-phase PV is statistically significant ($p <$ 0.001). These differences in the incidence of acute leukemia between patients with and without the spent phase observed for the total study population also were seen for each of the individual treatment arms (Tables 15–3 and 15–4). The higher incidence of leukemia among ^{32}P- or chlorambucil-treated patients with spent-phase PV reflects the influence of these myelosuppressive regimens as leukemogenic agents in all patients in the study, both with and without spent-phase PV.

If acute leukemia and myelofibrosis with myeloid metaplasia are independent outcomes of PV, the incidence of patients having both complications should be equivalent to the product of the relative frequencies of the two endpoints independently. As indicated in Table 15–4, this was not the case; the overall incidence of cases with both acute leukemia and myelofibrosis with myeloid metaplasia (2.1 percent) was 2.8 times that predicted from the incidences of the two endpoints separately (0.74 percent). The incidence of acute leukemia among patients who developed myelofibrosis with myeloid metaplasia following chlorambucil or ^{32}P therapy was 35 percent (8 of 23); in phlebotomy-treated patients who developed myelofibrosis with myeloid metaplasia, the incidence of acute leukemia was only 1 in 15 (6.7 percent). These data suggest that caution should be exercised in giving or continuing to give either ^{32}P or alkylating agent therapy to polycythemic patients in whom the development of myelofibrosis with myeloid metaplasia has been documented.[34]

Nonhematologic Malignancies

Although the documentation that both chlorambucil and ^{32}P therapy are leukemogenic confirms the results of earlier studies, there were no prior data that suggested that myelosuppressive therapy was associated as well with an increase in the inci-

TABLE 15–4. PVSG PROTOCOL 01: OCCURRENCE
OF ACUTE LEUKEMIA IN POLYCYTHEMIA VERA AS
A FUNCTION OF THERAPY AND DEVELOPMENT
OF SPENT PHASE

	PHLEB	CHLOR	^{32}P	TOTAL	PERCENT
AL and MM/MF	1	5	3	9	2.1
Total AL	2	19	15	36	8.4
Total MM/MF	15	11	12	38	8.8
Total randomized	134	141	156	431	—

Note: (A) Overall incidence of combined AL + MM/MF = 2.1 percent (9 of 431);
(B) Incidence of AL alone × incidence of MM/MF alone: 0.084 × 0.088 = 0.0074,
or 0.74 percent; A/B = 2.8.

dence of nonhematopoietic malignancies. However, in 1981, the PVSG began to be aware of a possible increased frequency of nonhematologic malignancies in patients receiving either chlorambucil or radioactive phosphorus.[35] Since the late 1970s, the incidence of reported cancers and leukemias on the study has been compared with that predicted from data for an age- and sex-matched population developed by the National Cancer Institute (NCI).[36] In an analysis performed in 1986 (Table 15–5), the incidence of nonhematopoietic malignancies occurring in chlorambucil-treated patients at 7, 9, and 14 years after entry into the study ranged from 2.0 to 2.4 times that expected in a control population; in ^{32}P-treated patients the ratio of observed to expected cases ranged from approximately 1.8 to 1.9, based on NCI data. These results suggested an increased incidence of cancer in the chlorambucil- and ^{32}P-treated patient populations at each of these time points ($p \leq 0.01$ in each case). By contrast, the incidence of nonhematopoietic neoplasms in phlebotomy-treated patients ranged from 1.1 to 1.5 times expected, values that were not statistically significantly increased ($p = 0.16$ to 0.82).

As of January 1, 1987, a total of 62 nonhematopoietic neoplasms had developed in patients on active study, of which 22 were gastrointestinal cancers and 14 were skin cancers (Table 15–6). Only 8 breast cancers, 10 genitourinary carcinomas, and 5 lung cancers, as well as 3 miscellaneous malignancies, were reported. Hence the distribution of cancers seems unusually weighted toward those of the skin and gastrointestinal tract. Although differences in the overall incidences of nonhematopoietic neoplasms among the three treatment arms of the study were not statistically significantly different, there was significantly more gastrointestinal cancer or gastrointestinal plus skin cancer in patients treated with either of the two myelosuppressive regimens (chlorambucil, ^{32}P) than in phlebotomy-treated patients. By contrast, for all cancers other than skin and gastrointestinal cancer, differences among the three treatment groups were essentially random (see Table 15–6). Cancer-free cumulative survival curves for the three treatment groups are illustrated in Fig. 15–10.

TABLE 15–5. PVSG PROTOCOL 01: EXPECTED CANCERS BY TREATMENT GROUP ADJUSTED FOR AGE AND SEX: MALES AND FEMALES COMBINED (ON-STUDY EVENTS)

TREATMENT	7 YEARS	9 YEARS	14 YEARS
Phlebotomy (n = 134)			
Observed	7	7	12
Expected	5.4	6.4	8.0
O/E	1.29	1.09	1.49
Chlorambucil (n = 141)			
Observed	15	20	23
Expected	7.5	8.6	9.7
O/E	2.00	2.33	2.38
[32]P (n = 156)			
Observed	16	18	23
Expected	8.5	10.2	12.4
O/E	1.88	1.77	1.86

TABLE 15–6. PVSG PROTOCOL 01: INCIDENCE OF NONHEMATOLOGIC MALIGNANCIES (ON-STUDY EVENTS ONLY)

	TREATMENT GROUP				COMPARISON OF INCIDENCE		
	Phlebotomy	Chlorambucil	[32]P	Total	χ^2	Log rank (DF)	p
No. in group	134	141	156	431			
Cancers	15	24	23	62	3.6	(2)	0.16
		Phleb vs. (chlor + [32]P)			1.1	(1)	0.29
		chlorambucil vs. [32]P			2.0	(1)	0.16
Type of Cancer							
GI	1	11	10	22	7.7	(2)	0.02
Skin	4	6	4	14	2.4	(2)	0.30
GI + skin	5	17	14	36	8.0	(2)	0.02
		Phleb v. (chlor + [32]P)			4.5	(1)	0.03
		chlorambucil vs. [32]P			2.7	(1)	0.10
Other	10	7	9	26	0.9	(2)	0.64

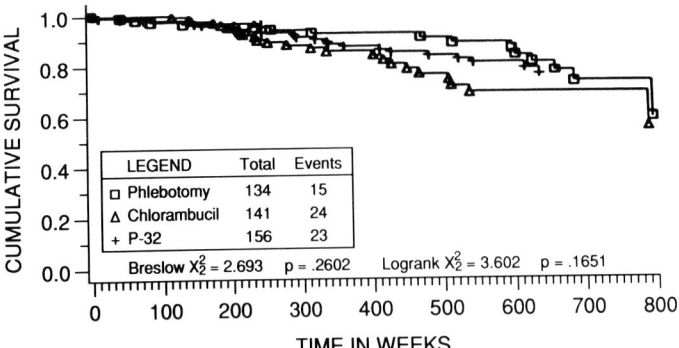

FIGURE 15–10. Cancer-free cumulative survival in PVSG protocol 01. Differences in the overall incidences of nonhematopoietic neoplasms among the three treatment arms of the study were not statistically significantly different. However, there was significantly more gastrointestinal cancer or gastrointestinal plus skin cancer in patients treated with either chlorambucil or ^{32}P than in phlebotomy-treated patients. For cancers other than skin and gastrointestinal cancer, differences among the three treatment groups were essentially random (see text).

Figure 15–11 provides a Kaplan-Meier analysis of all the malignant complications observed in PVSG protocol 01, including acute leukemia, lymphocytic lymphoma, and nonhematologic malignancies. There is a strikingly increased incidence of malignant complications in patients treated with ^{32}P or with chlorambucil compared with the incidence observed in phlebotomy-treated patients. The increased incidence of malignancies of bone marrow, lymphoid tissue, skin, and gastrointestinal tract highlights mutagenic effects of chronic myelosuppressive therapy with either radiation or radiomimetic alkylating agents when applied to the three most rapidly proliferating tissues of the body.

The Therapeutic Dilemma

As summarized in Table 15–7, each of the treatment regimens used in PVSG protocol

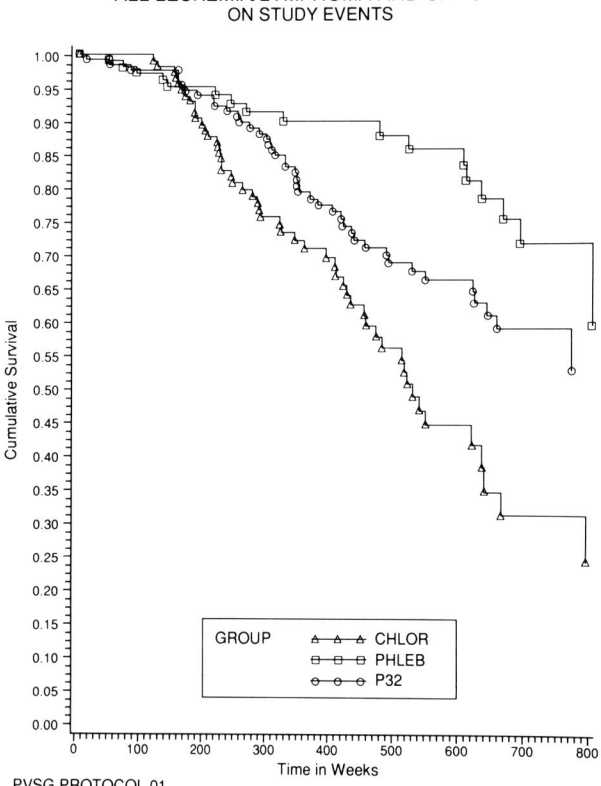

FIGURE 15–11. Malignancy-free cumulative survival in PVSG protocol 01. Curves reflect all leukemias, lymphomas, and nonhematologic malignancies that occurred on study and illustrate the highly significant excess of malignant disease observed in chlorambucil- and ^{32}P-treated patients.

TABLE 15-7. COMPLICATIONS OF POLYCYTHEMIA VERA: RELATIONSHIP TO THERAPY

	EARLY THROMBOSIS (FIRST 3 YEARS)	ACUTE LEUKEMIA	CANCER (SKIN, GI)
Phlebotomy	+	−	−
Chlorambucil	−	+	+
^{32}P	−	+	+

01 was found to be associated with a significantly increased incidence of some type of complication. Patients treated with phlebotomy alone were subjected to an unacceptably high incidence of early thrombotic events, often fatal or severely disabling cerebral vascular accidents, which occurred particularly during the first 3 years on study. These were most common in elderly patients, those with a previous history of a thrombotic event, or in patients with a high phlebotomy requirement. By contrast, patients treated with either chlorambucil or ^{32}P had a significantly increased risk of leukemia, lymphocytic lymphoma, or carcinoma of the skin or gastrointestinal tract. These tended to become apparent beyond the fifth year of the study. If these three were the only treatment regimens available, the therapeutic dilemma would be whether to avoid the risk of late malignant complications by treating all patients with phlebotomy alone, recognizing that this would cause an appreciable degree of morbidity and mortality early in the courses of many patients due to thrombotic events. Alternatively, should one ameliorate the risk of early thrombotic complications by using myelosuppression, thereby creating a risk for a later malignant complication?

One alternative suggested by the data of PVSG protocol 01 is that all patients should receive myelosuppression for the first 3 to 5 years after diagnosis in the hope that this would get them over a particularly thrombosis-prone period, following which they could then be treated with phlebotomy. This hypothesis has not been tested experimentally and, in the current climate for funding long-term clinical trials in chronic diseases, is unlikely to be tested in the foreseeable future. If, as some suspect, there is a thrombosis-prone subset of polycythemic patients, this approach might simply delay into the period

of phlebotomy treatment a group of complications that might otherwise have occurred earlier.

The results of PVSG protocol 01, as summarized above, point to the critical need for a means of reducing the incidence of thrombotic complications in patients treated with phlebotomy, as well as the need for a nonmutagenic myelosuppressive agent in those patients in whom phlebotomy alone poses an unacceptable risk. The PVSG examined the possibility of the former approach in PVSG protocol 05, a study in which the platelet antiaggregating agents aspirin and Persantine were used in conjunction with phlebotomy in an attempt to reduce the incidence of thrombotic complications in patients treated primarily with this therapeutic modality. In PVSG protocol 08, first the efficacy and then the long-term safety of the nonalkylating myelosuppressive agent hydroxyurea was examined. In the sections that follow, the design and results of each of these PVSG protocols will be described and summarized.

PVSG PROTOCOL 05: THE ROLE OF ASPIRIN AND PERSANTINE IN REDUCING THE RISK OF THROMBOTIC COMPLICATIONS IN PATIENTS TREATED WITH PHLEBOTOMY

Thrombotic complications are a well-recognized major cause of morbidity and mortality in patients with PV.[5, 6, 18–21, 37] In PVSG protocol 01, as described above, such complications were particularly prevalent early in the courses of patients treated with phlebotomy alone.[18] Advanced age, a high phlebotomy requirement, and a history of a prior thrombotic event were all additional predictors of a high risk for thrombosis. However, detailed statistical analysis indicated that treatment with phlebotomy, in and of itself, was a significant risk factor, especially within the first 3 years.[18] Although myelosuppression with either radioactive phosphorus or chlorambucil reduced the risk of early thrombosis, these modalities were in turn associated with an increased incidence of late malignant transformation, including acute leukemia,[4, 18, 22, 23] lymphocytic lymphoma,[28] and nonhematologic malignancies.[35] Hence, in the 1970s, finding an alternative means of reducing the risk of thrombosis in phlebotomy-treated patients appeared to be highly desirable. Because the progressive increase in malignant complications of myelosuppression with long follow-up has made phlebotomy the treatment of choice in many patients, the need for a means of reducing the incidence of thrombosis in phlebotomy-treated patients is even more pressing today.

Because aspirin and/or dipyridamole (Persantine) had been proven effective in reducing thrombosis in several of other clinical settings, including early postoperative occlusion of coronary bypass grafts,[38-40] the PVSG initiated, in 1977, a randomized, controlled trial of phlebotomy supplemented by aspirin and Persantine in the management of PV (PVSG protocol 05). The control group received ^{32}P rather than phlebotomy alone, in part because of concern by some investigators that it would be unethical to assign patients to a regimen associated with a high incidence of serious thrombotic events.

Diagnostic Criteria and Patient Eligibility

Patients older than 21 years of age in whom the diagnosis of PV had been made within the preceding 4 years and who had received no treatment other than phlebotomy were eligible for entry into the study if they met two additional criteria. These were absence of any chronic disorder, e.g., arthritis, requiring long-term aspirin therapy and, for patients under 40 years of age, an expressed intent not to have additional children. In each patient, the diagnosis of PV was established initially according to the previously published criteria of the PVSG (see Table 15–1). These were the same criteria employed in PVSG protocol 01. After entry into the study, the diagnosis in all patients was confirmed by additional investigations that ruled out the various causes of secondary polycythemia (see Chap. 3).

Treatment Regimens

All eligible patients were initially phlebotomized in 500-ml increments, at a frequency of up to three times per week, until a hematocrit of 40 percent or less was achieved. Patients were then treated with one of the following regimens, to which they were assigned at random. It was initially intended that the study be conducted for a period of 3 years.

Phlebotomy - Aspirin - Persantine. Patients in this group were phlebotomized as often as necessary to maintain a hematocrit of 40 percent or greater but less than or equal to 45 percent. Visits were initially scheduled at monthly intervals, but the interval between visits was lengthened to up to bimonthly as the phlebotomy requirement diminished. In addition, patients in this group took aspirin (300 mg) and dipyridamole (75 mg) in combination three times daily after meals.

Radioactive Phosphorus (^{32}P). This agent was administered intravenously in a dose of 2.7 mCi/m^2 of body surface area (limit 5 mCi per dose) as often as every 12 weeks. The frequency of administration depended on the response, criteria for which have been reported previously.[8] If there was no response to the initial dose, subsequent doses were increased by 25 percent. During ^{32}P treatment, supplemental phlebotomy was used as needed to maintain a hematocrit of less than 45 percent.

Method of Analysis

The primary objective of this study was to determine whether phlebotomy in conjunction with platelet function inhibitors could decrease the frequency of thrombotic complications in PV patients to the level observed in patients treated with ^{32}P. PVSG protocol 05 was designed to detect an improvement in the rate of thrombotic complications of 25 percent relative to the expected rate in patients treated with ^{32}P at a significance level of 5 percent (one-tailed) and a power of 50 percent. Follow-up data were submitted at 3-month intervals.

The primary analysis included all randomized eligible patients. Characteristics of patients randomized to the two treatment groups were compared using methods of descriptive chi-squared tests and t tests. The purpose of these analyses was to determine the comparability of patients in the two groups and to indicate possible areas of imbalance. The main endpoint of interest was the incidence of thrombotic complications, which was compared using the Kaplan-Meier product-limit method to estimate the distributions of time to thrombotic complication.[41] A similar comparison was carried out for the incidence of major hemorrhagic complications, defined as hemorrhagic episodes requiring hospitalization and the transfusion of at least 2 units of blood. The differences between the distributions for the two treatment groups were assessed using the generalized Wilcoxon test for comparing curves,[10, 11] which gives greater weight to early failures, and the log-rank test, which gives greater weight to late events.[12, 13] In addition, incidences of hemorrhage and death were compared using similar methods to assess the comparability of the two treatment regimens with regard to other endpoints. Other variables that might be related to thrombosis also were examined to determine whether this result was due to treatment or other factors. These variables were examined individually and jointly in Cox regression methods for censored data with a strategy similar to that described above and in a previous report.[14–16, 42]

Because of the excess incidence of thrombosis, hemorrhage, and death observed among the patients treated with phlebotomy, aspirin, and dipyridamole compared with both the randomized ^{32}P control group and the historical group of patients treated on PVSG protocol 01 with ^{32}P (described above), the study was stopped early (see below).

Results

Comparability of Treatment Groups. Table 15–8 reports on the status of all patients ever entered into the study (as of the close of the study in April of 1981). Of 178 fully eligible patients, 88 were randomized to the phlebotomy-aspirin-dipyridamole arm and 90 to the ^{32}P arm. A prior report,[42] based on data approved by the quality control committee as of April of 1981, noted 83 eligible patients in each group, excluding 12 whose data were late in arriving at the central office but who were subsequently found to have been fully eligible. The addition of these 12 cases to the present and final analysis does not alter any of the previously reported conclusions.[42] Because patients were randomized and initially entered into the study based on data developed at participating institutions without waiting for the quarterly meetings of the quality control committee, 10 patients initially randomized were subsequently found to be ineligible. These ineligible patients were already excluded from the earlier, published reports.

Patients within the two treatment groups were comparable with respect to age and sex at randomization (Table 15–9), principal hematologic parameters (Table 15–10), and disease duration. In particular, 50 percent of these patients entered the study within 2 weeks and 75 percent within 4 months of the initial diagnosis of PV. Twenty-seven percent of patients on phlebotomy-aspirin-dipyridamole had had a thrombosis prior to randomization, as had 13 percent of patients on ^{32}P. The incidence of other risk factors such as diabetes and hypertension was virtually identical in the two groups (Table 15–11). Although 21.6 percent of phlebotomy-aspirin-dipyridamole patients and 13.3 percent of ^{32}P patients had had a hemorrhage before randomization, this difference was not significant ($p > 0.10$).

Thrombosis. As of April of 1981, when the study was stopped, the phlebotomy-aspirin-dipyridamole and ^{32}P groups had been followed for a maximum of 3.1 and 3.4 years and a median of 1.5 and 2 years, respectively. There had been seven severe thrombotic complications on the phlebotomy-aspirin-di-

TABLE 15–8. PVSG PROTOCOL 05: STATUS OF PATIENTS BY TREATMENT GROUP AS OF STUDY CLOSE

	TREATMENT GROUP					
	Phleb*		^{32}P		Total	
STATUS	No.	Percent	No.	Percent	No.	Percent
Alive at last observation	67	76.1	83	92.2	150	84.3
Dead on study	2	2.2	0	0.0	2	1.1
Excluded	1	1.1	1	1.1	2	1.1
Terminated†	18	20.5	6	6.7	24	13.5
Total	88	100.0	90	100.0	178	100.0
Ineligible	2		8		10	

* Phleb: phlebotomy-aspirin-Persantine.
† Includes 21 cases terminated for reaching specified study endpoint and 3 cases for unauthorized aspirin use.

TABLE 15–9. PVSG PROTOCOL 05: DISTRIBUTION OF AGE AND SEX BY TREATMENT GROUP (ELIGIBLE PATIENTS)

AGE AND SEX	TREATMENT GROUP		
	Phlebotomy-Aspirin-Persantine (%)	^{32}P (%)	Total (%)
Male			
<50	7.95	6.67	7.3
50–70	43.18	38.89	41.01
≥70	10.23	10.00	10.11
Female			
<50	5.68	5.56	5.62
50–70	20.45	25.56	23.03
≥70	12.50	13.33	12.92
TOTAL	100.00	100.00	100.00
Number	88	90	178

pyridamole arm of the study compared with only two severe thrombotic complications among patients treated with ^{32}P.* While this difference in cumulative incidence is not quite statistically significant (Wilcoxon χ_1^2 = 2.84; p = 0.092; log-rank χ_1^2 = 3.09; p = 0.079), there is certainly no suggestion of benefit from the use of aspirin-dipyrida-mole. The average relative risk of thrombosis on the phlebotomy-aspirin-dipyridamole arm was 3.6 times that observed among patients treated with radioactive phosphorus. The nine severe thrombotic complications included one myocardial infarction, five cerebrovascular accidents, one additional major arterial thrombosis, and two cases of Budd-Chiari syndrome. When compared with corresponding data over the first 2 years of PVSG protocol 01 (Table 15–12), the incidence of thrombotic events during the initial 2 years of the study among patients receiving phlebotomy-aspirin-dipyridamole in PVSG protocol 05 was virtually identical to that among patients treated with phlebotomy alone in PVSG protocol 01. Hence there is no evidence, either within PVSG protocol 05 alone or in a comparison of this protocol with

---

*The diagnosis of *thrombosis* was applied to any obstruction to blood flow in the arterial or venous vascular tree leading to organ ischemia or prevention of venous outflow. This includes cerebral vascular accidents, myocardial and pulmonary infarctions, arterial or venous occlusions, and hepatic vein thrombosis. A thrombosis was considered *severe* if the primary physician and/or a review committee of the PVSG considered the event to be potentially life-threatening, requiring hospitalization and immediate medical intervention. Other thrombotic events were considered moderate.

our earlier study, that aspirin-dipyridamole significantly reduced the incidence of thrombotic complications in patients with PV. The lower incidence of thrombotic complications observed among ^{32}P-treated patients during year 1 of PVSG protocol 05, compared to PVSG protocol 01, has not been explored in detail and remains unexplained.

Hemorrhage. Furthermore, although there was no apparent benefit with respect to thrombotic complications from aspirin and dipyridamole therapy, there was a significant increase in hemorrhagic complications. Thus six of the patients receiving phlebotomy-aspirin-dipyridamole had severe gastrointestinal hemorrhages requiring hospitalization and transfusion.† There were no such events

TABLE 15–10. PVSG PROTOCOL 05: COMPARISON OF TREATMENT GROUPS BY BLOOD VALUES AT INITIAL EVALUATION (ELIGIBLE PATIENTS)

	TREATMENT GROUP	
	Phlebotomy-Aspirin-Persantine	^{32}P
Number of patients	88	90
Blood value		
Hct (%)		
Number	87	88
Mean	57.45	58.0
SD	6.37	7.4
Median	57	58.35
Range	40.6–76.2	41.2–78.5
RBC × 10^6		
Number	81	84
Mean	6.91	6.90
SD	0.89	0.94
Median	6.88	6.90
Range	4.9–9.9	3.5–8.9
Ln (platelets × 10^3)		
Number	84	87
Mean	6.19	6.08
SD	0.49	0.62
Median	6.19	6.13
Range	5.0–7.6	4.6–7.8
Ln (WBC × 10^3)		
Number	85	87
Mean	2.54	2.54
SD	0.37	0.37
Median	2.51	2.56
Range	1.5–3.3	1.4–3.8

---

† A *major hemorrhage* was defined as a bleeding event requiring hospitalization and blood transfusion, as judged by the primary physician and/or a review committee of the PVSG. Other hemorrhages were considered moderate.

**TABLE 15–11. PVSG PROTOCOL 05: COMPARISON
OF INITIAL ENTRY CHARACTERISTICS
BY TREATMENT GROUP**

	PHLEBOTOMY-ASPIRIN-PERSANTINE		^{32}P	
Total no. of patients	88		90	
Complication*	**No.**	**Percent**	**No.**	**Percent**
Myocardial infarction	6	6.8	10	11.1
Hypertension	32	36.4	35	38.9
Stroke	5	5.7	6	6.7
Diabetes	35	5.7	9	10.0
Prior thrombosis	13	14.8	11	12.2
Prior hemorrhage	19	21.6	12	13.3

* History of prior event.

among patients treated with ^{32}P. The difference in the incidence of hemorrhagic complications is statistically significant with the Wilcoxon test ($\chi^2_1 = 5.9$, $p = 0.015$) but not the log-rank test ($\chi^2_1 = 6.2$, $p = 0.13$). The incidence of severe hemorrhage in the phlebotomy-aspirin-dipyridamole group in PVSG protocol 05 also was significantly increased when compared with corresponding data in phlebotomy-treated patients over the first 2 years of PVSG protocol 01.

The overall cumulative failure rate, including severe thrombotic complications, hemorrhage, and death, was eight times greater on the phlebotomy-aspirin-dipyridamole arm than among patients treated with ^{32}P (Wilcoxon $\chi^2_1 = 9.4$, $p = 0.002$; log-rank $\chi^2_1 = 9.5$, $p = .002$). Figure 15–12 shows the failure-free cumulative survival curves (including toxicities). The results of exploratory analyses using multivariate Cox models

**TABLE 15–12. PVSG PROTOCOL 05:
INCIDENCE OF THROMBOSIS
BY STUDY YEAR, PROTOCOL,
AND TREATMENT GROUP**

	TREATMENT GROUP	
STUDY YEAR AND PROTOCOL	**Phleb-Asp-Persant* Cum% ± SE**	**^{32}P Cum% ± SE**
Year 1		
01	8.7 ± 2.5	7.1 ± 2.1
05	7.0 ± 3.1	1.2 ± 1.2
Year 2		
01	14.0 ± 3.2	9.1 ± 2.3
05	9.4 ± 3.8	4.2 ± 3.2

* Phleb-Asp-Persant: Phlebotomy (01) or Phlebotomy + Aspirin/Persantine (05).

suggest that the increased failure rate on the phlebotomy-aspirin-dipyridamole arm could not be accounted for by any characteristic of the two treatment groups other than the treatment regimen itself. Furthermore, an examination of the proportion of patients on the phlebotomy-aspirin-dipyridamole arm with specific risk factors, including diabetes, hypertension, prior stroke, myocardial infarction, or other thrombosis, or prior hemorrhage who subsequently failed did not suggest any prior factor that might explain the result.

Role of the Platelet Count. The relationship between the platelet count and the development of thrombotic and hemorrhagic complications also was examined.[42] In PVSG protocol 05, of the seven patients on the phlebotomy-aspirin-dipyridamole arm who had thrombotic complications, two suffered these events with normal platelet counts; of the two thromboses on ^{32}P, one occurred with a normal and one with a moderately elevated platelet count.[42] By contrast, the six patients in PVSG protocol 05 who experienced a major hemorrhage were all on the phlebotomy-aspirin-dipyridamole arm of the study, and four of these six had elevated platelet counts ranging from 930,000 to 1,935,000/ml at the time of the event.[42]

Discussion

This randomized, controlled clinical trial demonstrates that aspirin and dipyridamole, administered at doses of 300 and 75 mg tid, respectively, to patients undergoing phlebotomy therapy for PV, failed to reduce the

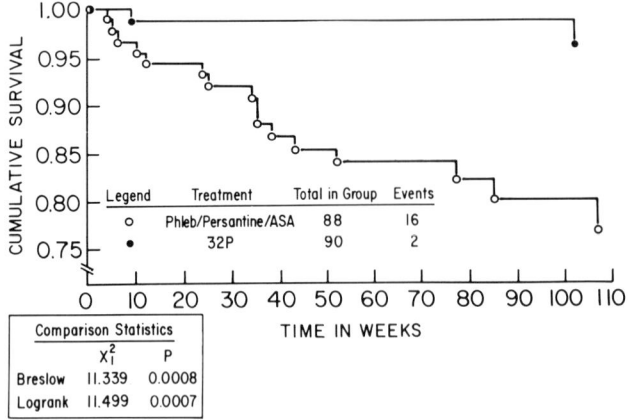

FIGURE 15-12. Failure-free cumulative survival in PVSG protocol 05. See text for discussion.

incidence of thrombotic complications typical of this disease. Not only were there more thromboses among patients on this regimen than among the randomly selected group receiving myelosuppression with ^{32}P, but there also was no difference in the incidence of thrombotic complications in the phlebotomy-aspirin-dipyridamole group in this study (PVSG protocol 05) and in a quite similar historical control group receiving phlebotomy alone, without antiplatelet agents, in an earlier study (PVSG protocol 01).[18,42] While aspirin and dipyridamole failed to protect against thrombosis, their administration at the dosage employed was associated with a significantly increased incidence of gastrointestinal hemorrhage of a severity sufficient to require hospitalization and transfusion as compared with both the ^{32}P treatment group and the patients in the previous study who had been treated with phlebotomy alone. As a result of these hemorrhagic complications, the study was terminated early. The use of aspirin and dipyridamole *at doses employed in this study* would appear to be contraindicated in patients with PV.

The availability of patients to enter this study required that we choose a single antithrombotic regimen for the phlebotomy arm of the study in order for the study to be feasible. Although the doses of aspirin utilized in our study may, in retrospect, be considered high, the arguments that are currently offered to support the use of lower doses of aspirin to prevent thrombosis were not at all clear in 1977, when the clinical protocol on which the current study is based was written. Hence the study was initiated with what, at that time, were totally conven-

tional doses of aspirin and dipyridamole. In fact, several other major trials of platelet function inhibitors (Paris AM, Canadian TIA) ongoing at that time utilized aspirin doses in the same range as those employed in PVSG protocol 05. Even today, despite both the theoretical arguments and in vitro studies suggesting a beneficial effect from lower-dose aspirin therapy, the results with respect to clinical efficacy remain a morass.[39,40,43-45] Although some studies, in fact, report benefit in a variety of clinical settings from low-dose aspirin regimens, several recent critical reviews conclude that in settings in which aspirin-containing antiplatelet regimens are effective, there is no demonstrated difference in efficacy between regimens containing 325 mg daily and those containing three or more times as much (reviewed in ref. 43). Hence the failure of the aspirin-dipyridamole regimen selected by the PVSG to prevent thrombosis cannot be dismissed out of hand as a clinically inappropriate choice even today. The advantage of the lower-dose regimens is in a lesser incidence of gastrointestinal toxicity, especially bleeding.[43,45] The failure to prevent thrombosis in a myeloproliferative disorder (MPD) by a regimen that is clearly effective in other settings must surely be a reflection of the uniquely disordered pathophysiology in PV that predisposes to thrombosis in the first place. These predisposing factors remain poorly understood.

The failure of aspirin-dipyridamole, as employed in this study, to prevent thrombotic complications when given prophylactically in asymptomatic patients must be contrasted with their apparent efficacy in attenuating neurologic and peripheral vascular complications when administered acutely to MPD patients with symptomatic evidence of local ischemia.[46] Again, an understanding of these differences requires a more detailed appreciation of the underlying pathophysiologic disturbances. In the abnormal MPD platelet, these may include alterations in arachidonic acid metabolism, of which only limited studies have thus far been reported.[47,48]

The data of PVSG protocol 05 indicate that aspirin and dipyridamole at the doses employed in this study *should not be used* prophylactically in patients with PV to prevent thrombosis. They do not establish that alternative drug or dosage regimens might not be both safe and effective for this purpose. In this regard, Gilbert and Hanna[49] have recently reported in abstract form a retrospective analysis of the efficacy of a phlebotomy-aspirin regimen in 32 patients with PV; 16 were newly diagnosed, 6 were established cases previously treated only with phlebotomy, and 10 were established cases with a history of prior myelosuppressive therapy discontinued at least 6 months earlier. Several aspirin doses were employed. During 69 patient-years of follow-up on regimens containing 325 mg aspirin per day or less, there were no thrombotic and no hemorrhagic complications. Unfortunately, patient characteristics in this study were appreciably different from those in PVSG protocols 01 or 05. Aside from appreciable differences in age, sex, and hematologic parameters, the average duration of disease in this retrospective study, 3.8 years (range 0 to 27.5 years), was appreciably greater than in PVSG protocol 01 (mean 0.7 years, range 0 to 3.8 years) or protocol 05 (mean 0.47 years, range 0 to 3.8 years). This raises the possibility that many of the reported patients were beyond the early years after diagnosis when, as suggested by the results of PVSG protocol 01, the risk of thrombosis may be especially high. Hence, although low-dose aspirin regimens may be less likely to cause hemorrhagic complications than the regimen employed in PVSG protocol 05, their efficacy in preventing thrombosis remains unproven.

This issue is of considerable importance. After 10 calendar years and more than 5000 patient-years of follow-up, the results of PVSG protocol 01 clearly indicate that phlebotomy is the treatment of choice in *many* patients with PV.[18,35,37] The major drawback to the phlebotomy regimen is the excessive incidence of severe thrombotic complications, principally strokes, within the first few years of treatment. Development of an effective regimen to prevent thrombosis in phlebotomized patients thus continues to merit a very high priority.

PVSG PROTOCOL 08: MANAGEMENT OF PV WITH THE NONALKYLATING MYELOSUPPRESSIVE AGENT HYDROXYUREA

Because of the obvious need for a nonmutagenic myelosuppressive agent for the management of PV, the PVSG explored a number of potential candidates. Ultimately, attention focused on hydroxyurea. This nonalkylating agent inhibits DNA synthesis, and hence cell replication, by blocking the enzyme ribonucleoside diphosphate reductase.[50] It had previously been utilized effectively in the treatment of other hematologic malignancies, notably chronic myelogenous leukemia,[51] and less often in combination with other chemotherapeutic agents in the treatment of nonhematologic "solid" tumors[52] or as an adjunct to radiotherapy for carcinoma of the cervix.[53] There is also some experience with its use in nonmalignant disorders of cellular proliferation such as psoriasis.[54] Although there was some laboratory experience suggesting that the drug was not entirely free of mutagenic potential, when PVSG protocol 08 was initiated, it had not been shown clinically to be leukemogenic in any of the settings in which it had been used previously.

PVSG protocol 08 was initially designed to be a short-term, phase II efficacy trial to establish the proportion of patients with PV whose hematocrits and platelet counts could be controlled effectively with only minimal use of supplemental phlebotomy and without unacceptable hematologic toxicity. By the time these limited goals were accomplished and the short-term efficacy of the drug established,[55] restrictions in funding markedly hampered the PVSG's ability to proceed with further randomized trials. Instead, the decision was made to maintain patients already enrolled in PVSG protocol 08 on hydroxyurea in order to establish its long-term efficacy and the risks of various complications, including both thrombotic events and the development of acute leukemias associated with its chronic use.

Diagnostic Criteria and Patient Eligibility

All patients in whom the diagnosis of PV was established according to the conventionally accepted PVSG criteria (see Table 15–1 and Chap. 3) were eligible for PVSG protocol 08, irrespective of their prior treatment history. However, patients were stratified into two groups: those previously untreated or treated with phlebotomy alone and those who had received any form of myelosuppressive treatment. In the latter group, a minimum waiting period of 4 months since the last myelosuppressive therapy was required prior to initiation of hydroxyurea.

Treatment Regimen

The initial goal of the study was to estimate the proportion of cases in which a hematocrit of less than 50 percent and a platelet count of less than 1,000,000/ml could be achieved and maintained with hydroxyurea alone, with only minimal and highly restricted use of supplemental phlebotomy. All patients initially received hydroxyurea 30 mg/kg per day for 1 week, followed by 15 mg/kg per day. The dose was subsequently modified downward for cytopenia and upward, in increments of 5 mg/kg per day every 4 weeks, for inadequate control of the hematocrit, according to predefined criteria.[55] Patients who required more than six phlebotomies of 500 ml each within any 12-month period while taking hydroxyurea were considered treatment failures.

Patient Evaluation

Patients were assessed for both initial response and long-term control. Because virtually all patients had received at least limited phlebotomy therapy prior to entry into the study, initial hematocrit response to hydroxyurea was assessed only in 21 patients with an elevated hematocrit on entry into the study who did not require early supplemental phlebotomy; similarly, initial platelet response was assessed only in the 26 patients whose pretreatment platelet counts were 1,000,000/µl or greater. In these patients, a good initial response was defined as reduction of the hematocrit to less than 50 percent and reduction in the platelet count to less than 600,000/µl within 12 weeks of starting hydroxyurea.[55]

All eligible patients were assessed for achievement of long-term disease control.[55, 56] Patients were considered treatment failures if, while receiving hydroxyurea, their hematocrits reached or exceeded 50 percent or their platelet counts reached or exceeded 1,000,000/µl for 12 weeks or more or if they required more than six phlebotomies in any 52-week period, if they developed major disease-related complications such as thrombosis, leukemia, cancer, myelofibrosis with myeloid metaplasia, or death, or if they developed an untoward reaction to the drug that precluded its continued administration.[56] All patients who did not fail therapy according to these criteria were considered to have achieved good control.

Results

Initial Responses and 1-Year Control. As already noted, 50 percent of the patients entered into the protocol had received no prior myelosuppressive therapy at the time hydroxyurea was initiated; the remaining half had been treated previously with ^{32}P and/or other myelosuppressive agents. The ability of hydroxyurea to achieve and maintain control of the peripheral blood counts of patients was determined in both groups.

Equivalent initial responses to hydroxyurea were observed in both groups of patients. In the 26 patients from both groups with pretreatment platelet counts of 1,000,000/µl or greater, 65 percent had achieved platelet counts of less than 600,000/µl within 3 weeks, and 88 percent responded by 12 weeks. Control of hematocrit in the 21 patients with elevated pretreatment levels occurred somewhat more slowly, no doubt related to the longer red blood cell life span, but by 12 weeks, 80 percent had achieved normal values.[55]

Long-term efficacy also was demonstrated.[56] Sixty-three percent of evaluable and previously untreated patients and 51 percent of previously treated patients remained well controlled on hydroxyurea. The cumulative 1-year failure-free survival (as previously defined) was 73 percent in previously untreated patients and 59 percent in those previously treated with other my-elosuppressive modalities. Thus hydroxy-urea was demonstrated to be an effective treatment modality in the armamentarium that may be used in the treatment of PV. In fact, many clinicians now consider hydroxy-urea to be the treatment of choice for pa-tients with myeloproliferative disorders who require bone marrow suppression.[57]

The majority of toxicities observed in both groups of patients occurred within 8 weeks of starting therapy. Cytopenias at the dosing level employed occurred not infrequently but were typically dose-dependent and clini-cally of no consequence. Thrombocytopenia and leukopenia tended to occur early after the initial loading dose. However, subsequent off-protocol experience has shown that by reducing or eliminating the loading dose and using supplemental phlebotomy therapy in addition to hydroxyurea to achieve control of the hematocrit, the incidence of toxicity can be decreased significantly. Indeed, we now recommend that hydroxyurea therapy be initiated at a dose of 15 to 20 mg/kg per day.

Patient requirements for hydroxyurea are quite variable and must be determined em-pirically in each individual. Average daily doses are in the 500 to 1000 mg/d range.[55] However, some patients require only 1500 to 2000 mg of hydroxyurea per *week*, along with occasional phlebotomies, to maintain con-trol, whereas others require from 1500 to more than 2000 mg per *day*.

For hydroxyurea to be effective, it must be used continuously. If the drug is discon-tinued, unmaintained remissions are ex-tremely short, and thrombocytosis com-monly occurs within 7 to 10 days in those patients who presented initially with a high platelet count. The requirement for contin-uous hydroxyurea therapy and the potential occurrence of significant myelotoxicity ne-cessitate frequent and conscientious patient monitoring. It is recommended that the blood count be monitored at least bimonthly for the first 3 months of therapy, with the dosage of hydroxyurea being adjusted ap-propriately. Following this initial period, the blood count should be followed every 4 to 6 weeks, and appropriate adjustments, if any, in dosage should be made as indicated. Thus this agent may not be suitable for unreliable or noncompliant patients. Nevertheless, when hydroxyurea is used judiciously and in com-bination with phlebotomy to minimize the

doses employed, and patients are monitored carefully, excellent long-term responses are achieved.

Hydroxyurea also can be used effectively when a rapid reduction of the platelet count is required, although faster control of this particular parameter has been reported with both anagrelide[58] and interferon.[59, 60] Some patients also report alleviation of severe pru-ritus during hydroxyurea myelosuppression. Shrinkage of symptomatic and massive sple-nomegaly also has been noted with this agent. Others have confirmed the efficacy of hydroxyurea in the management of PV.[51]

Long-Term Management

Encouraged by these results, the PVSG elected to continue the patients on PVSG protocol 08 or on long-term hydroxyurea management with careful monitoring of the frequency of the well-recognized long-term complications of PV, specifically thrombotic disease and leukemic transformation. Pa-tients with PV who were treated with hydrox-yurea and phlebotomy on the protocol 08 study and who previously received no other myelosuppressive therapy were compared for the incidence of these complications with a group considered to be the best available historical control population, namely, PV pa-tients treated with phlebotomy alone on pro-tocol 01.

Comparison of Groups At presentation, the age and sex distributions of the two pa-tient groups [protocol 08 hydroxyurea not previously treated (NPT) and protocol 01 phlebotomy] were similar (Table 15–13). The major differences between the two groups were that (1) a history of a prior thrombotic event (thrombophlebitis, pulmo-nary embolism, completed stroke, transient ischemic attack, or myocardial infarction) was more frequent in the hydroxyurea-treated group (35.3 versus 14.2 percent), (2) the mean hematocrit and red cell count of phlebotomy-treated patients exceeded those of hydroxyurea-treated patients, and (3) hy-droxyurea-treated patients had higher plate-let counts at presentation.

Effect on Thrombotic Complications. As discussed previously, one of the important findings of PVSG protocol 01 was the in-creased incidence of thrombosis in phlebot-omy-treated patients, which occurred pri-marily during the first 3 years after

TABLE 15–13. PVSG PROTOCOL 08: CLINICAL AND LABORATORY CHARACTERISTICS AT INITIAL EVALUATION BY TREATMENT AND PROTOCOL

CHARACTERISTIC	01—PHLEBOTOMY	08—HYDROXYUREA: NO PRIOR THERAPY
Number	134	51
Male (%)	54.5	52.9
Age: <50	11.2	11.8
50–70	31.3	31.4
>70	11.9	9.8
Female (%)	45.5	47.1
Age: <50	9.7	15.7
50–70	25.4	25.5
>70	10.4	5.9
Prior thrombosis (%)	14.2	35.3
Hematocrit (%)	61.7 ± 7.5*	52.9 ± 8.1
RBC ($\times\ 10^{-8}/\mu l$)	7.16 ± 1.09*	6.60 ± 0.86
Platelets ($\times\ 10^{-3}/\mu l$)	505 ± 24.6+	778 ± 63.6
Percentage with platelets:		
<600,000	76	47
600,000–1,000,000	17	31
>1,000,000	7	22

*Mean ± SE.
+Mean ± SD.

randomization. Accordingly, the incidence of thrombosis in the PVSG protocol 01 phlebotomy group was compared with the incidence of thrombosis in hydroxyurea-treated patients in PVSG protocol 08. Hydroxyurea was highly effective in decreasing the propensity for thrombosis during the first few years of therapy, when the incidence of thrombosis in phlebotomy-treated patients is highest[18] (Table 15–14). In an analysis conducted at 378 weeks on study, thrombosis was the first manifestation of treatment failure in 32.8 percent of PVSG protocol 01 patients treated with phlebotomy, compared with only 9.8 percent of patients in the hy-

TABLE 15–14. PVSG PROTOCOL 08: COMPARATIVE INCIDENCE OF THROMBOSIS BY STUDY YEAR, BY PROTOCOL, AND BY TREATMENT GROUP

	CUMULATIVE %, ± SE	
PROTOCOL	Year 1	Year 2
On-study events		
HU (08 NPT*)	2.8 ± 4.0	6.6 ± 3.7
Phlebotomy (01)	8.7 ± 2.5	14.0 ± 3.2
All Events		
HU (08 NPT)	5.9 ± 3.3	7.9 ± 3.8
Phlebotomy (01)	9.0 ± 2.5	15.8 ± 3.2

*HU: hydroxyurea; NPT: no prior myelosuppressive therapy.

droxyurea group.[56] Thus, during the first 7.5 years of study, thromboembolic events occurred significantly less frequently in patients treated with hydroxyurea (PVSG protocol 08) than in those managed by phlebotomy alone (PVSG protocol 01).[56] In a further analysis conducted after 591 weeks (11.4 years) on study, with a median treatment interval of 6.2 years, the incidence of thrombosis remains appreciably less in patients treated with hydroxyurea than in those treated with phlebotomy alone (Table 15–15).

Leukemia. These data indicate that hydroxyurea can play a major role in minimizing the thrombotic complications of PV. The critical question is whether it is safe for long-term use. PVSG protocol 01 confirmed that patients with PV have a small but significant background incidence of leukemic transformation when treated with phlebotomy therapy alone. This incidence of leukemic transformation is influenced by the therapy employed[18] and increases significantly when the myelosuppressive agents chlorambucil or ^{32}P are used. The incidence of leukemic transformation in patients managed with long-term hydroxyurea therapy was investigated. Fifty-one hydroxyurea-treated patients with no prior exposure to other myelosuppressive agents have been followed for up to 591 weeks (11.4 years) with a median treatment interval of 6.2 years (Table

TABLE 15–15. PVSG PROTOCOL 08: COMPARATIVE INCIDENCE OF THROMBOSIS BY PROTOCOL AND TREATMENT

PROTOCOL	TOTAL NO. OF PATIENTS	NO. OF EVENTS	PERCENT
On-study events, first 591 weeks of study			
HU (08 NPT)	51	11	21.6
Phlebotomy (01)	134	50	37.3
Wilcoxon $\chi_1^2 = 3.986, p = 0.0459$			
Log-rank $\chi_1^2 = 3.354, p = 0.0670$			
All events, first 591 weeks of study			
HU (08 NPT)	51	13	25.5
Phlebotomy (01)	134	54	40.3
Wilcoxon $\chi_1^2 = 3.671, p = 0.0554$			
Log-rank $\chi_1^2 = 2.954, p = 0.0857$			

15–16). Three patients (5.9 percent) have developed acute leukemia, compared with 1.5 percent of the PVSG protocol 01 historical control group treated by phlebotomy for the same time interval. The difference in the incidence of leukemia between patients treated with hydroxyurea and supplemental phlebotomy (PVSG protocol 08) versus those treated with phlebotomy alone (PVSG protocol 01) does not reach statistical significance at the 0.05 level. Moreover, one of the hydroxyurea-treated patients who developed leukemia received the agent for only 2 months and developed acute leukemia 2

TABLE 15–16. PVSG PROTOCOL 08: COMPARATIVE INCIDENCE OF ACUTE LEUKEMIA BY PROTOCOL AND TREATMENT

PROTOCOL	TOTAL NO. OF PATIENTS	NO. OF EVENTS	PERCENT
On-study events, first 591 weeks of study			
HU (08 NPT)	51	3	5.9
Phlebotomy (01)	134	2	1.5
Wilcoxon $\chi_1^2 = 1.811, p = 0.1783$			
Log-rank $\chi_1^2 = 2.709, p = 0.0998$			
All events, first 591 weeks of study			
HU (08 NPT)	51	4	7.8
Phlebotomy	134	4	3.0
Wilcoxon $\chi_1^2 = 2.190, p = 0.1389$			
Log-rank $\chi_1^2 = 2.154, p = 0.1422$			

TABLE 15–17. PVSG PROTOCOL 01: LEUKEMIA BY TREATMENT GROUP

TREATMENT GROUP	TOTAL NO. OF PATIENTS	NO. OF EVENTS	PERCENT
On-study events, first 591 weeks of study			
Chlorambucil	141	15	10.6
^{32}P	156	13	8.3
Phlebotomy	134	2	1.5
$\chi_2^2 = 20.5, p < 0.0002$			
All events, first 591 weeks of study			
Chlorambucil	141	16	11.3
^{32}P	156	15	9.6
Phlebotomy	134	4	3.0
$\chi_2^2 = 6.8, 0.025 < p < 0.05$			

years after the agent was discontinued. In a parallel analysis that included all PVSG protocol 08 patients treated with hydroxyurea, including those off-study due to another complication of their disease, a protocol violation, or treatment failure, the incidence of leukemia was not statistically different from that in PVSG protocol 01 patients treated with phlebotomy alone (7.8 versus 3.0 per cent, respectively) (see Table 15–16, all events).

Although the data available to date thus suggest that long-term treatment with hydroxyurea does not result in a statistically significantly increased risk of developing acute leukemia, it should be emphasized that the number of events in both treatment groups is small. Accordingly, only one additional leukemia in the hydroxyurea group would render the increased leukemia incidence in this group significant, whereas a single additional case of leukemia in the phlebotomy group would render the differences comfortably nonsignificant. By contrast to the results with hydroxyurea, in patients treated with either chlorambucil or ^{32}P, the incidence of leukemic transformation at 591 weeks was highly significantly greater than with phlebotomy therapy alone (Table 15–17), whether the analysis was restricted to on-study events only or included all events.

Conclusions

Hydroxyurea in combination with phlebotomy is an effective agent in controlling the peripheral blood abnormalities in patients with PV. Optimal therapy requires that peripheral blood counts be monitored frequently and the dose of drug adjusted accordingly. In a subset of patients, hydroxyurea may minimize the very debilitating symptom of generalized pruritus. It also can be effective in decreasing symptomatic splenomegaly. Myelosuppression with this agent decreases the incidence of life-threatening thrombosis that occurs in patients with PV who are managed with phlebotomy alone. After being employed and studied for over 11 years in patients with PV, it appears not to significantly increase the risk of leukemic transformation in this population. However, these patients continue to be monitored to help determine its ultimate safety. Obviously, the question of long-term safety is crucial as the clinical role of hydroxyurea is being expanded with studies in such nonmalignant disorders as sickle cell disease.[61]

REFERENCES

1. Modan B, Lilienfeld AM: Polycythemia vera and leukemia—The role of radiation treatment: A study of 1222 patients. Medicine 44:305–344, 1965
2. Tinney WS, Hall BE, Giffen HZ: Hematologic complications of P. vera. Proc Staff Meet Mayo Clin 18:227–230, 1943
3. Chievitz E, Thiede T: Complications and causes of death in polycythemia vera. Acta Med Scand 172:513, 1962
4. Landaw SA: Acute leukemia in polycythemia vera. Semin Hematol 43:156–165, 1986
5. Thomas DJ, Marshall J, Ross Russell RW, et al: Cerebral blood-flow in polycythemia. Lancet 2:161–163, 1977
6. Pearson TC, Wetherley-Mein, G: Vascular occlusive episodes and venous hematocrit in primary proliferative polycythemia. Lancet 2:1219–1222, 1978
7. Thomas DJ, Marshall J, Ross Russell RW, et al. Effect of hematocrit on cerebral blood flow in man. Lancet 2:941–943, 1977
8. Wasserman LR: Treatment of polycythemia vera. Semin Hematol 13:57–77, 1976
9. Donovan PB, Landaw SA, Dresch C, et al: Resistance to therapy of acute leukemia developing in the course of polycythemia vera. Nouv Rev Fr Hematol 23:187–192, 1981
10. Gehan EA: A generalized Wilcoxon test for comparing arbitrarily singly-censored samples. Biometrika 52:203–334, 1965
11. Breslow N: A generalized Kruskal-Wallis test for comparing K samples subject to unequal patterns of censorship. Biometrika 56:579–594, 1970
12. Mantel N: Evaluation of survival data and two new rank order statistics arising in its consideration. Cancer Chemother Rep 50:163–70, 1966
13. Peto R, Pike MC, Armitage P, et al: Design and analysis of randomized clinical trials requiring prolonged observation of each patient: II. Analysis and examples. Br J Cancer 35:1–39, 1977
14. Cox DR: Regression models and life-tables. J R Soc Surg [B] 34:187–220, 1972
15. Breslow N: Covariance analysis of censored survival data. Biometrics 30:89–99, 1974
16. Breslow N: Analysis of survival data under the proportional hazards mode. Int Stat Rev 43:45–58, 1975
17. Byar DR, Corle DK: Selecting optimal treatment in clinical trials using covariate information. J Chronic Dis 30:445–459, 1977
18. Wasserman LR, Balcerzak SP, Berk PD, et al: Influence of therapy on causes of death in polycythemia vera. Trans Assoc Am Physicians 44:30–38, 1981
19. Valla D, Casadevall N, Lacombe C, et al. Primary myeloproliferative disorder and hepatic vein thrombosis. Ann Intern Med 103:329–334, 1985
20. Levy VG, Ruskone A, Baillou C, et al: Polycythemia and the Budd-Chiari syndrome: Study of serum

erythropoietin and bone marrow erythroid progenitors. Hepatology 5:858–861, 1985

21. Tartaglia AP, Goldberg JD, Berk PD, Wasserman LR: Adverse effects of antiaggregating platelet therapy in the treatment of polycythemia vera. Semin Hematol 23:172–176, 1986

22. Berk PD, Goldberg JD, Silverstein MN, et al: Increased incidence of acute leukemia in polycythemia vera associated with chlorambucil therapy. N Engl J Med 204:441–447, 1981

23. Weinfeld A, Westin G, Ridell B, Swolin B: Polycythemia vera terminating in acute leukemia. Scand J Haematol 19:255–272, 1977

24. Hoffman R, Estren S, Kopel S, et al: Lymphoblastic-like leukemic transformation of polycythemia vera. Ann Intern Med 89:71, 1978

25. Marks SM, Baltimore D, McCaffrey RP: Terminal transferase as a predictor of initial responsiveness to vincristine and prednisone in blastic chronic myelogenous leukemia. N Engl J Med 298:812–814, 1978

26. Preisler HD, Bjornsson S, Henderson E: Chemotherapy for acute myelogenous leukemia (AML) with cytosine arabinoside (Ara-C) and Adriamycin (ADR) (abstract). Blood 48:982, 1976

27. Capizzi RL, Davis R, Powell B, et al: Synergy between high-dose cytarabine and asparaginase in the treatment of adults with refractory and relapsed acute myelogenous leukemia: A Cancer and Leukemia Group B study. J Clin Oncol 6:499–508, 1988

28. Peterson P, Ellis JT, Geller SA, Rappoport H: Occurrence of non-Hodgkin's lymphoma in treated polycythemia vera (abstract). Lab Invest 52:51A, 1985

29. Laszlo J: Myeloproliferative disorders (MPD): Myelofibrosis, myelosclerosis, extramedullary hematopoiesis, undifferentiated MPD, and hemorrhagic thrombocythemia. Semin Hematol 12:409–432, 1975

30. Berk PD: Myeloproliferative disorders. In Wyngaarden JB, Smith LH, Bennett JC (eds): Cecil Textbook of Medicine, 19th ed. Philadelphia, Saunders, 1991, pp 929–933

31. Silverstein MN: Post-polycythemia myeloid metaplasia. Arch Intern Med 134:113–120, 1974

32. Silverstein MN, Brown AL: Idiopathic myeloid metaplasia. Arch Intern Med 132:709–712, 1973

33. Lawrence JH, Winchell HS, Donald WG: Leukemia in polycythemia vera: Relationship to splenic myeloid metaplasia and therapeutic radiation dose. Ann Intern Med 70:763–771, 1969

34. Ellis JT, Peterson P, Geller SA, Rappaport H: Studies of the bone marrow in polycythemia vera and the evolution of myelofibrosis and second hematologic malignancies. Semin Hematol 23:144–155, 1986

35. Berk PD, Goldberg JD, Donovan PB, et al: Therapeutic recommendations in polycythemia vera based on Polycythemia Vera Study Group protocols. Semin Hematol 23:132–143, 1986

36. Cancer Expected Rates: National Cancer Institute Monograph No. 41. Third National Cancer Survey: Incidence Data. DHEW publication no. (NIH) 75-787. Bethesda, Md, US Department of Health, Education and Welfare, National Institutes of Health, National Cancer Institute, 1975

37. Berk PD: Erythrocytosis and polycythemia. In Wyngaarden JB, Smith LH, Bennett JC (eds): Cecil Textbook of Medicine, 19th ed. Philadelphia, Saunders, 1991, pp 920–929

38. Ekeström SA, Gunnes S, Brodin UB: Effect of dipyridamole (Persantin) on blood flow and patency of aortocoronary vein bypass grafts. Scand J Thorac Cardiovasc Surg 24:191–196, 1990

39. Chesebro JH, Webster MWI, Zoldhelyi P, et al: Antithrombotic therapy and progression of coronary artery disease: Antiplatelet versus antithrombins. Circulation 86 (suppl III):S100–S111, 1992

40. Coller BS: Antiplatelet agents in the prevention and therapy of thrombosis. Annu Rev Med 43:171–180, 1992

41. Kalbfleisch JD, Prentice RL: The Statistical Analysis of Failure-Time Data. New York, Wiley, 1980

42. Tartaglia AP, Goldberg JD, Berk PD, Wasserman LR: Adverse effects of antiaggregating platelet therapy in the treatment of polycythemia vera. Semin Hematol 23:172–176, 1986

43. Harker LA: Antithrombotic therapy. In WJ Williams, E Beutler, AJ Erslev, MA Lichtman (eds): Hematology, 4th ed. New York, McGraw-Hill, 1990, pp 1569–1581

44. Antiplatelet Trialists Collaboration: Secondary prevention of vascular disease by prolonged antiplatelet treatment. Br Med J Clin Res 396:320–331, 1988

45. Hirsh J, Salzman EW, Harker L, et al: Aspirin and other platelet active drugs: Relationship among dose, effectiveness, and side effects. Chest 95:128–185, 1989

46. Jabaily J, Iland HJ, Laszlo J, et al: Neurologic manifestations of essential thrombocythemia. Ann Intern Med 99:513–518, 1983

47. Schafer AI: Essential thrombocythemia. Progr. Hemost Thromb 10:69–96, 1991

48. Frenkel EP: Southwestern Internal Medicine Clinical Conference: The clinical spectrum of thrombocytosis and thrombocythemia. Am J Med Sci 301:69–80, 1991

49. Gilbert HS, Hanna MM: Low-dose aspirin/low-hematocrit regimen: A safe and efficacious treatment for polycythemia vera. Blood 68:223a, 1986

50. Frenkel EP, Arthur C: Induced ribotide reductive conversion defect by hydroxyurea and its relationship to megaloblastosis. Cancer Res 27:1016–1019, 1967

51. Kennedy BJ: Hydroxyurea therapy in chronic myelogenous leukemia. Cancer 29:1052, 1972

52. Constanzi JJ, Vaitkevicius VR, Quagliana JM, et al: Combination chemotherapy for disseminated malignant melanoma. Cancer 35:342, 1975

53. Piver MS, Barlow J, Vongtama V, Blumenson L: Significantly improved five-year survival in women with stage IIB cervical cancer treated with hydroxyurea plus radiation as compared to placebo plus radiation. Proc ASCO 2:146, 1983

54. Yarbro JW: Hydroxyurea in the treatment of refractory psoriasis. Lancet 2:846, 1969

55. Donovan PB, Kaplan ME, Goldberg JD, et al: Treatment of polycythemia vera with hydroxyurea. Am J Hematol 17:329–334, 1984

56. Kaplan ME, Mack K, Goldberg JD, et al: Long-term management of polycythemia vera with

hydroxyurea: A progress report. Semin Hematol 23:167–171, 1986

57. Zuckerman K, Bagby G, Emanuel P, et al: Myeloproliferative Disorders. Education Program, American Society of Hematology Annual Meeting, 1992

58. Anagrelide Study Group: Anagrelide, a therapy for thrombocythemic states: Experience in 577 patients. Am J Med 92:69–76, 1992

59. Gisslinger H, Ludwig H, Linkesh W, et al: Long-term interferon therapy for thrombocytosis in myeloproliferative diseases. Lancet 1:634–637, 1989

60. West WO, Ruff JD, Yarbro JW: Response of polycythemia vera to treatment with interferon. J Lab Clin Med 74:1022–1023, 1969

61. Rogers GP, Dover GJ, Noguchi CT, et al: Hematologic responses of patients with sickle disease to treatment with hydroxyurea. N Engl J Med 322:1037–1045, 1989.

ACKNOWLEDGMENTS: Preparation of the chapter was supported by Grant CA-10728 from the National Institutes of Health to the Polycythemia Vera Study Group and by generous gifts from the Polly Annenberg Levee Charitable Trust, the Albert A. List Research Fund, and the Shirley B. Kellner Memorial Polycythemia Vera Research Fund.

16

Secondary Polycythemia

EDWARD A. COPELAN *and* STANLEY P. BALCERZAK

Secondary polycythemia may be defined as an absolute increase in red cell mass caused by enhanced stimulation of red cell production. Enhanced stimulation results most often from the physiologic signal of generalized inadequate tissue oxygenation, such as occurs with decreased arterial oxygen tension, reduced capacity for oxygen transport, or impaired oxygen delivery by hemoglobin. Less frequently, stimulation of red cell proliferation does not occur as a physiologic response to decreased systemic oxygen supply but instead results from secretion of erythropoietin or other erythroid-stimulating substances by neoplasms or areas of local renal ischemia. The former group of disorders has been labeled *physiologic* or *compensatory* and the latter *nonphysiologic* or *inappropriate*.[1–3]

ERYTHROPOIETIN

The role of erythropoietin in the regulation of red cell replication has been reviewed in detail in Chap. 5. In humans, the kidney is the chief site of the oxygen sensor and the major organ producing erythropoietin. The liver is normally responsible for production of a small portion of erythropoietin. Although the precise nature of the renal oxygen sensor has not been defined, it appears to detect tissue oxygen concentration and to stimulate erythropoietin secretion when the tissue oxygen concentration falls below a threshold level. When an isolated kidney from a dog is perfused with hypoxic blood,[4] the kidney responds by increasing erythropoietin release. The localization of the oxygen sensor in the kidney permits sensible regulation of red cell mass. While alteration of blood flow to many organs profoundly affects their extraction of oxygen, small fluctuations in renal blood flow do not dramatically change oxygen extraction by the kidney. Renal oxygen consumption decreases proportionately with moderate reductions in renal blood flow because sodium reabsorption and, therefore, work by the kidney decreases.[5,6] The oxygen sensor is therefore relatively insensitive to modest changes in regional blood flow in the kidney. When flow is more substantially reduced, the isolated dog kidney increases erythropoietin production. Unlike the carotid and aortic body sensors, the renal oxygen sensor is not cyanide-sensitive, suggesting that its response is not related to its mitochondrial energy metabolism.[7] The mechanism by which the oxygen sensor detects deficient oxygen supply, however, has not been defined. A rapid erythropoietin response occurs when severe anemia is induced in animals[8] or when animals or humans are made hypoxemic by exposure to high altitude.

A number of methods have been used to measure erythropoietin levels. In vivo bioassays in mice transfused to hematocrits in excess of 60 percent or made plethoric by hypoxia measure radioactive iron incorporation several days after injection of test plasma. This assay detects erythropoietin levels that are moderately elevated (lower limit approximately 20 to 50 mU) but does not detect levels in the normal range of 10 to 20 mU/ml of erythropoietin.[9,10] In addition, the bioassay method is expensive and laborious. Erythropoietin cell culture assays, which measure radioactive iron incorporation or erythroid colony formation, detect 1 to 5 mU of erythropoietin. However, the cells are influenced by a variety of factors in human serum and may fail to detect activity demonstrable in the whole-animal assay. Also (asialo)erythropoietin, though devoid of in vivo activity, is active in vitro. A hemagglutination inhibition assay has been developed and is commercially available. However, this assay kit has been found to be of little value for erythropoietin determination and in the differential diagnosis of polycythemia.[11] The isolation of human erythropoietin in pure form has led to development of the erythropoietin radioimmunoassay. Radioimmunoassay (RIA) provides a simple rapid technique that is both sensitive and specific. The RIA can detect 2 mU of erythropoietin in 0.1 ml.[12] This sensitivity permits measurement not only of normal but also of depressed erythropoietin levels. The RIA shows good correlation with the polycythemia mouse bioassay. Erythropoietin concentrations in plasmas from secondary polycythemia patients are markedly increased over the levels in normal subjects and polycythemia vera (PV) patients as measured by RIA.[13]

Discrepancies between the RIA and biologic assays of erythropoietin occur in patients with anemia of chronic renal disease, in whom a biologically inactive but immunologically reactive fragment of erythropoietin may exist.[14] Similar discrepancies may exist in other diseases. In patients with PV, bioassay and radioimmunoassay of plasma generally demonstrate erythropoietin titers that are below normal. In secondary polycythemia, levels are high.

OXYGEN TRANSPORT

Transport in the Lung

The adequacy of tissue oxygen supply is determined by the effectiveness of oxygen transfer from the air to the tissues. Approximately 21 percent of the air at sea level is oxygen; the partial pressure of O_2 is 0.21×760 mmHg, or 160 mmHg. As air is saturated with water in the upper airways and mixed with CO_2-containing air from the alveoli, the air P_{O_2} drops to 95 mmHg. Alveolar O_2 tension ($P_{A_{O_2}}$) may be markedly decreased when ambient O_2 tension is low, as at high altitude, when hypoventilation leads to an increased P_{CO_2} and displacement of O_2 in alveoli, or when another gas such as CO is inspired and displaces O_2.[15, 16]

The $P_{A_{O_2}}$ is influenced by the O_2 content of pulmonary capillary blood and by alveolar ventilation. $P_{A_{O_2}}$ will approach the partial pressure of O_2 in the air as alveolar ventilation increases. The quantity of oxygen transported across the capillary membrane is determined by the gradient between $P_{A_{O_2}}$ and the oxygen tension of capillary blood and by the diffusing capacity of the membrane. The membrane of surfactant, alveolar epithelium, basement membrane, interstitial tissue, and capillary endothelium is between 0.1 and 0.3 μm thick. Only when the membrane is markedly thicker does a detectable difference occur between alveolar and arterial P_{O_2} at the level of the individual gas exchange unit. Uneven distribution of ventilation and perfusion, however, reduces the P_{O_2}.

Normally, the right ventricle transmits a systolic pressure of approximately 25 mmHg to the pulmonary artery. While the right ventricle pressure falls to zero, a diastolic pressure of approximately 9 mmHg is maintained in the pulmonary artery by closure of the pulmonic value. The mean pulmonary artery pressure is approximately 14 mmHg, 6 mmHg greater than the mean left atrial pressure. This drop in pressure across the pulmonary vascular bed is caused by the resistance of the bed. Gravity is the most important determinant of the distribution of blood flow in the lung. The pressure at a specific point in a pulmonary vessel is related to the height of the blood column above or below the location of the main pulmonary artery. The pressure in the vascular bed increases by 1 cmH_2O (1 cmH_2O is equal to 0.735 mmHg) for every centimeter below the level of the main pulmonary artery. If the mean pressure in the pulmonary artery is 20 cmH_2O, the pressure in a vessel 10 cm below the main pulmonary artery is 30 cmH_2O. The pressure in a vessel 10 cm above the main pulmonary artery is 10 cmH_2O (Fig. 16–1). Higher intravascular pressure dilates the pulmonary blood vessels, decreases pulmonary vascular resistance, and increases blood flow. In upright individuals, pulmonary blood flow is greatest at the lung bases and decreases from base to apex. Local capillary blood flow depends on the arterial-to-venous pressure

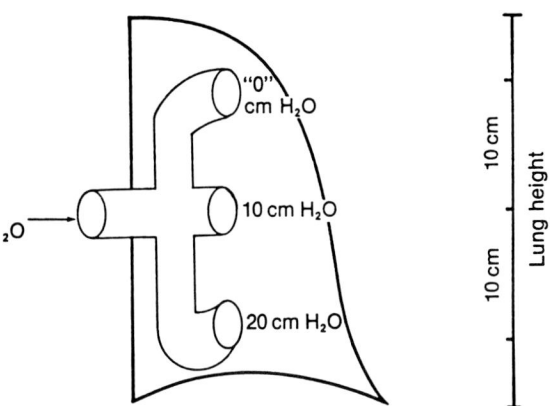

FIGURE 16-1. The effect of gravity on the perfusion pressure in the pulmonary arterial system of the upright lung. The mean pressure in pulmonary arteries varies from the mean pressure in the main pulmonary artery by height of the blood column at the point of measurement above or below the main pulmonary artery. *(Used with permission from Whitcomb M: The Lung: Normal and Diseased. St Louis, Mosby, 1982, p 206.)*

across the capillary bed. Near the apex of the normal upright lung, alveolar pressure exceeds venous pressure. This transmural pressure tends to collapse vessels and further decreases flow.[17]

Ventilation also varies in different regions, being lowest in the apex and highest in the base. This is related to differences in pleural pressure and in transpulmonary pressures for alveoli in different lung zones. Greater transpulmonary pressure in the apex results in less ventilation. While ventilation and perfusion are lowest in the apices and highest at the bases, the relative change differs. The ratio of ventilation to perfusion is high (>1) at the apex and low (<1) at the base. In normal lungs, most alveoli have $\dot{V}/\dot{Q}$ ratios of approximately 1, but $\dot{V}/\dot{Q}$ ratios range between 0.3 and 3.0. Neuromuscular abnormalities, alterations in the mechanical properties of airways or alveoli, and changes in distribution of blood flow may decrease the proportion of alveoli with normal ratios, and hypoxemia may result.

In order to understand the mechanism by which ventilation/perfusion ($\dot{V}/\dot{Q}$) abnormalities lead to hypoxemia, the effect of mixing of blood from individual gas exchange units must be understood. Most of the oxygen in blood is bound to hemoglobin in red cells. When fully saturated, a gram of hemoglobin binds 1.39 ml of O_2. The degree of saturation is related to the P_{O_2}, as depicted by the oxyhemoglobin dissociation curve (Fig. 16-2). Above 100 mmHg, hemoglobin is nearly completely saturated. Higher P_{O_2} values, therefore, result in little additional oxygen being bound to hemoglobin. In contrast, small changes in oxygen tensions between 20 and 50 mmHg produce large changes in hemoglobin oxygen saturation.

While most O_2 is bound to hemoglobin, a small amount of oxygen is dissolved in cells and plasma. If the concentration of hemoglobin is 15 g/dl, the volume of O_2 bound to hemoglobin is 65 times that dissolved in plasma. Because of variations in $\dot{V}/\dot{Q}$ ratios, blood leaving individual gas exchange units has a wide range of partial pressures of oxygen. The P_{O_2} of blood leaving individual alveoli reflects the $\dot{V}/\dot{Q}$ ratio of that gas exchange. Areas with high $\dot{V}/\dot{Q}$ ratios result in

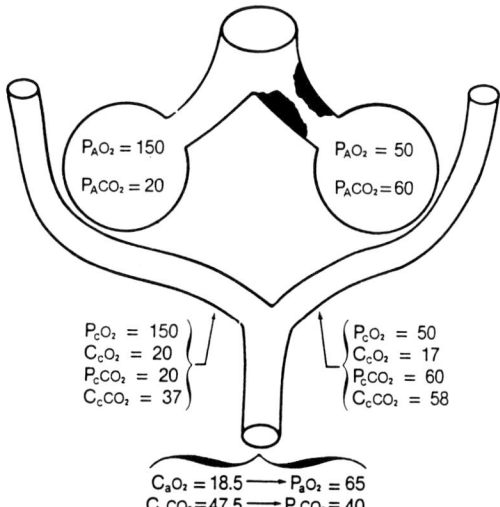

FIGURE 16-2. Two gas exchange units with equal blood flow but markedly different $\dot{V}/\dot{Q}$ ratios. Since the relationship between content and partial pressure is essentially linear for carbon dioxide, a normal arterial carbon dioxide tension can be maintained despite marked abnormalities in regional $\dot{V}/\dot{Q}$ ratios. However, increasing oxygen tension does not cause a proportional increase in oxygen content, thus resulting in a low arterial oxygen tension. Representative values for alveolar gas tensions (PA), pulmonary-capillary gas tensions (Pc), contents (Cc), arterial gas tensions (Pa), and contents (Ca) are given. *(Used with permission from Whitcomb M: The Lung: Normal and Diseased. St. Louis, Mosby, 1982, p 263.)*

blood leaving the area with high P_{O_2} values and low ratios lead to low P_{O_2} values. When blood from individual units is mixed, the partial pressure of the mixture is *not* the mean of the individual partial pressures. Rather, the O_2 content of the mixture is the mean of the individual O_2 contents. The significance of this principle is depicted in Fig. 16–3. Oxygen content of blood with high P_{O_2} values is not proportionately increased and does not compensate for blood with low O_2 content from low $\dot{V}/\dot{Q}$ areas. Thus variations in $\dot{V}/\dot{Q}$ ratios in individual gas exchanging units can lead to hypoxemia, even if the $\dot{V}/\dot{Q}$ ratio for the entire lung approaches 1.

Hypoxemia is produced by decreased oxygen tension in the inspired air, alveolar hypoventilation, mismatching of ventilation and perfusion, impaired diffusion of oxygen across the alveolar membrane, or increased intrapulmonary shunt volume. Normally, the alveolar-arterial oxygen (A–a) gradient is less than 20 mmHg. This difference results largely from the small portion of cardiac output that is shunted across the lung without oxygenation. As this mixes with oxygenated blood from pulmonary capillaries, the mean O_2 content of arterial blood falls.

In alveolar hypoventilation, a decreased $P_{A_{O_2}}$ leads to a decreased $P_{a_{O_2}}$ without abnormal oxygen exchange across the lung. As alveolar ventilation decreases with perfusion constant, O_2 is removed more rapidly from the alveoli than it is supplied by ventilation. Since the partial pressure of oxygen in blood leaving the alveolar capillary is nearly identical to the partial pressure in the alveolus, the $P_{a_{O_2}}$ decreases as the $P_{A_{O_2}}$ decreases.

In $\dot{V}/\dot{Q}$ mismatching, a large percentage of pulmonary blood flow is distributed to gas exchange units with $\dot{V}/\dot{Q}$ ratios less than 1. Blood leaving the pulmonary capillaries of these units has a low O_2 content and results in hypoxemia in the mixed blood from multiple gas exchange units.

In patients with severe interstitial pulmonary disease, equilibrium between alveolar and capillary O_2 tension may not occur. This contributes to an increased A–a gradient P_{O_2} difference and hypoxemia.

Increases in shunt fraction occur when blood perfuses nonventilated capillary beds. The partial pressure of O_2 leaving the capillaries is identical to the entering blood, which is the mixed venous P_{O_2}. As the fraction of shunted blood increases, it progressively decreases the $P_{a_{O_2}}$.

In recumbency, the functional residual capacity of the lung decreases, resulting in closure of some airways and, therefore, poor ventilation of perfused areas of the lung. In airways disease or obesity, recumbency may result in considerable areas of poorly ventilated alveoli.

Transport in the Blood

The transport of O_2 to tissues is determined by the hemoglobin concentration, the blood flow to the specific tissue, and the effectiveness by which O_2 is transferred from hemoglobin to the tissue. Under normal conditions, hemoglobin is nearly fully saturated with O_2 in the lungs. As blood flows through systemic capillaries, it is exposed to low O_2 tensions. O_2 is unloaded from hemoglobin as predicted by the oxyhemoglobin dissociation curve. O_2 released from hemoglobin diffuses into plasma and tissues along a gradient that is a function primarily of the P_{O_2} in the specific tissue and the distance of the tissue from the capillary.

The oxyhemoglobin dissociation curve has a sigmoidal shape because the affinity of each binding site of the hemoglobin tetramer is altered by binding at the other O_2 binding sites of the tetramer. This property of the hemoglobin tetramers has been labeled *heme-*

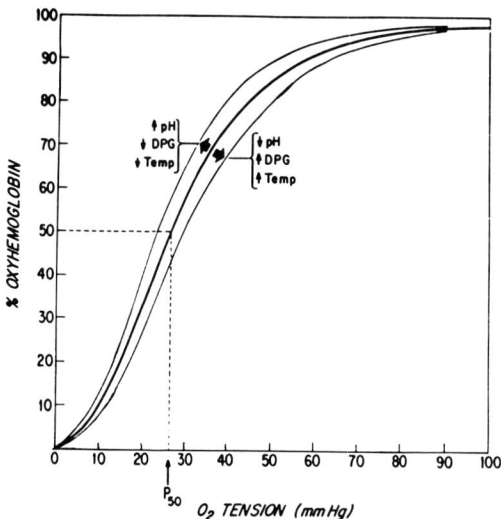

FIGURE 16–3. The oxyhemoglobin dissociation curve and the principal factors that influence the position of the curve. *(Used with permission from Bunn HF, Forget BG: Oxygen and Carbon Dioxide Transport in Health and Disease. In Hemoglobin: Molecular, Genetic and Clinical Aspects. Cambridge, Saunders, 1986, p. 95.)*

heme interaction. The partial pressure of O_2 at which hemoglobin is 50 percent oxygenated is the P_{50} (see Fig. 16–2). The P_{50} is one measure used to describe the oxygen affinity of hemoglobin.

The affinity of hemoglobin for oxygen is primarily determined by the structure of hemoglobin but is also influenced by temperature, pH, and red cell 2,3-diphosphoglycerate (2,3-DPG) level. The affinity of hemoglobin for O_2 is inversely related to temperature. Thus, in hypothermia, where metabolic demands are low, less O_2 is released to tissues. Increased hydrogen ion concentration decreases the affinity of hemoglobin for O_2. Thus, when the red cell interior becomes more acidic, as occurs with CO_2 diffusion into the cell, hemoglobin affinity for O_2 decreases due to H^+ and CO_2 allosteric modification of the reactivity of the heme groups.[18] In the tissues where CO_2 is taken up by red cells, O_2 is made more readily available. The level of 2,3-DPG is the third important determinant of the O_2 affinity of whole blood and is covered in detail elsewhere. Since 2,3-DPG is highly charged, it has a dual effect in lowering O_2 affinity. It interacts directly with deoxyhemoglobin as an allosteric modifier to decrease its O_2 affinity, and it also lowers intracellular pH.

The flow of blood to tissues is influenced by blood viscosity. Viscosity describes the resistance of a liquid to flow. As a liquid flows, its adjacent layers move in parallel (shearing), and resistance develops from friction between adjacent layers. For simple (newtonian) fluids, viscosity is independent of the rate of flow. Blood is a nonnewtonian fluid. Its viscosity is influenced by interactions of blood cells and plasma proteins. Blood viscosity depends on flow rate, hematocrit, vessel caliber, and the deformability and orientation of the red cells. The term *apparent viscosity* is applied to the value for viscosity measured by available techniques. Blood viscosity varies inversely with shear rate (the gradient of velocity across a sheared fluid). The shear-rate dependence of blood viscosity is related in part to red cell aggregation at low shear rates and red cell deformability at high shear rates.[19] At high shear rates, red cell aggregates are dispersed, and blood flows in parallel streamlines. At low shear rates, red cells are no longer deformed from their resting biconcave disk shape and are aggregated by large plasma globulins.[20] The resistance of blood to flow is therefore greater under conditions of slow flow. Lowe and Forbes[19] have compared blood to nondrip paint, which when stirred (application of high shear forces) is diaggregated, made less viscous, and now may drip.[19]

Apparent viscosity progressively increases as the number of red cells in plasma increases[21] (Fig. 16–4). At high shear rates, blood with a hematocrit of 55 percent is twice as viscous as blood with a hematocrit of 35 percent. With decreasing shear rate, red cell interaction increases, and the effect of hematocrit or blood viscosity is more pronounced. The normal circulation tends to minimize blood viscosity. High shear rates in large vessels ensure minimum viscosity. In small vessels, red cells migrate toward the center of the vessel (axial migration) and travel in the central, rapidly flowing zone, while low-viscosity plasma forms a lubricating outer zone. Still, when organs isolated from animals are perfused with blood of varying hematocrits, increased blood viscosity at high hematocrits leads to decreased blood flow.[22] When blood flow is decreased locally for any reason, the fall in shear rate will increase red cell aggregation and blood viscosity, further reducing blood flow.

The effects of hematocrit on cerebral blood flow have been studied extensively. An inverse relationship between cerebral blood flow and hematocrit has been demonstrated within the normal range of hematocrit,[23] in primary or secondary polycythemia,[24,25] in relative polycythemia,[26] and in anemia.[27] Decreased cerebral blood in patients with increased viscosity due to high hematocrit impairs cerebral function. Objective testing reveals impaired alertness in patients with hematocrits over 46 percent.[28] A significant rise in cerebral blood flow follows reduction in hematocrit in patients with high hematocrits.[23,24] Patients whose alertness is impaired in association with an increased hematocrit improve with phlebotomy. Since cerebral blood flow is regulated primarily by arterial oxygen content, decreased cerebral blood flow in polycythemia might be a physiologic response to increased arterial O_2 content. Brown et al.[25] have demonstrated that cerebral blood flow correlates inversely with arterial O_2 content within the range of hematocrits studied. No patient with a hemoglobin greater than 19.1 g/dl was studied, however, and no mention is made of patients with hy-

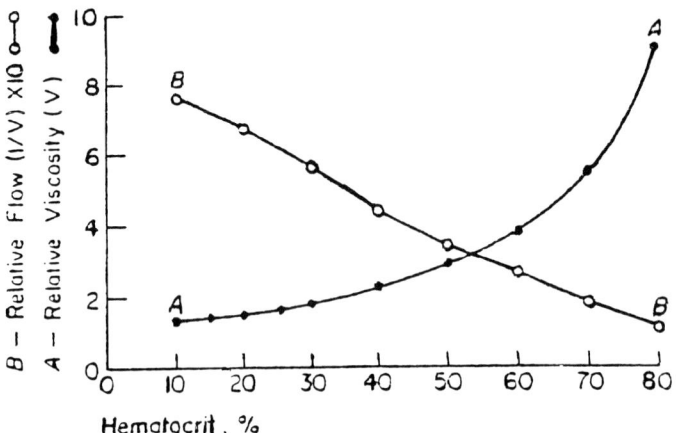

FIGURE 16–4. Relative viscosity (curve A) and relative flow through a capillary tube (curve B) of blood of various hematocrits. *(Used with permission from Castle WB, Jandl JH: Semin Hematol 3:193–198, 1966.)*

poxemic polycythemia. A crucial factor that appears to improve O_2 transport in polycythemic individuals is increased cardiac output. The marked increase in blood volume that accompanies absolute polycythemia results in increased venous return and increased cardiac output. The tendency to increase cardiac output is opposed by increased blood viscosity. The net result may depend on the relative benefits and strains on specific organ systems induced by these changes. For example, atherosclerotic lesions in the cerebral vessels of older individuals might limit flow to slow rates where viscosity becomes a more important factor than the carrying capacity of hemoglobin.

Compromised blood flow and oxygen delivery to the brain, gastrointestinal tract, and muscles have been demonstrated in polycythemic animals.[29] In general, total blood volume of these animals was not expanded. The effects of hypervolemia-induced increased cardiac output and higher blood oxygen content might outweigh the effects of increased blood viscosity, which is reduced by high flow rates. Maximal oxygen transport in dogs can be achieved under conditions of hypervolemia and polycythemia[30–32] (Fig. 16–5). Further complicating the issue is the underlying cause of polycythemia in an individual. The rise in hematocrit may be useful in increasing work capacity in circumstances where polycythemia occurs as an adaptation to hypoxia. In that same individual, however, the effects of cerebrovascular disease may be exacerbated by polycythemia. Thus the effects of polycythemia might differ not only between individuals but between different organ systems in a single individual.

COMPENSATORY ERYTHROCYTOSIS

Low Atmospheric Pressure

In 1890, the French physician Viault, after residing at 4392 m in the Peruvian Andes, described an increased number of red cells in his blood compared with his prior sea-level red cell count.[33] Because barometric pressure is reduced progressively at high altitude, the P_{O_2} in the air is reduced. Alveolar and arterial hypoxia results. Several adapta-

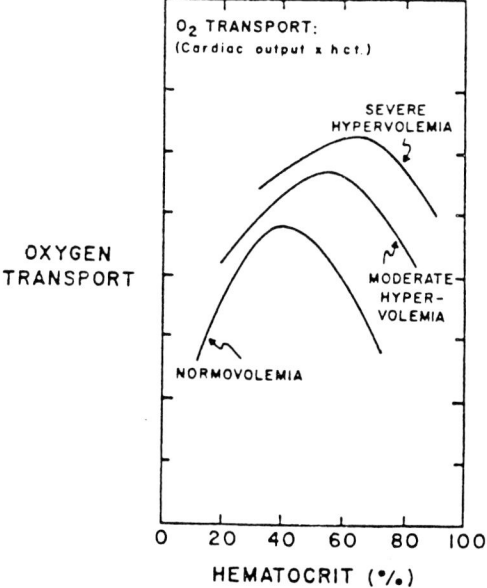

FIGURE 16–5. Calculated oxygen transport in dogs under normovolemic and hypervolemic conditions following red cell transfusions. *(Used with permission from Castle WB: The Polycythemia. In Beck WS (ed): Hematology. Cambridge, Mass, MIT Press, 5th ed. 1991, p 305.)*

tions occur at high altitude.[34,35] Chronic hypercapnia results from carotid and aortic chemoreceptor recognition of reduced Pa_{O_2}. Increased ventilation minimizes the oxygen gradient between atmospheric and alveolar air. The beneficial effect of increased ventilatory activity is counterbalanced by the metabolic cost. Chronic hyperventilation leads to an increased vital capacity due to a stretching effect on the lung.[36] An increased diffusing area results, and the A–a gradient is reduced, enhancing arterial oxygen tension.

Acute exposure to high altitude results in hyperventilation alkalosis, shifting the oxygen dissociation curve to the left, impairing oxygen release from hemoglobin, and causing tissue hypoxia.[37] Alkalosis and hypoxia promote red cell 2,3-DPG synthesis, shifting the curve to the right.[38] This rightward shift has been thought to be an important short-term benefit for unclimatized individuals,[39,40] but comparison of altitude adaptation between normal subjects and those with hemoglobins possessing high oxygen affinity demonstrates that the subjects with the abnormal hemoglobins have much better short-term physiologic responses to altitude.[41] High-altitude–dwelling llamas have left-shifted O_2 dissociation curves,[42] as do individuals with the high oxygen affinity hemoglobin Andrew-Minneapolis,[41] who appear to be better adapted to high altitude by virtue of their left-shifted O_2 dissociation curve. These findings suggest that the normal human response to altitude of a slightly decreased hemoglobin oxygen affinity is disadvantageous. In chronically acclimatized individuals, the O_2 dissociation curve is only slightly shifted to the right.

Although the llama does not develop erythrocytosis,[43] in humans, erythrocytosis is the most prominent physiologic adaptation to prolonged high-altitude living. Faura et al.[44] demonstrated markedly enhanced erythropoietin release in sea-level dwellers within 6 hours of exposure to high altitudes. Increased erythropoietin release in response to tissue hypoxia causes increased plasma iron turnover, reticulocytosis, and a gradual rise in the hematocrit.

Weil and colleagues[45] studied normal males who had lived in either Los Angeles (sea level), Denver (1600 m), or Leadville, Colorado (3100 m) for at least 2 years. Between sea level and 1600 m, the mean Pa_{O_2} fell from 85.6 to 69.0 mmHg. The percent-

age saturation of arterial hemoglobin with O_2 (Sa_{O_2}) fell only from 96.4 to 93.9 percent because of the minimal slope of the oxyhemoglobin dissociation curve in that range. The red cell mass, plasma volume, blood volume, and hematocrit were not significantly different at these altitudes. Between 1600 and 3100 m, the mean Pa_{O_2} fell by a similar amount, from 69.0 to 57.2 mmHg, but the steeper slope of the oxyhemoglobin dissociation curve resulted in a greater fall in Sa_{O_2} from 93.9 to 89.9 percent. The red cell mass, hematocrit, plasma volume, and blood volume were all significantly higher at this elevation. When individual values were examined, Pa_{O_2} values greater than 67 mmHg showed no significant relationship between Pa_{O_2} and red cell mass, while Pa_{O_2} values less than 67 mmHg showed a significant correlation with red cell mass (Fig. 16–6). This biphasic relationship between Pa_{O_2} and red cell mass contrasts with the linear relationship between Sa_{O_2} and red cell mass, as depicted in Fig. 16–7. Since 67 mmHg is on the shoulder of the oxyhemoglobin dissociation curve, changes in Pa_{O_2} above this level have little

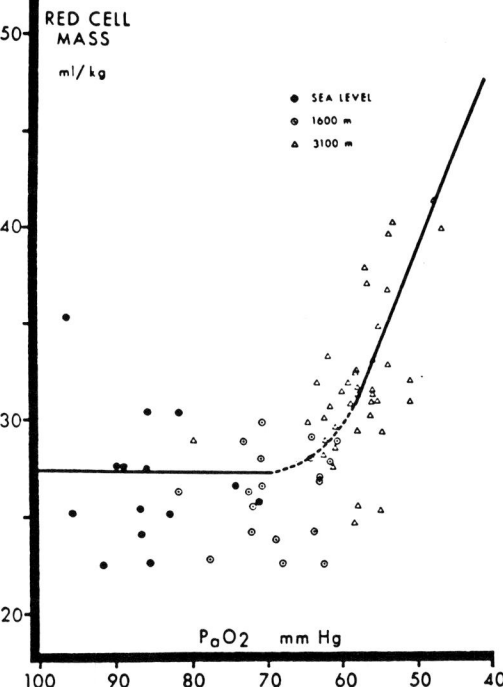

FIGURE 16–6. The relationship between red cell mass and PaO_2 in normal men residing at sea level and 1600 and 3100 m (● = sea level; ☉ = 1600 m; △ = 3100 m). (Reproduced from the *Journal of Clinical Investigation*, 1968, 47, 1627–1638 by Copyright permission of the American Society for Clinical Investigation.)

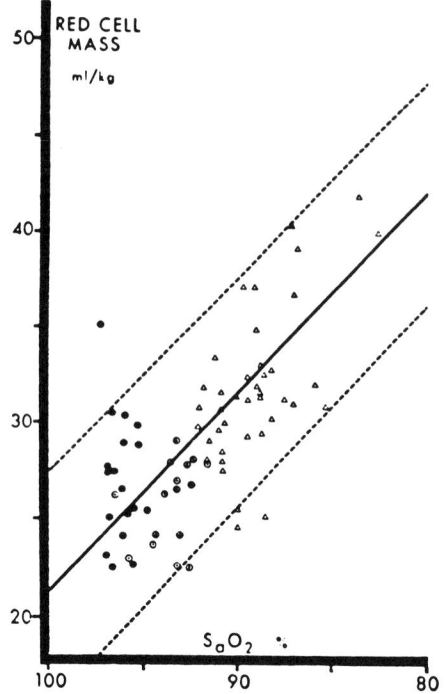

FIGURE 16-7. Red cell mass–SaO₂ relationship in normal men residing at sea level and 1600 and 3100 m. Broken lines represent 95 percent confidence limits on individual estimates. (Reproduced from the *Journal of Clinical Investigation*, 1968, 47, 1627–1638 by Copyright permission of the American Society for Clinical Investigation.)

impact on Sa_{O_2}. Below a Pa_{O_2} of 67 mmHg, Sa_{O_2} is more dramatically affected because of the steepness of the curve. The Pa_{O_2} appears to alter red cell mass only through its effect on Sa_{O_2}. The change in hematocrit associated with a decrease in Sa_{O_2} is consistently smaller than the change in red cell mass.[45–47] Since the hematocrit is the ratio of red cell volume to the sum of the red cell volume and plasma volume, a doubling of red cell mass with no change in plasma volume results in only a 33 percent rise in hematocrit.[45] The rise in hematocrit is lessened further if the plasma volume increases.

Many studies of Andean natives who dwell at altitudes in excess of 4200 m demonstrate about a 30 percent increase in hematocrit[44, 48–50] over sea-level dwellers. The increased O_2 carrying capacity of blood associated with this degree of polycythemia is negated at least in part by the detrimental effects of increased blood viscosity, increased peripheral resistance, decreased blood flow, and increased cardiac workload.[51–53] Many investigators have felt that these extreme de-

grees of erythrocytosis would be deleterious. Garruto and Dutt,[54] in reviewing earlier investigations, noted that these studies were largely performed on adult residents of recently established mining communities, where the incidence of chronic respiratory disorders was high. For example, a study of high-altitude Andean miners demonstrated increasing degrees of polycythemia with increased severity of silicosis.[50] Some studies included a high number of smokers as well. Garruto and Dutt[54] evaluated 303 male Quechua Indians with a mean age of 34.7 years (range 6 to 57 years) born and raised at a mean altitude of 4200 m who lived as traditional pastoralists and horticulturalists. The mean hematocrit for adult males was 51.4 percent, the mean hemoglobin concentration 17.3 g/dl, and the mean red blood cell concentration was $5.63 \times 10^6/mm^3$. These values contrast markedly with the previously described values for mining community residents. Between the ages 6 and 21 years, the hematocrit was 10 percent higher than in sea-level populations and increased with age in a pattern similar to sea-level rates. These values are similar to those reported in studies from nonmining communities in Peru[55] and Bolivia[56] and similar to Sherpa and Tibetan populations in the Himalayas.[57–59] Thus, supported by their belief that a 20 to 38 percent increase in hematocrit is not a beneficial adaptive mechanism, a number of investigators have presented evidence that the degree of adaptive polycythemia that exists in high-altitude residents is less than was once thought. When more dramatic polycythemia does occur, it may result from a combination of altitude and some form of pulmonary insufficiency. Such a response is pathologic rather than adaptive. These individuals are exemplified by a markedly obese patient with probable sleep hypoventilation, who at 2000 m had dramatic erythrocytosis and severe mountain sickness which resolved when she was placed at sea level.[60]

Chronic mountain sickness was described by Monge[61] as a pathologic decompensation in humans with prolonged high-altitude exposure. The manifestations of this disorder include headaches, fatigue, poor exercise tolerance, cyanosis, plethora, clubbing, and prominent signs of right ventricular failure in association with hematocrit and red cell mass values far in excess of those in acclimated individuals. Excessive erythrocytosis and high blood viscosity are important in the pathogenesis of this disorder. Tissue hypoxia may be aggravated by the excessive erythrocytosis perpetuating excessive red cell proliferation through increased erythropoietin release. Therapeutic phlebotomy may give symptomatic improvement, providing further evidence of the role of high red cell mass in the pathogenesis of this syndrome. Winslow[62] studied oxygen transport in high-altitude natives of the Andes. One individual had chronic mountain sickness with a hematocrit of 62 percent at 4250 m. This hematocrit is well outside the normal distribution of healthy natives (mean Hct 52 percent). With reduction of hematocrit to 42 percent and no change in total blood volume, the patient reported better sleep, better concentration at work, and fewer headaches. Cardiac output improved markedly at rest and with exercise. Reduced O_2 carrying capacity of blood following hemodilution appears to be balanced by increased cardiac output. Maximal work, as measured by bicycle ergometry, however, was not improved significantly.

While erythrocytosis contributes to many manifestations of altitude illness, other contributing factors are present. Acute exposure to high altitude with consequent hypoxia leads to pulmonary vasoconstriction, which, when sustained, leads to pulmonary hypertension.[63-67] In chronic hypoxia, morphologic changes occur in the pulmonary circulation, notably pulmonary arterial muscularization.[68-71]

An important distinction must be made between sojourners and natives of high altitude. While high hematocrits are observed in both situations, the etiology, effects on tissue O_2 delivery, and clinical consequences may vary considerably. Many of the physiologic studies performed on lowlanders exposed to high altitudes were performed on high-altitude climbers. Although increased hematocrit in these individuals is generally attributed to hypoxemia-induced erythropoiesis, this is probably not the principal explanation. Zink et al.[72] have demonstrated excessive water loss in high-altitude expeditioners. Most of this water is needed to humidify the cold inspired air and is lost in expiration. In a group of climbers in whom the mean hematocrit rose from 44 to 57 percent, the increasing hematocrit was associated with decreasing plasma volume. Furthermore, a significant fall in plasma volume occurs for less clear reasons in nonclimbers transported to high altitude. Sea-level dwellers transported to an altitude of 4500 m develop a 10 percent rise in hemoglobin concentration within 1 day due to a fall in plasma volume of uncertain cause.[73] Plasma volume in sea-level residents transported to high altitudes is reduced for 6 to 8 months and returns to normal by 1 year.[50] On the eve of his departure for the Andes, Viault found that his blood contained 5 million cells/mm³. After 15 days in the Andes, there were 7.1 million cells/mm³.[33] In retrospect, it seems likely that decreased plasma volume may have been largely responsible for this historic observation of an increased red cell concentration at high altitude.

True acclimation may require years of residence at high altitudes. Animal models demonstrate capillary proliferation and increased efficiency of O_2 utilization at high altitudes[74,75] similar to that which occurs with endurance training. Prolonged high-altitude exposure has been compared with endurance training. Distance runners who train at moderate altitudes have offered subjective evidence of its increased effectiveness. In this context, an elevated hematocrit could be beneficial to high-altitude climbers. High-altitude climbers with polycythemia due to decreased plasma volume, however, may not have the increased blood volume needed to overcome the detrimental effects of increased viscosity on blood flow. In acclimated individuals, increases in red cell mass are generally accompanied by increased plasma volume and markedly increased total blood volume, with venous return maximizing cardiac output.

In high-altitude climbers, however, with decreased plasma volume and total blood volume, maximal O_2 consumption is decreased, indicating reduced tissue O_2 extraction due to reduced flow.[76] Individuals from lowlands exposed to high altitudes are subject to deep venous thrombosis, pulmonary infarction, retinal hemorrhage, and frostbite, all of which may be caused in part by increased blood viscosity.[77] Cerebral venous thrombosis has recently been reported as a complication of polycythemia in a previously healthy young man climbing at high altitudes.[78] Hemodilution by intravenous infusion of isotonic solution is commonly employed by high-altitude mountain climbers.[79]

Although controlled studies are not available, Zink et al.[72] reported that on a Himilayan expedition, climbers with diluted blood were less symptomatic than other climbers.

Chronic Obstructive Pulmonary Disease (COPD)

Patients with COPD frequently suffer from arterial hypoxemia. The alveolar-arterial difference for P_{O_2} is increased in patients with obstructive lung disease. Large amounts of ventilation occur in gas exchange units with high ventilation-to-perfusion ratios (physiologic dead space) and are wasted. Large amounts of blood flow to gas exchange units with low $\dot{V}/\dot{Q}$ ratios (physiologic shunt) and account for severe hypoxemia.[9] Reduction of the Pa_{O_2} below 67 mmHg occurs as a result of marked impairment of lung mechanics, as evidenced by markedly reduced airflow rates during forced expiration.

The red cell mass is generally increased in hypoxemic COPD patients and correlates more closely with the level of Sa_{O_2} than does the hemoglobin and hematocrit,[80,81] which are less dramatically increased. Some individuals with COPD have markedly increased plasma volume, especially patients with cor pulmonale. Hematocrits above 65 percent in COPD are unusual,[81,82] but levels as high as 75 percent have been reported.[83] When compared with individuals with similar Sa_{O_2} values due to altitude hypoxia or cyanotic congenital cardiac disease, patients with COPD have lower levels of hemoglobin and hematocrit. The role of increased plasma volume has been questioned in some studies that have found variable mean plasma volumes[83–85] in patients with COPD.

Relatively low red cell mass values have been found in some studies of hypoxemic COPD patients.[86] Since many of these patients had infections or chronic inflammatory disorders with low plasma iron and low total iron-binding capacity, the variability of the erythropoietic response may be related to the effects of inflammation. Red cell life span may be decreased for unknown reasons in the majority of patients with COPD,[86,87] but this finding has been contested.[88] When Weil et al. compared patients with obstructive airway disease with patients at high altitudes, the former group demonstrated a steeper increase for red cell mass for a given Sa_{O_2}.

The measured Sa_{O_2}, however, may not be representative of the average Sa_{O_2}.

One difficulty in attempting to correlate red cell mass with the degree of hypoxemia is the variability of Sa_{O_2} in an individual. Posture is an important variable affecting Sa_{O_2}. Some patients with COPD develop decreased Sa_{O_2} during sleep.[89–91] During recumbency, portions of perfused lung are poorly ventilated, thus lowering Sa_{O_2}. Some patients also have sleep apnea or hypopnea, both of which decrease ventilation and Sa_{O_2}. Exercise is a second variable. Many severely hypoxemic patients develop a further fall in Pa_{O_2} with exercise. A third variable is exposure to carbon monoxide. Many studies have failed to recognize the potential additional influence of carbon monoxide on tissue hypoxia. A large number of patients with severe obstructive lung disease continue to smoke. Calculation of Sa_{O_2} from Pa_{O_2} values without realization that the patient has a significant level of carboxyhemoglobin underestimates the degree of hypoxemia present.

Some have suggested that a shift in the oxygen dissociation curve modulates the erythropoietin response to hypoxemia, but Lenfant et al.[92] found that patients with COPD-induced hypoxemia (mean Pa_{O_2} of 47.5 mmHg) demonstrated a positive correlation between P_{50} and hematocrit. Patients with high P_{50} values also had high hematocrits.[92] A similar correlation was not detected in high-altitude dwellers, sea-level natives transiently at high altitude, or patients with congenital cyanotic cardiac disease. The response of red cell 2,3-DPG to hypoxemia in COPD is less than that in altitude hypoxia or cyanotic heart disease. This has been attributed to the acidosis of COPD patients. The buffering capacity of deoxyhemoglobin reduces the degree of intraerythrocyte acidosis, permitting a modest increase in 2,3-DPG synthesis[93] due to hypoxemia. The combined effects of decreased blood pH, increased P_{CO_2}, and increased intraerythrocyte 2,3-DPG result in a rightward shift in the oxygen dissociation curve. The adaptive value of a rightward shift of the oxygen dissociation curve in patients with COPD and hypoxemia is questionable because of impaired O_2 loading in the pulmonary capillaries.

The effectiveness of increased red cell mass as an adaptation to hypoxemia in COPD is also unclear. Certainly, increased blood volume serves to increase cardiac output and tissue oxygen delivery, but factors in addition to a high hematocrit may increase viscosity. Acidosis and hypoxia both increase the rigidity of red cells. An increase in hematocrit from 45 to 65 percent at normal pH causes a twofold increase in viscosity at a low shear rate. In the presence of acidosis, a similar increase in hematocrit may increase viscosity fivefold.[94] Thus unique characteristics of the blood in COPD increase the viscosity to a greater extent than would occur with polycythemia alone.

Chronic O_2 therapy is beneficial in hypoxemic polycythemia patients with COPD.[95, 96] O_2 dilates pulmonary arterioles, decreasing pulmonary vascular resistance.[97] If used for 6 weeks, O_2 therapy reportedly reduces the hematocrit and blood viscosity, thus further decreasing pulmonary vascular resistance. These effects of O_2 therapy produce clinical improvements and a reduced incidence of cor pulmonale requiring hospitalization.[98]

Other studies have demonstrated only modest changes in hematocrit with chronic O_2 therapy. A clinical trial by the Nocturnal Oxygen Therapy Group randomly allocated patients with hypoxic chronic obstructive lung disease to either continuous oxygen therapy (most $\geq$ 19 h/d) or 12-hour noctural O_2 therapy for at least 12 months.[99] The hematocrit and pulmonary vascular resistance showed statistically significant changes dependent on treatment regimen. Hematocrit values fell more in patients on continuous O_2 and were significantly different at 12 and 18 months. At 18 months, the hematocrit fell an average of 9.2 percent in the continuous O_2 therapy group but only 2 percent from baseline in the nocturnal therapy group. Mortality in the nocturnal O_2 group was nearly twice that in the continuous O_2 group.

Phlebotomy is a more direct and rapid method of reducing red cell mass. Following phlebotomy and replacement of blood volume with dextran 40 to decrease mean hematocrit from 63 to 48 percent, Harrison et al.[100] demonstrated improved work capacity in individuals with COPD. Systemic O_2 delivery during exercise was maintained with increased cardiac output, diminished pulmonary arterial pressure, and decreased calculated pulmonary vascular resistance. These changes were attributed to decreased blood viscosity. No changes in arterial blood gases occurred, but the arteriovenous O_2 content difference was greater during exercise after phlebotomy. Increased tissue oxygen extraction was attributed to improved tissue capillary perfusion. This study suggests that impaired tissue perfusion limits work capacity in individuals with polycythemia secondary to COPD. Other studies have shown improvement in cerebral blood flow with reduction of packed cell volume.[101, 102] Wade and colleagues[102] reduced hematocrits from a mean of 61.3 to 49.5 percent by weekly venesection in 12 patients with polycythemia secondary to hypoxic lung disease. Reduced blood viscosity and increased cerebral blood flow resulted. A marked improvement in mental alertness occurred in four patients, and two others described resolution of headaches. Interestingly, cerebral blood flow in patients with hypoxic lung disease is higher than in patients with similarly elevated hematocrits but normal lung function, suggesting that cerebral vessels are dilated, perhaps related to hypercapnea.[102] Despite a marked reduction in apparent viscosity with phlebotomy, cerebral blood flow improved only modestly (average 21 percent) in Wade's study. Oxygen carriage did not generally improve because of the lowered hematocrit. The authors speculated that symptomatic improvement in the absence of improved O_2 carriage might result from the influence of other factors, e.g., pH or Pa_{CO_2}, on cerebral metabolism. Nevertheless, low cerebral blood flow may predispose to intravascular thrombosis in diseased vessels, and improving cerebral blood flow without improving O_2 carrying capacity may prevent strokes. Patients with PV have an increased incidence of cerebral infarction and other vascular occlusive episodes which is related to the level of the hematocrit.[103]

Evaluation of the value of lowering hematocrit in patients with COPD is complicated by the use of different techniques. Simple phlebotomy has been shown to be effective, but even a small reduction in blood volume may acutely decrease cardiac output, and fatalities have been reported.[104] Additionally, only relatively small quantities of blood can be removed safely on one occasion, and in some studies, an average of 7 weeks have been required to reduce the hematocrit to the normal range.[102] To avoid problems of reduced blood volume with simple venesection, colloids such as dextran 40 can be exchanged easily isovolumetrically for red cells.

Wedzicha and colleagues[105] used the technique of erythrophoresis (the removal of red cells using a cell separator) to reduce hematocrit in patients with polycythemia secondary to hypoxic lung disease. This technique was used because of the rapidity of reduction of hematocrit and the decreased risk of acute changes in blood volume. In four men, erythrophoresis reduced hematocrit from a mean of 64 to 48 percent and in six women from 56 to 41 percent. Significant reduction in blood viscosity at high and low shear rates was demonstrated. Although spirometric volumes and blood gases were not significantly different, distance walked in 6 minutes was improved after treatment in all patients. Tests of mental alertness similarly showed significant improvement. Significant subjective improvement in shortness of breath, sadness, and mood were noted within 24 hours. Two months after erythrophoresis, hematocrits remained within normal limits, and symptomatic benefit was maintained. The procedure was well tolerated by all patients, and no complications of the procedure were noted. A subsequent study by Wedzicha et al.[106] compared erythrophoresis with placebo apheresis, whereby venous blood circulated through the blood processor and then was reinfused into the patient with no red cell removal. Results demonstrated no significant placebo effect on exercise tolerance. Erythrophoresis is favored by some as a rapid and effective technique of reducing hematocrit and viscosity to normal in patients with polycythemia secondary to COPD. Advantages over multiple venesections include convenience with reduced hospital visits and safety with minimization of sudden changes in cardiac output due to replacement of red cells with equal volumes of isotonic fluid. Disadvantages include expense and availability of the necessary apparatus. While it is not practical for all patients with erythrocytosis secondary to lung disease to undergo erythrophoresis, erythrophoresis may be considered for patients who would require a prolonged period of venesection to reduce their red cell mass or for those in whom potentially adverse hemodynamic changes of phlebotomy might be exceptionally undesirable.[107]

Alveolar Hypoventilation

Periodic breathing and oxygen desaturation during sleep are not unique to COPD but occur in normal subjects as well.[108] The greater degree of desaturation in patients with severe lung disease reflects their lower baseline arterial oxygenation. Block et al.[108] used ear oximetry to monitor the oxygen saturation of 45 normal subjects in a sleep laboratory. Seventeen of 30 males but none of 19 females experienced episodes of oxygen desaturation (defined as a 4 percent fall in O_2 saturation) associated with hypopnea or apnea. Episodes of desaturation correlated significantly with increasing weight-to-height ratio. The more obese the person, the more likely he or she was to experience hypopnea, apnea, and oxygen desaturation. The maximum fall in O_2 saturation was 29 percent, to a saturation level of 68 percent. Four subjects experienced desaturation to levels of 72 percent or below. All were men who snored heavily and who weighed more than 90 kg. These findings are useful in understanding noctural desaturation in the syndrome of hypersomnolence with periodic breathing (the pickwickian syndrome). This syndrome is characterized by obesity, alveolar hypoventilation, hypersomnolence, and secondary polycythemia. A disturbance of ventilatory control characterized by depression of both hypoxic and hypercapnic ventilatory drives characterizes these patients. Marked obesity may lead to severe hypoxemia during sleep in some patients, and eventually, this hypoxemia may depress hypoxic ventilatory drive.[109] Weight loss clearly improves many patients. The four obese asymptomatic males in the study by Block et al. might, with increasing weight and the cumulative effect of years of oxygen desaturation with sleep, be potential pickwickians. The marked difference in sex distribution of desaturation during sleep has been attributed to the presence in women of progesterone, a respiratory stimulant. Progestational agents have been beneficial in the treatment of some patients with the pickwickian syndrome.[110,111] Substantial improvements in hypoxia and hypercapnia with reduction of polycythemia and improvement of cor pulmonale have resulted. Disordered breathing during sleep has been reported in patients with altitude sickness with polycythemia,[112] who may have a blunted hypoxemic ventilatory response as an adaptation to altitude and later respiratory center desensitization to carotid body output leading to hypercapnia.[60] Excessive polycythemia of high altitude has been reversed by progesterone treatment.[113]

Erythrocytosis Secondary to Cardiovascular Disease

The red cell mass in congenital heart diseases with a right-to-left shunt increases linearly as resting Sa_{O_2} falls.[114] The red cell mass may exceed 100 ml/kg, and the hematocrit may reach 85 percent. The plasma volume generally diminishes with increasing hematocrit. Patients usually do not exhibit symptoms of high viscosity, but thrombosis in the lungs, central nervous system, and kidneys and bleeding problems can occur and are sometimes precipitated by dehydration.[115,116] Lethargy, headaches, fatigue, and difficulty concentrating are common. A recent report described myocardial infarction in two patients with erythrocytosis and cyanotic heart disease.[117] One patient had a hematocrit of 75 percent; the other, 80 percent. Thrombotic occlusion of a coronary artery with myocardial infarction and death had been described previously in a young man with undiagnosed tetralogy of Fallot.[118] Myocardial oxygen demand may be increased in these patients because of the congenital defects and the hypervolemia caused by secondary erythrocytosis. O_2 supply is reduced because of the markedly increased viscosity of blood, especially when the hematocrit exceeds 60 percent. Erythrophoresis in the two patients presenting with myocardial infarctions lowered hematocrit and promptly terminated chest pain. Periodic erythrophoresis was performed to maintain hematocrits at levels close to 60 percent, and both patients remained well during more than 3 years of follow-up. Judicious lowering of the hematocrit appears to be indicated in circumstances where viscosity problems develop. Normalization of the hematocrit has not been attempted commonly, and reduction to the 55 to 60 percent range is generally advocated. Erythrophoresis or phlebotomy with replacement of volume with plasma expanders for acute blood volume reduction is generally preferable to venesection alone, although careful venesection may be employed. Reduction of erythrocytosis also has been carried out in patients with right-to-left shunts, who did not have acute symptoms. Oldershaw and Sutton[119] reduced hematocrits from a mean of 66 to 58 percent with venesection and isovolumic infusion of plasma. The mean hematocrit value remained at 58 percent for 14 days after venesection. Cardiac output and peripheral oxygen uptake were both significantly increased during exercise in these patients.[119] Using phlebotomy with isovolumic replacement with plasma or 5 percent albumin, Rosenthal et al.[120] demonstrated markedly increased cardiac output and systemic oxygen transport when polycythemic patients with congenital cyanotic heart disease had hematocrits reduced from a mean of 73.5 to 62 percent. The improvement was attributed to decreased blood viscosity and vascular resistance. The authors emphasized the importance of maintaining hypervolemia. As in the other hypoxemic states, the "optimal" level of hematocrit and red cell mass has not been well defined. Clearly, where possible, surgical correction is the treatment of choice. Erythrocytosis will abate in individuals following surgical correction of the defect responsible for hypoxemia.

Some patients with cirrhosis have cyanosis and polycythemia due to pulmonary arteriovenous anastomoses[121] or vascular communication between portal and pulmonary veins.[122] In both circumstances, right-to-left shunting causes hypoxemia, which leads to erythrocytosis.

Hemoglobin Abnormalities

Erythrocytosis due to defects in oxygen transport by hemoglobin occurs in a variety of disorders, including high-oxygen-affinity hemoglobinopathies and congenitally decreased red cell 2,3-DPG. These conditions are discussed in Chap. 3. Chronic exposure to carbon monoxide (CO) from smoking or from environmental pollutants is also an important cause of polycythemia due to defective oxygen transport.

Under physiologic conditions, CO binds to hemoglobin with an affinity more than 200 times that of oxygen.[123] When CO binds to a single heme group of a hemoglobin molecule, the O_2 affinity of the remaining heme groups is markedly increased. Because of the influence of CO on the unbound heme groups on the tetramer, an individual with 50 percent carboxyhemoglobinemia is more hypoxic than one with a 50 percent reduction in hemoglobin.

Carbon monoxide is generated by incomplete combustion. Excessive exposure is common and can occur in a variety of settings, most commonly with exposure to industrial wastes or automobile exhaust and with smoking. CO is absorbed across the alveolar membrane as a function of the partial pressure of CO in alveolar air, the diffusing capacity, the rate of ventilation, and the match between perfusion and ventilation. Absorbed CO is almost totally bound to hemoglobin.

The effect of smoking on tissue oxygen supply was studied by Sagone and colleagues[124] in 1973. Previous reports of increased hematocrits in smokers[125, 126] had been published, but red cell mass had not been studied. Morning (the minimum) levels of carboxyhemoglobin were between 4 and 6.8 percent in eight individuals smoking one to two packs of cigarettes per day and 9.2 percent in an individual smoking two to three packs per day. Individuals smoking more than one pack of cigarettes per day had an increased red cell mass and elevated hematocrit. Normal blood gases in the three patients with the highest red cell masses excluded hypoxic pulmonary disease as the cause of erythrocytosis. Subsequently, Sagone and Balcerzak[127] identified five smokers with red cell masses between 39 and 47 ml/kg of body weight. Two of the five patients stopped smoking with return of their hematocrits and red cell masses to normal within 3 months.

Smith and Landow[128] more recently studied 22 polycythemic patients who had elevated carboxyhemoglobin levels and no demonstrable cause for their polycythemia except smoking. Several carboxyhemoglobin levels of 20 percent or more were documented. These higher levels were generally in inhaling cigar smokers or cigarette smokers who used three to four packs daily. The decrease in the P_{50} in patients with 15 to 20 percent carboxyhemoglobin was of a similar magnitude to that of some abnormal hemoglobins having increased O_2 affinity. Reduced plasma volume in the majority of patients was an additional contributor to elevated hematocrit. The CO yield of unventilated filter cigarettes is 25 percent higher than that of plain cigarettes. Other factors that significantly affect the CO-hemoglobin levels in smokers include the pattern of smoking (higher peak levels when more cigarettes are smoked in a short period) and the level of physical activity (shorter half-life of CO-hemoglobin with increased activity).[129]

Increased hematocrit values have been estimated to occur in 3 percent of all cigarette smokers.

Since the Sa_{O_2} is calculated from the measured Pa_{O_2} and the standard oxyhemoglobin dissociation curve in most clinical laboratories, the decreased O_2 carrying capacity of blood in smokers is not detected by standard techniques. The investigation of erythrocytosis in smokers requires direct measurement of arterial oxygen saturation. Alternatively, carboxyhemoglobin can be measured. Using these techniques, the Sa_{O_2} can be demonstrated to be decreased. This decrease in Sa_{O_2} and the effect of CO on the oxygen dissociation curve combine to increase red cell mass in smokers.

Carboxyhemoglobinemia with secondary erythrocytosis also occurs in nonsmokers exposed to carbon monoxide from a variety of sources, most commonly automobile and airplane exhaust or industrial processes such as printing and welding. Highway toll booth workers, miners, and welders are prone to CO exposure due to high concentrations of CO in inhaled air. Since the half-life of carboxyhemoglobin is nearly 4 hours at rest, high CO levels are maintained in these individuals long after they leave the area of high CO concentration. Individuals with chronic carboxyhemoglobinemia may have neuropsychiatric dysfunction and cardiac toxicity.

Two patients with smoker's polycythemia who had cerebral thrombosis as the initial manifestation of their disorder were reported recently.[130] Both patients were young (42 and 45) and had high hematocrits (68 and 59 percent), high red cell mass (58.8 and 53.8 ml/kg), and high carboxyhemoglobin levels (12.2 and 16 percent). Both patients were phlebotomized to maintain hematocrits below 55 percent and experienced no further thrombotic complications. Patients with COPD or other hypoxic states are especially susceptible to the effects of chronically elevated CO levels. Figure 16–8 demonstrates the mechanism responsible for exaggerated reduction of arterial P_{O_2} in patients with pulmonary disease and carboxyhemoglobinemia. When ventilation and perfusion are badly mismatched, as in patients with COPD, the oxygen gradient between alveoli and systemic arteries is widened by elevated CO-hemoglobin. O_2 from fully ventilated and perfused alveolar vessels is transferred to partially unsaturated CO-hemoglobin in

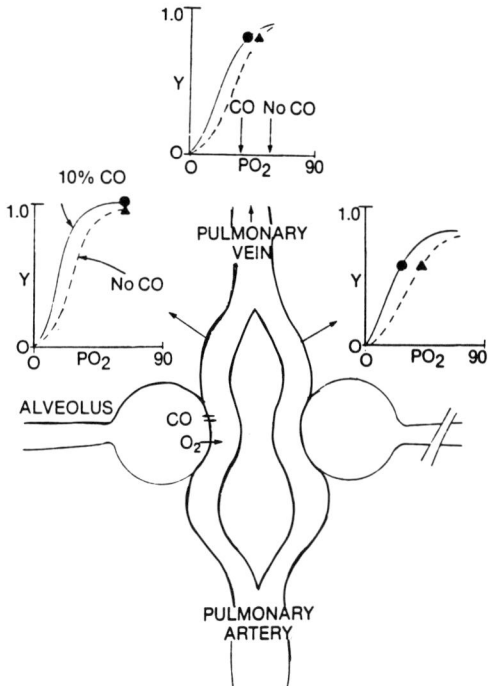

FIGURE 16–8. The mechanism of dramatic reduction of PaO$_2$ in patients with carboxyhemoglobinemia and $\dot{V}/\dot{Q}$ mismatch. The alveolus on the left is ventilated and perfused. The alveolus on the right is perfused but not ventilated. Patients with 10 percent HbCO (——) have a significantly lower arterial PO$_2$ compared with those with minimal HbCO (----). *(Used with permission from Bunn HF, Forget BG: Carboxyhemoglobin and carboxyhemoglobinemia. In Hemoglobin: Molecular, Genetic and Clinical Aspects. Cambridge, Saunders 1986, Chap 17, pp 663–675.)*

shunted blood when they admix and is, therefore, less readily available at the tissue level. The combination of chronic lung disease and CO exposure markedly compromises exercise tolerance.[123] Together they are also potent inducers of erythrocytosis.

INAPPROPRIATE ERYTHROCYTOSIS

Since the demonstration that erythropoietin production is nearly abolished in bilaterally nephrectomized rats,[131] abundant evidence has accumulated that the kidney is the chief source of erythropoietin. In the just-described syndromes associated with secondary erythrocytosis, erythropoietin production in the kidney is signaled by the renal O$_2$ sensor, which accurately senses systemic hypoxia. In some circumstances, however, localized renal ischemia occurs in the absence

of systemic hypoxia yet stimulates erythropoietin secretion and erythrocytosis. The erythropoietin response is thus inappropriate for systemic oxygen requirements.

Erythrocytosis Secondary to Renal Ischemia

Patients with arteriosclerotic narrowing of the renal arteries who developed secondary erythrocytosis have been reported.[132, 133] Patients with hypertension with renal artery disease have a higher incidence of erythrocytosis than similarly hypertensive patients without renal artery disease.[134] Nevertheless, the incidence of erythrocytosis in vascular disease of the kidney is low. Secondary erythrocytosis following renal transplantation is of special interest. Posttransplant erythrocytosis has occurred in association with renal artery stenosis[135, 136] and with acute and chronic rejection[137–140] of transplanted kidneys and has been thought by some to indicate impending rejection. Narrowing and occlusion of small renal arteries that develop as part rejection have been proposed to cause ischemia and increased erythropoietin production.

Clearly, however, erythrocytosis may occur in transplanted patients with no vascular compromise. In some patients, increased production of erythropoietin by native kidneys has been reported,[141–143] and erythrocytosis has resolved following removal of native kidneys.[141] In all, 5 to 13.5 percent of renal allograft recipients develop erythrocytosis. Many of these patients, however, have not been documented to have elevated red cell mass. Decreased plasma volume secondary to diuretic use or alterations in water and sodium handling in the posttransplant period may contribute to the elevated hematocrits in some transplanted patients.[144]

Lamperi and Carozzi[145] reported a progressive rise in hemoglobin and hematocrit despite diminution of serum erythropoietin levels in six transplanted patients. In vitro burst forming units-erythroid (BFU-E) cultures from these individuals demonstrated increased erythropoietin sensitivity and the capacity to grow in the absence of erythropoietin.[145, 146]

Thrombotic events, including stroke, deep vein thrombosis, and pulmonary embolism, have been reported in transplanted patients with high hematocrits. These have occurred in patients with elevated red cell mass as well as in patients with elevated hematocrits with normal red cell mass and decreased plasma volume.[144] Measurement of both red cell mass and plasma volume in posttransplant patients with high hematocrits is useful to better define the contributing factors. In situations of elevated red cell mass, measurement of erythropoietin may help to determine whether erythrocytosis is a result of erythropoietin production from transplanted or native kidneys or whether red cell proliferation and maturation occur relatively independently of erythropoietin.

Erythrocytosis Due to Benign Renal Lesions

The mechanism by which a variety of renal lesions such as hydronephrosis and cysts provoke erythrocytosis is not clear. Angiographic studies in rabbits show decreased renal blood flow within 24 hours of ureteral ligation.[147] Intraparenchymal and intrapelvic pressure in hydronephrosis results in compromised blood flow by compressive and vasoconstriction mechanisms (Fig. 16–9). When renal blood flow is reduced suffi-

ciently to cause ischemia, erythropoietin production is stimulated.[148] The initial burst of erythropoietin production in experimental hydronephrosis in animals is shortly interrupted by parenchymal destruction, and thus this process is self-limiting.[148, 149] Similarly, high-pressure hydronephrosis in animals is not associated with erythrocytosis, most likely because of rapidly progressive renal atrophy.[150] Backpressure must stimulate erythropoietin before advanced renal atrophy develops in order to expand red cell mass. The degree of renal parenchymal destruction and erythropoietin production do not appear to absolutely correlate. In experimental animals, normal erythropoiesis occurs despite destruction of 80 percent of renal tissue.[151] In 12 cases of erythrocytosis accompanied by unilateral hydronephrosis, elevated serum erythropoietin levels and erythrocytosis resolved after resolution of hydronephrosis, usually by nephrectomy.[148] Preoperative hematocrit ranged from 57 to 71 percent (mean 64.5 percent). Postoperatively, hematocrits fell to a mean of 45 percent.

Erythrocytosis also has been described in patients with solitary renal cysts and polycys-

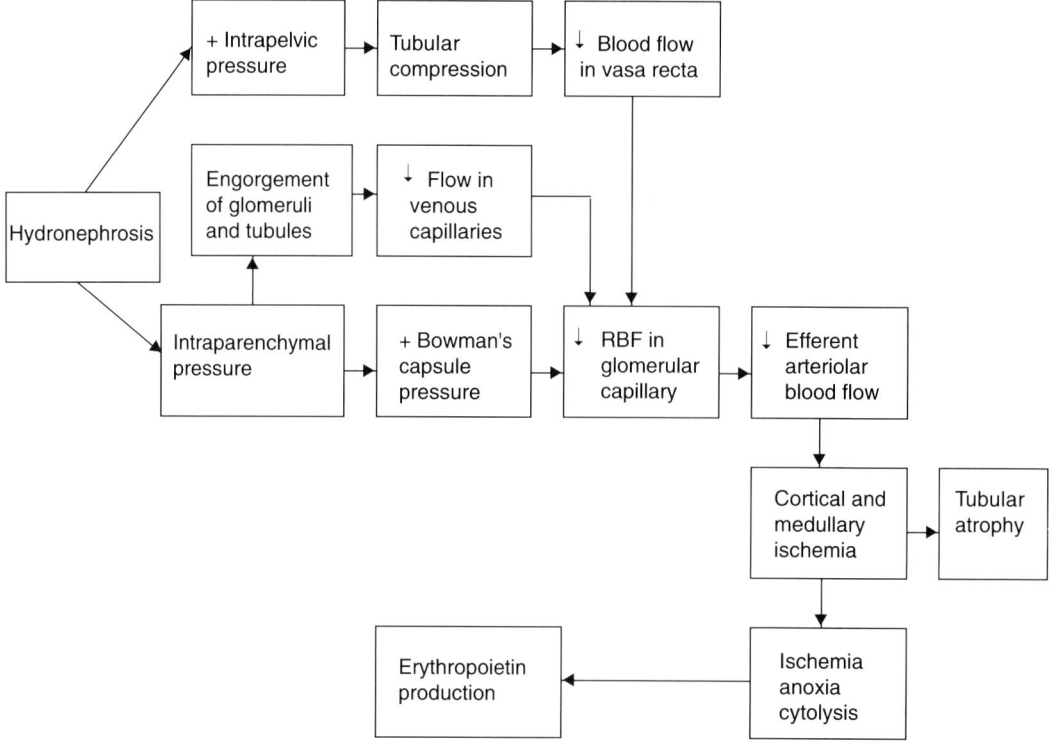

FIGURE 16–9. The mechanism of erythropoietin production in hydronephrosis. (*Used with permission from Hirsch I, Leiter E: Urology 21:345–350, 1983.*)

tic renal disease. Although erythropoietin has been detected in renal cysts from erythrocytotic individuals, similar concentrations have been found in cyst fluid from patients without erythrocytosis.[152–154] Whether the cysts make erythropoietin or whether the erythropoietin found in cysts is responsible for erythrocytosis is unclear. Decompression of a renal cyst without removal of the cyst wall decreased the red cell mass in one individual.[155] Most likely cysts cause increased red cell mass by a mechanism similar to hydronephrosis, with intrarenal pressure causing tissue hypoxia that triggers erythropoietin production.[156] Patients with polycystic renal disease generally have significant renal injury that reduces the mass of erythropoietin-producing tissue. Patients with polycystic disease have higher hematocrits than would be expected for their degree of uremia.[157]

Polycythemia has been observed infrequently with diffuse renal parenchymal lesions, including chronic glomerulonephritis, nephrosclerosis, and pyelonephritis.[158] Expansion of red cell mass in these disorders often occurs concomitantly with elevation of plasma volume. Reliance on the hematocrit alone may underestimate the incidence of polycythemia. Increased intrarenal pressure seems unlikely in these disorders. Functional glomerular ischemia due to capillary basement membrane thickening causing increased erythropoietin activity has been proposed as a mechanism. Experimental nephritis in rabbits results in capillary basement membrane thickening and erythrocytosis in some, although erythropoietin levels were not measured.[159] Red cell mass elevation in patients with diffuse parenchymal renal lesions is generally moderate. The hematocrit almost always remains less than 60 percent because of the relatively modest increase in red cell mass (perhaps related to decreased functional renal parenchyma) and concomitant increases in plasma volume. Secondary polycythemia accompanying increased erythropoietin levels also has been reported in Bartter's syndrome and in juxtaglomerular apparatus hyperplasia.[160,161]

Polycythemia Secondary to Tumors

Renal Carcinoma

Secondary polycythemia has been reported in association with many neoplasms, but tumors of the kidney account for more than a third. Polycythemia occurs in more than 1 percent of patients with hypernephromas.[162] Erythropoietin production has been demonstrated in cultures of human renal carcinoma cells.[163–166] The erythropoietin detected in the medium of a renal carcinoma cell culture was found to be immunologically similar to that of highly purified human urinary erythropoietin.[167] When a renal tumor from a patient with polycythemia and hypernephroma was transplanted into nude mice, the mice became polycythemic and demonstrated elevated serum erythropoietin levels.[168] When mRNA was extracted from renal tumor cells and microinjected into oocytes, translated products had a molecular weight identical to erythropoietin and stimulated erythropoiesis;[169] indicating that hypernephroma cells can produce erythropoietin. Disappearance of erythrocytosis and decreased erythropoietin levels after resection of tumor occur commonly in patients with renal carcinoma.[170,171] Erythrocytosis may again develop in patients who have metastatic recurrence.[154]

Cerebellar Hemangioblastoma

Cerebellar hemangioblastomas are associated with erythrocytosis in 9 to 20 percent of patients.[172–174] Erythrocytosis probably occurs as a result of increased erythropoietin production by this tumor,[174] and erythrocytosis disappears after tumor removal.[173] Alternative explanations of the mechanism of erythrocytosis with cerebellar hemangiomas have included neurogenic hypoventilation due to tumor injury of the nearby respiratory center, but arterial blood gas studies have been normal where studied.

Hepatoma

Hepatomas are associated with erythrocytosis in up to 10 percent of patients.[175,176] A number of mechanisms, including defective catabolism of erythropoietin[177] and local liver anoxia[178] with stimulation of hepatic erythropoietin production, have been proposed. The demonstration that a hepatocellular carcinoma transplanted into nude mice evokes erythrocytosis and that media from cultures of the transplanted tumor have high erythropoietic activity indicates that the tumor cells produce erythropoietic stimulatory activity.[179]

Uterine Fibroma

Uterine fibromas, especially when very large, have been associated with polycythemia. Production of erythropoietin by the tumor has been demonstrated.[180,181] Removal of the tumor has resulted in resolution of the polycythemia.[182] Leiomyomas of the esophagus[183] and the skin[184,185] have similarly been associated with secondary erythrocytosis, with the smooth-muscle cell the most likely source of excess erythropoietin production in these tumors.

Other Tumors

Several additional tumors have been described in association with erythrocytosis. Patients with pheochromocytomas and aldosterone-producing adenomas with erythrocytosis and elevated erythropoietin titers have been reported.[186,187] Both polycythemia and erythropoietin normalized when these tumors were excised. The mechanism of erythrocytosis is not clear, although a number of mechanisms, including compromised renal vascular supply and secretion of erythropoietin by the tumor, have been suggested.

Certain tumors produce erythropoietin-stimulating substances distinct from erythropoietin. Adrenal cortical tumors and virilizing ovarian tumors may produce androgens, which have erythropoietic effects.[188] Androgens increase erythropoiesis by direct stimulation of marrow stem cells and by increasing production of erythropoietin. Erythropoietin due to excess androgens may result not only from tumors but also from therapeutic administration, as in treatment of refractory anemia, where the red cell response occasionally "overshoots" into the polycythemic range.[2]

Erythrocytosis Achieved Through Autologous Blood Transfusions

Erythrocytosis achieved through blood transfusions (usually autologous), commonly referred to as "blood doping," is of interest because of physiologic consideration as well as the increasing use of this procedure by endurance athletes. Evidence that the optimal hematocrit for O_2 delivery is approximately 45 percent is derived largely from studies of resting anesthetized animals.[189,190]

In these animals, anemia or polycythemia resulted in a fall in O_2 transport (i.e., cardiac output × oxygen content). The application of these determinations to exercising athletes is of questionable value.

At rest, the volume of oxygen necessary to meet the body's metabolic requirement is between 150 and 250 ml/min. The maximally exercising, well-trained athlete may require more than 3 liters/min. A number of adjustments occur with physical conditioning, some of which maximize O_2 delivery. Maximal cardiac output improves substantially. Vascular proliferation in active tissues occurs, and the diversion of blood to active muscles makes maximal use of cardiac output. In addition, it has been suggested that endurance-trained individuals may have decreased plasma viscosity at rest and with exercise related to lower fibrinogen levels compared with normal controls.[191] A recent carefully performed study failed to confirm this observation.[192] The study found no differences in plasma viscosity with aerobic conditioning. It demonstrated substantial increases in whole-blood viscosity due to loss of plasma volume and hemoconcentration with strenuous exercise which was not influenced by endurance training.

Aerobic work capacity depends on the amount of O_2 transported to tissue. Increased maximal cardiac output augments O_2 delivery and substantially improves aerobic capacity. Increased O_2 content of blood could potentially result in more O_2 for tissue use and more aerobic capacity. Infusion of packed red cells to accomplish this has been performed. Many studies of red cell reinfusion have been flawed by failure to achieve substantial increase in hemoglobin concentration for various reasons and defects in experimental design. Buick and colleagues[193] reinfused 900 ml of autologous frozen red cells 6 weeks after removal in 11 well-trained runners. Mean hemoglobin increased from 15.1 to 16.3 g. Maximum O_2 consumption and running time to exhaustion were significantly increased posttransfusion. Thus an increase in the concentration of hemoglobin resulted in improved aerobic performance of highly conditioned runners.

These are several reasons why erythrocytosis might not be disadvantageous during exercise. Muscle pumping improves venous return and may overcome the effects of increased viscosity. Vasodilation in exercising muscle may improve flow despite increased viscosity. Increased flow associated with exercise minimizes the effects of viscosity. Conscious, chronically instrumented dogs trained to run on a treadmill were studied before and after their hematocrit was increased by isovolumic exchange transfusion with packed red cells. While cardiac output fell linearly as hematocrit was increased to 65 percent, increasing arterial O_2 content resulted in constant systemic oxygen transport.[194] Previous investigations had demonstrated minimal effects of elevation of hematocrit on in vivo viscosity in a vasodilated vascular bed in exercising muscle.[195]

It appears that the optimal hematocrit for the exercising, well-trained athlete may be higher than 45 percent. In Buick's exercising, transfused patients, a hematocrit of 49 percent improved performance. Whether higher hematocrits would be better or whether the increased viscosity would outweigh potential benefits is not clear. It must be appreciated, though, that the unique features of superbly trained, intensely exercising athletes make conclusions from these studies unique to this population.

DIAGNOSIS

When repeated hematocrit levels exceed 52 percent in males and 47 percent in females, red cell mass and plasma volume should be measured. The diagnosis of secondary erythrocytosis requires documentation of an increased red cell mass using ^{51}Cr as a red cell label. If red cell mass is normal but plasma volume is reduced, relative polycythemia exists. If red cell mass is elevated (≥ 36 ml/kg in men, ≥ 32 ml/kg in women), absolute polycythemia is present. The diagnosis of PV is discussed in detail elsewhere in this book. The secondary polycythemias generally lack the distinguishing features of PV, such as splenomegaly, leukocytosis, and thrombocytosis. If the criteria for PV are not met, secondary polycythemia should be suspected.

In evaluating the etiology of secondary erythrocytosis, an organized approach must be taken. Polycythemia associated with arterial hypoxia (due to altitude, pulmonary disease, heart disease, or hypoventilation) occurs only when the Pa_{O_2} is less than 67 mmHg. Significant increase in red cell mass occurs only when the arterial oxygen saturation is less than 92 percent. As discussed previously, O_2 saturation may vary with time of day and position, and multiple measurements, including during sleep, may be required. In smokers or those with occupational exposure to carbon monoxide, the carboxyhemoglobin level is valuable. The Sa_{O_2} must be measured directly and not calculated from the Pa_{O_2}. Also, because the half-life of carboxyhemoglobin is about 4 hours, an individual removed from CO exposure for a prolonged period may have a low carboxyhemoglobin level. A normal Pa_{O_2} and Sa_{O_2} does not exclude tissue hypoxia, since a hemoglobin with increased O_2 affinity is not excluded without measurement of the oxyhemoglobin dissociation curve, as discussed by Adamson. Where systemic hypoxia is excluded, local renal hypoxia from an impaired vascular supply or the presence of renal cysts or hydronephrosis can be evaluated with radiographic studies. When an etiology is not defined easily, the measurement of erythropoietin is helpful. Except for rare adrenal and ovarian tumors, serum erythropoietin is elevated in secondary polycythemia.

TREATMENT

The development of secondary erythrocytosis in response to the stimulus of tissue hypoxia is probably beneficial to many individuals. Expansion of the red cell mass may partially or totally restore tissue oxygen supply to a normal level. Studies of hypertransfused animals demonstrate that modest increases in hematocrit, when accompanied by expansion of blood volume, maximize O_2 tension in subcutaneous and intraperitoneal air pockets.[196] Oxygen transport is compromised with elevation of the hematocrit above 60 to 65 percent depending on the degree of hypervolemia. Determination of blood viscosity and determinations of blood flow have generally supported optimal hematocrits in a lower range. Why the red cell mass expands beyond an optimal level has been a crucial issue. One model proposes that if a rise in red cell mass in response to tissue hypoxia does not restore tissue O_2 supply to normal, erythropoietin secretion remains elevated. The subsequent continued rise in hematocrit and viscosity further impairs tissue oxygen delivery and leads to greater secretion of erythropoietin and higher hematocrits. This positive-feedback loop may play an important role in some individuals with extreme and harmful degrees of erythrocytosis. Such a system, however, should provide a continuously expanding red cell mass. In most individuals at high altitude or with hypoxic pulmonary disease, hematocrits remain reasonably stable. Erythropoietin production may not increase in response to the tissue hypoxia that accompanies extreme elevation of the hematocrit. Studies of mice and of individuals with PV suggest that hematocrits of 75 to 80 percent are not accompanied by stimulation of erythropoietin production despite evidence of tissue hypoxia.[5] Increased viscosity and decreased blood flow in the kidney probably do not dramatically affect oxygen tension in the kidney due to the proportional decrease in glomerular filtration rate and work by the kidney. Thus the relative insensitivity of the kidney to moderate reductions in blood flow may prevent the positive-feedback loop of progressive expansion of the red cell mass in most individuals with secondary polycythemia. Still, it is clear that many patients have degrees of red cell mass expansion that are not optimal.

Patients with extreme degrees of secondary polycythemia often have impaired alertness, dizziness, headaches, and compromised exercise tolerance. They may be at increased risk of thrombotic events, including strokes, myocardial infarction, and deep vein thrombosis. The role of the underlying disease, the level of the hematocrit, and the plasma volume are each of importance, yet it is usually difficult to define the specific role of each in causing symptoms or in placing the patient at risk. Measures used to treat the underlying problem clearly are most important, and these measures often correct the polycythemia through correction of the physiologic stimulus for red cell production. Patients with severe COPD should be treated with O_2 therapy. Patients with obesity-hypoventilation will benefit from weight loss. Individuals with high carboxyhemoglobin levels should be encouraged to stop smoking or be removed from industrial exposure to CO. Patients with right-to-left shunt who can have surgical correction will similarly correct their polycythemia.

Two questions of clinical importance in the treatment of secondary polycythemia are

1. Which patients, if any, with secondary polycythemia will benefit from reduction of hematocrit?
2. How should the hematocrit be lowered?

Neither question can be answered adequately from available data. In fact, there are no accepted criteria for hematocrit reduction in secondary polycythemia. Certain guidelines, however, can be inferred. Patients with COPD and hematocrits in excess of 60 percent clearly improve subjectively and in work capacity when the hematocrit is reduced to about 50 percent.[100, 116] Whether further reduction of hematocrit is beneficial is not clear. Some patients with hematocrits between 50 and 60 percent appear to improve symptomatically and objectively with hematocrit reduction, but improvement is not as consistent, and the decision to reduce hematocrit should depend on the individual's clinical status. Patients with erythrocytosis due to residence at high altitude should be treated in the presence of the symptoms of high-altitude illness or other clinical problems.

In patients with cyanotic congenital heart disease, careful reduction of hematocrit to approximately 55 percent probably benefits the majority, especially if hypervolemia is maintained. In patients with chronic carboxyhemoglobinemia due to smoking, the best treatment is cessation of smoking, which, depending on the degree of pulmonary disease, may result in the return of the red cell mass to normal. For patients who continue to smoke, the hematocrit should be reduced to 50 percent. The decision to lower the hematocrit in an individual must depend on careful clinical evaluation of that individual. Clearly, even in individuals with similar etiologies for secondary polycythemia, optimal hematocrits will vary depending on symptoms attributable to polycythemia, level of activity, complicating illnesses, and other factors. Since tissue tension of oxygen varies from organ to organ despite the common source of oxygenated blood,[5] compromised function of a specific organ may require attempts to optimize hematocrit for that organ. When polycythemia occurs as a result of a physiologic stimulus and potentially improves O_2 carrying capacity, decisions are more difficult than when polycythemia is "inappropriate." In the latter situation it is clear that the polycythemia has no benefit, and the hematocrit should be maintained in the normal range. Potential benefits of lowering hematocrit in polycythemic individuals include improved cerebral blood flow and resolution of CNS symptoms, improved exercise ability, and perhaps prevention of strokes and myocardial infarction in certain individuals.

The technique by which the hematocrit is lowered must be considered in each individual. Simple phlebotomy of 200 to 500 ml of blood can be performed simply and safely up to three times weekly until the desired hematocrit is obtained. In most individuals, this simple and inexpensive technique is efficient and safe and should be used. Reports of sudden death, including a case of fatal pulmonary thrombosis, have led to phlebotomy with volume replacement, called *manual exchange transfusion*. Red cell mass is measured, and the volume to be removed to reduce the red cell mass to the desired value is calculated. As blood is removed from one arm, half the volume of removed blood is replaced during phlebotomy in the other arm using dextran 40 or 5 percent dextrose. The identical volume of dextran is infused over the next 8 to 12 hours.[116] The hypertonic dextran draws approximately an equal volume of fluid from the extravascular space into the intravascular space. This technique reportedly allows removal of up to 3 liters of blood at once. Anaphylactic reactions to dextran can occur. Plasma is an alternative solution. This technique avoids the precipitous fall in cardiac output that follows phlebotomy alone and is generally effective and safe. However, when large amounts of blood are removed, the procedure is cumbersome and time-consuming.

Cell separator devices permit large-volume isovolumetric exchange without difficulty. In acute, potentially lethal situations, such as myocardial infarction in a patient with congenital cyanotic cardiac disease and polycythemia, automated erythrophoresis offers an effective, rapid method of reducing hematocrit. In individuals with precarious cardiac disease, it should be considered as an alternative to manual exchange transfusion. The perception that phoresis procedures are virtually risk-free is not accurate, and in most situations, the expense and risks are not justified. Thrombosis, stroke, gangrene, and fatal perforation of the heart have occurred following intravascular catheterization. Hypo- and hypervolemia, cardiac arrhythmia, and anaphylactic reaction to replacement fluids have occurred. The overall mortality of a phoresis procedure has been estimated at 3 per 10,000 procedures.[197]

In patients treated with repeated phlebotomies, iron deficiency may be induced. It has been suggested that polycythemic patients whose symptoms resolve following phlebotomies may develop identical symptoms at lower hemoglobin concentrations after phlebotomy. This has been attributed to increased viscosity of blood associated with iron deficiency. It has been demonstrated previously that at low shear rates, whole-blood viscosity increases with decreasing cell size (and increasing cell number). Additionally, with iron deficiency, changes in the red cell membrane occur that increase cell rigidity.[198] Evidence that strokes in children with tetralogy of Fallot might be related to iron deficiency was initially published nearly 20 years ago.[199,200] Patients with polycythemia secondary to hypoxia were reported to benefit symptomatically from simultaneous oral iron therapy (40 to 60 mg elemental iron daily) and phlebotomy accompanied by isovolumic replacement.

These effects of iron deficiency on whole-blood viscosity have been corroborated.[201] However, others have attributed the effect of iron deficiency on whole-blood viscosity to the method of measurement of hematocrit. Coulter counters significantly underestimate the hematocrit when there are iron-deficient red cells.[202,203] It has been recommended that centrifuged hematocrit volume be used to follow such patients. Others have found no correlation between whole-blood viscosity and iron deficiency when the hematocrit is maintained around 45 percent.[203] Until this issue is clarified, it does not seem reasonable to supplement iron in individuals in whom the hematocrit is maintained at less than 50 percent. In patients with right-to-left shunt whose hematocrit may be maintained between 55 and 60 percent, 40 to 60 mg of oral supplemented elemental iron is reasonable.

REFERENCES

1. Balcerzak SP, Bromberg PA: Secondary polycythemia. Semin Hematol 12:353–382, 1975
2. Erslev AJ: Secondary polycythemia (erythrocytosis). *In* Williams WJ, Beutler E, Erslev AJ, Lichtman MA (eds): Hematology. New York, McGraw-Hill, 1983
3. Hocking WG: Pathophysiology. Ann Intern Med 95:71–87, 1981

4. Fisher JW, Langston JW: The influence of hypoxemia and cobalt on erythropoietin production in the isolated perfused dog kidney. Blood 29:114–125, 1967

5. Erslev AJ, Caro J: Secondary polycythemia: A boon or a burden? Blood Cells 10:177–191, 1984

6. Fisher JW, Samuels AI: Relationship between renal blood flow and erythropoietin production in dogs. Proc Soc Exp Biol Med 125:482–485, 1967

7. Necas E, Thorling EB: Unresponsiveness of erythropoietin-producing cells to cyanide. Am J Physiol 222:1187–1190, 1972

8. Necas E, Neuwist J: Feedback regulation by red cell mass of the sensitivity of the erythropoietin-producing organ to hypoxia. Blood 36:754–763, 1970

9. Golde DW, Hocking WG, Koeffler HP, et al: Polycythemia: Mechanisms and management. Ann Intern Med 95:71–87, 1981

10. Erslev AJ, Caro J: Pure erythrocytosis classified according to erythropoietin titers. Am J Med 76:57–61, 1984

11. Gibson J, Yuen E, Rickard KA, et al: An evaluation of serum erythropoietin estimation by a hemagglutination inhibition assay in the differential diagnosis of polycythemia. Pathology 16:155–156, 1984

12. Koeffler HP, Goldwasser E: Erythropoietin radioimmunoassay in evaluating patients with polycythemia. Ann Intern Med 94:44–47, 1981

13. Garcia JF, Ebbe SN, Hollander L: Radioimmunoassay of erythropoietin: Circulating levels in normal and polycythemic human beings. J Lab Clin Med 99:624–635, 1982

14. Koeffler HP: Chemistry and metabolism. Ann Intern Med 95:71–87, 1981

15. West JB: Pulmonary Pathophysiology. Baltimore, Williams & Wilkins, 1982

16. Bunn HF, Forget BG: Oxygen and carbon dioxide transport in health and disease. In Hemoglobin: Molecular, Genetic and Clinical Aspects. 1986, Cambridge, Saunders, Chap 5, pp 91–125

17. Whitcomb M: The Lung: Normal and Diseased. St. Louis, Mosby, 1982

18. Kilmartin JV, Rossi-Bernardi L: Interaction of hemoglobin with hydrogen ions, carbon dioxide, and organic phosphates. Physiol Rev 53:836–890, 1973

19. Lowe GDO, Forbes CD: Blood rheology and thrombosis. Clin Haematol 10:343–367, 1981

20. Chien S: Biophysical behavior of red cells in suspensions. In Surgenor DM (ed): The Red Blood Cell, vol 2, 2d ed. New York, Academic Press, 1975, pp 1031–1133

21. Castle WB, Jardl JH: Blood viscosity and blood volume: Opposing influences upon oxygen transport in polycythemia. Semin Hematol 3:193–198, 1966

22. Skovborg F, Nielsen AV, Schlichtkrull J: Blood viscosity and vascular flow rate. Scand J Clin Lab Invest 21:83–88, 1968

23. Thomas DJ, du Boulay GH, Marshall J, et al: Effect of haematocrit on cerebral blood-flow in man. Lancet 2:941–943, 1977

24. Thomas DJ, du Boulay GH, Marshall J, et al: Cerebral blood flow in polycythaemia. Lancet 2:161–163, 1977

25. Brown MM, Wade JPH, Marshall J: Fundamental importance of arterial oxygen content in the regulation of cerebral blood flow in man. Brain 108:81–93, 1985

26. Humphrey PRD, du Boulay GH, Marshall J, et al: Cerebral blood flow and viscosity in relative polycythaemia. Lancet 2:873–877, 1979

27. Scheinberg P: The effects of postural changes, stellate ganglion block and anaemia on the cerebral circulation. J Clin Invest 28:808–809, 1949

28. Willison JR, Thomas DJ, du Boulay GH, et al: Effect of high haematocrit on alertness. Lancet 1:846–848, 1980

29. Dunn SP, Gross KR, Scherer LR, et al: The effect of polycythemia and hyperviscosity on bowel ischemia. J Pediatr Surg 20:324–327, 1985

30. Murray JF, Gold P, Johnson BL Jr: The circulatory effects of hematocrit variations in normovolemic and hypervolemic dogs. J Clin Invest 42:1150–1159, 1963

31. Thorling EB, Erslev AJ: The "tissue" tension of oxygen and its relation to hematocrit and erythropoiesis. Blood 31:332–343, 1968

32. Castle WB: The Polycythemia. In Beck WS, (ed): Hematology. Cambridge, Mass, MIT Press, 1985, pp 305–322

33. Viault F: On the large increase in the number of red cells in the blood of the inhabitants of the high plateau of South America. In West JB, Hutchinson R, Stoudsberg (eds): High Altitude Physiology. Stroudsberg, PA, Hutchinson Ross, 1981 p. 333–334

34. Winslow RM: High Altitude Polycythemia and Man. Bethesda, Md, American Physiological Society, 1984

35. Erslev AJ: Blood and mountains. In Wintrobe MM (ed): Blood, Pure and Eloquent. New York, McGraw-Hill, 1980, p 257

36. Frisancho AR: Functional adaptation to high altitude hypoxia. Science 187:313–319, 1975

37. Miller ME, Rorth M, Parving HH, et al: pH effect on erythropoietin response to hypoxia. N Engl J Med 288:706–710, 1973

38. Lenfant C, Torrance J, English E, et al: Effect of altitude on oxygen binding by hemoglobin and on organic phosphate levels. J Clin Invest 47:2652–2656, 1968

39. Torrance JD, Lenfant C, Cruz J, et al: Oxygen transport mechanisms in residents at high altitude. Respir Physiol 11:1–15, 1970/71

40. Lenfant C, Torrance JD, Reynafarje C: Shift of the O_2-Hb dissociation curve at altitude: Mechanism and effect. J Appl Physiol 30:625–631, 1971

41. Hebbel RP, Eaton JW, Kronenberg RS, et al: Human llamas: Adaptation to altitude in subjects with high hemoglobin oxygen affinity. J Clin Invest 62:593–600, 1978

42. Hall FG, Dill DB, Barron ESG: Comparative physiology in high altitudes. J Cell Comp Physiol 8:301–313, 1936

43. Reynafarje C, Faura RJ, Villavicencio D: Erythrokinetics in altitudes camelides. In Proceedings of the XIII Congress of the International Society for Hematology. New York, Springer-Verlag, 1968, p 79

44. Faura J, Ramos J, Reynafarje C, et al: Effect of altitude on erythropoiesis. Blood 33:668–676, 1969

45. Weil JV, Jamieson G, Brown DW, et al: The red cell mass: Arterial oxygen relationship in normal man. J Clin Invest 47:1627–1639, 1968
46. Shaw DB, Simpson T: Polycythemia in emphysema. Q J Med 30:135–152, 1961
47. Vanier T, Dulfano MJ, Wu C, et al: Emphysema, hypoxia and the polycythemia response. N Engl J Med 269:169–178, 1963
48. Barcroft J, Binger CA, Bock AV, et al: Observations upon the effect of high altitude on the physiological processes of the body, carried out in the Peruvian Andes, chiefly at Cerro de Pasco. Philos Trans R Soc Lond [Biol] 211:351–480, 1923
49. Hurtado A: Studies at high altitude: Blood observations on the indian natives of the Peruvian Andes. Am J Physiol 100:487–505, 1932
50. Reynafarje C: Physiological patterns: Hematological aspects. In Life at High Altitudes, Scientific Publication No. 140. Washington, Pan American Health Organization, 1966, pp 32–35
51. Balke B: Cardiac performance in relation to altitude. Am J Cardiol 14:796–810, 1964
52. Banchero N, Sime F, Penaloza SD, et al: Pulmonary pressure, cardiac output and arterial oxygen saturation during exercise at high altitude and sea level. Circulation 33:249–262, 1966
53. Smith EE, Crowell JW: Role of an increased hematocrit in altitude acclimatization. Aerospace Med 38:39–43, 1967
54. Garruto RM, Dutt JS: Lack of prominent compensatory polycythemia in traditional native Andeans living at 4200 meters. Am J Phys Anthropol 61:355–366, 1983
55. Frisancho AR: Altitude and growth: A study of the patterns of physical growth of a high altitude Peruvian Quechua population. Am J Phys Anthropol 32:279–292, 1970
56. Quilici JC, Vergnes H: The hematological characteristics of high altitude populations. In The Biology of High Altitude People. Cambridge, Cambridge University Press, 1978, pp 189–218
57. Adams, WH, Strang LJ: Hemoglobin levels in persons of Tibetan ancestry living at high altitude. Proc Soc Exp Biol Med 149:1036–1039, 1975
58. Morpurgo G, Arese P, Bosia A, et al: Sherpas living permanently at high altitude: A new pattern of adaptation. Proc Natl Acad Sci USA 73:747–751, 1976.
59. Samaja M, Veicsteinas A, Cerretelli P: Oxygen affinity of blood in altitude Sherpas. J Appl Physiol 47:337–341, 1979
60. Gronbeck C, Maj MC: Chronic mountain sickness at an elevation of 2000 meters. Chest 85:577–578, 1984
61. Monge C: High altitude disease. Arch Intern Med 59:32–40, 1937
62. Winslow RM: Red cell mass and O_2 transport at altitude. In Sutton JR, Jones NL, Houston CS (eds): Hypoxia: Man at Altitudes. New York, Thieme-Stratton, 1982, pp 57–61
63. Kryger M: Breathing at high altitude: Lessons learned and application to hypoxemia at sea level. Adv Cardiol 27:11–16, 1980
64. Fishman AP: Hypoxia on the pulmonary circulation: How and where it acts. Circ Res 38:221–231, 1976
65. Penaloza D, Sime F: Chronic cor pulmonale due to loss of altitude acclimatization (chronic mountain sickness). Am J Med 50:728, 1971
66. Bohr DF: The pulmonary hypoxic response: State of the field. Chest 71(suppl):244–246, 1977
67. Tucker A, Migally N, Wright ML, et al: Pulmonary vascular changes in young and aging rats exposed to 5486 m altitude. Respiration 46:246–257, 1984
68. Abraham AS, Kay JM, Cole RB, et al: Haemodynamic and pathological study of the effect of chronic hypoxia and subsequent recovery of the heart and pulmonary vasculature of the rat. Cardiovasc Res 5:95–102, 1971
69. Murray JF, Gold P, Johnson BL: The circulatory effects of hematocrit variations in normovolemic and hypervolemic dogs. J Clin Invest 42:1150–1159, 1968
70. Hunter C, Barer GR, Shaw JW, et al: Growth of the heart and lungs in hypoxic rodents: A model of human hypoxic disease. Clin Sci Mol Med 46:375–391, 1974
71. Tucker A, McMurtry IF, Reeves JT, et al: Lung vascular smooth muscle as a determinant of pulmonary hypertension at high altitude. Am J Physiol 228:762–767, 1975
72. Zink RA, Schaffert W, Messmer K, et al: Hemodilution: Practical experiences in high altitude. In Brendel W, Zink RA (eds): High Altitude Physiology. New York, Springer-Verlag, 1982, pp 291–297
73. Huff RL, Laurence JH, Siri WE, et al: Effects of changes in altitude on hematopoietic activity. Medicine 30:197–217, 1951
74. Opitz E: Increased vascularization of the tissue due to acclimatization to high altitude and its significance for oxygen transport. Exp Med Surg 9:389–403, 1951
75. Tenney SM, Ou LC: Physiological evidence for increased tissue capillarity in rats acclimatized to high altitude. Respir Physiol 8:137–150, 1970
76. Cerretelli P: Oxygen transport on Mount Everest: The effects of increased hematocrit on maximal O_2 transport. Adv Exp Med Biol 75:113–119, 1976
77. Houston CS: Disease of the respiratory system. In Wilkerson JA (ed): Medicine for Mountaineering. Seattle, Mountaineers, 1975, pp 203–206
78. Fujimaki T, Matsutani M, Asai A, et al: Cerebral venous thrombosis due to high-altitude polycythemia. J Neurosurg 64:148–150, 1986
79. Zink RA, et al: Hemodilution in high altitude mountain climbing: A method to prevent or treat frostbite, high altitude pulmonary edema, and retinal hemorrhage. Chicago, Abstracts of Scientific Papers, Am. Soc. Anesthesiol. Annual Meeting, 1978, p 93
80. Cocking JB, Darke CS: Blood volume studies in chronic obstructive nonspecific lung disease. Thorax 27:44–51, 1972
81. Gallo R, Fraimow W, Cathcart R, et al: Erythropoietic response in chronic pulmonary disease. Arch Intern Med 113:559–568, 1964
82. Wilson RH, Borden CW, Ebert RV: Adaptation to anoxia in chronic pulmonary emphysema. Arch Intern Med 88:581–590, 1951
83. Hume R, Goldberg A: Actual and predicted-normal red cell and plasma volumes in primary and

secondary polycythaemia. Clin Sci 26:499–508, 1964

84. Hume R: Blood volume changes in chronic bronchitis and emphysema. Br J Haematol 15: 131–139, 1968

85. Harrison BDW: Polycythaemia in a selected group of patients with chronic airways obstruction. Clin Sci 33:563–570, 1973

86. Tura S, Pollycove M, Gelpi A: Erythrocyte and iron kinetics in patients with chronic pulmonary emphysema. J Nucl Med 3:110–127, 1962

87. Vanier T, Dulfano M, Wu C, et al: Emphysema, hypoxia and the polycythemic response. N Engl J Med 269:169–178, 1963

88. Hammarsten JF, Whitcomb WH, Johnson PC, et al: The hematologic adaptation of patients with hypoxia due to pulmonary emphysema. Am Rev Resp Dis 78:391–398, 1958

89. Pierce AK, Jarrett CE, Werkle G Jr, et al: Respiratory function during sleep in patients with chronic obstructive lung disease. J Clin Invest 45:631–636, 1966

90. Trask CH, Cree EM: Oximeter studies on patients with chronic obstructive emphysema, awake and during sleep. N Engl J Med 266: 639–642, 1962

91. Flick MR, Block AJ: Continuous in vivo monitoring of arterial oxygenation in chronic obstructive lung disease. Ann Intern Med 86:725–730, 1977

92. Lenfant C, Ways P, Aucutt C, et al: Effect of chronic hypoxic hypoxia on the O_2-Hb dissociation curve and respiratory gas transport in man. Respir Physiol 7:7–29, 1969

93. Gerlach E, Duhm J: 2,3-DPG metabolism of red cells: Regulation and adaptive changes during hypoxia. In Astrup P, Roth M (eds): Oxygen Affinity of Hemoglobin and Red Cell Acid Base Status. New York, Academic Press, 1972, p 552

94. Dintenfass L, Read J: Pathogenesis of heart failure in acute or chronic respiratory failure. Lancet 1:570–572, 1968

95. Levine BE, Bigelow DB, Hamstra RD, et al: The role of long-term continuous oxygen administration in patients with chronic airway obstruction with hypoxemia. Ann Intern Med 66: 639–650, 1967

96. Chamberlain DA, Millard FJC: The treatment of polycythaemia secondary to hypoxic lung disease by continuous oxygen administration. Q J Med 32:341–50, 1963

97. Abraham AS, Cole RB, Bishop JM: Reversal of pulmonary hypertension by prolonged oxygen administration to patients with chronic bronchitis. Circ Res 23:147–157, 1968

98. Petty TL, Finigan MM: Clinical evaluation of prolonged ambulatory oxygen therapy in chronic airway obstruction. Am J Med 45:242–252, 1968

99. Nocturnal Oxygen Therapy Trial Group: Continuous or nocturnal oxygen therapy in hypoxemic chronic obstructive lung disease: A clinical trial. Ann Intern Med 93:391–398, 1980

100. Harrison BDW, Davis J, Madwick RG, et al: The effects of therapeutic decrease in packed cell volume on the responses to exercise of patients with polycythemia secondary to lung disease. Clin Sci Mol Med 45:833–847, 1973

101. York EL, Jones RL, Menon D, et al: Effects of secondary polycythemia on cerebral blood flow in chronic obstructive pulmonary disease. Am Rev Respir Dis 121:813–818, 1980

102. Wade JPH, Pearson TC, Ross Russell RW, et al: Cerebral blood flow and blood viscosity in patients with polycythaemia secondary to hypoxic lung disease. Br Med J 283:689–692, 1981

103. Pearson TC, Wetherley-Mein G: Vascular occlusive episodes and venous haematocrit in primary proliferative polycythaemia. Lancet 2:1219–1222, 1978

104. Constantinidis K: Venesection fatalities in polycythaemia secondary to lung hypoxia. Practitioner 222:89–91, 1979

105. Wedzicha JA, Rudd RM, Apps MCP, et al: Erythrophoresis in patients with polycythaemia secondary to hypoxic lung disease. Br Med J 286: 511–514, 1983

106. Wedzicha JA, Cotter FE, Rudd RM, et al: Erythrophoresis compared with placebo aphoresis in patients with polycythaemia secondary to hypoxic lung disease. Eur J Respir Dis 65:579–585, 1984

107. Wedzicha JA, Newland AC, Empey DW: Apheresis procedures in polycythaemia. Br Med J 289:1072, 1984

108. Block AJ, Boysen PG, Wynne JW, et al: Sleep apnea, hypopnea and oxygen desaturation in normal subjects. N Engl J Med 300:513–517, 1979

109. Zwillich CW, Sutton FD, Pierson DJ, et al: Decreased hypoxic ventilatory drive in the obesity-hypoventilation syndrome. Am J Med 59: 343–348, 1975

110. Lyons HA, Huang CT: Therapeutic use of progesterone in alveolar hypoventilation associated with obesity. Am J Med 44:881–888, 1968

111. Sutton FD Jr, Zwillich CW, Creagh CE, et al: Progesterone for outpatient treatment of pickwickian syndrome. Ann Intern Med 83: 476–479, 1975

112. Kryger M, Weil J, Grover R: Chronic mountain polycythemia: A disorder of the regulation of breathing during sleep? Chest 73(suppl): 303–304, 1978

113. Kryger M, McCullough RE, Collins D, et al: Treatment of excessive polycythemia of high altitude with respiratory stimulant drugs. Am Rev Respir Dis 117:455–464, 1978

114. Rosenthal A, Button LN, Nathan DG, et al: Blood volume changes in cyanotic congenital heart disease. Am J Cardiol 29:162–167, 1971

115. Rosenthal DS, Braunwald E: Hematologic-oncologic disorders and heart disease. In Braunwald E (ed): Heart Disease: A Textbook of Cardiovascular Medicine. Philadelphia, Saunders, 1980, pp 1782–1783

116. Harrison BDW, Stokes TC: Secondary polycythemia: Its causes, effects and treatment. Br J Dis Chest 76:313–340, 1982

117. Yeager SB, Freed MD: Myocardial infarction as a manifestation of polycythemia in cyanotic heart disease. Am J Cardiol 53:952–953, 1984

118. Kulkarni H, Nair KG, Kmare SG, Pinto IJ. Congenital pulmonary outflow tract obstruction and myocardial infarction. Ind Heart J 28:177–182, 1976

119. Oldershaw PJ, St John Sutton MG: Haemodynamic effects of haematocrit reduction in patients with polycythaemia secondary to cyanotic

congenital heart disease. Br Heart J 44: 584–588, 1980

120. Rosenthal A, Nathan DG, Marty AT, et al: Acute hemodynamic effects of red cell volume reduction in polycythemia of cyanotic congenital heart disease. Circulation 42:297–307, 1970

121. Hutchison DC, Sapru RP, Sumerling MD, et al: Cirrhosis, cyanosis and polycythemia: Multiple pulmonary arteriovenous anastomoses. Am J Med 45:139–151, 1968

122. Wolfe JD, Toshkin DP, Holly FE, et al: Hypoxemia of cirrhosis: Detection of abnormal small pulmonary vascular channels by a quantitative radionucleide method. Am J Med 63:746–754, 1977

123. Bunn HF, Forget BG: Carboxyhemoglobin and carboxyhemoglobinemia. *In* Hemoglobin: Molecular, Genetic and Clinical Aspects. 1986, Chap 17, pp 663–675

124. Sagone AL, Lawrence T, Balcerzak SP: Effect of smoking on tissue oxygen supply. Blood 41:845–851, 1973

125. Eisen ME, Hammond ED: The effect of smoking on packed cell volume, red cell counts, hemoglobin and platelet counts. Can Med Assoc J 75:520–523, 1956

126. Isager H, Hagerup L: Relationship between cigarette smoking and high packed cell volume and haemoglobin levels. Scand J Haematol 8:241–244, 1971

127. Sagone AL Jr, Balcerzak SP: Smoking as a cause of polycythemia. Ann Intern Med 82:512–515, 1975

128. Smith JR, Landaw SA: Smokers' polycythemia. N Engl J Med 298:6–10, 1978

129. Wald N, Idle M, Smith PG: Carboxyhaemoglobin levels in smokers of filter and plain cigarettes. Lancet 1:110–112, 1977

130. Doll DC, Greenberg BR: Cerebral thrombosis in smokers' polycythemia. Ann Intern Med 102: 786–787, 1985

131. Jacobson LO, Goldwasser E, Fried W, et al: Role of the kidney in erythropoiesis. Nature 179:633–635, 1957

132. Hudgson P, Pearce JM, Yeates WK: Renal artery stenosis with hypertension and high hematocrit. Br Med J 1:18–21, 1967

133. Luke RG, Kennedy AC, Stirling WB: Renal artery stenosis, hypertension and polycythemia. Br Med J 5428:164–166, 1965

134. Tarazi RC, Frohlich ED, Dustan HP, et al: Hypertension and high hematocrit. Am J Cardiol 18:855–858, 1966

135. Bacon BR, Rothman SA, Ricanati ES, Rashad FA: Renal artery stenosis with erythrocytosis after renal transplantation. Arch Intern Med 140: 1206–1211, 1980

136. Schramek A, Adler O, Hashmonai M, et al: Hypertensive crisis, erythrocytosis, and uremia due to renal-artery stenosis of kidney transplants. Lancet 1:70–71, 1975

137. Jepson JH, de Leeuw NKM, Gault MH, et al: Characteristics of erythropoiesis following human renal homotransplantation. Transplant Proc 3:353–357, 1971

138. Nellans R, Otis P, Martin DC: Polycythemia following renal transplantation. Urology 6:158–163, 1975

139. Westerman MP, Jenkins JL, Dekker A, et al: Significance of erythrocytosis and increased eryth-

ropoietin secretion after renal transplantation. Lancet 2:755–757, 1967

140. Nies BA, Cohn R, Schrier SL: Erythremia after renal transplantation. N Engl J Med 15:785, 1975

141. Dagher FJ, Ramos E, Erslev A, et al: Erythrocytosis after renal allotransplantation: Treatment by removal of the native kidneys. South Med J 73: 940–942, 1980

142. Dagher FJ, Ramos E, Erslev A, et al: Are the native kidneys responsible for erythrocytosis in renal allorecipients? Transplantation 28:496–498, 1979

143. Ianhez LE, DaFonseca JA, Chocair PR, et al: Polycythemia after kidney transplantation. Urol Int 32:382–392, 1977

144. Obermiller LE, Tzamaloukas AH, Avasthi PS, et al: Decreased plasma volume in post-transplant erythrocytosis. Clin Nephrol 23:213–217, 1985

145. Lamperi S, Carozzi S: Erythroid progenitor growth in erythrocytotic transplanted patients. Artif Organs 9:200–204, 1985

146. Lamperi S, Carozzi S, Manca F, et al: Erythropoietin-independent erythropoiesis in polycythemic transplanted patients. Transplant Proc 17: 86–88, 1985

147. Herdman JP, Jaco NT: The renal circulation in experimental hydronephrosis. Br J Urol 22: 52–55, 1950

148. Hirsch I, Leiter E: Hydronephrosis and polycythemia. Urology 21:345–350, 1983

149. Mitus WJ, Toyama K: Experimental renal erythrocytosis: Role of the juxtaglomerular apparatus. Arch Pathol 78:658–664, 1965

150. Toyama K, Mitus EJ: Experimental renal erythrocytosis: III. Relationship between the degree of hydronephrotic pressure and the production of erythrocytosis. J Lab Clin Med 68:740–752, 1966

151. Osnes S: Experimental study of an erythropoietic principle produced by the kidney. Br Med J 2:650–658, 1959

152. Waldmann TA, Rosse WF, Swarm RL: The erythropoiesis-stimulating factors produced by tumors. Ann NY Acad Sci 149:509–515, 1968

153. Plzak LF Jr: Erythropoietin and renal cyst fluid (abstract). Clin Res 13:281, 1965

154. Murphy GP, Kenny GM, Mirand EA: Erythropoietin levels in patients with renal tumors or cysts. Cancer 26:191–194, 1970

155. Vertel RM, Morse BS, Prince JE: Remission of erythrocytosis after drainage of a solitary renal cyst. Arch Intern Med 120:54–58, 1967

156. Rosse WF, Waldmann TA, Cohen P: Renal cysts, erythropoietin and polycythemia. Am J Med 34:76–81, 1963

157. Friend D, Hoskins RG, Kirkin MW: Relative erythrocythemia (polycythemia) and polycystic kidney disease with uremia: Report of a case with comments on frequency of occurrence. N Engl J Med 264:17–19, 1961

158. Hoppin CH, Depner T, Yamuchi H, Hopper J: Erythrocytosis associated with diffuse parenchymal lesions of the kidney. Br J Haematol 32:557–563, 1976

159. Davies SW: Erythraemia in experimental nephritis. Br J Haematol 15:237–243, 1968

160. Erkelens DW, Status Van Eps LW: Bartter's syndrome and erythrocytosis. Am J Med 55:711–719, 1973

161. Jepson J, McGarry EE: Polycythemia and increased erythropoietin production in a patient with hypertrophy of the juxta-glomerular apparatus. Blood 32:370–375, 1968

162. Ways P, Huff JW, Kosmaler CH, et al: Polycythemia and histologically proven renal disease. Arch Intern Med 107:154–162, 1961

163. Murphy GP, Brendler H, Mirand EA: Erythropoietin release from renal carcinomas grown in tissue culture. Res Commun Chem Pathol Pharmacol 1:617, 1970

164. Kazal LA, Erslev AJ: Erythropoietin production in renal tumors. Ann Clin Lab Sci 5:98–109, 1975

165. Sherwood J, Goldwasser E: Erythropoietin production by human renal carcinoma cells in culture. Endocrinology 99:504–510, 1976

166. Katsuoka Y, Baba S, Hata M, et al: Transplantation of human renal cell carcinoma to the nude mice: As an intermediate of in vivo and in vitro studies. J Urol 115:373–376, 1976

167. Hagiwara M, Chen I-L, McGonigle R, et al: Erythropoietin production in a primary culture of human renal carcinoma cells maintained in nude mice. Blood 63:828–835, 1984

168. Tamaoki N, Hata J, Izumi S, et al: Systemic effects of human renal cell carcinoma on nude mice: Polycythemia, anemia, hypovolemia and hepatomegaly. In Nomura T, Ohsawa N, Tamaoki N, Fujiwara K (eds): Proceedings of the Second International Workshop on Nude Mice. Tokyo, University of Tokyo Press, 1977, p 417

169. Saito T, Saito K, Trent DJ, et al: Translation of messenger RNA from a renal tumor into a product with the biological properties of erythropoietin. Exp Hematol 13:23–28, 1985

170. Damon A, Holub DA, Melicow MM, et al: Polycythemia and renal carcinoma: Report of 10 new cases, two with long hematologic remission following nephrectomy. Am J Med 25:182–197, 1958

171. Hammond D, Winnick S: Paraneoplastic erythrocytosis and ectopic erythropoietin. Ann NY Acad Sci 230:219–227, 1974

172. Doll DC, Weiss RB: Neoplasia and the erythron. J Clin Oncol 3:429–446, 1985

173. Hammond D, Winnick S: Paraneoplastic erythrocytosis and ectopic erythropoietins. Ann NY Acad Sci 230:219–227, 1974

174. Waldmann TA, Levin EH, Baldwin M: The association of polycythemia with a cerebellar hemangioblastoma: The production of an erythropoiesis stimulating factor by the tumor. Am J Med 31:318–324, 1961

175. McFadzean AJS, Todd D, Tsang KC: Polycythemia in primary carcinoma of the liver. Blood 13:427–435, 1958

176. Davidson CS: Hepatocellular carcinoma and erythrocytosis. Semin Hematol 13:115–119, 1976

177. Gordon AS, Zanjani ED, Zalusky R: A possible mechanism for the erythrocytosis associated with hepatocellular carcinoma in man. Blood 35:151–157, 1970

178. Tso SC, Hua ASP: Erythrocytosis in hepatocellular carcinoma: A compensatory phenomenon. Br J Haematol 28:497–503, 1974

179. Okabe T, Urabe A, Kato T, et al: Production of erythropoietin-like activity by human renal and hepatic carcinomas in cell culture. Cancer 55:1918–1923, 1985

180. Wrigley PMF, Malpas JS, Turnbull AL, et al: Secondary polycythemia due to a uterine fibromyoma producing erythropoietin. Br J Haematol 21:551–555, 1971

181. Ossias LA, Zanjani ED, Zulusky R, et al: Case report: Studies on the mechanism of erythrocytosis associated with uterine fibromyoma. Br J Haematol 25:179–185, 1973

182. Morton ED, Evans EF, Daines WP: Polycythemia and uterine myomata. JAMA 200:149, 1967

183. Fried W, Ward HP, Hopeman AR: Leiomyoma and erythrocytosis: A tumor producing a factor which increases erythropoietin production. Report of a case. Blood 31:813–816, 1968

184. Eldor A, Even-Paz Z, Polliack A: Erythrocytosis associated with multiple cutaneous leiomyomata: Report of a case with demonstration of erythropoietic activity in the tumor. Scand J Hematol 16:245–249, 1976

185. Venenci PY, Puissant A, Boffa GA, et al: Multiple cutaneous leiomyomata and erythrocytosis with demonstration of erythropoietic activity in the cutaneous leiomyomata. Br J Dermatol 107:483–486, 1982

186. Bradley JE, Young JD, Lentz G: Polycythemia secondary to pheochromocytoma. J Urol 86:1–6, 1961

187. Mann DL, Gallagher NJ, Donati RM: Erythrocytosis and primary aldosteronism. Ann Intern Med 66:335–340, 1967

188. Walmann TA, Rosse WF, Swarm RL: The erythropoiesis-stimulating factors produced by tumors. Ann NY Acad Sci 149:509–515, 1968

189. Richardson TQ, Guyton AC: Effects of polycythemia and anemia on cardiac output and other circulatory factors. Am J Physiol 197:1167–1170, 1959

190. Stone HO, Thompson HK Jr, Schmidt-Nielsen K: Influence of erythrocytes on blood viscosity. Am J Physiol 37:658–664, 1974

191. Litcher RL, Pickering TG, Shien S, et al: Plasma viscosities in athletes and sedentary normal subjects. Clin Cardiol 4:172–179, 1981

192. Martin G, Ferguson EW, Wigatoff S, et al: Blood viscosity responses to maximal exercise in endurance-trained and sedentary female subjects. J Appl Physiol 59:348–353, 1985

193. Buick FJ, Gledhill N, Froese AB, et al: Effect of induced erythrocythemia or aerobic work capacity. J Appl Physiol 48:636–642, 1980

194. Lindenfeld J, Weil JV, Travis VL, et al: Hemodynamic response to normovolemic polycythemia at rest and during exercise in dogs. Circ Res 56:793–800, 1985

195. Gustafsson L, Appelgren L, Myrvold HE: The effect of polycythemia on blood flow in working and nonworking skeletal muscle. Acta Physiol Scan 109:143–148, 1980

196. Thorling EB, Erslev AJ: The "tissue tension" and its relation to hematocrit and erythrocytosis. Blood 31:332–343, 1968

197. Urbaniak SJ: Therapeutic plasma and cellular apheresis. Clin Haematol 13:217–251, 1984

198. Hutton RD: The effect of iron deficiency on whole blood viscosity in polycythaemic patients. Br J Haematol 43:191–199, 1979

199. Martelle RR, Linde LM: Cerebrovascular accidents with tetralogy of Fallot. Am J Dis Child 101:206–209, 1961

200. Iolster NJ: Blood coagulation in children with cyanotic congenital heart disease. Acta Paediatr Scand 59:551–557, 1970

201. Milligan DW, MacNamee R, Roberts BE, et al: The influence of iron-deficient indices on whole blood viscosity in polycythaemia. Br J Haematol 50:467–473, 1982

202. Pearson TC, Guthrie DL, Slates NGP, et al: Method of PCV measurement and the effect of iron deficiency on whole blood viscosity in polycythaemia. Br J Haematol 52:166–168, 1982

203. Birgegard G, Carlsson M, Sandhagen B, et al: Does iron deficiency in treated polycythaemia vera affect whole blood viscosity. Acta Med Scand 216:165–169, 1984

17

Familial Myeloproliferative Disease

HARRIET S. GILBERT

The myeloproliferative disorders (MPDs) have been shown to arise from clonal expansion of a pluripotential hematopoietic precursor cell (PHPC) that possesses a growth advantage over other polyclonally derived PHPCs but still retains its pluripotentiality. The clonal expansion results in increased and abnormal hematopoiesis and produces an array of interrelated syndromes, each variant being named according to the phenotypic expression of the myeloproliferative clone.[1] MPD variants are usually classified by the hematic cell type predominantly involved in the proliferation and the syndromes include polycythemia vera (PV), essential thrombocythemia (ET), and myeloid metaplasia (MM). Myelofibrosis is a secondary phenomenon and may occur in any MPD. Changes in phenotype of the PHPC are not uncommon and result in transitions among the syndromes during the course of MPD. Since the phenotype of MPD determines the course and complications of each syndrome, much attention has been devoted to establishing diagnostic criteria by which to classify a given patient with MPD. However, "hybrid" phenotypes presenting simultaneously or sequentially sometimes present difficulties in establishing a clear-cut diagnosis. Insofar as the underlying disorder in MPD involves the PHPC, the interrelatedness of MPD phenotypes is not surprising. This is an important consideration in studies of familial occurrence of MPD and one that has been overlooked in the past.

MPD is an uncommon hematologic malignancy, with an annual incidence of 0.5 to 1 per 100,000 for each of the syndromes. Numerous reports of familial polycythemia have appeared, but most cases do not fulfill the diagnostic criteria for primary PV and are better classified as secondary polycythemia. Documented cases of familial MPDs other than PV are rare and insufficient to implicate a common genetic defect or basis of inheritance. However, some compelling evidence of familial occurrence of PV was provided by a systematic study of patients enrolled in the Polycythemia Vera Study Group (PVSG) in which an increased prevalence of PV in parents of these patients was demonstrated.[2] In a subsequent report, PV in four members of one family was described[3] and the literature was reviewed. Thirteen kindreds with familial PV in 31 members were felt to have adequate documentation. In view of these findings, it appears that familial PV is not a rare occurrence.

Reports and reviews of familial involvement with other phenotypes of MPD are sparse.[4–6] They include rare instance of familial ET, myelofibrosis, and osteosclerosis. The paucity of cases may be due to the lack of a collective patient population, such as that made available by the PVSG. Appreciation of a familial occurrence of MPD is facilitated by prolonged contact with a sufficiently large patient population in whom family history data are obtained initially and monitored prospectively. During such an experience, I have encountered 12 kindreds in whom 2 or more members developed MPD. One striking feature of this series is the phenotypic variation of the MPD that occurred in some of the kindreds. This experience is presented and compared with the existing body of literature on familial MPD in which phenotypic homogeneity of the MPD has been observed.

Twelve kindreds with 26 patients exhibiting an MPD have been observed by me. The diagnosis was confirmed personally in the 12 index cases from each family and in 1 additional involved family member of 5 families, all of whom were under my care. The presence of MPD in the remaining 9 family members was documented by records obtained from attending physicians and/or hospitals. Instances in which other family members were alleged to have MPD but for which documentation was lacking were not included. The classification of the MPD phenotype was based on published criteria.[1]

Table 17–1 summarizes the findings in 12 families with familial MPD involving 26 patients. Ten families had 2 involved members, and 2 families had 3 involved members. In 4 of the families, MPD developed in a family member subsequent to its diagnosis in the propositus and was reported to me after the initial family history of the propositus was obtained. The MPD involved siblings in 7 families and parent-child combinations in 7 families.

There were 8 families in this series in which 1 or more family member had PV. Eight of the 12 patients with PV (67 percent) in 7 families developed MM, and this transformed to acute leukemia in 2 patients (16 percent). In the eighth family, the patient with PV did not develop MM or leukemia, but the other involved family member had MM. The high incidence of MM and leukemic transformation in the patients with PV in the present series is further confirmation that the diagnosis of familial PV was correct and that the series does not include families with secondary polycythemia. There was no known exposure to toxic agents that have been implicated in the etiology of MPD[7] and have been suggested as the etiology of "familial PV" reported in 2 families.[8]

The phenotype of the MPD was the same in 5 families: 3 with PV, 1 with ET, and 1 with

TABLE 17–1. SUMMARY DATA ON 12 KINDREDS WITH FAMILIAL MYELOPROLIFERATIVE DISEASE

FAMILY	AGE AT DIAGNOSIS YEARS/SEX	TYPE OF MPD*	TREATMENT†	SURVIVAL FROM DIAGNOSIS (YEARS)	OUTCOME	COMMENTS
Case 1	45/M	PV	Phleb, cyclophosphamide	19	Died, MM, acute leukemia	
Brother	60/M	PV	Phleb	—	Not known	
Case 2	37/F	PV	Phleb, interferon	>15	Still active PV with MM	PV in 2 great
Father	52/M	PV	Phleb, 32P, splenectomy	8	Died, MM of liver, hepatitis	aunts and great grandfather
Case 3	60/F	PV	Phleb, interferon	8	Died, MM, acute leukemia	
Daughter	39/F	PV	Phleb	>10	Still active PV	
Case 4	50/M	PV	Phleb, aspirin	>0.5	Still active PV	
Father	67/M	MM,MF	None	3	Died, diabetic complications	
Case 5	54/M	PV	Phleb, aspirin	>5	Transformed to MM,MF	
Father	72/M	MM,MF	None	12	Died, congestive heart failure	
Case 6	46/F	PV	Phleb, hydroxyurea, interferon	>18	Still active PV with MM	
Brother	53/M	MM,MF	Splenectomy	6	Died, acute leukemia	
Father	60/M	PV	Phleb	13	Died, suicide	
Case 7	66/F	ET	Aspirin	>3	Still active ET	
Brother	65/M	ET	Aspirin	>1.5	Still active ET	
Case 8	63/F	ET	Anagrelide	>8	Still active ET	
Mother	35/F	PV	Phleb, hydroxyurea	25	Died, MM	
Case 9	39/F	ET	Aspirin	>2.5	Still active ET	Acute leukemia, 2
Brother	44/M	MM,MF	Hydroxyurea	3	Died, acute leukemia	paternal aunts
Father	49/M	MM,MF	Splenectomy	3	Died, MM of liver	and 2 cousins
Case 10	55/M	MM,MF	Interferon	>3	Still alive	Son, acute leuke-
Sister	47/F	PV	Phleb	11	Died, MM, acute leukemia	mia, age 15
Case 11	53/F	MM	Interferon	>3	Still alive	
Sister	58/F	MM	Interferon	1	Died, sepsis	
Case 12	73/M	MM	Hydroxyurea, procrit	>2	Still alive	Sister, acute leu-
Sister	75/F	ET	Hydroxyurea	>5	Still active ET	kemia, age 61

*MPD abbreviations: PV = polycythemia vera; ET = essential thrombocythemia; MM = myeloid metaplasia; MF = myelofibrosis.
† Treatment abbreviations: Phleb = phlebotomy.

agnogenic MM. In 7 families, the MPD phenotype of the involved family members differed. Combinations of PV and MM occurred in 4 families, ET and MM in 2 families, and ET and PV in 1 family. In the family of case 2, family members with PV were reported in four generations. In addition to PV in her father, there were 3 additional members with PV in the two generations preceding her father's. Two great aunts died in their eighth decade with PV documented by hospital records, and a great-grandfather is reputed to have had PV. Since the details of these cases are not available, they have not been tabulated but are listed under Comments. Also noted under Comments is the occurrence of de novo acute leukemia in family members of 3 other kindreds with MPD.

The presentation of mixed phenotypes of MPD in families has not been reported previously. The PVSG searched the records of 652 cases for a family history of polcythemia but made no mention of other forms of MPD in family members.[2] In all the case reports of familial PV or familial MPD, only one MPD phenotype was observed at presentation, although transformation to another MPD phenotype or acute nonlymphocytic leukemia occurred during the course of some patients.

There is no clear mode of inheritance in the kindreds reported here. There was no history of consanguinity in the involved families. The previous analysis of 13 kindreds with familial PV in 31 members[3] supported a genetic predisposition for PV but failed to reveal a clear-cut mode of inheritance. The studies of a kindred with familial MPD involving the megakaryocytic cell line and presenting as thrombocytosis[4] suggested an autosomal dominant transmission with variable penetrance based on its presence in more than one generation and in both sexes. A similar mode of inheritance was reported in another family with ET in 5 members of both sexes from 2 to 62 years of age in three successive generations.[5] In the 2 kindreds in my series in which 3 family members were affected, MPD occurred in a father and 2 children, one male and one female. None of the 7 pairs of involved siblings were twins. Five pairs were of different genders, one pair was female, and one was male.

The occurrence of mixed phenotypes in familial MPD is entirely consistent with the accepted theory of MPD as a disease of the pluripotential hematopoietic precursor cell that manifests phenotypic heterogeneity of the expanded clone. Transformations from one phenotypic variant to another during the course of MPD are common, and it would be surprising if only a single MPD variant were to appear in all involved members of a family with MPD. The absence of reports of mixed phenotypes from the literature is striking but unexplained. Clearly, if I was able to observe a dozen families with familial MPD, 7 of which exhibited mixed phenotypes, this cannot be a rare occurrence. One deterrent to detection of such cases may be the patient's lack of understanding of the nature of MPD and the diagnostic terminology. Unless the patient is introduced to the concept of MPDs as a group of syndromes, the occurrence of a different but related syndrome in a relative might go unreported. Familiarization of the patient with the terminology of MPD has elicited a family history in more than one case in my series. Another deterrent to the detection of MPD kindreds is dismissal by the physician of a possible familial occurrence and failure to explore the family history with this in mind because of its perceived rarity.

Although almost every type of cancer has been reported to occur in a familial form, evidence of hereditary and familial influences exists in only a few percent of cases.[9] An awareness of the importance of molecular genetic events in the development of familial cancer has evolved through the evaluation of clinical observations, genetic epidemiology, and molecular biology of the rare but important family cancer syndrome, the Li-Fraumeni syndrome (LFS). Alterations of the p53 tumor suppressor gene are the most frequently encountered genetic events in human malignancy.[10] Analysis of the DNA of 5 LFS families identified base-pair mutations of the gene encoding p53 in the germ line of all affected members.[11] This demonstration has resulted in analysis of large populations of patients for constitutional abnormalities of the p53 gene and the finding that certain high-risk patients and their families carry germ-line p53 mutations that presumably predispose them in some manner to the development of their respective malignancies.

Chromosomal abnormalities involving the pluripotential hematopoietic stem cell are present with regularity in chronic myelocytic leukemia and with some frequency in non-

CML MPD. These are the result of somatic mutations arising in the hematopoietic precursor cell. The familial occurrence of MPD cannot be explained by mutations that arise spontaneously in somatic tissues over the organism's life span. Familial incidence would require the presence of a germ-line mutation that is vertically transmitted and predisposes family members to the development of MPD. As molecular biologic techniques become more sophisticated and more genes involved in cancer promotion are identified, cases of familial MPD will become increasingly important as subjects for studies of somatic and germ-line DNA. An awareness of the familial occurrence of MPD will lead to identification of "MPD families" that will be added to existing cases and lead to better characterization of the genetic aspects of the syndromes that comprise MPD.

REFERENCES

1. Gilbert HS: Diagnosis and treatment of polycythemia vera, agnogenic myeloid metaplasia, and essential thrombocythemia. *In* Wiernik PH, Canellos GP, Kyle RA, Schiffer CA (eds): Neoplastic Diseases of the Blood. New York, Churchill Livingstone, 1991, pp 123–136

2. Brubaker LH, Wasserman LR, Goldberg JD, et al: Increased prevalence of polycythemia vera in parents of patients on Polycythemia Vera Study Group protocols. Am J Hematol 16:367–373, 1984

3. Miller RL, Purvis JD III, Weick JK: Familial polycythemia vera. Cleve Clin J Med 56(8):813–818, 1989

4. Slee PH, van Everdingen JJ, Geraedts JP, et al: Familial myeloproliferative disease: Hematological and cytogenetic studies. Acta Med Scand 210(4):321–327, 1981

5. Eyster ME, Saletan SL, Rabellino EM, et al: Familial essential thrombocythemia. Am J Med 80(3):497–502, 1986

6. Randi ML, Fabris F, Visentin I, Girolami A: Low incidence of familial occurrence of thrombocythaemia and/or thrombocytosis. Folia Haematol (Leipz) 115(5):695–699, 1988

7. Modan B: Polycythemia: A review of epidemiological and clinical aspects. J. Chronic Dis 18: 605–645, 1965

8. Ratnoff WD, Gress RE: The familial occurrence of polycythemia vera: Report of a father and son, with consideration of the possible etiologic role of exposure to organic solvents, including tetrachloroethylene. Blood 56(2):233–236, 1980

9. Li FP: Genetic and familial cancer: Opportunities for prevention and early detection. Cancer Detect Prev 9:41, 1986

10. Levin AJ, Momand J, Finlay CA: The p53 tumor suppressor gene. Nature 351:453, 1991

11. Malkin D, Li FP, Strong LC, et al: Germ-line p53 mutations in a familial syndrome of breast cancer, sarcomas, and other neoplasms. Science 250:1233, 1990

18

Relative Polycythemia

NEAL J. WEINREB

"Acquire for yourself a teacher" (Mishna Avoth). I have been fortunate to have encountered many esteemed teachers and colleagues, but none greater than Dr. Louis R. Wasserman, a true giant in hematology and medicine. It is a privilege to be counted among his students.

Individuals who are abnormal by virtue of having an increased hemoglobin concentration, increased venous hematocrit, and increased peripheral red blood cell count are, according to widely accepted, if imprecise, medical usage, *polycythemic*. More often than not, such persons will prove not to have *absolute polycythemia*, as defined as an increase in total-body red cell mass beyond the upper limits of statistically defined normal range.[1] The concept of *relative polycythemia*, which was originally promulgated by Osler[2] to describe a transient state of acute hemoconcentration associated with intravascular fluid depletion, is now commonly broadened to include all individuals in whom an elevated peripheral red blood cell concentration is not accompanied by a corresponding absolute increase in red cell mass.

Well-recognized causes for transient relative polycythemia include dehydration from, for example, protracted vomiting or diarrhea, loss of plasma as in extensive burns,[3] fluid shifts as in acute altitude adaptation,[4] sudden cold exposure[2] or protracted exercise,[5] insensible fluid loss as occurs in fever, sepsis, diabetic ketoacidosis,[3] and acute ethanol intoxication,[6] and endocrinologic disturbances such as Cushing's syndrome.[7] Although acute relative polycythemia usually resolves with appropriate medical management within hours or, at most, a few days, hemoconcentration associated with acute fluid depletion is sometimes of and by itself felt to be deleterious and causally associated with occlusive vascular complications.[8]

There is generally more interest in and greater controversy and less understanding about patients with chronic, sustained, relative polycythemia. Although it is now apparent that these patients do not constitute a single, unique, nosologic entity, in the past they have usually been conglomerated in the medical literature under a veritable plethora of nomenclature, including polycythemia hypertonica,[9] pseudopolycythemia,[10,11] Gaisbock's syndrome,[12] stress erythrocytosis,[12] benign polycythemia,[13] spurious polycythemia,[14] and apparent polycythemia.[8] None of these terminologies may be considered truly satisfactory. The use of adjectives such as *benign, spurious, pseudo,* and *apparent,* selected to convey the concept that absolute polycythemia is not present, has been criticized for seeming to minimize the significant morbidity experienced by at least some of the patients with chronic relative polycythemia. *Stress erythrocytosis* is controversial inasmuch as a causal relationship between emotional stress and hematocrit elevation, as initially postulated, has not yet been proven.[15,16] *Gaisbock's syndrome,* referring to an association between nonsplenomegalic polycythemia and hypertension, is insufficiently specific and noninclusive of the substantial number of patients with chronic relative polycythemia who are normotensive.

It follows, therefore, that a clearer understanding of the various disorders associated with chronic relative polycythemia is dependent on the development of a classification system based on pathogenetic mechanisms that is analogous to the scheme according to which the absolute polycythemias are meticulously defined. The basis for such a classification system is the recognition that patients with chronic relative polycythemia form two major groups based on plasma volume measurement. In hypovolemic relative polycythemia, the elevation in venous hematocrit is largely attributable to an absolute decrease in plasma volume. In the high normal red cell mass group (normovolemic relative polycythemia), the elevation in venous hematocrit is associated with a red cell mass in the higher range of normal with either normal or only modestly decreased plasma volume. Although some individuals in this latter group may represent a normal extreme[14] ("odd men out"[17]), some may have abnormal venous compliance with shifts in intravascular blood distribution.[18] Relative polycythemia in both the hypovolemic and normovolemic groups may, in many instances, be associated with, or possibly secondary to, smoking, hypertension, obesity, sleep apnea disorders, alcohol ingestion, or combinations thereof. Given the prevalence of these potential etiologic factors in Western society, it is likely that only occasionally will relative polycythemia of either variety prove to be truly idiopathic, provided that the primary causes are carefully sought.

The major clinical significance of chronic relative polycythemia lies in an increased risk for occlusive vascular complications, including coronary artery disease, myocardial infarction, cerebrovascular disease, and stroke. The propensity for vascular thrombotic events, which may equal that found in polycythemia vera (PV),[19] is usually attributed to the magnitude of hematocrit elevation, increased whole-blood viscosity, and consequent abnormal hemorrheology. Evidence concerning this proposed pathogenetic mechanism will be reviewed. Nevertheless, although patients with hypovolemic relative polycythemia do not seem to differ from those with high normal red cell mass polycythemia with respect to venous hematocrit, the increased risk of vascular occlusive events

seems primarily directed at the hypovolemic patients.[20, 21] Although it is not absolutely certain that the high normal red cell mass group is free of increased risk of thrombotic complications (a matter currently under prospective investigation[8]), one study suggests that morbidity and mortality in this group do not differ significantly from an age-matched, "normal" population.[21] This observation, if sustained, would suggest that hypovolemia per se and additional factors such as increased peripheral resistance may be as significant as the hematocrit level in the causation of clinical disease. The additional independent contribution to morbidity and mortality by smoking, hypertension, obesity, sleep apnea, and nocturnal hypoxemia also cannot be discounted. For example, an incidence of thromboembolic events of 41 percent was described in patients with smoker's polycythemia with absolute elevations in red cell mass compared with an incidence of 60 percent in comparable patients with PV, suggesting that smoker's polycythemia does not represent a hypercoagulable state equivalent to that of PV.[22] Patients with relative polycythemia were excluded from this study.

It is clear that both variants of relative polycythemia represent disorders in blood volume regulation rather than a primary hematologic disease. Treatment is usually directed at alteration in lifestyle, emphasizing weight loss, cessation of smoking, and control of hypertension. A possible role for phlebotomy in the management of chronic relative polycythemia remains uncertain and unsettled.

HISTORICAL PERSPECTIVE

From antiquity, plethora has been recognized as a prominent manifestation of disease. Classical Galenic doctrine finds its echo in the Talmudic statement that "an excess of blood is the main cause of all illness."[23] Plethora and headache are among the signs and symptoms for which phlebotomy was recommended in Talmudic times (1500 to 1800 years ago), and recognition of an association between plethora and pruritus ("much blood produces severe skin inflammation"[24]) may conceivably have alluded to ancient patients with PV. In what may be the earliest perception of the normal hematocrit and recognition of the dependence of blood concentration on the relationship between the red blood and plasma volumes, rabbinic literature states, "the body of a normal person is in equilibrium, having half blood and half water; when a person is healthy, the water does not exceed the blood, nor does the blood exceed the water. When he is ill [lit. "sins"], at times, the water increases relative to the blood causing 'hydrops'; in other circumstances, the blood may increase relative to the water, causing zara'at [a skin ailment usually mistranslated as leprosy]."[25] Surely this statement seems to hint at an awareness of a concept of relative polycythemia.

In more recent history, Andral[13] in 1843 commented on the association of plethora with polycythemia, described as increased quantity of "globules" in the blood, often associated with symptoms of vertigo and dizziness. Persistent polycythemia, as distinguished from transient states of hemoconcentration, was first described in 1892 by Vaquez.[26] Subsequently, in 1903, Osler[2] differentiated true polycythemia from chronic relative polycythemia occurring in patients with intravascular fluid depletion. Relative polycythemia was sometimes of high grade and persisted for months or even years.

Early classifications of polycythemia relied heavily on the presence or absence of splenomegaly. In 1905, Gaisbock[9] described the association of polycythemia with hypertension in 18 patients without splenomegaly. He regarded this syndrome of polycythemia hypertonica as a distinct clinical entity, with the presence of hypertension as the most important characteristic distinguishing his syndrome from PV. In a subsequent review of 149 reported cases of erythremia, Lucas[27] also commented on the frequency of hypertension in nonsplenomegalic erythremic patients and the infrequency of hypertension in polycythemic patients with splenomegaly. (This observation has, in fact, not been confirmed in later studies, and substantial numbers of patients with PV are indeed hypertensive.[1]) Unlike Gaisbock, however, Lucas did not clearly categorize nonsplenomegalic erythremia with hypertension as a specific entity distinct from PV, although he did differentiate erythremia from secondary absolute polycythemia caused by hypoxemia and from transient relative polycythemia associated with rapid fluid loss and decrease in blood volume. Lucas additionally observed that an increase in red blood cells also was seen at times in obesity, and he noted

an association between polycythemia and paralysis.

These early observations were recorded when accurate methods for the determination of blood volume were unavailable. In 1915, with the advent of dye dilution techniques for plasma volume measurement, 3 cases of hypovolemic polycythemia were reported in which elevations of hemoglobin and red blood cell count were not associated with an increased red cell mass but rather were attributed mainly to a decrease in the plasma volume.[28] In 1940, a further description of this entity, now called "pseudopolycythemia," was reported in 2 patients by Bassen and Abel.[10] However, a retrospective review of this paper confirms the contention of Kaung and Peterson[11] that, in actuality, both patients had absolute polycythemia, which in one case was secondary to either alveolar hypoventilation or sleep apnea syndrome.

Interest in relative polycythemia increased following the publication in 1952 by Lawrence and Berlin[12] of a series of 18 patients described as having "relative polycythemia— the polycythemia of stress.[12] Eighty-three percent of the patients were male and of a substantially younger age than the usual patient with PV. Obesity, hypertension, and significant anxiety were common associated findings. Although all these patients were considered to have relative polycythemia, the reported hematocrit was less than 52 percent in 9 of the 15 male patients described. Of the 6 male patients with unequivocal abnormal hematocrit elevations, one lived at an altitude of 6700 feet. Two of the remaining 5 patients were hypertensive, and 2 others were obese, one of whom having had a prior history of thrombosis. Smoking histories were not reported. Red cell mass measurements with radiophosphorus-labeled red blood cells were normal. Plasma volume was calculated from the red cell mass and measured venous hematocrit without correction for the body/ venous hematocrit ratio and was characteristically low.

These patients were felt to correspond in many respects to the group of patients described by Gaisbock.[9] The blood volume changes were presumed related to some form of emotional stress, suggesting that this condition might be a psychosomatic phenomenon. Previously, Allbutt, as cited by Lucas,[27] had associated polycythemia with nervous excitement and mental worry.

Osler[2] had related polycythemia to physiologic stress, noting that "the polycythemia of vasomotor disturbances such as after the cold bath and after violent exercise also comes in this class." It should be noted at this time, however, that this description of "stress polycythemia" is not related to the rapid transient erythrocytosis observed in some animal species when red blood cells are suddenly infused into the circulation from the splenic storage pool, a mechanism that does not occur in normal humans.[3]

In 1962, Kaung and Peterson[11] described 10 male patients with hematocrits ranging from 53 to 62 percent with normal red cell mass measurements and significant decreases in calculated plasma volume. Eight patients were age 60 or above, thus being quite different in age from the patients of Lawrence and Berlin. All were obese, and indeed, when red cell mass was corrected for lean body mass, 3 patients had modest absolute erythrocytosis. Six of 10 patients were hypertensive. Smoking history was not recorded. Only 1 of 10 patients was noted to be anxious, with all others calm, cooperative, and apparently well adjusted. A striking occurrence of vascular occlusive disease was reported in these patients, including three cerebral thromboses, four coronary thromboses, one venous thrombosis of the leg, and one arterial embolism to the leg. The authors stressed the possible importance of an elevated peripheral hematocrit in increasing blood viscosity and thrombotic potential.

In 1964, Russell and Conley[13] described 23 male patients, predominantly of early middle age, moderately overweight, and stocky, with tense, anxious personalities and hematocrits ranging from 54 to 65 percent. Red cell mass was measured in only 8 patients, with 3 patients having significantly elevated values. Of the 5 patients with normal red cell mass, 3 had significantly decreased plasma volumes. Nearly all patients smoked cigarettes. Only 4 consumed large quantities of alcohol, and 18 patients were consistently hypertensive. Manifestations of vascular disease occurred in 7 patients, including 4 with myocardial infarction, 1 with cerebrovascular accident, a saddle embolism, and 2 with thrombophlebitis. In contrast to patients with PV, these patients appeared to derive little subjective improvement in symptoms of lightheadedness, dizziness, or headache following phlebotomy, and it was therefore suggested that there was no cause-and-effect relationship between the increased hematocrit level and the vascular disease. Ten patients were followed for at least 5 years without developing evidence of PV, thus justifying, to the authors, the designation of this syndrome as "benign polycythemia." This syndrome was felt to correspond to that described by Gaisbock but was not considered to be a disease, but rather a manifestation of a genetically determined constitutional type. In subsequent practice, the terminology *benign polycythemia* or *benign erythrocytosis* is generally reserved to describe patients with an idiopathic absolute elevation in red cell mass who have insufficient additional criteria to establish a diagnosis of PV.[29]

In 1965, Hall[30] reported a series of 19 male patients with Gaisbock's disease. Ages range from 31 to 68 years, but only 3 patients were older than 60 years. Hematocrits ranged from 51 to 61 percent. Red cell mass was elevated in 3 patients. The plasma volume was decreased in half the patients but normal or low normal in the others. Of the 16 patients with relative polycythemia, 6 were obese. The incidence of hypertension is not given but is stated to be frequent, as was excessive nervousness or tension. Occurrence of smoking is not reported. A family predisposition was noted. Ten of 16 patients presented with either cardiac, cerebral, or peripheral vascular disease, including 2 with myocardial infarction, 1 with cerebrovascular accident, and 2 with peripheral arterial occlusions. Phlebotomies were performed in 7 patients, but good responses were few and minor. Three patients were treated with radiophosphorus with little effect on the blood count or on the clinical manifestations. Twelve patients were followed for an average of 5 years without any real change in their basic disorder, although with an increasing incidence of vascular disease.

The elevated hematocrits in the various studies described above were generally associated with chronic diminution in plasma volume. Much of the data supporting this conclusion were obtained indirectly as derived values from the measured red cell volume. This calculation is invalid and inappropriately low compared with plasma volume values determined with radioiodinated albumin unless corrected by a factor of 0.9, representing the normal value for the body/venous hematocrit ratio in humans.[5] The discrepancy between body and venous hematocrit is related to the concept that the distribution of erythrocytes and plasma is unequal in different organs and that the hematocrit in the microvasculature is considerably less than that of the macrocirculation.[31] Thus the hematocrit of blood drawn from arteries, veins, or the finger is not necessarily representative of the cell-to-plasma ratio of the entire circulating blood.

Blum and Zbar,[32] using direct measurement of both red cell mass and plasma volume, reported that albumin plasma volumes were normal or only minimally decreased in a series of 10 patients with relative polycythemia. Furthermore, the ratio of body-to-venous hematocrit was unusually low, suggesting that the elevation in venous hematocrit found in these patients might be attributed to a redistribution of blood cells from smaller to larger vessels. A decrease in the body/venous hematocrit ratio was not confirmed in one later extensive study of relative polycythemia.[21] In assessing the series of Blum and Zbar, it should be pointed out that of the 10 patients, 1 had chronic myelocytic leukemia, 1 had myeloid metaplasia with marked anemia, 1 had apparently significant chronic obstructive pulmonary disease, and there is no clinical information regarding 2 others. Three of the remaining 5 patients had recent or concurrent blood loss, and in 1 patient, a measured red cell mass of 24.5 ml/kg seems unlikely in the context of a venous hematocrit of 62 percent.[1]

In a recent study of 35 patients with spurious polycythemia, Watts and Lewis[18] found a lack of correlation between the red cell mass and the plasma volume, values for which were widely scattered, although generally 75 to 90 percent of predicted. The lowest plasma volumes were noted in 7 patients with coexistent peripheral vascular disease. Abnormally low body/venous hematocrit ratios were observed in a subset of 10 patients with hypertension. The initial abnormally high hematocrit in this subgroup returned to normal with antihypertensive therapy. These results, along with evidence for a decrease in compliance of the venous system with a shift of blood toward the central region in hypertensive patients,[33] suggests that an abnormally low body/venous hematocrit ratio may be a significant etiologic factor in relative polycythemia associated with hypertension. Parenthetically, defective venous tone was proposed as playing an important role in the pathogenesis of polycythemia 80 years ago by Anders.[27]

In the Watts and Lewis series, positive correlation was observed between hematocrit and red cell mass. The red cell mass was particularly influenced by smoking, with 7 of 9 smokers having red cell mass measurements in the high-normal range.[18] In earlier series, red cell volumes in relative polycythemia, particularly after correction for lean body mass in obese patients, were often in the higher range of normal.[11] This pattern suggested that relative polycythemia should be regarded not as a disease but rather as a normal extreme consisting of subjects at the outer limit of the normal frequency distribution curve for red cell and plasma volumes.[17] Such "odd men out" should not be regarded as necessarily abnormal, although, clearly, physiologic parameters whose levels are at the extreme edge of the normal distribution curve may contribute to pathologic events under appropriate circumstances. A cogent example is serum cholesterol concentration. Preliminary evidence in favor of this hypothesis in patients with relative ("spurious") polycythemia was reported by Brown et al.[14] in 1971. Thirty-two patients with spurious polycythemia were compared with 43 control subjects, admittedly drawn from a group of patients referred for evaluation for polycythemia but in whom an abnormally elevated hematocrit was not confirmed. Except for a higher incidence of mild hypertension, the patients with spurious polycythemia were indistinguishable from the control group. Normal physiologic variation, manifested by high-normal red cell volume and low-normal plasma volume, was the most common but not the exclusive alteration accounting for the elevation in hematocrit. The heterogeneity of findings in these patients suggested that spurious polycythemia did not constitute a true nosologic entity, leading the authors to the conclusion, previously espoused by Wintrobe,[34] that spurious polycythemia is a nonexistent disease.

This study was later extended by Weinreb and Shih,[21] although with a substantial influx of new patients replacing some studied years earlier and subsequently lost to follow-up. Forty-seven men with relative ("spurious") polycythemia were compared with 22 control subjects referred for evaluation for polycythemia but with hematocrits below 52 percent. Simultaneous red cell mass and plasma volume measurements were performed. Two patient groups were identified. In 21 patients, the elevated venous hematocrit was attributable to an absolute decrease in plasma volume. In 26 other patients, however, the values for the red cell and plasma volumes represented only opposite extremes of the normal range. Although these groups were indistinguishable with respect to hematocrit, they differed significantly in some clinical and laboratory findings and, most importantly, with regard to survival. The hypovolemic group had a significantly greater incidence of hypertension and a tendency to a greater incidence of hypercholesterolemia. Survival in this group was significantly poorer than in the high-normal red cell mass group, significantly poorer than the expected U.S. survival for age-matched patients, and even poorer than the survival in newly diagnosed patients with PV treated with radiophosphorus. Vascular occlusive complications, particularly myocardial infarction and stroke, represented the overwhelming cause of morbidity and mortality. Although 80 to 85 percent of all the patients on study were cigarette smokers, the hypovolemic group did not differ significantly from the high-normal red cell mass group with respect to the proportion of smokers, nor did the groups differ with respect to age, alcohol ingestion, obesity, or use of diuretics. Hypertension was associated with significant risk for morbidity and mortality for both groups with spurious polycythemia.

In 1975, Burge et al.[20] described initial findings and follow-up in 35 patients with pseudopolycythemia. All patients had a stable hematocrit of at least 50 percent, a normal red cell mass, and a simultaneously measured plasma volume of less than 36 ml/kg. The mean plasma volume was 31.7 ml/kg, a significantly decreased value comparable with the mean of 30.4 ml/kg found in the hypovolemic group of Weinreb and Shih.[21] Thirty-two patients were male, with a mean age of 49.8 years. Eighty percent were heavy smokers, and more than half the patients were believed to be anxious. Hypertension was found in 33 percent of the patients, and several of the patients were overweight. Twenty-seven patients were followed for up to 12 years, with a mean of 4 years of follow-up. Six patients died, 2 of sudden death, 1 of myocardial infarction, 1 of cerebral thrombosis, 1 of glioma, and 1 of unknown cause. Significant nonfatal vascular occlusive events also occurred with some frequency in the survivors. The death rate in this patient series was six times greater than expected.

The differentiation of patients with relative polycythemia into two groups based primarily on plasma volume measurement now seems well established. Wetherley-Mein[8] defines idiopathic (low plasma volume) polycythemia as an elevation in the hematocrit due to a reduction of plasma volume below 15 percent of the patient's normal predicted value in association with a normal red cell mass. This disorder is believed to carry a risk of occlusive vascular complications equal to that of absolute nonhypoxic polycythemia at equivalent hematocrit levels. The high-normal red cell mass group is referred to as having "apparent polycythemia." In a recent review, Pearson[35] describes the incidence of relative polycythemia as being approximately one-fourth that of apparent polycythemia. The natural history and indications for treatment for this group are a subject of prospective study by a research unit of the Royal College of Physicians (London),[8] but to my knowledge, results of this study have not yet been reported.

A retrospective study of 34 patients with either relative (low plasma volume) or apparent (normal red cell mass and plasma volume) polycythemia was reported by Pearson and Messinezy.[36] Male sex, smoking, hypertension, and diuretic therapy were found to be associated factors, and 15 percent had arterial hypoxemia. The two subgroups did not differ with regard to these probable contributory factors. Preliminary follow-up data indicated that the hematocrit abnormality reverted to normal in a third, persisted in a third, and recurred intermittently in a third. Further prospective studies are planned.

In a comprehensive review article, Isbister[37] convincingly reintroduces the nomenclature of "chronic stress polycythemia" to define a pathophysiologic syndrome of diverse and often multiple etiologies but whose unifying hallmark is chronic hemoconcentration associated with a contracted plasma volume. The centrality of stress to this definition is in its applicability to a variety of physiologic and psychological interactive processes whose combined effect is to promote stimulation of the sympathetic nervous system, decreased venous compliance, activation of hormones involved in blood volume and pressure control, and consequent plasma volume contraction and blood hyperviscosity. Illustrative provocative factors include hypoxia, smoking, cold exposure, alcohol, and mental stress. In applying this broad definition of stress to this syndrome, Isbister restores, in essence, the original definition of this entity by Lawrence and Berlin.[12]

DIAGNOSTIC CRITERIA

Blood Volume Measurement

The determination of the red cell mass and plasma volume is central to the diagnosis of relative polycythemia. In current practice, red cell mass and plasma volume are measured simultaneously but independently using reliable techniques employing radiochromate-labeled red blood cells and radioiodinated serum albumin. Lower plasma volume values have been found when plasma proteins of higher molecular weight than albumin (fibrinogen, gamma globulin) are used for the measurement of plasma volume.[38, 39]

Representative normal values for red cell mass (plus or minus standard deviation) are 28.2 ± 4.1 ml/kg, and normal plasma volume values are 39.7 ± 5.3 ml/kg.[21] The Polycythemia Vera Study Group (PVSG) criterion for absolute red cell mass elevation (red cell mass greater than 36 ml/kg in men) has achieved wide acceptance in the United States. Many investigators, however, have questioned the propriety of calculating blood volumes on a body-weight basis,[8, 11, 35, 40] pointing out that such practice causes underestimation of the red cell mass in obese individuals and may obscure a state of true erythrocytosis. Wetherley-Mein[8] recommends a method by which the actual red cell and plasma volumes are compared with the normal predicted values calculated from the Nadler height and weight formula.[8] This method yields equivalent values to those derived from surface area or lean body mass methods. In this system, an increase in actual red cell mass greater than 25 percent above the predicted value indicates absolute polycythemia, and a decrease in plasma volume of more than 15 percent below predicted is indicative of definite hypovolemia. Chien et al.[41] have suggested, however, that body height may be a better parameter than either weight or surface area for expressing blood volume measurements in normal subjects.

In normal, healthy individuals in a stable environment, red cell and plasma volumes remain essentially unchanged over many years despite changes in body weight.[41] The plasma volume, however, is subject to rapid change related to posture and physical activity.[5, 42] Seasonal variations and changes of 15 to 30 percent associated with shifts from cool to warm environments have been reported.[43] Diurnal variation in plasma volume is also well recognized.[44, 45] It is apparent, therefore, that diagnostic blood volume measurements must be obtained under controlled, standard conditions with respect to time of day, position, and activity if meaningful, comparative data are to be generated.

Hematocrit

Although measurements of red blood cell concentration are among the most elementary and commonplace laboratory procedures, the question as to what value represents an abnormally elevated hematocrit is not necessarily self-evident or simplistic. The traditional solution to this problem is based on a statistical analysis of an allegedly normal population and the arbitrary designation of all values in excess of 2 standard deviations from the mean as abnormal. According to this approach, the upper limit of normal for sea-level hematocrit in adult men ranges from 50 to 54 percent.[3, 11, 34, 41, 46–49] Despite considerable changes in laboratory methodology, normal hematocrit values have been relatively consistent for a period of over 50 years in a variety of geographic settings and populations.[34] Differences in altitude of over 1000 to 1500 m are, of course, associated with hematocrit differences of up to 5 percent.[34] Lower-normal mean hematocrits in African-Americans,[48] not attributable to socioeconomic factors,[48] may possibly reflect expression of α-thalassemic genes.[50] No significant difference in plasma volume or total blood volume has been found between the two racial populations.[51] In healthy, young adult men, the hematocrit appears to remain stable within narrow range. In 41 male subjects compared over a 16- to 17-year period, hematocrit values showed no significant change.[41] A tendency to lower hematocrit values after 50 to 60 years of age[52] has not been universally noted.[34] Diurnal variations in hematocrit, caused by fluctuations in plasma volume, occur, with decreases of up to 10 percent from morning to evening having been observed. The usual fall in hematocrit, however, is approximately 3 percent, and changes are rarely evident between morning and midday.[45] Variations in hematocrit associated with season and climate may have been obscured by the advent of climate-control systems, but the influence of sudden changes in ambient temperature and in body position should not be neglected in formulating investigative methodology.

There are, of course, potential problems in automatically translating the statistical limits of normalcy and abnormalcy to biologically equivalent states of health versus disease. For example, as previously discussed, it has not been conclusively shown that all individuals in whom the hematocrit mildly exceeds the statistical upper limit of normal are necessarily at risk for excess morbidity or mortality. Indeed, inasmuch as 2.3 percent of the population must, by definition of the normal frequency distribution, exceed the upper limit by chance, it is inherently unreasonable to assume that all such individuals are biologically abnormal.

Furthermore, the assumption that individuals in whom the hematocrit is *less* than the arbitrary upper limit of normal are indeed biologically normal with regard to that parameter needs to be validated experientially as well. In point of fact, in a study of 100 consecutive blood volume measurements in the PVSG laboratory at Mount Sinai Hospital,[1] the red cell mass was abnormally elevated in approximately 35 percent of patients with hematocrits less than 54 percent, and red cell mass elevations were found 10 percent of the time when the hematocrit was 48 to 49 percent. Cornesco et al.[53] also found elevated red cell mass values in male patients with hematocrits as low as 49 percent. Based on such data, were we to establish a normal upper limit for hematocrit as that at which less than 2 percent of the population would have elevated red cell mass determinations, one might arrive at a value of 47 to 48 percent.

Such lower than traditional values have been reported by some investigators[41, 46, 49] for relatively homogeneous populations. One explanation for the variability in results may lie in the criteria according to which individual subjects are selected for inclusion in a purportedly normal population. Cigarette smokers have significantly higher hematocrit values than nonsmokers, and hematocrit also has been found to be significantly associated with blood pressure, serum cholesterol level, and body weight.[48] Although individuals who smoke and/or are hypertensive, obese, or hypercholesterolemic are certainly all too common, their inclusion in an "ideal" population surely is misleading. It seems likely that when these confounding variables are eliminated, normal hematocrit values are indeed probably lower than those usually expected.

How, then, should one define a hematocrit value beyond which a male patient not otherwise suspected as having absolute polycythemia could be considered, for purposes of further investigation, as having a relative polycythemia? Based on the reasoning cited above, and in the absence of a universally accepted criterion, I propose a consistently demonstrated value of 49 percent as the upper limit of "normal." Hematocrits in excess of 49 percent have been associated with increased morbidity, as, for example, in primary polycythemia, where there is a linear increase in occlusive vascular complications as the hematocrit increases from 49 to 54 percent.[54] By this criterion, approximately 15 percent of the general population might be suspect, a figure that is roughly comparable with the incidence of hypertension in the U.S. adult population.[55] However, it is anticipated that after the subsequent exclusion of patients with relative polycythemia shown to be secondary to smoking, hypertension, obesity, and/or intermittent hypoxemia, the incidence of truly idiopathic relative polycythemia would be vastly less.

CLINICAL AND LABORATORY FINDINGS

Patients with chronic relative polycythemia are usually younger than patients with PV. The mean age at diagnosis ranges from 45 to 53 years, in distinction to a mean age at diagnosis of 60 years for patients with PV.[21] Based on statistical considerations, an elevated hematocrit in excess of 2 standard deviations of the norm should occur in approximately 2.5 percent of the general population. The elevated hematocrit may likely revert to normal in about a third of this group and fluctuate between normal and abnormal in another third.[36] However, patients with abnormally elevated hematocrits may be encountered more frequently than predicted. About 8 percent of regular volunteer blood donors in Milan, Italy, had hematocrit values in the range of 49 to 54 percent. Of the 81 males so identified in this series, nearly 4 percent were found to have early-stage PV, and 11 percent had secondary erythrocytosis associated with respiratory failure. Only 2.5 percent were found to have relative polycythemia associated with a decreased plasma volume,[56] a lower incidence than that described by Pearson.[36] Therefore, sustained relative polycythemia may be expected to occur in approximately 0.5 to 0.7 percent of the "normal" male population. In contrast, in a high-risk group of 117 patients with thrombotic strokes, 10 patients (8.5 percent) had relative polycythemia and 6 patients had PV.[57] In another study of 200 male patients in a hypertension clinic, 44 had hematocrits in excess of 50 percent, but the actual incidence of relative polycythemia is not known.[58]

The incidence of relative polycythemia in women is uncertain. In the literature, the vast majority of patients have been male, with only 13 of 158 reported cases being women.[12,13,20,21,36] However, a higher incidence is suggested in a more recent series,[18] which identified 6 women in a total of 35 patients despite diagnostic criteria that limited the investigation to women in whom the hematocrit exceeded 50 percent. Women with relative polycythemia appear comparable to their male counterparts with respect to a high frequency of smoking, hypertension, and obesity.

The common presenting symptoms are nonspecific and include fatigue, lethargy, lightheadedness, headache, dizziness, dyspnea, palpitations, sweating, and epigastric distress.[20,21] These symptoms often convey an impression of a high state of anxiety or emotional stress and are reminiscent of Gaisbock's observation of frequent complaints attributed to nervous tension or neurasthenia.[9] A striking incidence of spurious polycythemia was noted in 39 of 78 consecutive patients complaining of premature ejaculation.[59] The absence of comparable sexual disturbances in patients with PV and a lack of improvement after phlebotomy suggested that the high hematocrit was not the cause of the premature ejaculation. As is the case in PV, joint pain with a history of gout often

occurs in relative polycythemia, but pruritus and weight loss are considerably less common, and a history of hemorrhagic diathesis is rare.[21] Paresthesias[21] and peripheral neuropathy[60] also have been reported. Symptomatology associated with vascular occlusive disease is particularly significant and includes angina pectoris, transient ischemic attacks, neurologic deficits related to cerebrovascular accidents,[57,61] deep vein thrombosis,[20] intermittent claudication,[20] ischemia of the hand,[62] and other manifestations of peripheral vascular disease.[18]

Family histories are frequently relevant regarding disclosure of hypertension, cardiac disease, and diabetes mellitus, and the occurrence of relative polycythemia in multiple relatives has been reported.[13,21] The overwhelming number of patients with relative polycythemia are cigarette smokers, and moderate to heavy alcohol use has sometimes been noted.[6,20] Medication histories are often positive with regard to diuretics (usually thiazides), particularly in hypertensive patients with relative polycythemia,[20,36] but the best evidence suggests that these medications are not a significant causative factor.[8]

The most common physical findings are plethora and conjunctival suffusion.[21] Flushing, however, is rarely proportional to the elevation in hematocrit and sometimes persists even after the hematocrit decreases.[13] Hepatomegaly is occasionally noted,[21] but palpable splenomegaly is practically never found. Obesity and hypertension are commonly observed, with hypertension more frequently associated with those patients in whom decreased plasma volume is found.

There are no characteristic laboratory abnormalities other than the elevated red cell concentration. Platelet counts, serum B_{12} levels, serum transcobalamin levels, and serum iron and transferrin concentrations are usually normal.[21] Mild leukocytosis (WBC 10,000 to 12,000/μl) has been reported in up to a third of patients.[20] This finding may be a reflection of the known association between leukocyte count and smoking[63,64] and may be of prognostic significance in view of the reported relationship between leukocyte count and incidence of myocardial infarction[65,66] and increased mortality risk.[67] Leukocyte alkaline phosphatase scores are generally normal,[20] although a tendency to high-normal values was reported in patients with hypovolemic relative polycythemia.[21] Hypercholesterolemia is a common finding,[21] but hyperuricemia is relatively infrequent.[20, 21] Bone marrow biopsies are almost always normal with respect to cellularity, megakaryocyte numbers, and reticulin staining.[21] Bone marrow karyotype abnormalities occur much less frequently than in PV.[21] A distinction between relative polycythemia and "benign erythrocytosis" is suggested by the finding of a relatively high percentage of chromosomal aberrations in the latter.[29]

PATHOPHYSIOLOGY

Hemodynamic and Clinical Effects of Hyperviscosity

Hemodynamic Effects of Short-Term Polycythemia

Explanations of the pathophysiologic mechanisms through which the usually modest hematocrit elevations found in patients with chronic relative polycythemia translate into clinically evident occlusive vascular disease generally emphasize the interrelationship between increased hematocrit, increased blood viscosity, decreased cardiac output, increased vascular resistance, sluggish blood flow, and impaired systemic oxygen supply. Under ideal experimental conditions, when arterial oxygen saturation, arterial blood pressure, and vascular hindrance are constant, the rate of tissue oxygen supply is proportional to the ratio of hematocrit and blood viscosity. Thus, as shown in resting, anesthetized dogs, systemic oxygen supply is maximal at an "optimal hematocrit" and falls with either anemia or polycythemia.[68–70] A similar bell-shaped curve may be generated in vitro using capillary viscometry to calculate theoretical oxygen transport.[71, 72] There is a striking similarity between the optimal hematocrits thus calculated and the normal observed hematocrit values for a variety of species, including humans, for whom the optimal hematocrit is 35 to 40 percent.[73]

The properties of a red cell suspension observed in a viscometer do not necessarily fully relate to flow in the vascular bed in vivo,[74–76] nor are findings in anesthetized animals, in whom peripheral resistance is abnormally high and reflexes blunted,[77] necessarily representative of normal physiology. Blood is not a newtonian fluid, and with the possible exception of large vessels with high

shear rates,[78] the relationships expressed in the Poiseuille equation cannot be applied precisely to hemorrheology. Blood viscosity is not only determined by hematocrit but also varies inversely with shear rate, which is a function of blood vessel diameter and flow rate.[71] Additional factors of significance in determining blood viscosity in the macrocirculation include mean erythrocyte size,[71, 79] erythrocyte flexibility,[80] erythrocyte aggregation, platelet aggregation, and plasma viscosity.[81] Blood flow in the microcirculation is even more complex, being subject to all the preceding influences as well as to the Fahreus effect,[82, 83] an apparent decrease in viscosity and effective hematocrit in capillary-sized vessels which ceases and reverses as the vessel diameter approaches that of the erythrocyte.[84] Red blood cell flow in capillaries is additionally influenced by physiologic stimuli that alter the number of red blood cells within capillaries by modifying interactions between plasma and one or more components on the luminal surface of capillaries.[85] Although flow velocity is high in many capillaries, low flow or stasis may be observed in capillary systems such as those of brain and muscle.[86]

Clearly, therefore, blood viscosity will have many different values in different parts of the vascular system, and it is reasonable to expect that the optimal hematocrit in regional circulations should be a function of local hemodynamic factors and metabolic activities. Thus the range of optimal hematocrit for maximum transport in pentobarbitolized dogs was found to be 40 to 60 percent in the systemic circulation but much wider (20 to 60 percent) in the coronary circulation due to differences in vasoconstrictive properties.[87] A transfusion-induced increase in hematocrit from 41 to 55 percent in thiopental-anesthetized dogs was associated with a 35 percent decrease in blood flow and a 35 percent increase in blood viscosity in resting skeletal muscle, but polycythemia was associated with only negligible changes in blood flow and viscosity in working muscle, an effect attributed to flow facilitation by rhythmic muscle contractions.[88] In hamster striated muscle, hemoconcentration to a hematocrit of 65 percent resulted in little change in tissue oxygenation.[89] However, abnormal increases in blood viscosity responsible for major perturbations in blood flow and oxygen transport may occur in areas of focal ischemia where blood vessel radius is maximal and pressure autoregulatory mechanisms are lost. Factors that increase the contained volume of veins decrease shear rate significantly. Reduction in venous perfusion pressure due to decreased capillary pressure or venous distension accompanying polycythemia would be expected to decrease shear rate and to increase viscosity and stagnation of flow.[86]

Several studies suggest that short-term normovolemic polycythemia may not be detrimental. Severe polycythemia induced in rats by both altitude exposure and cobalt administration had no effect on sea-level exercise performance except in association with severe hypoxia.[90] In conscious dogs trained to run on a treadmill, normovolemic polycythemia to hematocrits as high as 65 percent was associated with a linear decrease in cardiac output, but this was balanced by an increasing blood oxygen content resulting in constancy of systemic oxygen transport.[77] The fall in cardiac output, which was due entirely to a fall in stroke volume, was much less in these animals than had been reported in anesthetized animals, suggesting that despite impressive polycythemia, changes in in vivo viscosity were quite small. The mechanism of the decrease in cardiac output is uncertain, and a major question remains as to whether it is homeostasis of mean arterial pressure, systemic oxygen transport, a combination of these, or an undefined factor that modulates cardiac output with polycythemia.[77] Similar considerations appear to pertain to regulation of cerebral blood flow in polycythemia.[91]

Several studies suggest that short-term polycythemia may improve exercise performance in humans as well. The work capacity of 9 healthy, nontrained male volunteers was studied during a 3-week sojourn on Pike's Peak (4300 m), during which time mean hematocrit increased from 46 to 54 percent. Despite a significant decrease in cardiac output, increased oxygen-carrying capacity afforded by hemoconcentration contributed significantly to increased systemic oxygen transport and increased oxygen consumption, leading to the conclusion that relative polycythemia is a major contributor to increased work capacity.[92] In a study of 11 highly trained runners, maximum oxygen consumption and running time to exhaustion significantly improved after infusion of 900 ml of autologous, freeze-preserved red blood cells so that the hematocrit was increased from a mean of 44 to 49 percent.[93] Emphasizing that during exercise there are changes in blood vessel diameter, blood flow, temperature, and distribution of blood volume, the authors conclude that "in humans, the optimal hematocrit for oxygen delivery is not the commonly observed value of 45 percent, but some value in excess of this." However, later studies suggest that the magnitude of increase in hemoglobin concentration after transfusion-induced erythrocythemia is not related to the magnitude of increase in maximal oxygen uptake but that the degree of increase in oxygen uptake is related to the individual's aerobic fitness.[94, 95] In a recent study of triathletes, it was reported that lower hematocrit values correlate with excellent competition results, since the competitors' hematocrit values could be elevated more effectively during exercise if their precompetition values were in the low-normal range.[96]

The applicability of these studies of "optimal hematocrit" to an older population with preclinical or overt atherosclerotic cardiovascular and/or cerebrovascular disease is, of course, questionable. In such a clinical setting, there is a substantial body of evidence that chronic, sustained increases in hematocrit and blood viscosity are associated with increased morbidity and mortality from occlusive vascular complications.[73] However, epidemiologic evidence that increased hematocrit is an independent variable for cerebrovascular and cardiovascular occlusive events is less convincing.

Hyperviscosity and Cardiovascular Morbidity

Evidence that patients with increased hematocrit due to absolute polycythemia are at substantial risk for thromboembolic complications is legion. Among the polycythemic disorders, only patients with polycythemia secondary to high-oxygen-affinity hemoglobinopathies appear to have a low incidence of occlusive vascular lesions.[8] Patients with secondary pulmonary polycythemia have been considered to be at less risk as well, perhaps because of compensatory hypervolemia.[97, 98] However, in two series, death due to occlusive vascular disease in patients with pulmonary polycythemia occurred in 10 to 15 percent.[8] Coronary blood flow is markedly decreased in secondary polycythemia,[99] myocardial infarctions and cerebrovascular accidents occur in patients polycythemic from cyanotic heart disease,[100, 101] cerebral thrombosis associated with smoker's polycythemia has been reported,[102] and bilateral central retinal vein thrombosis has been described as an initial manifestation of polycythemia secondary to alveolar hypoventilation.[103] Vascular occlusive events are, of course, common in patients with PV[54, 104] and idiopathic (benign) erythrocytosis.[19, 29] The frequency of cerebrovascular accidents in PV relative to the incidence of coronary artery disease distinguishes the pattern of arterial involvement in PV from that of arteriosclerotic cardiovascular disease.[105] In both PV and idiopathic erythrocytosis, the frequency of vascular occlusive events is linearly related to the magnitude of the hematocrit, even when the hematocrit is within the normal to high-normal range.[19, 54] These findings support the hypothesis that the risk of vascular occlusion is enhanced by even modest increases in hematocrit and attendant increases in whole-blood viscosity.

There is considerable additional evidence favoring this hypothesis. Diabetics with vascular complications were found to have higher hematocrit and blood viscosity levels than diabetics without complications.[106] The highest level of hematocrit and blood viscosity was found in patients with proliferative retinopathy. Increased blood viscosity, which was partly attributable to increased plasma viscosity as well as to increased hematocrit, predated the onset of clinically detectable vascular disease. Increased blood viscosity is an important factor in reduction of blood flow and genesis of symptoms in patients with peripheral vascular disease and intermittent claudication[107–110] and substantially increases the risk of postoperative deep venous thrombosis.[111] Hemoconcentration was associated with increased red cell trapping in the microvasculature of the ischemic rat kidney leading to long-term kidney damage.[112] Patients with definite evidence of ischemic heart disease had significantly higher blood viscosity than those with peripheral arterial disease alone. Increased blood viscosity is reported in patients with angina pectoris.[113] In patients with angiographically proven multivessel coronary artery disease, whole-blood viscosity was reported elevated due both to increased hematocrit and increased fibrinogen concentration.[114] In all the preceding studies, differences could not be attributed to differential smoking patterns.

Hematocrit and blood viscosity are often higher in patients with hypertension than in normotensive subjects.[48, 115] Increased blood viscosity in hypertension is associated both with increased hematocrit and with increased plasma viscosity caused by hyperfibrinogenemia,[116] which is itself a significant cardiovascular risk factor.[117] Hypertensive cardiac hypertrophy, the presence of which identifies subjects at high risk of cardiovascular complications,[118] is closely related to rheologic abnormalities. A strong correlation was observed between blood viscosity at high shear rate and left ventricular mass assessed by echocardiography,[119] whereas only weak correlations were found between left ventricular mass and systolic or diastolic blood pressure. However, it is not yet known whether increased blood viscosity is a determinant of or a response to hypertensive cardiac hypertrophy.

Considering the preceding body of evidence, it might be anticipated that epidemiologic studies would be likely to identify the hematocrit as a significant determinant of risk in cardiovascular and cerebrovascular disease. In fact, however, these studies do not generally confirm the hypothesis that relatively minor increases in hematocrit play a significant role in the expression of coronary artery disease. On the other hand, as regards cerebrovascular disease, the epidemiologic evidence is somewhat more convincing.

Any discussion based on the epidemiology of cardiovascular disease must be prefaced with a comment concerning changing long-term trends in cardiovascular morbidity and mortality.[120, 121] During the past 25 years, the United States has experienced an impressive decline in the overall death rate for cardiovascular diseases. The causes of this decreased mortality are as yet unproven. A particularly remarkable reversal in the death rate for coronary artery disease in American men has occurred over the same time frame that a substantial increase in the male death rate for coronary artery disease was observed in many western European countries.[120] In women, on the other hand, there has been a consistent multinational decline in coronary heart disease mortality.[121] Stroke mortality, which began to decrease in the 1950s,[121] has continued to markedly decelerate since

1972.[120] It is still unknown whether the decline is due to fewer new cases or there has been a change in severity or prognosis. Furthermore, "no one has yet established a convincing fit of trends for *any* risk factor with cardiovascular mortality trends."[120] Thus an assessment of the importance of increased hematocrit as a current risk factor for occlusive vascular disease based on historical epidemiologic surveys dating back two decades must be regarded with considerable caution. A reassessment of the role of hematocrit as a cardiovascular risk factor in elderly men and women is currently a project of the Dutch Nutrition Surveillance System.[122]

The early results of the Framingham Study suggested that increased hemoglobin concentration was associated with an increased frequency of coronary artery disease.[123] This relationship, also reported by Burch and De Pasquale,[124] was postulated to be due to increased blood viscosity, particularly within vessels with sluggish flow.[125] The relationship between hematocrit values and coronary artery disease was questioned by Conley et al.,[47] who did not find the hematocrit, unless markedly elevated, to be a significant factor in predisposition to acute myocardial infarction. Findings from McDonough et al.,[48] who studied populations from Evans County, Georgia, and from North Carolina Memorial Hospital, failed to support an association between hematocrit and coronary artery disease. Furthermore, hematocrit did not appear to have an appreciable influence on coronary heart disease case fatality. Hershberg et al.,[126] on the other hand, did find, in accord with Burch and De Pasquale,[125] Mayer[127] and Stables et al.,[128] that myocardial infarction patients tended to have statistically significantly higher hematocrit values than controls when age and other disease patterns are comparable. However, hospitalized infarction patients with higher hematocrit values tended to have prognoses that were at least as favorable as those with lower hematocrit values. No deaths occurred in this series in patients who had hematocrit values of more than 50 percent, although the number of such patients was small. In a study of 6222 middle-aged men in the Multiple Risk Factor Intervention Trial, total *white* blood cell count was found to be strongly and significantly related to risk of coronary heart disease independent of smoking status.[67] In univariate analysis, he-

matocrit was found to be related to the incidence of coronary heart disease. However, in multivariate analysis, the hematocrit value was of borderline or no significance and appeared to correlate with the white blood count as a risk factor.[129] Similar findings were reported by Lowik.[122] In the Stockholm Prospective Study, there was an increased risk of myocardial infarction among men less than 60 years of age who were in the highest quintile of blood hemoglobin concentration.[130] However, only weak associations between either high hemoglobin concentration or hematocrit and the risk of coronary heart disease were reported in two other studies,[131, 132] and according to Salonen et al.,[133] there was no significant association between blood hemoglobin and hematocrit and the risk of acute myocardial infarction when serum ferritin was allowed for. There was, however, a relationship between serum ferritin concentration and the risk of acute myocardial infarction, even after controlling for blood hemoglobin and hematocrit.[133] The question of a clinically significant association between high-normal hematocrit values and coronary heart disease seems to be most fairly stated as weak at best.

Hyperviscosity and Cerebrovascular Morbidity

With regard to cerebrovascular disease, however, evidence that hematocrit elevation plays a significant pathophysiologic role appears substantial, although not unequivocal. In young adults, hemoconcentration resulting from ethanol-induced diuresis may be associated with a risk of ischemic brain infarction.[134] There is an up to three- to fourfold greater incidence of cerebrovascular accidents relative to coronary artery disease in patients with PV.[105] The incidence of stroke in male patients with relative polycythemia is also striking. By combining data from previously reported literature, 125 subjects followed for an average of 5 years were reviewed. Eleven patients suffered cerebrovascular accidents, corresponding to an incidence of 17.6 per 1000 per year. The incidence of thrombotic brain infarction in 2270 men followed for 12 years in the Framingham Study was approximately 1 per 1000 per year.[135] In other studies,[136, 137] the incidence of cerebrovascular accidents and/or cerebral infarction in men is 2 to 3.5 per 1000 person years. The incidence of cerebrovascular occlusive disease in patients with relative polycythemia is, historically, therefore, at least 5 to 8 times that expected.

With regard to the potential risk of high-normal red cell concentrations, in the Framingham Study,[138] men with hemoglobin values of 15 g/dl or greater and women with values of 14 g/dl or greater had twice as many cerebral infarctions as did their cohorts with lower values. Within the normal range of hemoglobin values, the risk was proportional to the blood hemoglobin concentration in both sexes. Multivariate regression analysis suggested that much of the apparent relationship between hemoglobin concentration and acute brain infarction is accounted for by other related factors, namely, coexisting hypertension and cigarette smoking. Ott et al.[139] found that both whole-blood viscosity values, particularly at low shear rates characteristic of areas of sluggish blood flow, and mean hematocrit were significantly higher in 50 patients with recent cerebral infarction of the carotid system compared with an age-matched control group. Because the hematocrit values for the patients with stroke remained within the normal range, the authors attributed the increase in blood viscosity to factors other than changes in red cell concentration. In point of fact, however, the observed increases in blood viscosity in their report correspond to those expected from the reported differences in hematocrit between the cerebral infarction and control group based on experimental hematocrit viscosity curves.[140]

In a study of 432 Japanese necropsy patients over age 60, Tohgi et al.[141] found that the risk of cerebral infarction increased steeply in the elderly population when hematocrit values exceeded 45 percent. The risk of cerebral infarction with high hematocrit values was augmented by severe atherosclerosis and advancing age. High hematocrit values caused more risk for infarctions in deep structures of the brain than in cortical areas. Similar small deep cerebral infarctions (lacunar infarcts) have indeed been described in patients with PV and relative polycythemia[142] and also were found to be specifically associated with higher hematocrit values in patients with systolic hypertension.[143] No significant difference between stroke subtypes was found in normotensive patients.[139] In a prospective study of 16 years'

duration, Kiyohara et al.[61] found that the risk of cerebral infarction was greatest in men whose hematocrits exceeded 45 percent. A similar, although less clearly defined trend was noted in women.

In counterpoint, in a Japanese population in which 60 percent of the subjects were younger than 60 years old, neither hemoglobin nor hematocrit was found to be a significant risk factor for cerebral infarction.[133] It should be pointed out, however, that the influence of other generally recognized risk factors such as obesity, smoking, and abnormal lipid metabolism also was small in this study. However, Ozaita et al.,[144] in a study of 131 cerebral infarction cases, failed to find that higher hematocrit was indicative of a less favorable short-term outcome, and Kiyohara[145] found no relationship between smoking status, which might be expected to be correlated with a higher hematocrit, and the incidence of nonembolic cerebral infarction.

Although the contribution of high-normal red cell concentrations to cerebrovascular morbidity in apparently healthy individuals is still unresolved, even mildly elevated hematocrit values are an aggravating influence in both experimental and clinical cerebral ischemia. In spontaneously hypertensive rats, metabolic evidence of cerebral ischemia following carotid ligation was more pronounced when the hematocrit exceeded 50 percent,[146] and infarction volume in ischemic gerbils[147] and cats[148] correlates with hematocrit elevation. In 187 patients with transient ischemic attacks and minor strokes who underwent carotid angiography, a hematocrit of 50 percent or more was more common in those found to have carotid occlusions, and in 23 patients with completed strokes, computed tomography measurements showed a correlation between the size of the infarct and the height of the hematocrit.[149] There is a clear correlation between hematocrit and blood velocity in the middle cerebral artery as measured by Doppler ultrasonography,[150] and in patients with unilateral cerebral infarction, decreases in Doppler shift frequency associated with increasing hematocrit were more pronounced than in age-matched, presumed healthy controls.[151] In 11 patients with ischemic neurologic deficits and normal hematocrits, isovolemic hemodilution was associated with increased cerebral blood flow and rapid improvement in background EEG activity.[152] A pilot study of hemodilution in acute stroke indicated that the size of handicap following stroke is reduced by hemodilution.[153] A multicenter trial of hemodilution in ischemic stroke was restricted to patients with hematocrit levels between 38 and 50 percent in deference to a body of opinion that all patients with ischemic stroke and polycythemia should be hemodiluted.[154]

It is commonly postulated that the association between increased hematocrit and cerebrovascular ischemic disease is a manifestation of the interplay between blood viscosity and cerebral blood flow. Recommendations that patients with most forms of polycythemia are optimally maintained at hematocrit levels below 45 percent are largely based on observations of an inverse correlation between hematocrit and cerebral blood flow.[8] Cerebral blood flow is low in PV and rises to normal after lowering the hematocrit by phlebotomy.[155] In patients with relative polycythemia, regardless as to whether of the idiopathic hypovolemic or of the high-normal red cell mass variant, initially low cerebral blood flow rises significantly to normal values following either venesection[156] or hemodilution with dextran infusion.[157] A decrease in hematocrit and whole-blood viscosity following phlebotomy treatment of polycythemic patients was associated with a small, albeit significant, increase in oxygen transport to the brain.[158] The relative infrequency of occlusive vascular events in polycythemic patients with high-oxygen-affinity hemoglobinopathy is attributed to "compensatory" increases in cerebral blood flow sufficient to counterbalance the negative effects of hyperviscosity.[159]

Currently, however, a major role for blood viscosity as an independent determinant in the control of cerebral blood flow, in the absence of overt cerebrovascular damage, is often questioned. In anesthetized normal cats, an inverse correlation between hematocrit and cerebral blood flow was found, but cerebral blood flow responses were smaller than previously reported data suggested.[160] In the newborn lamb, cerebral blood flow decreases, and hematocrit, whole-blood viscosity, and arterial oxygen content increase following hypertransfusion. When arterial oxygen content was reduced by infusion of sodium nitrite, cerebral blood flow returned to normal values even though both the hematocrit and viscosity remained elevated. The reduction in cerebral blood flow in neonatal

polycythemia is therefore a physiologic response to increased arterial oxygen content rather than a result of hyperviscosity.[161] However, in a study of 7-day-old sheep rendered polycythemic by transfusion with either oxyhemoglobin-containing or methemoglobin-containing red blood cells, approximately 60 percent of the attendant fall in cerebral blood flow observed was attributed to the increase in red cell concentration alone.[162] Subsequently, it was demonstrated that there is no satisfactory single description of the effect of viscosity on cerebral blood flow. Rather, the effect of viscosity is contingent on baseline fractional oxygen extraction—that is to say, the ratio of oxygen demand to supply, which determines the intensity of homeostatic vasodilatation that occurs in response to perturbations of local oxygen availability.[163]

In humans, Paulson et al.[164] and Henriksen et al.[165] also found that low cerebral blood flow in patients with high hematocrits was determined primarily by increased oxygen availability rather than by increased blood viscosity. Mathew[166] also reported that in normal subjects, hematocrit was found to exert only minimal influence on the control of resting cerebral blood flow. Contrary to previous results,[167] in patients with high blood viscosity secondary to paraproteinemia or leukemia, changes in cerebral blood flow were significantly related to changes in arterial oxygen content but not to changes in blood viscosity.[168] Finally, in a study of 54 subjects with a very wide range of hemoglobin concentrations,[91] but excluding subjects with established cerebrovascular disease, multiple regression analysis identified arterial oxygen content as the major determinant of cerebral blood flow. There was no significant influence of blood viscosity, arterial P_{CO_2}, age, or mean arterial blood pressure. Therefore, the alterations in cerebral blood flow in patients with anemia and polycythemia are primarily physiologic.

Accordingly, in normal circumstances, regulatory mechanisms maintain normal cerebral oxygen transport despite increased plasma and whole-blood viscosity. In patients with cerebrovascular disease, however, physiologic regulatory mechanisms may be impaired[169,170] and vasodilatory reserve exhausted. If vessels are maximally dilated, then flow rates will be solely dependent on local pressure gradients and blood viscosity.[154] The deleterious effect of loss of auto-regulatory control is manifested in patients with multi-infarct dementia. Decreased cerebral blood flow preceded the onset of symptoms by 2 years with a consequent substantial increase in the risk of cerebral infarction.[171] An impairment in vasomotor adjustment was demonstrated in 27 patients with ischemic cerebrovascular disease, in whom hematocrit values ranged from 31 to 53 percent.[172] Cerebral oxygen delivery increased with hematocrit elevation, reached a maximum when the hematocrit was 40 to 45 percent, and then declined. The relationship of hematocrit to cerebral blood flow and oxygen transport was therefore analogous to that described in vitro in glass-tube models rather than to results observed in vivo, confirming the predicted loss of physiologic regulation in patients with cerebrovascular disease.

In summary, then, although there is ample clinical evidence that overt polycythemia, either absolute or relative, significantly increases the likelihood of thrombotic vascular complications and there is, at least, suggestive evidence that even a high-normal hematocrit may be a risk factor for occlusive vascular disease, proof that increased red cell concentration and resultant hyperviscosity are major determinants of clinical events, independent of other physiologic abnormalities and regulatory derangements, remains forthcoming. As an example, patients with hypovolemic relative polycythemia appear to be particularly at risk for occlusive vascular complications,[20, 21] although they differ not at all with respect to hematocrit from patients with normovolemic relative polycythemia, in whom morbidity and mortality seem much less pronounced.[21] Consequently, a potential role for hypovolemia as a significant determinant of the clinical manifestations of relative polycythemia also deserves examination.

Hemodynamic and Clinical Effects of Hypovolemia

Hemodynamic: Blood Volume and Blood Flow in Polycythemia

The significance of blood volume as a parameter determining systemic blood flow in polycythemic patients is reviewed in detail by Chien and Gallik (Chapter 10) in this volume.[81] Potential decreases in cardiac output

and systemic blood flow occasioned by increased blood viscosity in polycythemia are usually counterbalanced by a compensatory increase in blood volume (Fig. 18–1). Cardiac output is directly proportional to systemic blood pressure and inversely proportional to the peripheral resistance, which is itself directly proportional to blood viscosity and vascular hindrance. As the hematocrit increases, blood viscosity increases. If the blood volume simultaneously increases, as expected, the resulting vasodilatation is associated with a decrease in vascular hindrance and a restoration of total peripheral resistance toward normal baseline values. Blood flow in the microcirculation and venous return are facilitated, and stroke volume and cardiac output increase. Therefore, at a given hematocrit, cardiac output is directly related to blood volume, and oxygen transport is greater in hypervolemic polycythemia than in normovolemic polycythemia.

It follows, therefore, that in hypovolemic hemoconcentration, increases in peripheral resistance associated with hyperviscosity are not ameliorated by compensatory mechanisms but rather are exaggerated by vasoconstriction and increased vascular hindrance with a resulting decrease in systemic blood flow. Consequently, a sustained state of hypovolemic polycythemia must be accompanied by some combination of decreased cardiac output and/or increased systemic

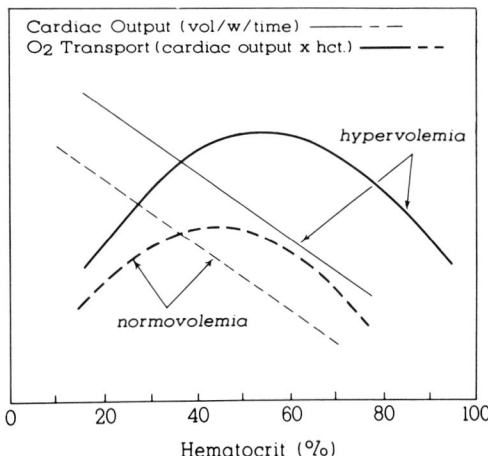

FIGURE 18–1. Effect of blood volume on systemic oxygen transport and cardiac output as functions of hematocrit. (*Reprinted with permission from Erslev AJ, Gabuzda TG: Pathophysiology of hematologic disorders. In Sodeman and Sodeman (eds): Pathologic Physiology: Mechanism of Disease, 5th ed. Philadelphia, WB Saunders Co, 1974, p 532.*)

blood pressure. In these circumstances, low blood flow potentiates hyperviscosity by reducing shear rates in the microvasculature, and increased transcapillary fluid loss secondary to elevated capillary hydrostatic pressure and the effect of atrial natriuretic peptide[173] may further adversely affect the plasma volume, thus creating a vicious circle that serves to perpetuate or even aggravate the abnormal hemodynamics. The expected clinical outcome of such altered hemodynamics would be a propensity for occlusive vascular disease, particularly when preexisting anatomic abnormalities render regional autoregulation inoperative. For example, cerebral small-vessel vasoconstriction induced in normal volunteers by graded lower body negative pressure (a model that reproduces the physiologic effects of hypovolemia) was felt to interfere with the autoregulatory response to a sudden fall in blood pressure and be a possible explanation for the common observation of neurologic deficit during hypovolemia even with a normal blood pressure.[174]

Abnormal hemodynamics, including decreased cardiac output and increased total peripheral resistance, were described in 11 patients with idiopathic hypovolemia, a syndrome associated with labile hypertension and orthostatic intolerance.[175] Symptoms were alleviated by volume expansion with a high-salt diet and long-term Florinef treatment. Hematocrit elevation was not reported in these patients, who also differ from patients with hypovolemic relative polycythemia in their favorable response to Florinef. Patients with relative polycythemia failed to respond to a 2-week course of fludrocortisone therapy.[176]

Hypovolemia and Hypertension

Evidence further supporting a role for hypovolemia in the pathophysiology of relative polycythemia may be adduced from observations in hypertensive patients. When hypertensives with elevated cardiac output and normal peripheral resistance are compared with age- and sex-matched patients with higher resistance and lower cardiac output, a significantly greater degree of concentric cardiac hypertrophy is observed in the group with increased resistance.[119] Plasma volume contraction, which is commonly observed in hypertensive patients, tends to be more pronounced with higher blood pressure and with higher peripheral resistance.[177,178] Obese, hypertensive patients are generally

found to have an expanded blood volume and elevated cardiac output compared with their lean counterparts, in whom raised total peripheral vascular resistance and contracted intravascular volume are characteristic.[179] In a population of 1727 men followed for 9 years, age-adjusted, all-cause cardiovascular and ischemic heart disease mortality rates were highest in the lean hypertensive subjects, suggesting that, in the presence of hypertension, obesity might be protective by virtue of its favorable influence on blood volume and peripheral resistance.[180] Similarly, it was proposed that mild obesity may protect a given patient from the deleterious effects of hypertension with regard to nephrosclerosis and cerebrovascular disease.[181] Significant hypovolemia, on the other hand, when associated with decreased cardiac output and increased peripheral resistance, thus emerges as a potential major determinant of increased risk for vascular occlusive disease.

A role for elevated blood pressure, independent of associated rheologic abnormalities, in the pathogenesis of vascular occlusive morbidity in relative polycythemia is less certain. Although even mild hypertension is associated with substantial morbidity and mortality in patients with relative polycythemia,[21] in a series of 23 patients with hypovolemic relative polycythemia, only 1 of 6 deaths occurred in patients who previously had been hypertensive.[20] Furthermore, in hypertensive disease, the level of blood pressure correlates only weakly with the incidence of cardiac hypertrophy, whereas the correlation with rheologic and hemodynamic abnormalities is much stronger.[119]

Increased plasma renin concentrations have been noted in some patients with hypovolemic relative polycythemia and hypertension,[182,183] prompting the suggestion that renin-associated vasculotoxicity may contribute to the observed increases in cardiovascular morbidity. Although there are extensive data suggesting that very high levels of renin are vasculotoxic,[184] the hypothesis that the renin mechanism may be implicated in the pathogenesis of vascular complications such as strokes or heart attacks in patients with essential hypertension with normal or mild increases in plasma renin activity[185] has not been generally accepted as proven.[186] Other potential pathogenetic mechanisms cited in patients with essential hypertension that might be of significance in patients with relative polycythemia include structural and biochemical changes in small blood vessels,[187,188] excessive central nervous system–mediated stimulation of the autonomic sympathetic system,[189] abnormalities in the vascular wall renin-angiotensin system,[190] and abnormalities in atrial natriuretic peptides.[191] Atrial natriuretic peptides (ANPs) also have been shown to play an important physiologic role during hypovolemia[192] and are at least one of the factors involved in hemoconcentration and hematocrit elevation associated with exercise.[193] Levels of ANPs and both basal and postexercise hematocrit levels increased significantly after administration of propranolol.[189] Infusion of ANPs in hypovolemic sheep is associated with decreased cardiac output and stroke volume,[194] findings commonly observed in chronically hypovolemic patients.[81] The effects of ANPs on hematocrit and blood volume appear to be independent of the effects of ANPs on blood pressure,[195,196] suggesting that ANPs may play a role even in normotensive patients with hypovolemic relative polycythemia. Additional mediator substances that may play a role in relative polycythemia include endothelin, whose effects appear to be modulated by ANPs,[192] and neurotensin and the related peptides neuromedin-N and xenopsin, which are potent stimulators of mast cell–mediated release of leukotrienes. IV injection of neurotensin in anesthetized rats produced a marked increase in hematocrit, labored breathing, and peripheral blood stasis.[197] Tissue plasminogen activator (t-PA) levels are significantly increased in patients with both spurious and secondary polycythemia, in contrast to patients with PV, in whom t-PA levels are decreased.[198] The extent to which these various mechanisms and substances are operative in relative polycythemia and serve to modify or augment the basic rheologic and hemodynamic derangements attributable to the interplay among altered blood viscosity, plasma volume, peripheral resistance, and systemic and regional blood and oxygen transport is a subject for continued investigation.

CLASSIFICATION AND ETIOLOGY

Classification

A proposed classification of chronic relative polycythemia into idiopathic and secondary categories based on etiologic considerations is presented in Fig. 18–2. Patients with relative polycythemia are initially divided into two subclasses: (1) those in whom a combination of high-normal red cell mass and normal or low-normal plasma volume creates an apparent polycythemia, and (2) those in whom the red cell mass is clearly not elevated, and hemoconcentration is attributed to an absolute decrease in plasma volume. It must be emphasized that the parametric criteria formulated to define these categories are, of necessity, arbitrary and are perhaps best

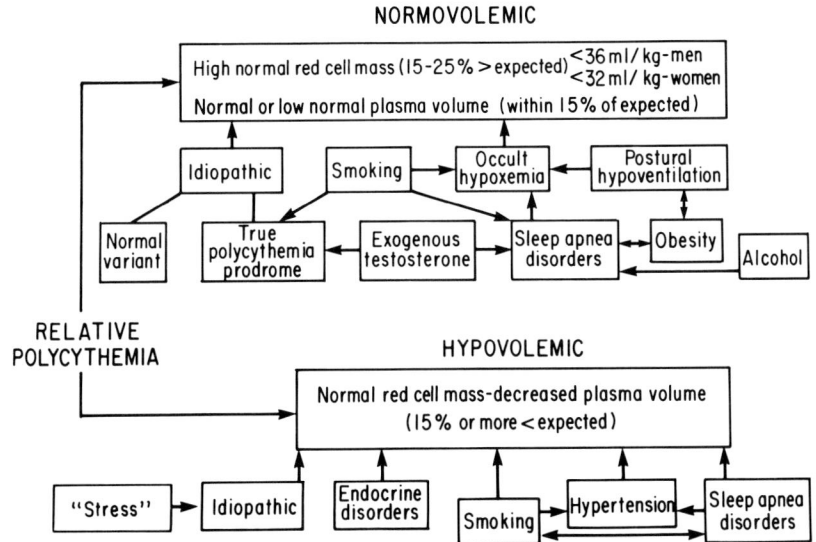

FIGURE 18–2. Classification of chronic relative polycythemia demonstrating potential etiologic interactions.

suited, as was indeed the intention in the formulation of the PVSG criteria, for defining unequivocal patient groupings for investigative purposes. An overly rigid application of these criteria in the clinical setting, ignoring the potential for overlapping circumstances, could be misleading, particularly when extended to prognostication. Thus, in defining the upper limits of red cell mass, beyond which conditions of absolute, rather than relative, polycythemia pertain, I have retained the PVSG criteria but also have incorporated those proposed by Wetherly-Mein, which are more accurately applied in obese patients. Furthermore, it should be noted that etiologic factors such as smoking and sleep apnea disorders may be of importance, via different mechanisms, in both subclasses. Lastly, a conclusion that polycythemia in any individual patient is secondary to a suspected etiology must be sustained by demonstrating a restoration of the blood count to normal when that factor is corrected or abolished.

Normovolemic Relative Polycythemia

Relative polycythemia associated with high-normal red cell mass and normal or low-normal plasma volume (normovolemic relative polycythemia) may be either idiopathic or secondary to conditions associated with intermittent hypoxemia, with the red cell mass increasing in response to oxygen deprivation yet not to levels of absolute erythrocytosis. The idiopathic category includes those patients previously described as "odd men out,"[17] the extreme normal variants,[14] but also includes patients destined to develop some type of unequivocal polycythemia who are passing through this apparent phase.[8] The ultimate status of these patients will be clear only after a perhaps lengthy period of observation. Although bone marrow karyotyping may disclose a cohort of patients in this category who are more likely to develop overt polycythemia,[29] the expense of this procedure and the absence of any known immediate therapeutic relevance suggest that it is best confined to a research, rather than to a standard, setting. The observation of spontaneous erythroid colony formation in the absence of erythropoietin should distinguish those patients in this group who will later develop clinically evident PV.[199] Reticuloendothelial scintigraphy, using the parameters of pelvic bone marrow activity, bone marrow extension, and splenic size, also can help in the discrimination of patients with PV from those with secondary or relative polycythemia.[200]

Smoking

Among the factors believed significant in the etiology of secondary normovolemic relative polycythemia, smoking may be preeminent. Smoking is additionally associated with plasma volume abnormalities and is therefore felt to be an important factor in the genesis of hypovolemic relative polycythemia as well. The vast majority of patients with relative polycythemia described in the literature have been smokers of either cigarettes or cigars.[201] Positive statistical correlations between hematocrit and cigarette consumption have been observed frequently,[202–204] even in the absence of impaired pulmonary function.[205] The hematocrits of blood donors who smoke are significantly higher than those of nonsmoking donors.[206] Cigarette smokers have a higher blood viscosity and fibrinogen concentration than nonsmokers,[207] and heavy smoking induces in otherwise healthy subjects under 30 years of age a distinct decrease in blood fluidity equal to that found in patients with chronic arterial occlusive disease.[208] Increases in hematocrit and hemoglobin in smokers relative to nonsmokers have been observed even in young adolescent women.[64] A failure to note a similar correlation in young adolescent men was felt to be attributable to a lower smoking rate in the male subjects compared with the female subjects. Absolute polycythemia secondary to cigarette and cigar smoking is now well recognized.[197,209,210]

The increase in hematocrit associated with smoking is caused by either an increase in red cell mass, a decrease in plasma volume, or some combination thereof.[206] Smoking-induced carboxyhemoglobinemia reduces the oxygen-carrying capacity of blood by as much as 30 percent,[206] presenting a significant hypoxic stimulus for erythropoiesis. Functional hypoxemia may be compounded by the left shift in the hemoglobin oxygen dissociation curve observed in carboxyhemoglobinemia,[197] although the clinical significance of this latter phenomenon has been questioned.[205] A possible further effect of smoking on bone marrow control was postulated to explain an increase in leukocyte and platelet count noted in adolescent smokers.[64]

Although it has been stated that the elevated hematocrit values in smokers appear to result from an increase in red cell mass rather than from decreased plasma volume,[97] reduced plasma volume was observed in 14 of 18 patients with smokers polycythemia, and rapid changes in hematocrit, attributable to plasma volume shifts, have been noted in nonpolycythemic college students after even first exposure to smoking.[197] Cessation of smoking restores the plasma volume to normal. The mechanism by which smoking decreases the plasma volume is uncertain. A direct effect of carbon monoxide was suggested by rapid increases in hematocrit observed in volunteers exposed to low concentrations of carbon monoxide gas,[211] but in contrast, significant changes in plasma volume were not observed in rats chronically exposed to increasing carbon monoxide concentrations.[212] Another postulate is that nicotine induces release of catecholamines,[213] resulting in chronically increased sympathetic tone, vasoconstriction, increased peripheral resistance and transcapillary pressure, with consequent increased transudation of intravascular fluid, leading to a decrease in plasma volume. Elevation in circulating catecholamines is also suspected as the cause for white blood cell count elevation in smokers, a phenomenon that has been correlated with increased risk of myocardial infarction.[65] Smoking is accompanied by a 20 percent increase in average heart rate and a 45 percent rise in urinary excretion of norepinephrine, with an increase in 24-hour energy expenditure of approximately 10 percent.[214] Cigarette-induced stimulation of energy expenditure ceases by the morning after a day of smoking,[210] and restoration of plasma volume and decrease in hematocrit may occur within 2 to 3 days of cessation of smoking.[197]

In light of the preceding, it is clear that the evaluation of any polycythemic patient should include a methodical smoking history, including details concerning frequency, amount, and inhalation patterns. Venous blood carboxyhemoglobin should be measured, preferably at the end of the day.[197] Nonsmoking status may be confirmed by measurement of serum thiocyanate concentration,[215] a procedure that may be useful in the initial evaluation of polycythemic patients claiming to be nonsmokers and in smokers in whom polycythemia fails to regress after alleged abstention from smoking.

Postural Hypoxemia and Sleep Apnea

Smoking, of course, may exacerbate coexisting respiratory disorders, which, of and by themselves, even in the absence of smoking may contribute to the development of normovolemic or hypovolemic relative polycythemia. Relative polycythemia, as well as true erythrocytosis, has been described in association with both postural hypoxemia and sleep apnea syndromes. When, as is often the case, these disorders are accompanied by hypertension, contracted plasma volume is frequently found as well. Obesity, which is frequently noted in patients with relative polycythemia, is also a common and contributing finding in patients with postural hypoxemia and sleep apnea. Ward et al.[216] described 7 patients with unexplained erythrocytosis, moderate obesity, and mild hypertension without splenomegaly in whom routine pulmonary studies were normal, but significant arterial hypoxemia was demonstrated in the supine position. Plasma volumes were generally decreased. Although 6 patients had absolute increases in red cell mass, and only 1, therefore, had relative polycythemia, all were residents of Denver, Colorado, and the ambient altitude of 5300 ft may have contributed to the absolute erythrocytosis. Nocturnal oxygen therapy and weight reduction restored the elevated hematocrit to the normal range. Similar patients with relative polycythemia, marked plasma hypovolemia, smoking history, hypertension, mild obesity, and supine hypoxemia were reported by Hamosh et al.[217] Hypoxemia is believed to be caused by abnormal expiratory airway closure with ventilation/perfusion mismatching and right-to-left shunting. Supine hypoxemia may occur frequently in elderly individuals but may be provoked in younger patients by smoking.[213]

The sleep apnea syndrome is now widely recognized and is thought to affect perhaps 1 percent of adults.[218] As in patients with relative polycythemia, patients with sleep apnea are usually male, frequently hypertensive and obese, and at significant risk for vascular occlusive disease. Habitual snoring, one of the hallmarks of the sleep apnea syndrome, is significantly associated with increased incidence of angina pectoris in men[219] and increased risk of cerebral infarction.[220] Other characteristic symptoms include daytime sleepiness, morning headaches, personality changes, and sexual dysfunction,[221] symptoms reminiscent of those described in patients with "stress erythrocytosis."[12] Sleeping is punctuated by loud, sonorous snoring and grunting, interrupted by apneic periods of as long as 1 to 2 minutes occurring several times an hour. Subjects may have nocturnal cardiac arrhythmias, significant hypoxemia, and transient arterial and pulmonary hypertension during sleep.[222] Abnormal upper airways with floppy pharyngeal walls and pharyngeal narrowing are common[214] but not invariable.[223]

Many patients with sleep apnea have either relative or absolute erythrocytosis. Evidence for this syndrome should be sought in patients with unexplained erythrocytosis, and inquiries concerning sleepiness, sleep patterns, and snoring should be part of routine history taking when evaluating polycythemic patients. If possible, the spouse should be questioned as well. If sleep apnea is suspected, polysomnography should be performed. For example, severe sleep breathing disorders and nocturnal oxygen desaturation were documented by polysomnography in 10 of 15 patients with heretofore unclassified erythrocytosis,[224] and prolonged nocturnal hypoxemia was demonstrated in 5 of 20 patients with unexplained polycythemia.[225] It is likely that patients with "Gaisbock syndrome" associated with decreased rapid eye movement (REM) sleep time[226] may have had an associated sleep respiratory disorder. The possibility of sleep breathing disorders should be considered even in asymptomatic patients with relative polycythemia, since otherwise asymptomatic, mildly to moderately obese men may have frequent, unsuspected breathing abnormalities during sleep, accompanied by arterial oxygen desaturation.[227] In one survey of 1000 moderately obese patients without significant lung diseases, 7 percent had evidence of polycythemia.[228]

Although the pathogenesis of relative polycythemia and true erythrocytosis in sleep apnea syndromes is most commonly related to hypoxic stimulation of erythropoiesis and increased red cell mass, other mechanisms may be operative as well. Androgenic male sex hormones promote obstructive

sleep apnea as well as polycythemia,[217] and sleep apnea and polycythemia have been induced by the exogenous administration of testosterone to a previously normal volunteer.[229] Alcohol increases the frequency and severity of sleep apnea, a phenomenon that may explain the occasional case reports of alcohol-induced erythrocytosis,[6, 230] as well as increased risk of ischemic brain infarction in adolescents and young adults associated with acute ethanol intoxication.[130] Hypovolemic relative polycythemia associated with sleep apnea may be related to the extraordinary incidence of hypertension in patients with sleep breathing disturbances, although acute hypoxemia itself can cause even marked decreases in plasma volume.[42, 231] Sustained systemic hypertension is seen in up to 90 percent of patients with the sleep apnea syndrome due, in part, to increased sympathetic discharge.[232] Sustained hypertension is frequently associated with plasma volume contraction and may play a major role in the etiology of hypovolemic relative polycythemia, as will be described below.

In summary, then, intermittent, occult hypoxemia appears to be the common final cause for secondary normovolemic relative polycythemia.[233] Contributory conditions that are often simultaneously present and mutually additive include smoking, postural hypoventilation, sleep breathing disorder, obesity, and possibly ethanol ingestion and excess androgenic stimulation. Some of these factors also may bring about plasma volume contraction and may therefore be relevant to the pathogenesis of hypovolemic relative polycythemia as well.

Hypovolemic Relative Polycythemia and Hypertension

Chronic hypovolemic relative polycythemia is either idiopathic or secondary to hypertension. As discussed earlier, smoking and sleep apnea syndromes also can induce plasma volume contraction, often in conjunction with hypertensive mechanisms. In a sense, even the decreased plasma volume associated with essential hypertension may be regarded as idiopathic, inasmuch as essential hypertension is itself a disorder of still uncertain etiology and ill-understood pathophysiology.[234]

As previously indicated (see pathophysiology), hematocrit and blood viscosity are positively correlated with diastolic blood pressure,[48,115] and multiple studies have demonstrated an increase in hematocrit associated with hypertension.[235-238] Plasma volume is significantly lower in hypertensive patients than in normotensive subjects, with the exception of renoprival hypertension, hypertension associated with acute glomerulonephritis, and hypertension in primary hyperaldosteronism, where expanded plasma volume is common.[173] The decrease in plasma volume in patients with uncomplicated hypertension is significantly more pronounced during and following exercise, suggesting an exaggerated and protracted sympathetic pressor effect in the hypertensive patients that causes increased transudation of plasma water into the extravascular space with a decrease in plasma volume and an increase in hematocrit, viscosity, and plasma protein level.[115] Despite increasing arterial blood pressure and increased total and renal vascular resistance associated with the contracted plasma volume, the increase in hematocrit in essential hypertension is not associated with an increase in red cell mass, which remains normal and stable until other complications ensue.[174]

Hypovolemic relative polycythemia associated with essential hypertension is often reversed with successful antihypertensive therapy, and previously low plasma volumes are restored to normal.[178] In 14 patients with relative polycythemia and essential hypertension, 4 weeks of therapy with α-methyldopa achieved a reduction in blood pressure associated with expansion of plasma volume and significant decreases in hematocrit, blood viscosity, and plasma renin activity.[179] Similarly, when prazosin successfully lowered the blood pressure level, blood viscosity was reduced largely because of hemodilution.[116] On the other hand, beta blockers such as propranolol, which appear to promote sensitivity to ANPs and decrease plasma volume and increase hematocrit,[192] might not be agents of choice for hypertensive patients with relative polycythemia. A theoretical role for calcium-channel blockers is also uncertain. Following sublingual administration of nifedipine, hematocrit, hemoglobin, and serum albumin concentration increased significantly, suggesting a decrease in plasma volume.[239] However, in patients with angina pectoris, hematocrit and blood viscosity at high shear rates were unaffected by nifedipine administration, but at low shear rates, blood viscosity and oxygen delivery were significantly increased.[240]

Why, then, if essential hypertension is so frequently associated with a contraction of plasma volume is it that most patients with essential hypertension do not have relative polycythemia? A number of possible answers come to mind. Decreases in plasma volume in essential hypertension are generally apparent only in those patients with moderately severe increases in blood pressure. Plasma volume contraction was not noted unless the diastolic blood pressure exceeded 100 to 105 mmHg,[173,174] suggesting that significant changes in plasma volume are not likely in the majority of the population with essential hypertension. The magnitude of plasma volume decrease in patients with even severe essential hypertension is usually relatively modest, generally less than 15 percent.[172,173] Assuming a normal body/venous hematocrit of 0.9 and a normal red cell mass of 28 ml/kg, even a plasma volume reduction of 15 percent would not be associated with a venous hematocrit greater than 51 to 52 percent, and polycythemia would not usually be suspected. Of course, if the body/venous hematocrit ratio is abnormally low, as has been reported in some patients with relative polycythemia,[18,32] smaller reductions in plasma volume would eventuate in larger hematocrit increases. Indeed, when body/venous hematocrit ratio is calculated for the 14 hypertensive patients with relative polycythemia reported by Chrysant et al.,[179] the mean value of 0.84 appears significantly lower than the normal value of 0.9 and similar to that reported by Watts et al.[18] in 10 hypertensive patients with relative polycythemia. The abnormality of the body/venous hematocrit ratio most likely reflects an abnormal distribution of red cells in the circulation, with a decrease in compliance of the venous system and a shift of blood toward the central region. Such an increase in resting venous tone and reduced venous distensibility has indeed been described in patients with hypovolemic relative polycythemia.[241] Abnormalities in venous compliance and elevated central venous pressure also have been observed in patients with essential hypertension in association with raised circulating levels of atrial natriuretic peptides.[187] Plasma volume contraction might tend to be perpetuated and exaggerated in these subjects, leading to overt manifestations of relative polycythemia. In this context, it is of interest that venous distensibility is decreased in some normotensive subjects with a family history of hypertension.[242] Venous distensibility is altered by high salt intake, but only in susceptible individuals.[243] Susceptibility to decreased venous distension and increased venous tone could define a population of hypertensive patients more likely to develop relative polycythemia.

Other than hypertension and its associated pathophysiologic derangements, no other mechanism is clearly proven to explain the diminution in plasma volume in hypovolemic relative polycythemia. Alcohol was proposed as a possible etiologic factor primarily on the basis of its ability to inhibit release of antidiuretic hormone.[6] Decreased nocturnal antidiuretic hormone-like activity with nocturnal water loss also has been postulated.[222] Plasma histamine, diurnal plasma cortisol, urinary hydroxycorticosteroids, and urine catecholamines were within normal limits in 2 patients with "Gaisbock syndrome."[222] Reduced aldosterone secretion, particularly after salt restriction, was reported in patients with relative polycythemia.[244] However, it is now known that such a response might be anticipated in 40 to 50 percent of the normal and high-renin essential hypertensive population who are termed *nonmodulators* because their adrenal and renal vascular responses to angiotensin II are not modified by changes in sodium intake.[245] A subsequent therapeutic trial of fludrocortisone did not accomplish an increase in plasma volume in patients with relative polycythemia.[153]

In summary, then, the etiology of the lowered plasma volume in hypovolemic relative polycythemia is still largely uncertain due to the number of systems that contribute to blood volume regulation: hormonal, vascular, renal, peripheral, and/or central adrenergic, and to the complex way in which these systems interact. There appears to be a close connection with abnormalities associated with essential hypertension, and control of hypertension may, in some circumstances, restore the plasma volume to normal and abolish the relative polycythemia.

TREATMENT

Based on the cumulative published experience heretofore cited, there seems little doubt that life expectancy is shortened and morbidity from vascular occlusive disease is heightened in some patients with chronic relative polycythemia, with particular risk extended to hypovolemic and hypertensive subjects.[20, 21] It is not at this time certain, however, whether this prediction of increased risk, based on historical observations 15 to 40 years old, may not require modification, given the impressive overall nationwide decline in cardiovascular and stroke mortality in the last 20 years.[120] Moreover, it is not yet evident to what extent the elevated hematocrit is an independent risk variable in relative polycythemia minus the confounding influences of smoking, hypertension, and obesity, which are themselves among the most highly prevalent major cardiovascular risk factors. In the absence of such information, the formulation of a therapeutic strategy becomes somewhat empirical.

It is certainly clear that relative polycythemia is not a primary hematologic disorder, and there is no evidence for uncontrolled erythroid proliferation. For this reason, myelosuppressive radiotherapy and/or cytotoxic chemotherapy is contraindicated in patients with relative polycythemia, being both scientifically senseless and potentially harmful. Ideally, therapy should be directed at underlying causes such as smoking, hypertension, obesity, and intermittent hypoxemia, to which relative polycythemia is often secondary. However, when such an approach is unsuccessful or untenable, usually due to patient noncompliance, or in those instances when, despite a methodical search for secondary causes, relative polycythemia is truly idiopathic, a venesection program may at times be advisable.

Modification of Lifestyle

There is little question that cessation of smoking is associated with normalization of hematocrit in patients with relative polycythemia.[197] The effect of smoking on catecholamine activity, vasomotor tone, platelet thrombus formation, and arterial endothelium indicate unequivocally that its elimination would be one great advance toward reducing cardiovascular morbidity and mortality.[121] The risk of myocardial infarction in cigarette smokers decreases within a few years of quitting to a level similar to that in men who have never smoked,[246] and even among subjects who already have coronary artery disease, stopping smoking markedly improves survival.[247] Cessation of smoking should be a constantly reinforced goal for all patients with relative polycythemia.

Correction of hypertension with antihypertensive medication also has been associated with normalization of the hematocrit in relative polycythemia.[116, 179] Hypertension in these patients is frequently severe,[179] and there is little doubt that control of severe hypertension reduces cardiovascular and cerebrovascular mortality. The importance of control of mild to moderate hypertension continues to be controversial, with some contending that the risk of pharmacotherapy outweighs the uncontrolled risk.[121] However, although some question whether control of hypertension reduces coronary mortality, it has been unequivocally demonstrated that morbidity and mortality from stroke and congestive heart failure are distinctly improved.[120] In planning antihypertensive regimens in patients with relative polycythemia, avoidance of diuretics has been advised.[248] Evidence now suggests that diuretics usually produce only a transient, unsustained, minimal increase in hematocrit and are therefore not necessarily contraindicated in patients with relative polycythemia.[8] A single dose of intravenous furosemide decreases venous resistance, lowers capillary hydrostatic pressure, and increases colloid osmotic pressure, replenishing intravascular volume at a rate equal to or in excess of the volume removed by diuresis.[249] This action of furosemide directly opposes the pathophysiologic abnormalities found in hypertensive patients with relative polycythemia. The effects of agents such as α-methyldopa, prazosin, beta blockers, and calcium-channel blockers such as nifedipine were discussed earlier. The role of angiotensin-converting enzyme inhibitors in the management of hypovolemic relative polycythemia has not yet been defined.

Weight control in patients with relative polycythemia is of benefit in reducing blood pressure,[250] in preventing left ventricular hypertrophy,[251] and in ameliorating intermittent nocturnal hypoxemia and sleep apnea.[217] Nocturnal oxygen therapy may be therapeutic in patients with relative polycythemia and postural hypoxemia,[212] and although previously felt to be hazardous, it may be of benefit as well in patients with sleep apnea.[217] Drug therapy for sleep apnea is of limited utility. Protriptyline is the drug of choice but is limited by anticholinergic side effects.[214] Progesterone, which is sometimes effective in the pickwickian syndrome, is less effective in sleep apnea.[217] Continuous positive airway pressure at night may help patients with severe symptoms. The role of surgical procedures is unclear. Tracheostomy has little or no role in the current treatment of sleep apnea.[214]

The efficacy of regular exercise as a component in the management of relative polycythemia has not been discussed previously. Forty minutes of exercise on a bicycle ergometer to a workload of 60 to 70 percent of maximum work capacity repeated three to seven times per week was associated with a reduction in blood pressure, decrease in total peripheral resistance, decrease in sympathetic activity, and decrease in plasma renin activity.[252] Exercise, therefore, might be expected to counter abnormalities operative in hypovolemic relative polycythemia. Moderation in the ingestion of caffeine-containing beverages also has been recommended.[253]

Treatments that directly attempt to increase plasma volume in patients with hypovolemic relative polycythemia have generally been unsuccessful. Dextran infusion was transiently effective in lowering the hematocrit and increasing cerebral blood flow, but the effects lasted less than 24 hours.[153] Fludrocortisone was given in a dosage of 0.1 mg daily for 1 week and increased to 0.2 mg daily for a second week without any significant effect on the hematocrit or whole-blood or plasma viscosity.[153] These results differ from those recently reported in patients with "idiopathic hypovolemia,"[171] in whom plasma volume increased significantly after 4 weeks of Florinef 0.1 mg twice a day and a high-sodium diet.

Phlebotomy

The success of the therapeutic strategy outlined above relies heavily on the desire of affected subjects to correct adverse lifestyle influences such as smoking and obesity. Unfortunately, "history records few instances in which disease has been prevented by motivating people to give up practices they like for future benefits in health."[120] For the patient with relative polycythemia who is unsuccessful at behavior modification or who continues to be polycythemic despite appropriate adjunctive management, a phlebotomy program may sometimes be indicated.

The indications for phlebotomy in patients with normovolemic relative polycythemia with high-normal red cell mass are unclear, since no study has objectively demonstrated that venesection improves either survival or quality of life in these patients. Patients in whom relative polycythemia is associated with occult intermittent hypoxemia should perhaps be managed similarly to patients with secondary pulmonary polycythemia, in whom no treatment is recommended for patients with minor elevations of hematocrit but in whom hematocrit reduction by phlebotomy is advised when the hematocrit exceeds 55 percent.[98] In patients with established occlusive cardiovascular and cerebrovascular disease, in whom the combination of increased blood viscosity, sluggish blood flow through partly obstructed blood vessels, and endothelial dysfunction, is likely to exacerbate a pathophysiologic hemostatic state,[121] initiation of a phlebotomy program when the hematocrit is 50 percent or greater is probably justifiable. As a cautionary note, however, when oxygen saturation is reduced, phlebotomy to the point of induction of iron-deficient red cell changes might be disadvantageous due to a reduction in oxygen-carrying capacity caused by a reduction in mean corpuscular hemoglobin.[254] A better definition of criteria for venesection in patients with normovolemic relative polycythemia should follow completion of an ongoing prospective study.[8]

In patients with idiopathic hypovolemic relative polycythemia, serial small-volume (250 ml) venesection was, contrary to expectation, effective in normalizing the hematocrit without apparent adverse reactions or side effects.[172] Following initial phlebotomies, blood viscosity decreased and cerebral blood flow returned from depressed to normal values. Venesection at 2-month intervals was generally sufficient to maintain a normal hematocrit.[172] Although it was feared that initially depressed plasma volumes might further decline after phlebotomy, in actuality, the plasma volume increased. Most likely, plasma volume expansion following venesection occurs for the same reason that plasma volume increases in successfully treated hypertensive patients[179] and in furosemide-treated patients with pulmonary edema.[245] Following phlebotomy, central venous pressure and mean pulmonary artery pressure decrease and systemic vascular resistance decreases, with a resulting increase in stroke volume and cardiac output.[255] By decreasing transcapillary hydrostatic pressure, a decrease in peripheral resistance favors plasma volume expansion. The increase in cardiac output after phlebotomy promotes increased exercise tolerance.[251]

Despite these preliminary favorable short-term results, there are as yet no published data indicating that a long-term phlebotomy program is effective in preventing the significant cardiovascular and cerebrovascular morbidity and mortality associated with hypovolemic relative polycythemia. Such a study, which also would address the safety of such a program, might well be advocated. Nevertheless, pending objective resolution of this question, might not a case be made in favor of routine venesection for patients with idiopathic relative polycythemia, particularly in the context of blood donation for transfusion purposes? In addressing this question, it should be remembered that a substantial incidence of thrombotic vascular complications was observed in patients with PV managed with a chronic venesection program,[256] and Kiraly et al.[257] reported that phlebotomy may not be free of hazard, particularly in patients with underlying cardiovascular disease. On the other hand, in a study of 14 healthy controls and 18 patients with coronary heart disease or hypertension, Thomas et al.[258] concluded that venesection can be performed safely without volume replacement in patients with stable cardiovascular disease. Furthermore, chronic phlebotomy is performed safely and is therapeutic in patients with hereditary hemochromatosis,[259] and there is ample anecdotal recognition of chronic multigallon blood donors who appear no worse the wear for their experience. Donation of up to 5 units of whole blood per year is not considered excessive,[260] and although iron stores are depleted, normal males are able to donate up to 2 liters per year without appreciable iron deficiency.[261] It also has been proposed that the greater incidence of heart disease in men and postmenopausal women compared with the incidence in premenopausal women results from higher levels of stored iron and that iron depletion by periodic phlebotomy might prevent cardiovascular disease[262] by virtue of strong antioxidant effects in vivo associated with iron deficiency and iron depletion.[263] In a preliminary study, a higher survival rate was found for blood donors than for non-blood donors, especially between 50 and 70 years of age.[264] Inasmuch as the adequacy of the control group in this study can be questioned, a randomized, prospective study of men who agree to give blood regularly has been proposed.[258,263] Such a trial could reasonably be extended to patients with idiopathic hypovolemic relative polycythemia.

CONCLUSIONS

Relative polycythemia continues to be the most common finding in patients who are referred for evaluation of an elevated hematocrit. The cumulative evidence clearly validates the position of those who have questioned the existence of relative polycythemia as a distinct primary disease entity, indicating rather that relative polycythemia is heterogeneous with respect to pathogenesis, pathophysiology, clinical manifestations, and prognosis. Nevertheless, particularly when in conjunction with hypovolemia and hypertension, relative polycythemia appears to be clinically disadvantageous and associated with a substantially increased morbidity and mortality from cerebrovascular and cardiovascular occlusive disease. The detection of relative polycythemia should alert both physician and patient to the existence of underlying abnormalities in physiology or in lifestyle, the correction of which should not only resolve the polycythemic state but also promote an improvement in overall health and longevity.

The formulation of a classification of the absolute polycythemias based on a recognition of disease entities and on physiologic considerations has been a key to a scientific understanding of these disorders and to the development of a rational diagnostic and therapeutic approach. The application of such a system to the relative polycythemias, as I have attempted herein, hopefully would be of equal value and a necessary first step toward a better definition of this heterogeneous group of disorders. A delineation of patient subsets based on blood volume measurement and incidence of smoking, transient hypoxemia, and hypertension offers a framework for future study while, from a pragmatic viewpoint, directing attention at those etiologic factors whose correction may lead to a resolution of the clinical disorder.

Until the completion of new long-term studies in which patients are stratified according to the incidence of the preceding pathogenetic factors, the optimal therapy for these patients will continue to be uncertain. Further information may be expected on completion of the British study of patients with "apparent" (normovolemic relative) polycythemia. In the interim, however, it is certainly difficult to take issue with a therapeutic approach that emphasizes cessation of smoking, control of hypertension, weight loss in the obese, dietary discretion, and appropriate exercise. In select circumstances, reduction in alcohol intake, nocturnal oxygen therapy, and nocturnal positive airway pressure also may be recommended. When, however, as is too often the case, lifestyle modification falls short of the mark and relative polycythemia persists, the propriety of a chronic phlebotomy program should be considered. Initial results suggest that periodic venesection can reduce the hematocrit successfully even in patients with hypovolemic relative polycythemia with preservation of or even improvement in the plasma volume. Patients with refractory relative polycythemia and established cardiovascular, cerebrovascular, or peripheral vascular disease, who have an inordinate risk of recurrence or extension of occlusive manifestations, would appear to be potential candidates for chronic phlebotomy management. The efficacy and safety of long-term venesection in patients with relative polycythemia would best be explored, however, in the context of a prospective, randomized trial.

REFERENCES

1. Berlin NI: Diagnosis and classification of the polycythemias. Semin Hematol 12:339–351, 1975
2. Osler W: Chronic cyanosis with polycythemia and enlarged spleen. Am J Med Sci 126:187–201, 1903
3. Wintrobe MM: Polycythemia: Erythrocytosis. In Wintrobe MM, Lee GR, Boggs DR, et al (eds): Clinical Hematology, 8th ed. Philadelphia, Lea and Febiger, 1981, pp 991–996
4. Lenfant C, Sullivan K: Adaptation to high altitude. N Engl J Med 284:1298–1309, 1971
5. Milnor WR: Blood Volume. In Mountcastle VB (ed): Medical Physiology, 13th ed. St Louis, Mosby, 1974
6. Smith JFB, Lucie NP: Alcohol—A cause of stress erythrocytosis. Lancet 1:637–638, 1973
7. Krauss S, Wasserman LR: Spurious (relative) polycythemia. In Williams WJ (ed): Hematol-

ogy. New York, McGraw-Hill, 1974, pp 555–558

8. Wetherley-Mein G: Erythrocytosis. *In* Brain MC, Carbone PP (eds): Current Therapy in Hematology-Oncology 1985–1986. Toronto, BC Decker, 1985, pp 46–50

9. Gaisbock F: Die bedentung der blutdruckmessung fur die arztliche praxis. Deutch Arch Klin Med 83:363–409, 1905

10. Bassen FA, Abel HA: Pseudopolycythemia. J Mt Sinai Hosp 6:322–326, 1940

11. Kaung DT, Peterson RE: "Relative polycythemia" or "pseudopolycythemia." Arch Intern Med 110:456–460, 1962

12. Lawrence JH, Berlin NI: Relative polycythemia— The polycythemia of stress. Yale J Biol Med 24:498–505, 1952

13. Russell RP, Conley CL: Benign polycythemia: Gaisbock's syndrome. Arch Intern Med 114:734–740, 1964

14. Brown SM, Gilbert HS, Krauss S, et al: Spurious (relative) polycythemia: A non-existent disease. Am J Med 50:220–227, 1971

15. Mathew RJ, Wilson WH: Hematocrit and anxiety. J Psychosom Res 30:307–311, 1986

16. Kitahara Y, Imataka K, Nakaoka H, et al: Hematocrit increase by mental stress in hypertensive patients. Jpn Heart J 29:429–435, 1988

17. Fessel WJ: Odd men out. Arch Intern Med 115:736–737, 1965

18. Watts EJ, Lewis SM: Spurious polycythemia—A study of 35 patients. Scand J Haematol 31:241–247, 1983

19. Pearson TC, Wetherly-Mein G: The course and complications of idiopathic erythrocytosis. Clin Lab Haematol 1:189–196, 1979

20. Burge PS, Johnson WS, Prankerd T: Morbidity and mortality in pseudopolycythaemia. Lancet 1:1266–1269, 1975

21. Weinreb NJ, Shih CF: Spurious polycythemia. Semin Hematol 12:397–407, 1975

22. Schwarcz TH, Hogan LA, Endean ED, et al: Thromboembolic complications of polycythemia: Polycythemia vera versus smokers' polycythemia. J Vasc Surg 17:518–522, 1993

23. Babylonian Talmud. Tractate Baba Bathra, p 58b

24. Ben Lakish S: Babylonian Talmud, Tractate Bechoroth, p 44b

25. Midrash Rabba. Leviticus 15:2

26. Vaquez H: Sur une forme speciale de cyanose s'accompant d'hyperglobulie excessive et persistente. C R Soc Biol 4:384–388, 1892

27. Lucas WSL: Erythremia or polycythemia with chronic cyanosis and splenomegaly. Arch Intern Med 10:597–667, 1912

28. Keith NM, Rountree LG, Geraghty JT: A method for the determination of plasma and blood volume. Arch Intern Med 16:547–576, 1915

29. Modan B, Modan M: Benign erythrocytosis. Br J Haematol 14:375–381, 1968

30. Hall CA: Gaisbock's syndrome: Redefinition of an old syndrome. Arch Intern Med 116:4–9, 1965

31. Ebert RV, Stead EA Jr: Demonstration that the cell plasma ratio of blood contained in minute vessels is lower than that of venous blood. J Clin Invest 20:317–321, 1941

32. Blum AS, Zbar MJ: Relative polycythemia. Arch Intern Med 104:385–389, 1959

33. London GM, Safar ME, Safar AL, et al: Blood pressure in the "low-pressure system" and cardiac performance in essential hypertension. J Hypertension 3:337–342, 1985

34. Wintrobe MM: Erythremia. *In* Wintrobe MM (ed): Clinical Hematology, 5th ed. Philadelphia, Lea and Febiger, 1961, p 796

35. Pearson TC: Apparent polycythaemia. Blood Rev 5:205–213, 1991

36. Messinezy M, Pearson TC: A retrospective study of apparent and relative polycythaemia: Associated factors and early outcome. Clin Lab Haematol 12:121–129, 1990

37. Isbister JP: The contracted plasma volume syndromes (relative polycythaemias) and their haemorheological significance. Ballieres Clin Haematol 1:665–693, 1987

38. Anderson SB: Simultaneous determination of plasma volume with ^{131}I-labeled gamma globulin, ^{131}I-labeled albumin and T-1824. Clin Sci 23:221–228, 1962

39. Larson OA: Studies of the body hematocrit phenomenon: Dynamic hematocrit of large vessel and initial distribution space of albumin and fibrinogen in the whole body. Scand J Clin Lab Invest 22:189–195, 1968

40. Huff R, Feller DD: Relationship of circulating red cell volume to body density and obesity. J Clin Invest 35:1–10, 1956

41. Chien S, Usami S, Simmon RL, et al: Blood volume and age: Repeated measurements on normal men after 17 years. J Appl Physiol 21:583–588, 1966

42. Castellini MA, Costa DP, Huntley A: Hematocrit variation during sleep apnea in elephant seal pups. Am J Physiol 251:R429–R431, 1986

43. Conley CL, Nickerson JL: Effects of temperature change on the water balance in man. Am J Physiol 143:373–384, 1945

44. Touitou Y, Touitou C, Bogdan A, et al: Differences between young and elderly subjects in seasonal and circadian variations of total plasma proteins and blood volume as reflected by hemoglobin, hematocrit, and erythrocyte counts. Clin Chem 32:801–804, 1986

45. Finlayson DC, Dagher FJ, Vandam LD: Diurnal variation in blood volume of man. J Surg Res 4:286–288, 1964

46. Watson C: Erythrocyte coproporphyrin. Arch Intern Med 86:797–809, 1950

47. Conley CL, Russell RP, Thomas CB, et al: Hematocrit values in coronary artery disease. Arch Intern Med 113:170–176, 1964

48. McDonough SR, Hames CG, Garrison GE, et al: The relationship of hematocrit to cardiovascular status of health in the negro and white population of Evans County, Georgia. J Chronic Dis 18:243–257, 1965

49. Hom BL, Arumanayagam M, Donnan SPB, et al: Blood cell values in normal Hong Kong Chinese adults. Blood 66(suppl):53a, 1985

50. Pierce HI, Kurachi S, Sofroniadou K, et al: Frequencies of thalassemia in American blacks. Blood 49:981–986, 1977

51. Messerli FH, DE Carvalho JGR, Christie B, et al: Essential hypertension in black and white subjects: Hemodynamic findings and fluid volume state. Am J Med 67:27–31, 1979

52. Miale JB: The blood. *In* Hematology. St Louis, Mosby, 1977, pp 426–432

53. Cornesco M, Karimeddini MK, Buat A, et al: Red blood cell mass determination: A cost-effectiveness analysis. Blood 66(suppl):172a, 1985
54. Pearson TC, Wetherly-Mein G: Vascular occlusive episodes and venous hematocrit in primary proliferative polycythaemia. Lancet 2:1219–1222, 1978
55. Weber MA, Laragh JH: Hypertension. In Conn HF (ed): Current Therapy. Philadelphia, WB Saunders Co, 1978, p 206
56. Zanella A, Silvani C, Banfi P, et al: Screening and evaluation of blood donors with upper-limit hematocrit levels. Transfusion 27:485–487, 1987
57. Jootar S, Withoonpanich R, Niramarnsakul S: Hematocrit in thrombotic stroke at Ramathibodi Hospital. J Med Assoc Thai 72:97–100, 1989
58. Kochar MS, Paka S, Kim MJ, et al: Relation between serum cholesterol and hematocrit (letter). JAMA 267:1071, 1992
59. Landau B, Benjamin D, Pinkhas J: Ejaculation praecox and spurious polycythemia (letter). JAMA 241:1791–1792, 1979
60. Martin J, Tomkin GH, Hutchinson M: Peripheral neuropathy in hypothyroidism—An association with spurious polycythemia (Gaisbock's syndrome). J R Soc Med 76:187–189, 1983
61. Kiyohara Y, Ueda K, Hasuo Y, et al: Hematocrit as a risk factor of cerebral infarction: Long-term prospective population survey in a Japanese rural community. Stroke 17:687–692, 1986
62. Nagendran I, Gaillard WE Jr: Ischemia of the hand secondary to Gaisbock's syndrome. Int Surg 65:179–181, 1980
63. Yeung MC, Buncio A: Leukocyte count, smoking, and lung function. Am J Med 76:31–37, 1984
64. Tell GS, Grimm RH, Vellar OD, et al: The relationship of white cell count, platelet count and hematocrit to cigarette smoking in adolescents: The Oslo Youth Study. Circulation 72:971–974, 1985
65. Zalokar JB, Richard JL, Claude JR: Leukocyte count, smoking and myocardial infarction. N Engl J Med 304:265–468, 1981
66. Ernst E, Hammerschmidt DE, Bagge U, et al: Leukocytes and the risk of ischemic diseases. JAMA 257:2318–2324, 1987
67. Grimm RH Jr, Neaton JD, Ludwig W, et al: Prognostic importance of the white blood cell count for coronary, cancer, and all-cause mortality. JAMA 254:1932–1937, 1985
68. Richardson TQ, Guyten AC: Effects of polycythemia and anemia on cardiac output and other circulatory factors. Am J Physiol 197:1167–1170, 1959
69. Murray JF, Gold P, John BL Jr: Systemic oxygen transport in induced normovolemic anemia and polycythemia. Am J Physiol 203:720–724, 1962
70. Kiel JW, Shepherd AP: Optimal hematocrit for canine gastric oxygenation. Am J Physiol 256:H472–H477, 1989
71. Stone HO, Thompson HK Jr, Schmidt-Nielson K: Influence of erythrocytes on blood viscosity. Am J Physiol 214:913–918, 1968
72. Pries AR, Neuhaus D, Gaehtgens P: Blood viscosity in tube flow: Dependence on diameter and hematocrit. Am J Physiol 263:H1770–H1778, 1992
73. Kiesewetter H, Jung F, Lazar H, et al: Hematocrit as a risk factor for vascular disease. Klin Wochenschr 64:974–978, 1986
74. Desjardins C, Duling BR: Microvessel hematocrit: Measurement and implications for capillary oxygen transport. Am J Physiol 252:H494–H503, 1987
75. Boyle J: Microcirculatory hematocrit and blood flow. J Theor Biol 131:223–229, 1988
76. Intaglietta M, Mirhashemi S, Tomkins WR: Capillary fluxmeter: The simultaneous measurement of hematocrit, velocity and flux. Int J Microcirc Clin Exp 8:313–320, 1989
77. Lindenfeld J, Weil JV, Travis VL, et al: Hemodynamic response to normovolemic polycythemia at rest and during exercise in dogs. Circ Res 56:793–800, 1985
78. Brookshier KK, Tarbell JM: Effect of hematocrit on wall shear rate in oscillatory flow: Do the elastic properties of blood play a role? Biorheology 28:569–587, 1991
79. Strumia MM, Phillips M: Effect of red cell factors on the relative viscosity of whole blood. Am J Clin Pathol 39:464–474, 1963
80. Yardin G, Meiselman HJ: Effects of cellular morphology on the viscoelastic behavior of high hematocrit RBC suspensions. Biorheology 26:153–175, 1989
81. Chien S, Gallik S: Personal communication, 1994
82. Fahreus R, Lindquist T: The viscosity of blood in narrow capillary tubes. Am J Physiol 96:562–568, 1931
83. Stadler AA, Zilow EP, Linderkamp O: Blood viscosity and optimal hematocrit in narrow tubes. Biorheology 27:779–788, 1990
84. Dreissen G, Scheidt H, Inhoffen W, et al: A comparative study: Perfusion of the micro- and macrocirculation as a function of the hematocrit value. Microvasc Res 35:73–85, 1988
85. Desjardins C, Duling BR: Heparinase treatment suggests a role for the endothelial cell glycocalyx in regulation of capillary hematocrit. Am J Physiol 258:H647–H654, 1990
86. Smith BD, Lacelle PL: Blood viscosity and thrombosis: Clinical consideration. Prog Hemost Thromb 6:170–201, 1982
87. Kung-Ming J, Chien S: Effect of hematocrit variations on coronary hemodynamics and oxygen utilization. Am J Physiol 223:H106–H113, 1977
88. Gustafsson L, Appelgren L, Myrvoid HE: The effect of polycythemia in blood flow in working and non-working skeletal muscle. Acta Physiol Scand 109:143–148, 1980
89. Kuo L, Pittman RN: Influence of hemoconcentration on arteriolar oxygen transport in hamster striated muscle. Am J Physiol 259:H1694–1702, 1990
90. Altland PD, Highman B: Effects of polycythemia and altitude hypoxia on rat heart and exercise tolerance. Am J Physiol 221:388–393, 1971
91. Brown MN, Wade JPH, Marshall J: Fundamental importance of the arterial oxygen content in the regulation of cerebral blood flow in man. Brain 108:81–93, 1985
92. Horstman D, Weiskoff R, Jackson RE: Work capacity during three week sojourn at 4300 m:

Effects of relative polycythemia. J Appl Physiol 49:311–318, 1980

93. Buick FJ, Gledhill N, Froese AB, et al: Effects of induced erythrocythemia on aerobic work capacity. J Appl Physiol 48:636–642, 1980

94. Sawka MN, Young AJ, Muza SR, et al: Erythrocyte reinfusion and maximal aerobic power: An examination of modifying factors. JAMA 257:1496–1499, 1987

95. Boutellier U, Deriaz O, di Prampero PE, et al: Aerobic performance at altitude: Effects of acclimatization and hematocrit with reference to training. Int J Sports Med 11(suppl):S21–S26, 1990

96. Nagao N, Imai Y, Arie J, et al: The Kaike triathletes' hematocrit values with relation to their competition results. J Sports Med Phys Fitness 32:201–205, 1992

97. Balcerzak SP, Bromberg PA: Secondary polycythemia. Semin Hematol 12:353–382, 1975

98. Gaminara E, Pearson TC: Should secondary polycythemia in COPD be treated? Pract Cardiol 11:106–113, 1985

99. Kershenovich S, Modiano M, Ewy GA: Markedly decreased coronary blood flow in secondary polycythemia. Am Heart J 123:521–523, 1992

100. Yeager SB, Freed MD: Myocardial infarction as a manifestation of polycythemia in cyanotic heart disease. Am J Cardiol 53:952–953, 1984

101. Martelle RR, Linde LM: Cerebrovascular accident with tetralogy of Fallot. Am J Dis Child 101:98–101, 1961

102. Doll DC, Greenberg BR: Cerebral thrombosis in smokers' polycythemia. Ann Intern Med 102:786–787, 1985

103. Rothstein T: Bilateral, central retinal vein closure as the initial manifestation of polycythemia. Am J Ophthalmol 74:256–260, 1972

104. Chievitz E, Thiede T: Complications and causes of death in polycythemia vera. Acta Med Scand 172:513–523, 1962

105. Barabas AP, Offen DN, Meinhard EA: The arterial complications of polycythemia vera. Br J Surg 60:183–187, 1973

106. Prentice CRM, Lowe GDO: Blood viscosity and the complications of diabetes. Adv Exp Med Biol 164:99–103, 1984

107. Dormandy JA, Hoare F, Colbey J, et al: Clinical, hemodynamic, rheological and biochemical findings in 126 patients with intermittent claudication. Br Med J 4:576–581, 1973

108. Hansen ES, Wethelund JO, Skajaa K: Hemoglobin and hematocrit as risk factors in below-the-knee amputation for incipient gangrene. Arch Orthop Trauma Surg 107:92–95, 1988

109. Hoffkes HG, Saeger-Lorenz K, Ehrly AM: Optimal hematocrit in patients with intermittent claudication. Acta Med Aust 18(suppl 1):16–19, 1991

110. Hoffkes HG, Ehrly AM: Hematocrit-dependent changes of muscle oxygen supply in the lower limb muscle of patients with intermittent claudication. Vasa 21:350–354, 1992

111. Dormandy JA, Edelman JB: High blood viscosity: An etiological factor in venous thrombosis. Br J Surg 60:187–190, 1973

112. Hellberg PO, Bayati A, Kallskog O, et al: Red cell trapping after ischemia and long-term kidney damage: Influence of hematocrit. Kidney Int 37:1240–1247, 1990

113. Nicolaides AN, Bowers R, Horbourne T, et al: Blood viscosity, red cell flexibility, hematocrit and plasma fibrinogen in patients with angina. Lancet 2:943–945, 1977

114. Lowe GDO, Drummond DMD, Lorimer AR, et al: Relation between extent of coronary artery disease and blood viscosity. Br Med J 1:673–674, 1980

115. Tibblin G, Bergentz SE, Bjure J, et al: Hematocrit, plasma protein, plasma volume and viscosity in early hypertensive disease. Am Heart J 72:165–176, 1966

116. Letcher RL, Chien S, Pickering TG, et al: Direct relationship between blood pressure and blood viscosity in normal and hypertensive subjects. Am J Med 70:1195–1202, 1981

117. Ernst E, Resch KL: Fibrinogen as a cardiovascular risk factor: A meta-analysis and review of the literature. Ann Intern Med 118:956–963, 1993

118. Casale PN, Milner M, Devereux RB, et al: Value of echocardiographic left ventricular mass in predicting cardiovascular morbid events in hypertensive men. Circulation 72(part 2):130, 1985

119. Devereux RB, Drayer JIM, Chien S, et al: Whole blood viscosity as a determinant of cardiac hypertrophy in systemic hypertension. Am J Cardiol 54:592–595, 1984

120. Kannel WB, Thom TJ: Declining cardiovascular mortality. Circulation 70:331–336, 1984

121. Oliver MF: Prevention of coronary heart disease: Propaganda, promises, problems and prospects. Circulation 73:1–9, 1986

122. Lowik MR, Odink J, Kok FJ, et al: Hematocrit and cardiovascular risk factors among elderly men and women. Gerontology 38:205–213, 1992

123. Dawber TR, Kannel WB: Susceptibility to coronary artery disease. Mod Concepts Cardiovasc Dis 30:671–676, 1961

124. Burch GE, De Pasquale NP: The hematocrit in patients with myocardial infarction. JAMA 180:63–65, 1962

125. Burch GE, De Pasquale NP: Hematocrit, blood viscosity and myocardial infarction. Am J Med 32:161–163, 1962

126. Hershberg PI, Wells RE, McGandy RB: Hematocrit and prognosis in patients with acute myocardial infarction. JAMA 219:855–860, 1972

127. Mayer GA: Blood viscosity in healthy subjects and patients with coronary heart disease. Can Med Assoc J 91:951–954, 1964

128. Stables DP, Rubenstein AH, Metz T, et al: The possible role of hemoconcentration in the etiology of myocardial infarction. Am Heart J 73:155–159, 1967

129. Grimm RH Jr: Personal communication, 1986

130. Bottiger LE, Carlson LA: Risk factors for ischaemic vascular death for men in the Stockholm Prospective Study. Atherosclerosis 36:389–408, 1980

131. Cullen KJ, Stenhouse NS, Waerne KL: Raised hemoglobin and risk of cardiovascular disease. Lancet 4:1288–1289, 1981

132. Knottnerus JA, Swaen GMH, Slangen JJM, et al: Haematologic parameters as risk factors for cardiac infarction in an occupational health care setting. J Clin Epidemiol 41:67–74, 1988

133. Salonen JT, Nyyssonen K, Korpela H, et al: High stored iron levels are associated with excess risk

of myocardial infarction in eastern Finnish men. Circulation 86:803–811, 1992

134. Hillbom M, Kaste M: Ethanol intoxication: A risk factor in ischemic brain infarction in adolescents and young adults. Stroke 12:422–425, 1981

135. Kannel WB, Dawber TR, Cohen ME, et al: Vascular disease of the brain, epidemiologic aspects: The Framingham Study. Am J Public Health 55:1355–1366, 1965

136. Alter M, Christoferson L, Resch J, et al: Cerebrovascular disease: Frequency and population selectivity in an upper midwestern community. Stroke 1:454–465, 1970

137. Tanaka H, Hayashi M, Date C, et al: Epidemiologic studies of stroke in Shibata, a Japanese provincial city: Preliminary report on risk factors for cerebral infarction. Stroke 16:773–780, 1985

138. Kannel WB, Gordon T, Wolfe PA, et al: Hemoglobin and the risk of cerebral infarction: The Framingham Study. Stroke 3:409–420, 1972

139. Ott EO, Lechner H, Aranibar A: High blood viscosity syndrome in cerebral infarction. Stroke 5:330–333, 1974

140. Wells RE, Merrill EW: The variability of blood viscosity. Am J Med 31:505–509, 1961

141. Toghi H, Yamanouchi H, Murakami M, et al: Importance of the hematocrit as a risk factor in cerebral infarction. Stroke 9:369–374, 1978

142. Pearce JMS, Chandrasekera CP, Ladersans EJ: Lacunar infarcts in patients with raised packed cell volumes. Br Med J 287:935–936, 1983

143. Larue L, Alter M, Lai SM, et al: Acute stroke, hematocrit, and blood pressure. Stroke 18:565–569, 1987

144. Ozaita G, Calandre L, Peinado E, et al: Hematocrit and clinical outcome in acute cerebral infarction. Stroke 18:1166–1168, 1987

145. Kiyohara Y, Ueda K, Fujishima M: Smoking and cardiovascular disease in the general population in Japan. J Hypertens Suppl 8:S9–S15, 1990

146. Kiyohara Y, Fujishima M, Ishitsuka T, et al: Effects of hematocrit on brain metabolism in experimentally induced cerebral ischemia in spontaneously hypertensive rats (SHR). Stroke 16:835–840, 1985

147. Pollock S, Tsitsopoulos P, Harrison NTG: The effect of hematocrit on cerebral perfusion and clinical status following carotid occlusion in the gerbil. Stroke 13:167–170, 1982

148. Sundt TM, Waltz AG, Sayre GP: Experimental cerebral infarction: Modification by treatment with hemodiluting, hemoconcentrating, and dehydrating agents. J Neurosurg 26:46–56, 1967

149. Harrison MTG, Kendall BE, Pollock S, et al: Effect of hematocrit on carotid stenosis and cerebral infarction. Lancet 2:114–115, 1981

150. Brass LM, Pavlakis SG, DeVivo D, et al: Transcranial Doppler measurements of the middle cerebral artery: Effect of hematocrit. Stroke 19:1466–1469, 1988

151. Titianova EB, Velcheva IV, Mateev PS: Effects of aging and hematocrit on cerebral blood flow velocity in patients with unilateral cerebral infarctions: A Doppler ultrasound evaluation. Angiology 44:100–106, 1993

152. Wood JH, Polyzoidis RS, Epstein CM, et al: Quantitative EEG alterations after isovolemic-hemodilutional augmentation of cerebral perfusion in stroke patients. Neurology 34:764–768, 1984

153. Thomas W: Hemodilution in acute stroke. Stroke 16:763–764, 1985.

154. Scandinavian Stroke Study Group: Multicenter trial of hemodilution in ischemic stroke—Background and study protocol. Stroke 16:885–890, 1985.

155. Thomas DJ, Marshall J, Russell RW, et al: Cerebral blood flow in polycythemia. Lancet 2:161–163, 1977

156. Humphrey PRD, DuBoulay GH, Marshall J: Cerebral blood flow and viscosity in relative polycythemia. Lancet 2:873–877, 1979

157. Humphrey PRD, Michael J, Pearson TC: Management of relative polycythemia: studies of cerebral blood flow and viscosity. Br J Haematol 46:427–433, 1980

158. Wade JPH: Transport of oxygen to the brain in patients with elevated hematocrit values before and after venesection. Brain 106:513–523, 1983

159. Wade JPH, DuBoulay GH, Marshall J, et al: Cerebral blood flow, hematocrit and viscosity in subjects with a high affinity hemoglobin variant. Acta Neurol Scand 61:210–215, 1981

160. Muizelaar JP, Bouma GJ, Levasseur JE, et al: Effect of hematocrit variations on cerebral blood flow and basilar artery diameter in vivo. Am J Physiol 262:H949–H954, 1992

161. Rosenkrantz TS, Stonestreet BS, Hansen NB, et al: Cerebral blood flow in the newborn lamb with polycythemia and hyperviscosity. J Pediatr 104:276–280, 1984

162. Massik J, Tang YL, Hudak ML, et al: Effect of hematocrit on cerebral blood flow with induced polycythemia. J Appl Physiol 62:1090–1096, 1987

163. Hudak ML, Tang YL, Massik J, et al: Baseline O_2 extraction influences cerebral blood flow response to hematocrit. Am J Physiol 254:H156–H162, 1988

164. Paulson OB, Parving HH, Olesen J, et al: Influence of carbon monoxide and of hemodilution on cerebral blood flow and blood gases in man. J Appl Physiol 35:111–116, 1973

165. Henriksen L, Paulson OB, Smith RJ: Cerebral blood flow following normovolemic hemodilution in patients with high hematocrit. Ann Neurol 9:454–457, 1981

166. Mathew RJ, Wilson WH, Tant SR: Determinants of resting regional cerebral blood flow in normal subjects. Biol Psychol 21:907–914, 1986

167. Humphrey PRD, DuBoulay GH, Marshall T, et al: Viscosity, cerebral blood flow and hematocrit in patients with paraproteinaemia. Acta Neurol Scand 61:201–209, 1980

168. Brown MM, Marshall J: Regulation of cerebral blood flow in response to changes in blood viscosity. Lancet 1:604–609, 1985

169. McHenry LC, West JW, Cooper ES, et al: Cerebral autoregulation in man. Stroke 5:695–706, 1974

170. Sakai F, Igarashi H, Suzuki S, et al: Cerebral blood flow and cerebral hematocrit in patients with cerebral ischemia measured by single-

photon emission computed tomography. Acta Neurol Scand 127(suppl):9–13, 1989

171. Rogers RL. Meyer JS, Mortel KF, et al: Decreased cerebral blood flow precedes multi-infarct dementia, but follows senile dementia of Alzheimer type. Neurology 36:1–6, 1986

172. Kusunoki J, Kimura K, Nakamura M, et al: Effects of hematocrit variations on cerebral blood flow and oxygen transport in ischemic cerebrovascular disease. J Cereb Blood Flow Metab 1:413–417, 1981

173. Fluckiger JP, Waeber B, Matsueda G, et al: Effect of atriopeptide III on hematocrit and volemia of nephrectomized rats. Am J Physiol 251: H880–883, 1986

174. Giller CA, Levine BD, Meyer Y, et al: The cerebral hemodynamics of normotensive hypovolemia during lower-body negative pressure. J Neurosurg 76:961–966, 1992

175. Fouad FM, Tadena-Thame L, Bravo EL, et al: Idiopathic hypovolemia. Ann Intern Med 104:298–303, 1986

176. Humphrey PRD, Michael J, Pearson TC: Red cell mass plasma volume and blood volume before and after venesection in relative polycythemia. Br J Haematol 46:435–438, 1980

177. Tarazi RC, Frohlich ED, Dustan HP: Plasma volume in men with essential hypertension. N Engl J Med 278:762–765, 1968

178. Kobrin I, Frohlich ED, Ventura HO, et al: Stable red cell mass despite contracted plasma volume in men with essential hypertension. J Lab Clin Med 104:11–14, 1984

179. Dustan HP: Obesity and hypertension. Ann Intern Med 103:1047–1049, 1985

180. Barrett-Conner E, Khaw K: Is hypertension more benign when associated with obesity? Circulation 72:53–60, 1985

181. Messerli FH: Obesity in hypertension: How innocent a bystander. Am J Med 77:1077–1082, 1984

182. Emery AC Jr, Whitcomb WH, Frohlich ED: "Stress" polycythemia and hypertension. JAMA 229:159–162, 1974

183. Chrysant SG, Frohlich ED, Adamopoulos PN, et al: Pathophysiologic significance of "stress" and relative polycythemia in essential hypertension. Am J Cardiol 37:1069–1072, 1976

184. Giese J: Renin, angiotensin, and hypertensive vascular damage: A review. Am J Med 55: 315–332, 1973

185. Brunner HR, Laragh JH, Baer L, et al: Essential hypertension: Renin and aldosterone, heart attack and stroke. N Engl J Med 286:441–449, 1972

186. Kaplan NM: The prognostic implications of plasma renin in essential hypertension. JAMA 231:167–170, 1975

187. Horwitz D, Patel W: Maximal hand blood flow in hypertensive and normal subjects. Am J Cardiol 55:418–422, 1985

188. Bohr DF, Webb AC: Vascular smooth muscle function and its changes in hypertension. Am J Med 77(4A):3–16, 1984

189. Ostman-Smith I: Cardiac sympathetic nerves on the final common pathway in the induction of adaptive cardiac hypertrophy. Clin Sci 61: 265–272, 1981

190. Dzau VS: Vascular wall renin-angiotensin pathway in control of the circulation—A hypothesis. Am J Med 77(4A):31–36, 1984

191. Sagnella GA, Shore AC, Markander ND, et al: Raised circulatory levels of atrial natriuretic peptides in essential hypertension. Lancet 1:179–181, 1986

192. Putensen C, Mutz N, Pomaroli A, et al: Atrial natriuretic factor release during hypovolemia and after volume replacement. Crit Care Med 20:984–989, 1992

193. Tsai RC, Yamaji T, Ishibashi M, et al: Role of atrial natriuretic peptide in hemoconcentration during exercise. Am J Hypertens 3: 833–837, 1990

194. Yates NA, Parkes DG, Coghlan JP, et al: The effect of hypovolemia on the renal and cardiovascular responses to atrial natriuretic factor (ANF) infusion. Life Sci 50:1905–1912, 1992

195. Aisaka K, Miyazaki T, Hidaka T, et al: Effects of nitric oxide–related compounds and carperitide on hemodynamics and hematocrit in anesthetized rats. Jpn J Pharmacol 59:489–492, 1992

196. Valentin JP, Gardner DG, Wiedemann E, et al: Modulation of endothelin effects on blood pressure and hematocrit by atrial natriuretic peptide. Hypertension 17:864–869, 1991

197. Carraway RE, Cochrane DE, Salmonsen R, et al: Neurotensin elevates hematocrit and plasma levels of leukotrienes, LTB4, LTC4, LTD4 and LTE4, in anesthetized rats. Peptides 12: 1105–1111, 1991

198. Cohen AM, Gelvan A, Kadour A, et al: Tissue plasminogen activator levels in different types of polycythemia. Eur J Haematol 45:48–51, 1990

199. Partenen S, Juvoneu E, Ikkala E, et al: Spontaneous erythroid colony formation in the differential diagnosis of erythrocytosis. Eur J Haematol 42:327–333, 1989

200. Rudberg U, Skarberg KO: RES scintigraphy in polycythemia vera and secondary or relative polycythemia. Acta Radiol 34:183–186, 1993

201. Smith JR, Landaw SA: Smoker's polycythemia. N Engl J Med 298:6–10, 1978

202. Helman H, Rubenstein LS: The effects of age, sex, and smoking on erythrocytes and leukocytes. Am J Clin Pathol 63:35–44, 1975

203. Lowe GDO, Gorbes CD, Barbanel JC: The effects of age and cigarette smoking on blood and plasma viscosity in men. Scott Med J 25:13–17, 1980

204. Eisen ME, Hammond EC: The effect of smoking in reduced cell volume, red blood cell counts, hemoglobin and platelet counts. Can Med Assoc J 75:520–523, 1956

205. Isager H, Hagerup L: Relationship between cigarette smoking and high packed cell volume and hemoglobin levels. Scand J Haematol 8: 241–244, 1971

206. Stewart RD, Baretta ED, Platte LR, et al: Carboxyhemoglobin levels in American blood donors. JAMA 229:1187–1195, 1974

207. Dintenfass L: Elevation of blood viscosity, aggregation of red cells, hematocrit values and fibrinogen levels in cigarette smokers. Med J Aust 1:617–620, 1975

208. Angelkort B, Kiesewetter H: Influence of risk factors and coagulation phenomena in the flu-

idity of blood in chronic arterial occlusive disease. Scand J Clin Lab Invest 41(suppl 156): 185–188, 1981

209. Sagone AL Jr, Balcerzak SP: Smoking as a cause of erythrocytosis. Ann Intern Med 82:512–515, 1975

210. Spiers ASD, Levine M: Smoker's polycythemia. Lancet 1:120, 1983

211. Ramsey JM: The time course of hematological response to experimental exposures of carbon monoxide. Arch Environ Health 18:323–329, 1969

212. Penney DG, Davidson SB, Gargulinski RB, et al: Heart and lung hypertrophy, changes in blood volume, hematocrit and plasma renin activity in rats chronically exposed to increasing carbon monoxide concentrations. J Appl Toxicol 8:171–178, 1988

213. Cryer PE, Haymond MW, Santiago JV, et al: Norepinephrine and epinephrine release and adrenergic mediation of smoking-associated hemodynamic and metabolic events. N Engl J Med 295:573–577, 1976

214. Hofstetter A, Schutz Y, Jequier E, et al: Increased 24 hour energy expenditure in cigarette smokers. N Engl J Med 314:79–82, 1986

215. Butts WC, Kuehneman M, Widdowson GM: Automated method for determining serum thiocyanate to distinguish smokers from nonsmokers. Clin Chem 20:1344–1348, 1974

216. Ward HP, Bigelow DB, Pelty TL: Postural hypoxemia and erythrocytosis. Am J Med 45:880–888, 1968

217. Hamosh P, Da Silva AMT: Supine hypoxemia and erythrocytosis due to airway closure at low lung volumes. Am J Med 55:80–85, 1973

218. Editorial: Snoring and sleepiness. Lancet 2:925–926, 1985

219. Koskenvuo M. Partinen M, Sarna S, et al: Snoring as a risk factor for hypertension and angina pectoris. Lancet 1:893–895, 1985

220. Partinen M, Palomaki H: Snoring and cerebral infarction. Lancet 2:1325–1326, 1985

221. Block AJ: Sleep apnea and related disorder. Dis Mon 31:6–56, 1985

222. Tikare SK, Chandhary BA, Bandisode MS: Hypertension and stroke in a young man with obstructive sleep apnea syndrome. Postgrad Med 78:59–66, 1985

223. Kamphinsen HAC: Sleep apnea syndrome (letter). Lancet 2:1304, 1985

224. Kryger MH, Mezon BJ, Acres JC, et al: Diagnosis of sleep breathing disorders in a general hospital. Arch Intern Med 142:956–958, 1982

225. Moore-Gillon JC, Treacher DF, Gaminara EJ, et al: Intermittent hypoxia in patients with unexplained polycythaemia. Br Med J (Clin Res Ed) 293:588–590, 1986

226. El Yousef MK, Makewell WE Jr: The Gaisbock syndrome. JAMA 220:864, 1972

227. Block AJ, Boysen PG, Wynne JW: Sleep apnea, hypopnea, and oxygen desaturation in normal subjects. N Engl J Med 300:513–517, 1979

228. Guilleminault C: Obstructive sleep apnea: The clinical syndrome and historical perspective. Med Clin North Am 69:1187–1203, 1985

229. Sandblom RE, Matsumoto AM, Schoene RB, et al: Obstructive sleep apnea syndrome induced by testosterone administration. N Engl J Med 308:508–510, 1983

230. Moore-Gillon J, Pearson TC: Smoking, drinking and polycythaemia (editorial). Br Med J (Clin Res Ed) 292:1617–1618, 1986

231. Pinder AW, Smits AW: Mechanisms of acute hemoconcentration in bullfrogs in response to hypoxemia. Am J Physiol 264:R687–R695, 1993

232. Fletcher EC, DeBehnke RD, Lovoi MS, et al: Undiagnosed sleep apnea in patients with essential hypertension. Ann Intern Med 103:190–195, 1985

233. Messinezy M, Aubry S, O'Connell G, et al: Oxygen desaturation in apparent and relative polycythaemia. Br Med J 302:216–217, 1991

234. Blake S, Carey M, McShane A, et al: Autoregulation of tissue blood flow in essential hypertension. Hypertension 7:1003–1007, 1985

235. Susic D, Mandal AK, Jovovic D, et al: The effect of acute and chronic hematocrit changes on cardiovascular hemodynamics in spontaneously hypertensive rats. Am J Hypertens 5:713–718, 1992

236. Lebel M, Grose JH, Blais R: Increased hematocrit with normal red blood cell mass in early borderline essential hypertension. Clin Exp Hypertens 11:1505–1514, 1989

237. Gobel BO, Schulte-Gobel A, Weisser B, et al: Arterial blood pressure: Correlation with erythrocyte count, hematocrit, and hemoglobin concentration. Am J Hypertens 4:14–19, 1991

238. Cirillo M, Laurenzi M, Trevisan M, et al: Hematocrit, blood pressure, and hypertension: The Gubbio Population Study. Hypertension 20:319–326, 1992

239. Takayama Y, Ichikawa S, Sakamaki T, et al: Increase in hematocrit by nifedipine in hypertensive patients. Tohoku J Exp Med 161:251–252, 1990

240. Kato T, Yoneda S, Kako T, et al: Effect of nifedipine on oxygen delivery in patients with angina pectoris: Relation between blood viscosity and hematocrit. J Clin Pharmacol 31:518–520, 1991

241. Velasquez MT, Schechter GP, McFarland W, et al: Relative polycythemia: a state of high venous tone. Clin Res 33:409a, 1974

242. Ito N, Takeshita A, Higuchi S, et al: Venous abnormality in normotensive young men with a family history of hypertension. Hypertension 8:142–146, 1986

243. Takeshita A, Ashihara T, Yamamoto K, et al: Venous response to salt loading in hypertensive subjects. Circulation 69:50–57, 1983

244. Prankerd TAJ: Polycythemia—Diagnosis and variants. Proc R Soc Med 59:1089–1091, 1966

245. Williams GH, Hollenberg NK: Are non-modulating patients with essential hypertension a distinct subgroup? Implications for therapy. Am J Med 79(3C):3–9, 1985

246. Rosenberg L, Kaufman DW, Helmrich SP, et al: The risk of myocardial infarction after quitting smoking in men under 55 years of age. N Engl J Med 313:1511–1514, 1985

247. Vlietstra RE, Krornnal RA, Oberman A, et al: Effect of cigarette smoking on survival of patients with angiographically documented coronary artery disease. JAMA 255:1023–1027, 1986

248. Weinreb NJ: Relative polycythemia. In Brain MC, McCulloch PB (eds): Current Therapy in He-

matology-Oncology 1983–1984. Toronto, BC Decker, 1983, p 62

249. Schuster CJ, Weil MH, Besso J, et al: Blood volume following diuresis induced by furosemide. Am J Med 76:585–592, 1984

250. Reisen E, Abel R, Modan M, et al: Effect of weight loss without salt restriction on the reduction of blood pressure in overweight hypertensive patients. N Engl J Med 298:1–6, 1978

251. MacMahon SW, Wikchen DEL, MacDonald GJ: The effect of weight reduction on left ventricular mass. N Engl J Med 314:334–339, 1986

252. Jennings G, Nelson L, Nestel P, et al: The effects of changes in physical activity on major cardiovascular risk factors, hemodynamics, sympathetic function and glucose utilization in man: A controlled study of four levels of activity. Circulation 73:30–40, 1986

253. Landaw SA: Polycythemia vera and other polycythemic states. Clin Lab Med 10:857–871, 1990

254. Van de Pette JE, Guthrie DL, Pearson TC: Whole blood viscosity in polycythaemia: The effect of iron deficiency at a range of haemoglobin and packed cell volumes. Br J Haematol 63:369–375, 1986

255. Chetty G, Brown SE, Light HW: Improved exercise tolerance of the polycythemia lung patient following phlebotomy. Am J Med 74:415–420, 1983

256. Wasserman LR, Balcerzak SY, Berlin NI, et al: Influence of therapy on causes of death in polycythemia vera. Trans Assoc Am Physicians 94:30–38, 1981

257. Kiraly JF III, Feldman JE, Wheby MS: Hazards of phlebotomy in polycythemic patients with cardiovascular disease. JAMA 236:2080–2081, 1976

258. Thomas SH, Smith SW, Slater NG, et al: The haemodynamic responses to venesection and the effects of cardiovascular disease. Clin Lab Haematol 14:201–208, 1992

259. Bomford A, Williams R: Long term results of venesection therapy in idiopathic hemochromatosis. Q J Med 45:611–623, 1976

260. Cohen MA, Oberman HA: Safety and long term effects of plasmapheresis. Transfusion 10:58–66, 1970

261. Finch CA, Cook JD, Labhe RF, et al: Effect of blood donation on iron stores as evaluated by serum ferritin. Blood 50:441–447, 1977

262. Sullivan JL: Iron and the sex difference in heart disease risk. Lancet 1:1293–1294, 1981

263. Sullivan JL: Blood donation may be good for the donor: Iron, heart disease, and donor recruitment. Vox Sang 61:161–164, 1991

264. Casale G, Rignamlni M, de Nicola P: Does blood donation prolong life expectancy? Vox Sang 45:398–399, 1983

ACKNOWLEDGEMENT: I am grateful to Eric Ottoway, Department of Computer Services, of Vitas Healthcare Corp. of Florida, for valued technical assistance.

19

Myeloid Metaplasia with Myelofibrosis (Agnogenic and Postpolycythemia Vera)

DAVID S. ROSENTHAL

Agnogenic myeloid metaplasia or myeloid metaplasia with myelofibrosis (MM-MF) is a disorder with many similarities to polycythemia vera (PV), essential thrombocythemia (ET), and chronic granulocytic leukemia (CGL). MM-MF is characterized by the presence of splenomegaly (often massive), a leukoerythroblastic blood film, teardrop red cell forms, and a varying degree of marrow fibrosis. Myeloid metaplasia (MM) or extramedullary hematopoiesis (EMH) is not a specific feature, since it is seen in a number of other disease states. Marrow fibrosis by itself is also not unique for MM-MF and is present in many disorders. The combination of myeloid metaplasia with myelofibrosis, however, is specific for this chronic myeloproliferative disorder. There is a subgroup of PV patients who transform or evolve into a clinical and laboratory picture indistinguishable from MM-MF, and this condition is referred to as *postpolycythemia myeloid metaplasia*. In addition, a small but significant number of CGL and ET patients may develop a similar picture with myelofibrosis. MM-MF is similar to other myeloproliferative disorders in that, with or without therapeutic intervention, conversion to acute leukemia or "blast crisis" may occur. However, the major causes of morbidity and mortality are cardiovascular in nature.

MM-MF and post-PV MM display an array of clinical, laboratory, and pathologic findings, and the course and the natural history of these disorders may be quite variable. Although a third of patients may be asymptomatic at presentation, the clinical problems that arise during the course of disease are many. Pancytopenia of varying degrees, thrombocytosis (with either increased bleeding or thrombosis), and symptomatic splenomegaly are the most common complications and often require difficult therapeutic decisions. Recent investigations into the nature of the nonhematopoietic proliferative cell, the fibroblast, have shed new light on the development of myelofibrosis, hopefully leading to better therapeutic approaches.

TERMINOLOGY AND HISTORICAL NOTES

A brief note must be made at the onset about the numerous titles that have been used to describe this disease over the 100 plus years since Heuck first reported the initial two cases.[1] Table 19–1 summarizes alphabetically the often descriptive terminology.

In 1879, Heuck first described two cases that differed from classical CGL on the finding of EMH and marrow fibrosis.[1] Askenazy[2] and Assman[3] demonstrated that the spleen was not the only site of EMH and that marrow fibrosis could progress to osteosclerosis. In 1907, Meyer and Heineke[4] demonstrated that extramedullary hematopoiesis occurred

TABLE 19–1. TERMINOLOGY

Agnogenic myeloid metaplasia
Aleukemic myelosis with osteosclerosis
Atypical myeloid leukemia
Atypical myelosis
Chronic erythroblastosis
Chronic nonleukemic myelosis
Idiopathic myeloid metaplasia
Leukanemia
Leukoerythroblastic anemia
Megakaryocytic myelosis with osteosclerosis
Megakaryocytic splenomegaly
Myelosis
Osteomyeloreticulosis
Osteosclerotic anemia
Osteosclerotic pseudoleukemia
Primary myelofibrosis

in sites where marrow naturally occurred in the embryo. In that same year, Donhauser[5] suggested that this disorder was primarily due to bone marrow failure with compensatory EMH. Hirschfeld[6] further demonstrated the uniqueness of this disorder from CGL on the basis of splenic histology, described below. In the 1930s, Vaughan and Harrison[7] theorized that the disease resulted from some marrow insult and involved the cell types derived from a primitive mesenchymal cell. Toxic exposure to chemicals such as benzol was suggested as directly causing this clinical entity, but there is a paucity of good scientific data to support this.[8]

In 1951, Dameshek[9] put forth his concept of "myeloproliferative disorders," which has, for the most part, stood up to the present time as a unifying theory linking MM-MF, PV, and CGL as primary marrow disorders. The 1960s brought forth large clinical studies and much further discussion of the rationale of "combining" or "splitting" all the myeloproliferative diseases.[10–15] The fact that MM-MF and post-PV MM could progress to acute leukemia became quite clear from a number of these studies.[12–15] MM-MF as a unique pathologic entity was further elucidated by Ward and Block[16] in 1971. From 1969 to 1978, it became clear from both glucose-6-phosphate dehydrogenase (G-6-PD) isoenzyme and cytogenetic studies that the fibroblast was the result of nonclonal proliferation.[17–20] These results implied that the fibroblast was a reactive cell and not a primary component of the hematopoietic proliferation. The 1980s brought even more refinement to this disorder with respect to pathogenesis and therapy of myelofibrosis.

Reversal of marrow fibrosis in MM-MF has been demonstrated to occur either as part of a natural conversion or metamorphosis of the disease or secondary to chemotherapy with alkylating agents alone or together with irradiation as part of marrow transplantation.[21–26] The marrow fiber content appears to be related to platelet number and, theoretically, platelet-derived growth factor (PDGF).[27–32] Histologic studies equate degree of megakaryocytopoiesis with degree of fibrosis.[16] Current evidence favors the theory that abnormal megakaryocytosis, morphologically evident in MM-MF, causes excessive release of PDGF, which promotes fibroblast proliferation and secretion of collagen. In turn, the normal process of degradation of newly formed collagen may be inhibited by a simultaneous release of platelet factor IV, inhibiting collagenase.[31,33] Finally, recent human embryonic studies fail to confirm the fetal spleen as a site of hematopoiesis.[34] This finding casts doubt on the theory that the spleen acts as a compensating organ for a damaged marrow and raises the possibility that the "diseased" marrow causes early release of hematopoietic precursors that find the splenic sinusoids an appropriate soil for cultivation.[35]

PATHOPHYSIOLOGY AND ETIOLOGY

Myeloid metaplasia is not difficult to produce in the experimental animal, nor is it unusual to see in a number of human disorders other than MM-MF. Myelofibrosis can be induced acutely by a number of toxic substances in animals, by some agents in humans, and can be seen as a secondary manifestation of a number of disease processes (Table 19–2). Although the etiology for most cases remains obscure, it is currently believed that a toxic insult(s) occurs in the marrow which suppresses the hematopoietic stem cells, causes a secondary increase in fibroblasts and osteoblasts, and allows for a selective advantage for certain myeloid clones. It has been theorized by Silverstein,[36] Ward and Block,[16] and others[35] that the marrow-proliferating cells, thus irritated, leave the marrow and begin to proliferate in extramedullary sites. In animals, it is known that chemicals, solvents, hormones, viruses, and ionizing irradiation may be toxic events lead-

TABLE 19-2. PROPOSED CAUSES OF MYELOID METAPLASIA

Experimental
1. Chemical
2. Solvents
3. Hormones
4. Viruses
5. Antigen-antibody complex
6. Ionizing radiation

Human
1. Chemical
2. Ionizing radiation
3. Chemotherapy
4. Immune complexes
5. Abnormal megakaryocytopoiesis

ing to MM-MF.[37-44] Chemicals such as lead and saponin, toxins such as benzene, the Rauscher and feline leukemia virus, antigen-antibody complexes, and ionizing radiation have all been demonstrated to cause myeloid metaplasia with myelofibrosis (MM-MF) in the experimental animal. It has been postulated that EMH results as a normal response of mesenchymal tissue to injury, that mesenchymal-derived cells differentiate and then migrate into a favorable environment.[45-47] In human beings, local myeloid metaplasia has been reported in a wide variety of tissues as a result of local inflammation and necrosis.[48] Generalized EMH in addition has been noted secondary to toxic substances such as benzene and irradiation, infections such as syphilis and tuberculosis, neoplasms, severe hemolytic or pernicious anemia, osteopetrosis or storage diseases (Gaucher's), and vitamin D-deficient rickets.[16,45,46,49-56] Chemicals and radiation have both been implicated as causative agents in humans. Benzene has been associated with a number of cases of MM-MF as well as with acute myelogenous leukemia (AMl).[57] In Hiroshima following the atomic blast, Anderson et al.[58] reported 12 to 13 cases of myelofibrosis in survivors; however, later reviews of the cases and histologic material failed to confirm these cases as consistent with the diagnosis of myelofibrosis, and no additional cases were discovered.[59]

The finding of a high frequency of immune abnormalities in patients with MM-MF and post-PV MM raises the possibility that immune complexes play a role in the pathogenesis of marrow fibrosis.[60-62] The types of immune abnormalities (discussed below) vary, but the incidence increases with degree of fibrosis.[62] It has been suggested that immune complexes could bind to platelets

through Fc receptors and stimulate platelet release of factors (e.g., platelet-derived growth factor, PDGF) that promote collagen synthesis by fibroblasts.

More recently, molecular biologists may have given us some insight into the pathogenesis of marrow fibrosis. The oncogene c-*sis* encodes PDGF and may stimulate fibroblast growth in vivo.[63,64] Conceivably, increased expression of this oncogene could have an etiologic role in the reactive myelofibrosis seen.

Historically, Ward and Block[16] had advanced three potential theories for the pathogenesis of MM-MF: (1) compensatory, (2) neoplastic, and (3) benign "myelostimulatory" theories. The compensatory theory was based on animal studies and suggested that a marrow insult preceded and led to EMH. The neoplastic theory places MM-MF in the arena of myeloproliferative disorders, and recent studies do support the clonal nature of this disease and its potential to progress or transform into an undifferentiated leukemia. The benign myelostimulatory theory suggests that the disorder is the result of a normal response of a normal stem cell to an unidentified abnormal stimulus. Current opinion and data strongly support the neoplastic theory. Results of studies in a few patients using G-6-PD isoenzymes indicate that MM-MF involves hematopoietic cells multipotent for granulocytes, erythrocytes, and platelets and that it is clonal at the time of diagnosis.[19] This clonal development cannot support the "compensatory" or benign "myelostimulatory" theory. As mentioned above, the marrow fibroblasts of MM-MF and those seen with CGL or PV have been studied and do not reveal monoclonality based on either G-6-PD isoenzyme studies or cytogenetics.[17-20] Castro-Malaspina and colleagues[31,65] developed a liquid culture system for cloning and growing bone marrow fibroblasts. They were able to conclude that the marrow collagen-producing cells in MM-MF and indeed from all patients with myeloproliferative disorders with or without fibrosis behave in vitro as do those cells from normal individuals and are nonclonal in origin. This confirmed the G-6-PD and cytogenetic studies on fibroblasts and supports the hypothesis that the marrow fibrosis in MM-MF and post-PV MM "results from a reactive process rather than from a primary disorder affecting the marrow collagen-producing cells."

There appears to be a direct relationship between megakaryocytes and/or platelets and myelofibrosis. The Polycythemia Vera Study Group (PVSG) demonstrated an initial increased incidence of myelofibrosis in PV patients when treated with phlebotomy alone as opposed to chlorambucil and radioactive phosphorus, although with the passage of time, the incidence became equivalent for all three therapies.[66] Although these data are preliminary, it is possible that phlebotomy stimulates further megakaryocytopoiesis. Bentley at al.,[29] using a digital imaging technique for estimating collagen and marrow fiber content, demonstrated a direct relationship between platelet number and fiber content (Fig. 19–1). Previously, Ward and Block[16] demonstrated a morphologic relationship between megakaryocytes and degree of myelofibrosis (Fig. 19–2). The relationship of increased platelets and megakaryocytes, fiber and collagen production, and levels of PDGF has led to a theory initiated by Groopman[30] and expanded by McCarthy.[67] The sequence of events explaining myelofibrosis might be megakaryocytes and/or platelets from MM-MF release inappropriately high levels of platelet-derived growth factor (PDGF), which stimulates fibroblasts to divide and secrete collagen. Castro-Malaspina[31,68] has shown that homogenates of normal human megakaryocytes can stimulate fibrogenesis, supporting this possibility. The rare "gray platelet syndrome" associated with myelofibrosis and elevated PDGF levels also lends evidence to this theory.[69,70] In addition, simultaneous release of platelet factor IV from the megakaryo-

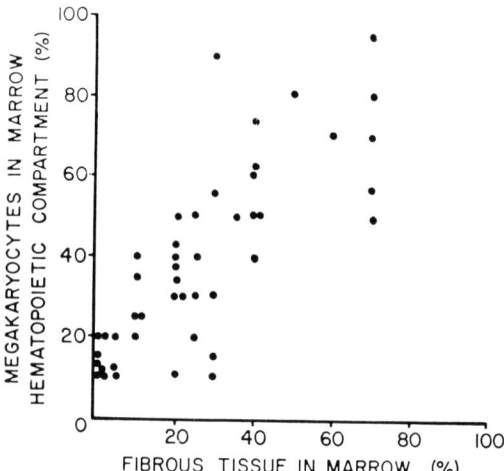

FIGURE 19–2. Relationship of marrow megakaryocytic number and degree of myelofibrosis. *(Adapted with permission from Ward HP, Block MH: Medicine 50:357–420, 1971.)*

cytes may inhibit breakdown of fibrosis by competing with collagenase activity, creating an imbalance between collagen production and degradation and thus excessive deposition of marrow collagen[33] (Fig. 19–3).

PATHOLOGY

The diagnosis of MM-MF is based on the simultaneous finding of myelofibrosis and extramedullary hematopoiesis. The latter in clinical practice may be demonstrated by direct histologic study of the liver or spleen or by the combination of an enlarged spleen and the typical peripheral blood smear described below. EMH has been described in practically every tissue site. Bone marrow findings are extremely variable at time of diagnosis, ranging from an aspirate revealing a "dry tap" and biopsy showing extensive fibrosis and bone sclerosis to a hypercellular aspirate and biopsy with a panmyelosis and only a trace of increased reticulin (Fig. 19–4). Bone marrow biopsies are essential in the diagnosis, and good histologic preparation cannot be overemphasized to aid in differentiating MM-MF from other clinical conditions that result in secondary myelofibrosis. In MM-MF, the majority of marrow biopsies are hypocellular at diagnosis, with a persistence of all three hematopoietic cell lines. Hickling[14] described seven grades of histologic change, ranging from slight hyper-

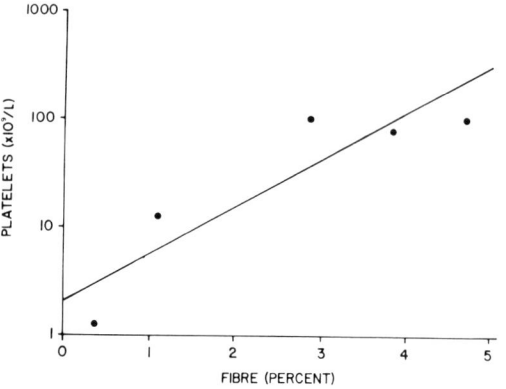

FIGURE 19–1. Relationship of platelet number and bone marrow fiber content. *(Adapted with permission from Bentley SA, Herman CJ: Br J Haematol 42:52–59, 1979.)*

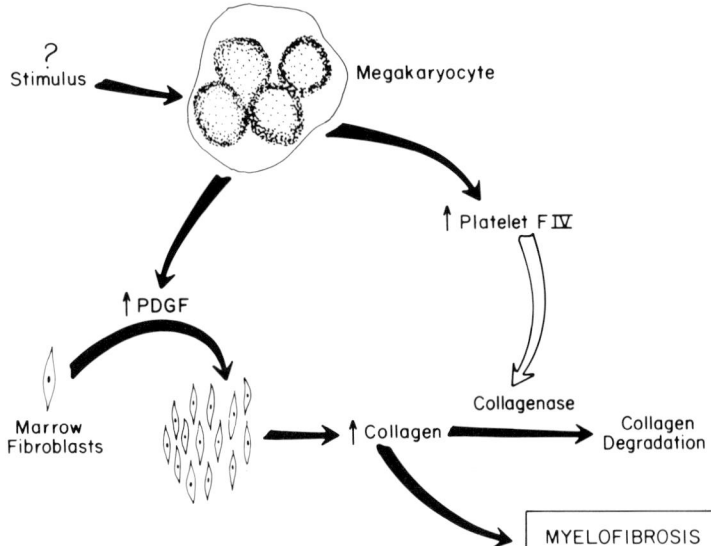

FIGURE 19–3. Possible mechanism for the development of myelofibrosis in MM-MF (black lines = increased activity, clear lines = inhibition).

cellularity without increased reticulin (grade I) to marked thickening and widening of bony trabeculae and few marrow cells, primarily megakaryocytes (grade VII). Ward and Block[16] simplified the marrow stages into three categories: (1) panhyperplasia, (2) myeloid atrophy and fibrosis, and (3) myelofibrosis and osteosclerosis. Panhyperplasia, noted in about 25 percent of patients,

consisted of a panmyelosis, with marrow cellularity greater than 70 percent and the trilineage comprising over 95 percent of the cells, and a slight increase in reticular fibers, as demonstrated by special stains. Approximately 40 percent of patients in their series presented with myeloid atrophy and myelofibrosis. There remained islets of residual hyperplastic trilineage separated by "an

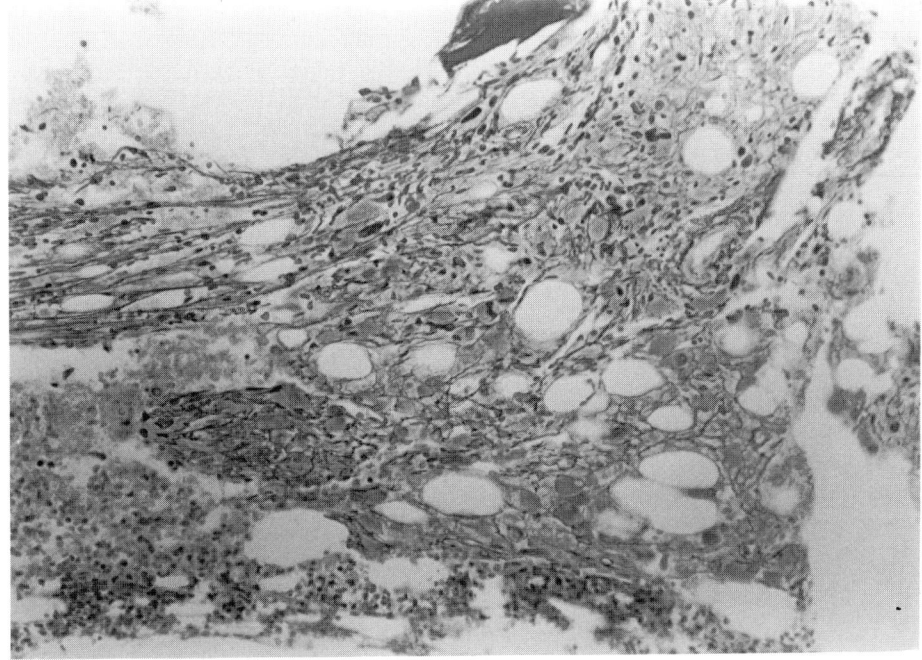

FIGURE 19–4. Bone marrow biopsy in severe myelofibrosis ($\times$ 1000).

amorphous ground substance with a network of reticular fibers, collagen fibers, plasma cells, and poorly defined stromal cells." The remaining 35 percent of patients presented with severe cellular depletion and bone trabeculation comprising 30 percent or greater of the bone biopsy sections. The reduced marrow cells consisted primarily of megakaryocytic clumps, and the remainder of the marrow consisted of myelofibrotic and osteosclerotic tissue. There appears to be a direct relationship between the degree of marrow fibrosis and marrow megakaryocytes[16] (see Fig. 19–2). In summary, the marrow generally demonstrates increased cellularity, a normal to slightly increased myeloid-to-erythroid ratio, normal to slightly increased granulopoiesis with maturation, variable erythropoiesis but with complete maturation, markedly increased megakaryocytes in clusters and with dysplastic forms, slight to markedly increased hemosiderin, and slight to markedly increased reticulin (Table 19–3).

The spleen enlargement may be the presenting complaint in the majority of patients, and its pathology confirms the diagnosis. Splenic weights may range from 1500 to 3000 g, but a 7000-g spleen is not unusual. Just a few decades ago splenic aspiration was a diagnostic procedure that would demonstrate the trilineage on Wright and Giemsa staining. Grossly, the spleens at surgery appear red and often have multiple adhesions and areas of infarction. The diagnostic histology is the evidence of the trilineage hematopoiesis largely confined to the sinuses with no appreciable predominance of any one cell type (Fig. 19–5A). There does not appear to be any direct relationship between the size of the spleen, the degree of EMH, and the amount of myelofibrosis. Histology of a CGL spleen is different with EMH in pulp cords as well as sinuses and a predominance of myeloid cells.

TABLE 19–3. MARROW FINDINGS IN MM-MF

Cellularity	Usually increased
M:E ratio	Usually within normal limits
Myeloid series	Normal to increased, with maturation, increased basophils
Erythroid series	Decreased, normal, or increased
Megakaryocytes	Usually moderate to marked increase, in clusters and dysplastic
Hemosiderin	Slight to marked increase
Reticulin	Slight to marked increase

Hepatomegaly may be evident in 70 percent of patients due to both congestion and EMH. Liver biopsies also may be diagnostic, with EMH in the hepatic sinusoids and prominent atypical megakaryocytes (Fig. 19–5B). Kupffer cell hyperplasia is common. Rarely will any parenchymal injury be demonstrated, and its occurrence or the progression to cirrhosis and portal hypertension would be more likely related to a Budd-Chiari syndrome or chemotherapy.

EMH has been described in lymph nodes, brain, dura, adrenal gland, kidney, breast, heart, pericardium, testis, ovary, bladder, lung, skin, thymus, and gastrointestinal tract and may even form tumor masses in these organs.[11,16,36,46,71,72] Spinal cord compression, obstructive liver disease, and pericardial tamponade have all been reported as complications of EMH.[73–76]

CLINICAL PRESENTATION

MM-MF is an infrequent disease, and like all other myeloproliferative disorders, there is a clear increase in incidence with age. The median age of most series is in the 60s, with little sex difference.[10–16,36] This disorder is rare in infancy and poses special problems in the young because of the numbers of years at risk for complications and transformations. The symptoms and physical findings at presentation of disease are listed in Table 19–4. Thirty percent or more may be totally asymptomatic when first presenting. Presenting complaints are generally referable to the degree of splenomegaly, anemia, bleeding, or thrombosis. Splenic enlargement may cause local or referred pain, fever, early satiety, or diarrhea. Anemia, a result of hypersplenism, marrow suppression, or blood loss, frequently will cause malaise, dyspnea, and worsening of underlying cardiovascular disease. Interestingly, as with PV, both bleeding and thrombotic complications are seen. Gout and renal stones, a manifestation of the high turnover of the hematopoietic cells, frequently may be elicited in the immediate history. The classic physical presentation is that of mild to moderate pallor, moderate to marked splenomegaly, and hepatomegaly. In addition, ecchymosis, monarthritis, and lymphadenopathy may occur at onset; ascites and jaundice may be a presenting finding indicating portal hypertension. The spleen

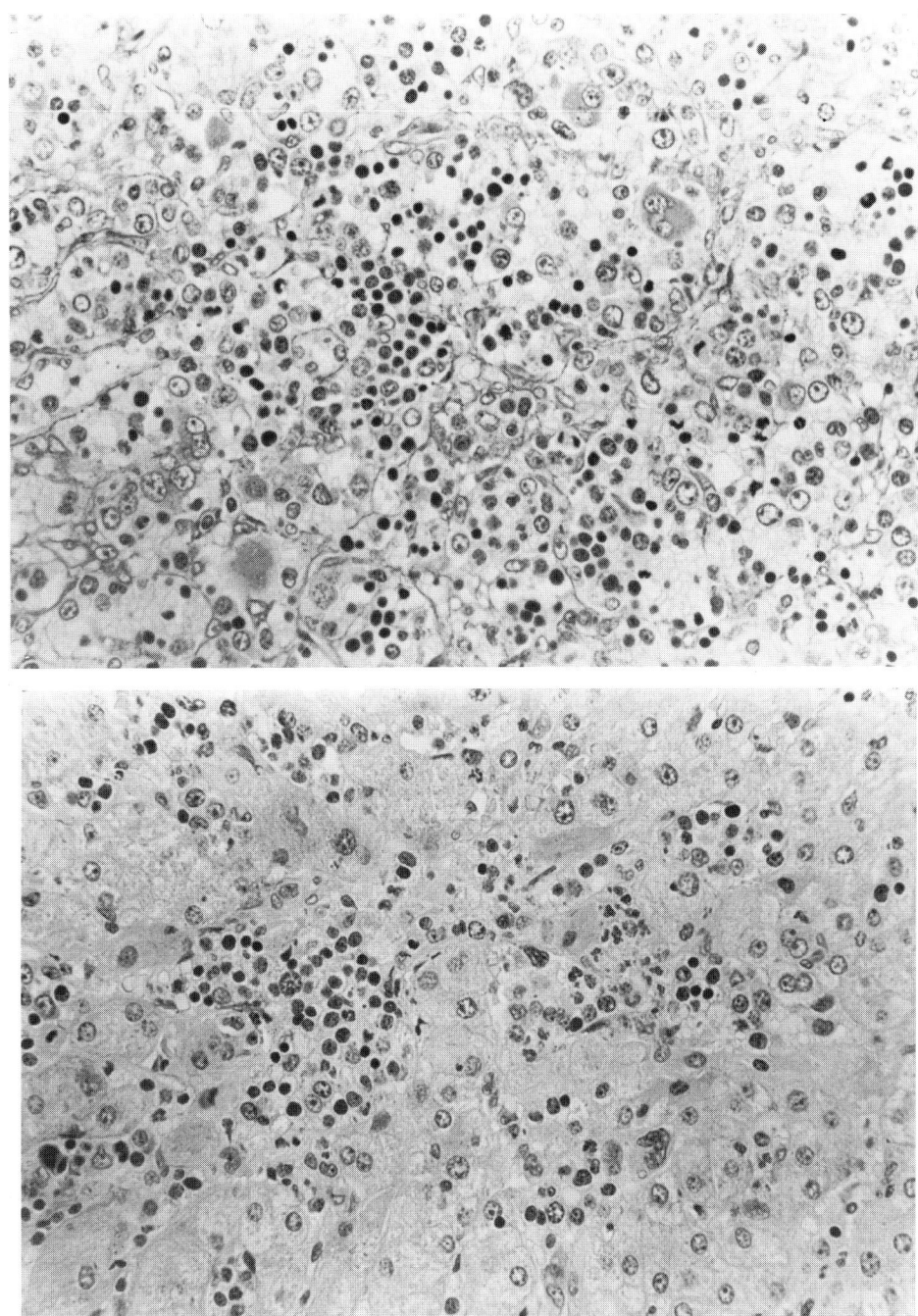

FIGURE 19-5. (A) Splenic histology demonstrating trilineage in red pulp and sinusoids. (B) Liver histology also demonstrating trilineage hematopoiesis in hepatic sinusoids.

size is usually greater than 5 cm below the left costal margin and in 25 percent of patients may be 10 cm or more.

The course of disease may be quite variable and poses many problems for the clini-cian. The major complications of MM-MF are listed in Table 19–5. Massive splenomeg-aly with compressive symptoms and develop-ment of portal hypertension is common. The pathogenesis of portal hypertension is

TABLE 19-4. CLINICAL PRESENTATION OF MM-MF

SYMPTOMS	PHYSICAL EXAMINATION
Asymptomatic	Pallor
Anemia	Splenomegaly
Weakness	$1/3$ < 5 cm
Fatigue	$1/3$ 5–10 cm
Dyspnea	$1/3$ > 10 cm
Angina	Hepatomegaly
Splenomegaly	Ecchymosis
Early satiety	Monarthritis
Pain	Lymphadenopathy
Diarrhea	Ascites
Bleeding	Jaundice
Thrombosis	
Hypermetabolic	
Weight loss	
Fever	
Gout	

unclear but is suspected to be related to increased portal blood flow, functional intrahepatic obstruction due to EMH, and perhaps increased sludging of blood through the portal and hepatic veins, all leading to periportal fibrosis and possible cirrhosis and ascites. Splenic pain secondary to infarcts may be severely uncomfortable but is usually transient as the spleen progressively enlarges. Anemia may be progressive due to development of myelofibrosis, increased phagocytic activity of the enlarging spleen, or blood loss. In addition, much of the erythropoiesis in MM-MF has been demonstrated to be ineffective. Bleeding and thrombosis are major causes of morbidity and mortality in MM-MF, as they are in PV and the other myeloproliferative conditions.[77–79] Estimates in various studies suggest that nearly 50 percent of patients with MM-MF have significant morbidity from bleeding and 10 to 25 percent will die from bleeding.[12, 16, 80, 81] Thrombotic complications may occur in almost 40 to 45 percent of patients, with 10 to 20 percent of all patients succumbing to this type of complication. The type of bleeding complications are characteristic of platelet and vascular dysfunction. Easy bruisability, epistaxis, and gastrointestinal mucosal bleeding are quite frequent, whereas deep tissue and visceral bleeding is rare. Thrombotic events appear to increase with age and may occur in customary sites such as deep veins of the legs, pulmonary arteries, and cerebral, coronary, or peripheral arteries. In addition, mesenteric artery thrombosis and hepatic vein oc-

clusion (Budd-Chiari syndrome) are often seen. In fact, the most frequent disorders underlying the Budd-Chiari syndrome are the chronic myeloproliferative diseases (MPDs). The hepatic or portal vein thrombosis is due to the combination of the massive splenomegaly with tremendously increased blood flow and the EMH in the hepatic sinusoids. The pathogenesis of increased thrombosis is unclear and not solely related to the absolute thrombocytosis. Patients with perfectly normal platelet counts, either spontaneously or therapeutically induced, may still have an increased susceptibility to increased clotting. Qualitative platelet defects commonly reported in all MPDs may be the cause.[82–84] Schafer[77] recently reviewed the specific qualitative platelet abnormalities in MPD patients. These are discussed below.

Leukemia has been reported as a final complication of this disease, and incidence varies from as low as 5 percent to as high as 25 percent.[10, 12, 13, 15, 21, 85] Although some believe that therapy with alkylating agents induces leukemic transformation, there are well-documented reports of acute leukemia occurring in patients treated by either androgen therapy or splenectomy alone.[16, 21] The acute leukemia may fit into any of the subtypes of the FAB classification or may even be lymphoid. The majority will be myeloid or myelomonocytic. As mentioned above, EMH can be found in any organ site, and a resulting mass effect can cause obstructive symptoms such as pericardial tamponade or spinal cord compression.[73, 75, 76] Skin and breast in-

TABLE 19-5. COMPLICATIONS OF MM-MF

Progressive splenomegaly
  Compressive symptoms
  Portal hypertension
  Ascites
  Splenic infarction
Bleeding
  Thrombocytopenia
  Abnormal platelet function
Thrombotic problems
  Deep vein thrombophlebitis
  Pulmonary embolism
  Arterial occlusion—cerebral, coronary, or peripheral
  Mesenteric vein thrombosis
  Budd-Chiari syndrome
Leukemic or blast transformation
Extramedullary hematopoiesis
  Organ infiltration, e.g., lymph nodes, skin, breast
Monarticular arthritis
Peptic ulcer disease

volvement may mimic tumor involvement and may only be distinguished by biopsy with specific histochemical staining.[12, 14, 72]

In general, about a third of patients with MM-MF will be asymptomatic at presentation, and the majority may remain so for over 5 to 10 years. Of the symptomatic patients, most will complain of symptoms related to anemia, others will complain of symptoms related to splenomegaly, and a smaller percentage will present with abnormal bleeding or thrombosis. From long-term follow-up of large series of cases, the median survival is 4 to 5 years but varies considerably, with asymptomatic patients having a better prognosis than symptomatic ones. Approximately 50 percent of patients will succumb to cardiovascular or thrombotic complications, 15 percent to bleeding problems, 10 to 15 percent to acute leukemia, and the remainder to various disorders, including infections and cancer.[10–16, 86]

LABORATORY STUDIES

The laboratory findings present many fascinating aspects (Table 19–6). The abundance of information may sometimes obscure rather than clarify the clinical situation. The leukoerythroblastic peripheral smear is

TABLE 19–6. LABORATORY FINDINGS IN MM-MF

Peripheral blood
  Anemia—Teardrops, stippled cells, NRBC
  Leukocytosis—Left shift, Pelger-Huet anomaly
  Basophilia—Poorly granulated
  Thrombocytosis—Megakaryocytic fragments, large forms
Clotting studies
  Factor deficiencies secondary to liver disease
  Abnormal platelet function
  Disseminated intravascular coagulation
Leukocyte alkaline phosphatase (LAP) score
  Usually elevated, 10 percent
Serum studies
  Increased B_{12}, unbound B_{12} binding capacity
  Increased lysozyme
  Increased histamine
  Increased uric acid
  Increased LDH and alkaline phosphatase
  Hypo- or hypergammaglobulinemia
  Monoclonal gammopathy (rare)
  Positive ANA, rheumatoid factor, immune complexes
    Pseudohyperkalemia
    Decreased cholesterol (LDL and HDL)

the hallmark of MM-MF. Significant numbers of teardrop cells, basophilic stippling, nucleated red cells, immature myeloid cells, basophilia, large platelets, and occasionally megakaryocytic fragments are the impressive features. The teardrop formation is thought to be a result of the EMH occurring in the spleen, caused by partial red cell membrane loss as the red cells traverse through the sinusoids. Although a wide range of routine blood levels have been reported (Fig. 19–6), patients will generally present with mild anemia (Hct in low 30s), moderate leukocytosis (WBC 15 to 20.0 × 10^9 liter), and moderate to marked thrombocytosis (platelets 500 to 2000 × 10^9 liter with a mean of about 800 × 10^9 liter). The anemia is generally normochromic and normocytic. Ferrokinetic studies have demonstrated decreased iron incorporation despite normal plasma iron clearance, compatible with ineffective erythropoiesis.[87–90] Radioactive chromium—labeled red cells, when infused back into the patient with MM-MF, may demonstrate a significantly shortened half-life compatible with the degree of splenomegaly. Rarely, the hemolytic or hypersplenic anemia will be associated with a positive antiglobulin test. A defect in the red cells of MM-MF patients similar to the PNH abnormality has been reported.[91–93] A positive acid-hemolysin test or sugar-water test may occur in as many as 10 percent of patients.

The leukocytosis is usually modest and helps distinguish MM-MF from CGL. In addition, the percentage of immature cells is less dramatic than in CGL, with only a few blast forms and primarily adult myeloid cells. Alternatively, as many as 15 percent of patients may have neutropenia, which may be secondary to ineffective granulocytopoiesis or increased splenic sequestration. Pelger-Hüet cells, poorly granulated basophils, and hypersegmented neutrophils may be noted. Basophilia is common and may lead to increased histamine levels in serum and urine and occasionally may result in a clinical flushing and hypotension. The myeloid cells appear normal but may have abnormal biologic behavior. They may demonstrate increased adherence, increased Fc-receptor activity, increased hexose monophosphate shunt activity, and increased release of specific granules.

The majority of patients will have thrombocytosis with megakaryocytic fragments in

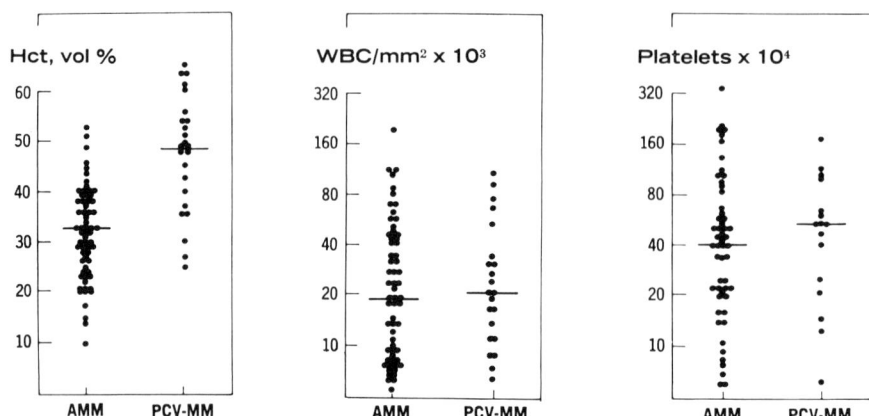

FIGURE 19-6. Laboratory findings at presentation in 98 patients with MM-MF and post-PV MM. *(Adapted with permission from Rosenthal DS, Moloney WC: Postgrad Med J 45:136-142, 1969.)*

the blood film along with large platelets, but about 15 percent present with thrombocytopenia, and more will develop this complication during the course of disease. The mechanisms of thrombocytopenia may include both ineffective production or hypersplenic activity.

Platelet function defects of all kinds have been reported in MM-MF. Abnormally prolonged bleeding times with normal or increased platelet counts have suggested varying types of platelet function defects. In addition, increased platelet reactivity has been described with decreased, normal, or increased platelet counts. Platelet counts by automated counter alone may be deceivingly low due to excessive platelet clumping and platelet size. Both abnormalities will result in underestimating total platelet count, which should be verified by peripheral blood smear or phase counting. A recent review has stressed the high incidence of either platelet hypoaggregability or hyperaggregability that has been described in patients with MM-MF.[77] In addition, a number of biochemical and metabolic abnormalities occur. Acquired platelet storage pool disease, platelet membrane abnormalities, and abnormal arachidonate metabolism in platelets have all been described but correlate poorly with clinical bleeding or thrombosis. Some of these abnormalities are aggravated by aspirin, and some are partially alleviated. As better understanding of the platelet membrane and its interactions are known, many of these laboratory abnormalities may become explainable.

Other abnormal bleeding and clotting parameters may be observed. Many patients will have prolongation of both prothrombin time and partial thromboplastin time due to liver disease or deficiency in factor V.[94] Silverstein[36] has noted that 12 to 25 percent will have a syndrome simulating disseminated intravascular coagulation (DIC), characterized by elevated fibrin split products, progressive thrombocytopenia, and decreased levels of factors V and VIII.[36] This syndrome has been seen as a complication surrounding the postsplenectomy period and may be related to a number of other factors. Various chemistry abnormalities have been seen, notably hyperuricemia, elevated serum lactate dehydrogenase (LDH), and elevated alkaline phosphatase. Elevated serum uric acid is quite frequent and is a consequence of purine catabolism caused by excessive intramedullary and intrasplenic blood cell destruction. Uric acid turnover rates are markedly increased in most patients studied. This partially explains the monarticular arthritis frequently reported as well as the occurrence of nonopaque renal stones. Ward and Block[16] believe that an excellent correlation exists between the elevated uric acid level and the amount of EMH and degree of ineffective erythropoiesis. Serum LDH probably is elevated for the same reasons. Elevated alkaline phosphatase levels in serum may be bone-related and correlate with the degree of myelofibrosis or liver-related and reflect EMH or superimposed liver disease. Serum protein levels have not been helpful in diagnosis but are not infrequently abnormal.[12, 16, 36, 95] Hypogammaglobulinemia as well as hypergammaglobulinemia with or without a monoclonal M spike have been reported.

Rondeau et al.[60] have reported that even in the absence of any cytotoxic or transfusion therapy, nearly 50 percent of all patients with MM-MF have a variety of immune abnormalities. Antinuclear antibodies, serum IgM rheumatoid factor, circulating immune complexes, M spikes, cryoglobulinemia, and positive direct Coombs' testing have all been reported. The incidence appears to increase with the severity of the disease and the lymphoid cellular infiltration of the marrow. This clinical presentation may be a variant of MM-MF or may indeed suggest that there may be a role for an immune mechanism in the pathogenesis.

Leukocyte alkaline phosphatase (LAP) levels clearly aid in the differential diagnosis.[15] The levels are usually elevated with a mean of just greater than 100 (normal values 15 to 80). However, the range of values is quite large, and approximately 10 percent of patients will have very low levels characteristic of CGL. A similar percentage will have elevations characteristic of PV. When LAP scores are low or absent, it is usually associated with low white blood counts and in some instances is an early sign of transformation to acute leukemia. Cytogenetic studies from peripheral blood or marrow aspirates, if possible, can aid in the differential diagnosis from CGL when these low LAP values are noted.

Serum vitamin B_{12} and vitamin B_{12}–binding protein levels have been shown to be elevated in all myeloproliferative disorders, and some believe that measurements of both the transcobalamin proteins help to differentiate one myeloproliferative disorder from another.[96] Transcobalamin I and II are two serum proteins that bind to serum B_{12}; one travels with the alpha and the other with beta globulin fraction on serum electrophoresis. Each is suspected to have a different function. One serves as a transport protein; the other as a storage or reserve compartment. Gilbert et al.[97] have demonstrated that the elevated B_{12} levels in myeloproliferative disorders are due to excessive binding of the vitamin by the greatly increased levels of the transcobalamins. There appears to be a direct correlation between the white blood cell count and levels of transcobalamins, with mature granulocytes producing a higher B_{12} binding capacity than immature myeloid cells. It is not surprising, then, that CGL has been associated with the highest B_{12} and unsaturated B_{12} binding capacity ($UB_{12}BC$). PV and MM-MF will both be associated with elevated levels, and the tremendous variability seems to be related to the wide range of WBCs found in these disorders. In MM-MF, the range of serum B_{12} has been reported as 250 to 1727 pg/ml (normal 258 to 584 pg/ml), with alpha $UB_{12}BC$ from 243 to 1490 pg/ml (normal 119 to 301 pg/ml) and beta $UB_{12}BC$ from 370 to 4206 pg/ml (normal 731 to 1093 pg/ml). The abnormally increased levels of the vitamin and its transport proteins may obscure the diagnosis of pernicious anemia, and clinical judgment should not be swayed by these laboratory studies.

Serum lysozyme (muramidase), shown to lyse certain bacterial cell walls, is produced by mature myeloid cells and monocytes and thus may be significantly elevated in the myeloproliferative disorders. Similar to vitamin B_{12}, there does appear to be a direct correlation of total granulocyte count and serum lysozyme level.[98] Enzyme levels would then be more elevated in CGL than in MM-MF or PV. Serial serum levels occasionally have been helpful in predicting the development of blast crisis, primarily when the undifferentiated cell turns out to be of myelomonocytic or monocytic origin.[99] In addition, markedly elevated lysozyme levels in serum and urine have been associated with hypokalemia as a result of renal potassium loss; this is due to a "Fanconi-like" tubular defect caused by deposition of the enzyme in tubular cells.[100] Control of the WBC count is necessary to prevent further potassium loss. Hyperkalemia is not an uncommon laboratory finding in MM-MF, as well as in ET and PV, and is usually factitious, associated with thrombocytosis. When platelet counts surpass 700,000/mm[3] and blood drawn for chemistry profiles is allowed to clot, the platelets release their intracellular potassium, leading to falsely elevated serum K levels. Drawing heparinized samples, centrifuging at high speeds, and performing a plasma potassium level will verify the pseudohyperkalemia. This phenomenon also will be noted with WBC counts greater than 100,000/mm[3]. Reduced plasma total cholesterol levels frequently occur in MM-MF patients.[101] These low levels appear to be due to significant reductions in both low-density and high-density lipoprotein.[102, 103] Reduced levels appear to correlate clinically with spleen size; that organ may act as a catabolic site for lipoprotein. Splenectomy has corrected the low levels, supporting this hypothesis.

**TABLE 19–7. CYTOGENETIC
FINDINGS**

Not specific
Abnormalities (40–50 percent)
Documented clonal abnormalities
   Trisomy 1q or 1q-
   Trisomy 8
   Trisomy 9
   Trisomy 21
   Iso 17q

Cytogenetic studies have proved quite useful in leukemia, lymphoma, and the myelodysplastic syndromes. The finding of a specific cytogenetic abnormality (t9:22) certainly has solidified the diagnostic criteria for CGL. Because of the hypercellularity and the often excessive amounts of reticulin and fibrosis in MM-MF, it may be difficult to obtain direct or short-term cultures from the marrow. As a result, very few reports of cytogenetics are available despite the marked improvement in culture, banding, and staining techniques. In cases with dry taps, attempts at cytogenetics have been partially successful in using blood, splenic aspirates, and occasionally biopsy material (Table 19–7). Whang-Peng et al.[104] reviewed 87 patients from the literature and found that 53 percent had abnormal karyotypes. Pierre[105] studied 28 patients either with the use of short-term cultures of the blood or careful attempts at marrow aspiration; he was able to evaluate 23 cases.[105] Fourteen of the 23 (61 percent) were normal. Of the 9 (39 percent) abnormal studies, there does not appear to be any specific marker chromosome for MM-MF. Similar findings have been reported for PV.[106] Trisomy 1q, trisomy 8, and trisomy 9 have been described in both MM-MF and PV.[107–110] In addition, trisomy 21 and iso (17q) have been found in both MM-MF and acute non-lymphocytic leukemia. To date, these cytogenetic abnormalities have not been predictive of blast transformation or prognosis in general. In one patient, a translocation involving 1q was associated with loss of the Rh antigen and acquired Rh antibodies.[111] When possible, exhaustive efforts should be made to obtain cytogenetic material from MM-MF marrow, peripheral blood, or tissue containing EMH. The major purpose in these studies would be to differentiate MM-MF from CGL. Prospective studies utilizing newer techniques hopefully will produce some valuable data.

Roentgenographic studies have demonstrated an incidence of osteosclerosis of from 30 to 70 percent. Vaughn and Harrison[7] in 1939 first correlated the abnormal bone films with the bone pathology. The variable incidence of findings most likely is related to the definition of stage of disease and the degree to which clinical investigators have prospectively studied this issue. Ward and Block[16] found a 40 percent incidence of osteosclerosis, and they commented that the degree of radiologic change was severe enough to produce a recognizable abnormality on chest x-ray in 32 percent of cases.[16] In addition, there appeared to be a correlation between the amount of fibrosis on histology, the degree of osteosclerosis, and the roentgenographic appearance of the pelvis (Fig. 19–7). The majority of radiologic abnormal-

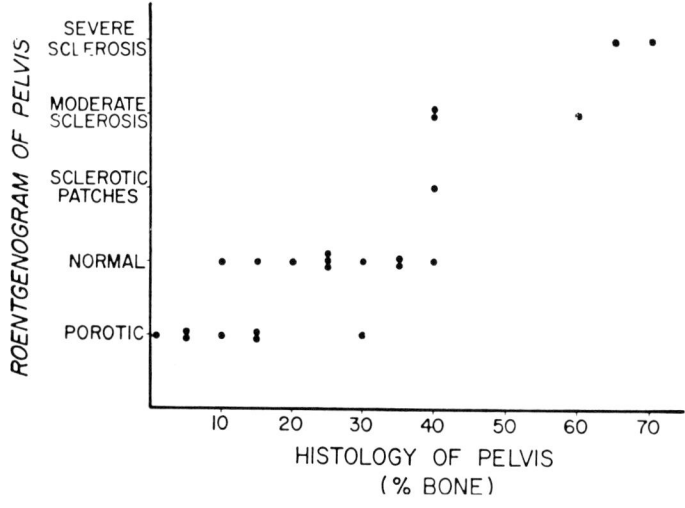

FIGURE 19–7. Comparison of roentgenogram pelvic appearance with percentage of marrow occupied by bony trabeculae. *(Adapted with permission from Ward HP, Block MH: Medicine 50:357–420, 1971.)*

ities were primarily in the axial skeleton, with vertebrae, ribs, clavicles, pelvis, scapula, and metaphyseal ends of the femur and humerus affected. Spared of changes were the bones distal to the elbow and knee. The classic radiologic findings are osteosclerosis with intact bone contour and no periosteal elevation (Table 19–8). The films show a "ground glass" appearance with gradual loss of individual trabeculae. There are gradual coalescing bony areas of increased density, which in the rib films give the picture of "jail bars." Ward and Block,[16] in their review, could demonstrate no serial progression in radiologic changes with time; neither Pettigrew and Ward[112] nor Silverstein[36] could correlate bone changes with age, sex, duration of disease, or degree of splenomegaly. Osteolytic disease is rarely seen and, if noted, should suggest the possibility of metastatic carcinoma or metabolic disease.

Nuclear scans, marrow scintigraphy, and ferrokinetic and chromium studies have all been utilized.[87, 88, 113–116] Technetium bone scans are not diagnostic and do not help in estimating the degree of fibrosis or sclerosis beyond the routine radiologic findings. Iron-52 and indium-111 have been evaluated as marrow scintigraphic agents[115, 117, 118] (see Chap. 6). Both agents can combine with transferrin and be transported to erythropoietic sites. Iron-52 is a more reliable agent, but because of its short half-life, it may be difficult to use in clinical practice. Indium-111, although it does not become incorporated into hemoglobin, has been shown to give results equivalent to iron-52 in myeloproliferative disorders.[115] Both radioisotopic studies correlate well with bone marrow activity but do poorly in estimating sites of EMH such as the liver and spleen. Figure 19–8 illustrates the results of indium scintigraphy in aplasia, MM-MF, and normal individuals. Although serial studies have not been routinely performed in MM-MF, mar-

row reversibility in treated aplasia has confirmed the usefulness of this procedure.[119] The indium isotope becomes a colloid and is phagocytozed by the reticuloendothelial cells in liver and spleen. Positive imaging in these organs therefore does not correlate with EMH.[115, 117, 118] Ferrokinetic studies have been used to determine sites of erythropoiesis, iron turnover, and utilization. Of 40 patients studied by Button et al.,[116] the results of interest were the plasma iron clearance, iron incorporation, and organ scanning over the sacrum, liver, and spleen. Simultaneous studies can be performed measuring red cell survival and splenic sequestration using a pulse height spectrometer, which can differentiate ^{59}Fe and ^{51}Cr activities. Patients can be divided into early stages of disease by near-normal iron clearance, greater than 50 percent incorporation, and abundant counts over the sacrum (greater than 150 cpm/μCi of iron injected). Those with advanced myelofibrosis with massive splenomegaly are characterized by normal to reduced iron clearance, markedly reduced iron incorporation (ineffective erythropoiesis), sacral counts less than 100 cpm/μCi, and markedly shortened red cell survival with significant splenic sequestration. These studies may be helpful in evaluating the course of disease, candidates for splenectomy, or the results of other therapeutic interventions.

Computed tomography (CT) is a sensitive detector for bone mineralization and may serve as a useful device in following subtle changes in the bone in patients with MM-MF.[120, 121] The radiologic studies described above change very slowly in patients from year to year. Subtle changes of progression or regression may be detected by CT study, aiding clinicians in their therapeutic options.

DIFFERENTIAL DIAGNOSIS AND ATYPICAL PRESENTATIONS

Variability in clinical presentation as well as degree of splenomegaly and myelofibrosis may cause difficulty in differentiating MM-MF from other diseases. Table 19–9 reviews the various disorders confused with MM-MF. The most common myeloproliferative disorder that mimics MM-MF is CGL. Leukemoid reactions, tuberculosis, hairy cell leukemia, metastatic carcinoma, and primary liver disease with portal hypertension may be dif-

TABLE 19–8. ROENTGENOGRAPHIC STUDIES

APPEARANCE	BONES INVOLVED
Osteosclerosis	Vertebrae
Intact bone contour	Ribs
No periosteal elevation	Clavicles
"Ground glass" appearance	Pelvis
Trabecular loss	Scapula
	Metaphyseal ends

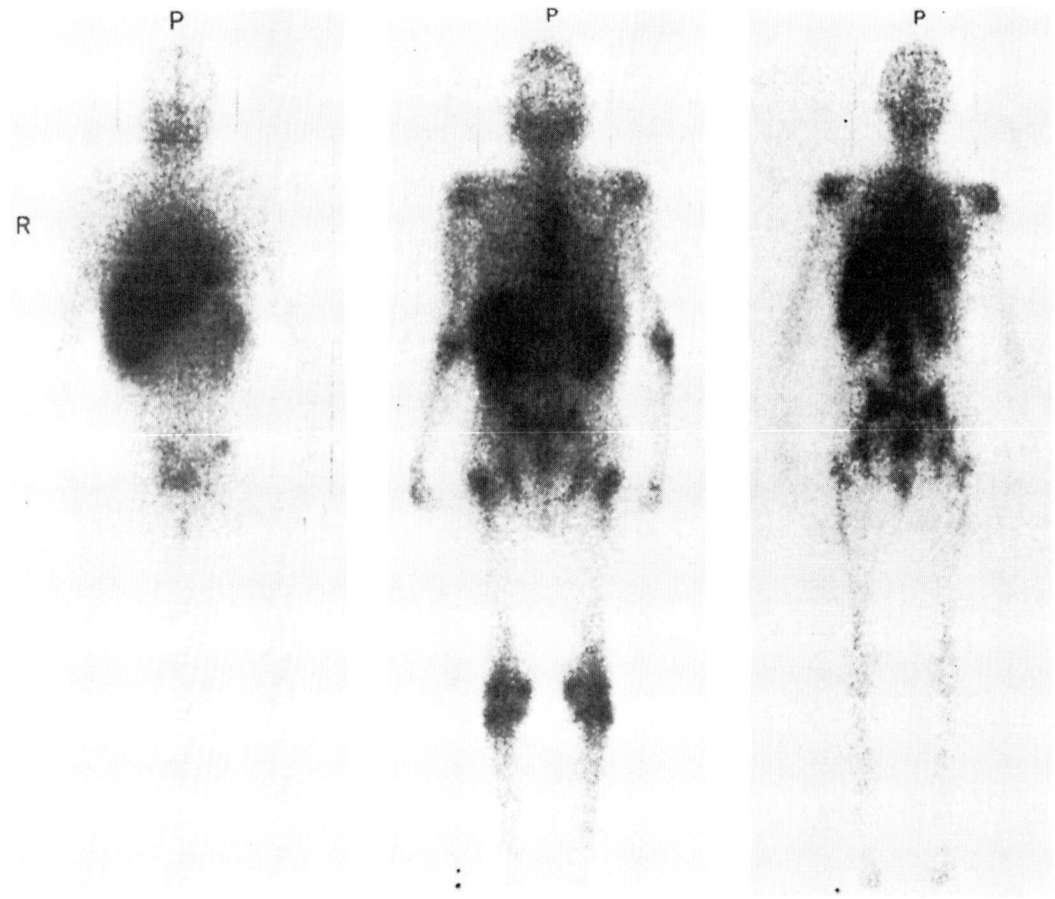

FIGURE 19-8. Marrow scintigraphy with indium-111 chloride in patients with aplasia (*far left*), MM-MF (*center*), and normal individuals (*far right*). (*Used with permission from McNeil BJ, et al: J Nucl Med 8:647–651, 1974.*)

ficult to distinguish from the variable presentations of MM-MF. The marked splenomegaly and abnormal peripheral blood smear will clearly differentiate MM-MF from most leukemoid reactions and the pattern of myelofibrosis from most other disorders causing fibroblastic marrow proliferation. Perhaps the most difficult differential diagnosis is between CGL, MM-MF, and other myeloproliferative disorders.

Because of the variable features of MM-MF, it has been helpful to describe classic as well as atypical presentations. It is possible on the basis of clinical symptoms, laboratory data, and degree of marrow fibrosis and splenomegaly to stage the disease as early, classic, and late. These stages may be demonstrated easily by ferrokinetic studies or marrow imaging as described above. Patients described as "early" are generally asymptomatic with

minimal anemia, mild splenomegaly, slight leukocytosis, and minimal marrow fibrosis. This stage of disease may easily be confused with leukemoid reactions or CGL. Cytogenetics and LAP score may help in the distinction (Table 19–10). The "late" stage of MM-MF, characterized by massive splenomegaly, pancytopenia, and marked myelofibrosis with

TABLE 19-9. DIFFERENTIAL DIAGNOSIS

Tuberculosis	Lymphoma
Chronic granulomatous disease	Hairy cell leukemia
	Metastatic carcinoma
Liver disease with portal hypertension	Polycythemia vera
	Chronic granulocytic leukemia
Leukemoid reaction	
Lipid storage disease	Primary thrombocytosis
Osteopetrosis	Acute myelosclerosis
Felty's syndrome	

TABLE 19–10. LABORATORY ASSISTANCE IN DIFFERENTIAL DIAGNOSIS

	LEUKEMOID	ET	CGL	MM-MF
WBC	+ to + +	nl to +	+ + to + + + +	+ to + +
Immaturity	Slight	None	Moderate to marked	Slight
Red cell	nl to −	nl	nl	− to − −
Morphology	nl to +	nl	nl	Teardrops, stippling
Platelets	nl to +	+ + to + + + +	nl to +	+ to + + + +
Basophils	nl	nl to +	+ to + +	+ to + +
LAP	+ to + +	nl to +	nl to −	+ to + +
Marrow-asp	nl to hyper	nl to hyper + + + megas	Hyper	Dry tap Dysplastic megas
Reticulin	0	tr to +	Rare	+ + to + + + +
Cytogenetics	nl	nd*	Ph′ +	nd

*nd = nondiagnostic.

sclerotic bone formation, must be distinguished from various storage diseases, hairy cell leukemia, and primary splenic malignancies such as non-Hodgkin's lymphoma that also may cause myelofibrosis. The intermediate or "classical presentation" may mimic disorders at either end of the spectrum and distinguished by specific laboratory data findings outlined in Tables 19–6 and 19–10.

The variable proliferative presentations have led others to further divide MM-MF into three categories: (1) myelofibrosis with marrow hyperplasia, (2) myelofibrosis with marrow dysplasia, and (2) myelofibrosis with an aplastic or hypoproliferative marrow.[122] This classification also may be helpful in determining therapeutic options. Myelofibrosis with marrow hyperplasia is essentially the "classic" (early to intermediate stage) presentation. It is characterized by marrow fibrosis of varying degree with excess megakaryocytes, hyperplasia of one or more hematopoietic cell lines, with maintenance of normal maturation and differentiation. It is certainly the most common presentation and must be differentiated from the other myeloproliferative disorders: PV, ET, and CGL. The essential feature of marrow fibrosis with marrow dysplasia is marrow fibrosis with an excess of megakaryocytes, normal or increased proliferation of one or more hematopoietic stem lines, and "abnormal" differentiation and maturation. The abnormal characteristics include ineffective hematopoiesis with intramedullary cell death and

resulting variable cytopenias (anemia with or without ringed sideroblasts, neutropenia, and/or thrombocytopenia). This presentation may be difficult to distinguish from the myelodysplastic disorders and "preleukemia." The third category, myelofibrosis with aplastic or hypoproliferative marrow, is characterized by generalized fibrosis, residual small clusters of atypical megakaryocytes, hyperplasia and immaturity of all marrow stem-cell lines, and a resulting marked decrease or absence of normal hematopoiesis. Extramedullary hematopoiesis is either unable to compensate for marrow hypofunction or is nonexistent. This presentation may be confused with the rare entity acute myelosclerosis.

Acute myelosclerosis, first described by Lewis and Szur in 1963, has been referred to as malignant myelosclerosis, subacute myelosclerosis, acute megakaryocytic myelofibrosis, and acute myelofibrosis.[123–126] This entity can be distinguished from MM-MF and other myeloproliferative disorders on clinical and pathologic findings. Although not definitively proven, acute myelosclerosis may best be described as a variant of acute nonlymphocytic leukemia of a megakaryocytic subtype.[127–129, 129a] The presentation is a sudden onset of pancytopenia, minimal to absent morphologic red cell changes, minimal to absent splenomegaly, a bone marrow with hyperplasia, immaturity of all three cell lines, a marked increase in reticulin or fibrosis, and a rapidly progressive downhill clinical course lasting a few weeks to months. The initial cases of acute myelosclerosis had no morphologic evidence of acute leukemia at autopsy, and thus it became a distinct entity.[123] Because of the marrow immaturity, the short survival, and the sudden presentation, most feel that the disorder is most compatible with acute leukemia, subclassified as acute megakaryoblastic leukemia or acute myelogenous leukemia with secondary fibrosis. It is now referred to as M7 leukemia in the FAB classification.

CGL, the spent phase of PV, and ET remain the most difficult disorders to separate from MM-MF. All these myeloproliferative disorders have overlapping laboratory data and clinical findings. As mentioned earlier, specific points of difference rest primarily with cytogenetic studies and marrow biopsy findings but occasionally may require histologic study of the spleen and/or liver. Table 19–10 summarizes the similarities and differences between these myeloproliferative disorders and leukemoid reactions.

THERAPY

General Comments

At the present time, as with all myeloproliferative disorders, there is no recognized cure. With so many variable clinical problems and presentations, it is impossible to recommend a universal therapy. In this regard, many past therapies reflected the historical concepts of the disease. If the marrow was "failing," then stimulate it with androgens; if the spleen was bothersome or the major cause of the anemia or thrombocytopenia, then remove it or shrink it with chemotherapy or irradiation. As is often the case in uncurable diseases, the modalities of therapy in the literature are numerous. The extreme clinical variability makes it difficult to evaluate the effects of these therapies and subsequent survival data. At the onset, however, it must be remembered from reviews of large series that almost 30 percent of patients are asymptomatic and require no initial therapy.[13, 15, 16, 86] In our own initial series of 71 cases, 24 patients, or 34 percent, required no intervention.[15] As therapies are discussed in this section, they will be considered as to the major symptoms being managed. Table 19–11 outlines the various therapeutic problems encountered. Major problems include

TABLE 19–11. THERAPEUTIC PROBLEMS IN MM-MF

Anemia
  Decreased production
  Ineffective erythropoiesis
  Iron deficiency
  Folate deficiency
  Autoimmune hemolytic
  Hypersplenism (dilutional)
  PNH
Thrombocytopenia
  Immune
  Ineffective megakaryocytopoiesis
  Hypersplenism
Symptomatic splenomegaly
Hypermetabolic symptoms
Thrombocytosis
  Increased bleeding
  Increased thromboses
Myelofibrosis and pancytopenia
Secondary leukemia

(1) anemia secondary to hypoplasia, nutritional deficiency, blood loss, ineffective erythropoiesis, hemolysis, or hypersplenism, (2) moderate to marked thrombocytopenia secondary to immune destruction, hypersplenism, or ineffective megakaryocytopoiesis, (3) complications of markedly enlarged spleens causing pain, weight loss, pancytopenia, or ascites, (4) hypermetabolic symptoms associated with elevated WBC counts or splenomegaly, (5) thrombocytosis with potential hypercoagulable or bleeding state, (6) pancytopenia or bone pain secondary to myelofibrosis, and (7) the development of an undifferentiated myeloproliferative disorder or acute leukemia. Each problem will be considered under a separate heading; however, specific therapies may accomplish more than one purpose.

Anemia is a characteristic finding in the majority of patients. In large series, the mean hematocrit or hemoglobin is in the low 30 percent and 10 g/dl range.[13, 15] Approximately 20 to 25 percent of presenting patients are symptomatic due to anemia. Nutritional deficiencies of iron or folate are easily diagnosed by serum levels and therapeutic responses. The causes for these deficiencies are probably related to the gastrointestinal or other blood loss and increased folate requirement noted in many of the myeloproliferative disorders. The low folate levels may, however, be artifactual because of the rapid folate clearance demonstrated in many of these patients.[130] Autoimmune hemolytic anemias response to glucocorticoids have been reported but are extremely rare.[11, 131, 132] The major cause of hemolysis is the massive splenomegaly. Chromium-51 red blood cell survival curves are markedly shortened with or without increased splenic sequestration. Therapeutic considerations for hypersplenism include chemotherapy, radioactive ^{32}P, splenic irradiation, and splenectomy. These alternatives will be discussed below under the category of symptomatic splenomegaly.

The vast majority of patients will have a normochromic, normocytic anemia and be unable to respond to iron or folate therapy. With the help of ferrokinetics, most will illustrate ineffective erythropoiesis, a normal to shortened plasma iron clearance with only a 15 to 70 percent red blood cell incorporation of the iron.[16, 133–135] Therapeutic decisions for anemia in these patients may be aided by the simultaneous use of ^{51}Cr and ^{59}Fe studies determining red cell mass, red cell survival, plasma iron clearance, iron turnover, and red cell iron utilization. Examples of these studies for a normal donor and a patient with

ineffective erythropoiesis secondary to MM-MF are shown in Fig. 19–9A. During these studies, organ ^{59}Fe scanning may be of help in determining the degree of residual marrow erythropoiesis within the myelofibrosis (Fig. 19–9B) and aid in elucidating the mechanism of the anemia. Marrow scintigraphy may be of similar help (see Fig. 19–8).

If ineffective erythropoiesis appears to be the primary cause of anemia, androgen therapy may be of benefit. The benefits of androgen therapy depend on residual marrow erythropoiesis.[89] In vitro, marrow hematopoietic cell lines are stimulated to proliferate by steroids and androgen therapy.[136, 137] Therapeutic responses occur in a variety of clinical settings and with a variety of different agents. Rosenthal and Erf[51] were the first to note a favorable but transient response to androgens after a 4-month trial. Gardner and colleagues[135] predicted a 10 to 20 percent response rate to either oral or intramuscular androgen therapy. Increased erythropoiesis and a decreased transfusion requirement were noted beginning after 2 months of ther-

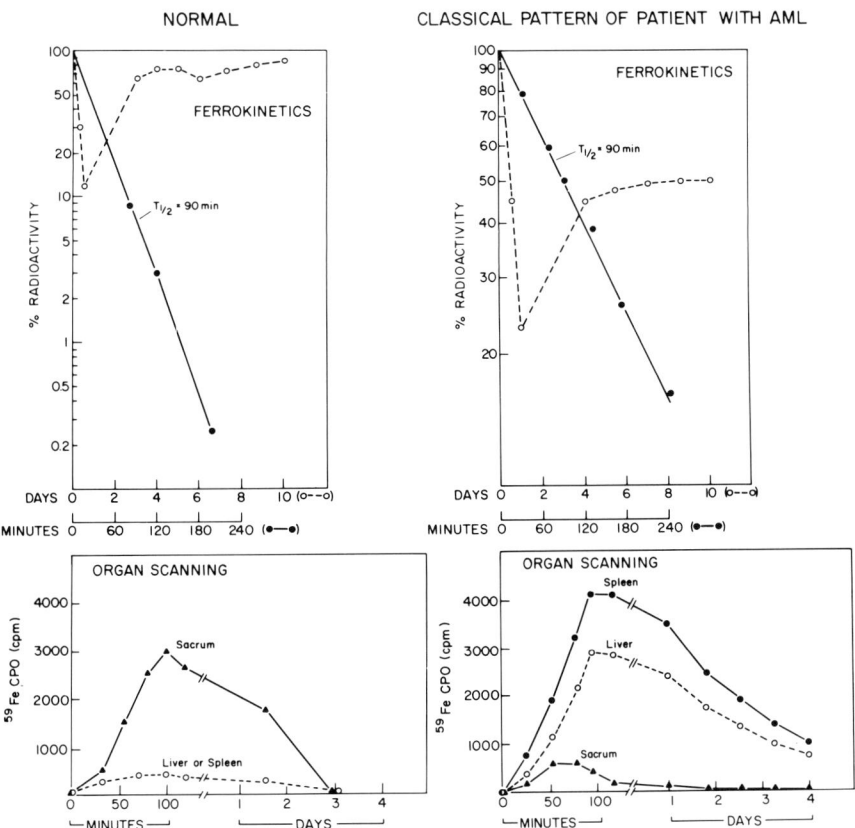

FIGURE 19–9. Ferrokinetic studies in a volunteer and in a patient with severe hypoplastic MM-MF (example).

apy. Progressive splenomegaly was noted during the course of therapy. Others confirm beneficial results in 10 to 40 percent of patients but associated with toxicity such as increasing spleen size, fluid retention, increased libido, hirsutism, and abnormal liver function, the latter with *oral* androgens.[16] In those patients with a good response, early relapse of the anemia was frequent following cessation of therapy. From some series there seemed to be an association of poor response to androgens and the presence of severe anemia, massive splenomegaly, and a long history of disease.[16, 36, 138]

The PVSG began a study in 1970 to compare the use of Halotestin versus transfusion therapy (PVSG protocol 04). A total of 27 eligible patients with anemia were randomized.[89] Patients were stratified as to the degree of myelofibrosis, those having greater than one-third of a cross-sectional area of marrow biopsy filled with collagen being classified as having "myelofibrosis," while those with less collagen being identified as having "unclassified myeloproliferative disease." Of 14 patients randomized to receive Halotestin, 4 good responses were noted. Of the 10 evaluable patients randomized to transfusional support therapy, there was only one partial response. In this series, all the responders had myelofibrosis and none were in the "unclassified" category. Ferrokinetics were of prognostic value in that all responders had a day 10 red cell iron utilization greater than 50 percent. None of the nonresponders demonstrated a greater than 50 percent ^{59}Fe utilization, and most had moderately severe ineffective erythropoiesis. Unfortunately, Halotestin toxicity included congestive heart failure in 3 and jaundice in 2. These results are similar to those seen in aplastic anemia; androgen therapy will cause a red cell response if there is a sufficient amount of residual effective erythropoiesis.[139] Brubaker[140] and the PVSG followed up with a study comparing high-dose oral with high-dose parenteral androgen therapy (PVSG protocol 11). With only 10 patients in each arm, there did not appear to be any discernible difference in response.

In summary, the causes of anemia in MM-MF are usually multifold. Nutritional deficiencies of folate and B_{12} are infrequent. Iron deficiency is more common and particularly occurs in post-PV MM patients. Hemolytic anemia is usually due to hypersplenism, but

occasional patients may have an autoimmune mechanism responsive to glucocorticoids. Most frequently, the anemia is secondary to ineffective erythropoiesis, and androgen responsiveness may be predicted by ferrokinetics.

Thrombocytopenia may occur in as many as 45 percent of patients in some series.[15] Although platelets may be found to have immunoglobulin or complement attached to the platelet membrane, immune destruction is usually not the mechanism of thrombocytopenia. A trial of glucocorticoids has been recommended in patients with symptomatic thrombocytopenia, and in one study of 16 patients, 50 percent had a partial response.[36] Hypersplenism and ineffective megakaryocytopoiesis are the most common reasons for significantly low platelet counts. Splenectomy with platelet coverage may be necessary in those patients with life-threatening thrombocytopenia. Silverstein[36] has reported several cases of disseminated intravascular coagulation (DIC) as a cause of severe thrombocytopenia; this syndrome was recognized in relatively asymptomatic patients because of simultaneous abnormal PTs and PTTs.[36] In some patients, the DIC was noted during or immediately after splenectomy and may have occurred as a result of operation-related hypotension. Qualitative platelet defects, as mentioned earlier, have been described in MM-MF as well as in other MPDs.[77] Platelet transfusion therapy with avoidance of aspirin and related medicines may temporarily alleviate increased bleeding.

Splenomegaly can be the most difficult clinical problem faced by the hematologist. Not only can the spleen cause local and compressive symptoms, it also can lead to a variety of significant cytopenias. The splenic enlargement may be massive and its size matched only by patients who have hairy cell leukemia or storage diseases (e.g., Gaucher's disease). There has been controversy over many years regarding the best approach to the symptomatic patient, and therapies include medical management with alkylating agents,[32]P, hydroxyurea, splenic irradiation, splenectomy, and recently, interferon. *Medical management* was first demonstrated to be of value by Dameshek and colleagues.[141] Busulfan (Myleran) therapy was able to reduce spleen size and in some instances improve blood counts.[16, 138] Bouruncle and Doan[11] noted clinical improvement that lasted in some cases for several months to years. Others confirmed these palliative responses and observed that the doses required to cause these beneficial results were lower than those necessary in CGL.[10, 142] However, there are just as many reports demonstrating unimpressive results and increased toxicity with alkylating agents. Spleen size and blood counts were reduced but at the expense of symptomatic anemia and thrombocytopenia. The discrepancy between these uncontrolled studies is probably due to the variability of the patients studied. Laszlo[86] has speculated that the best results would be expected in patients who have cellular marrows (the hypercellular marrow with myelofibrosis, CGL-like), whereas those patients with extensive fibrosis (myelofibrosis with pancytopenia or severe ineffective erythropoiesis) would be more sensitive and more difficult to manage with chemotherapy. Although there are very little data on MM-MF, the experience from managing CGL suggests that there is probably very little difference among the various alkylating agents in controlling splenomegaly. Because of the increased incidence and earlier onset of blast crisis or acute leukemia in PV patients treated with any alkylating agents, many investigators have preferred hydroxyurea to medically control symptomatic splenomegaly.[86, 143, 144] The overall results in long-term control of painful splenomegaly have been unsuccessful with medical therapy, and this therapy is usually reserved for the management of hypermetabolic symptoms and complications of thrombocytosis, as described below.

Splenic irradiation has been used in treating splenic pain since the 1950s. Hickling[145] and Videbaek[146] were the first to report favorable results with decreased splenic size and pain. Others noted either no response or only a transient response.[11, 147–149] Silverstein et al.,[13] employing this therapy early in the disease process, noted a decreased total survival compared with other forms of therapy. Ward and Block[16] irradiated 8 patients because of hypersplenism, abdominal discomfort, and an elevated WBC count. They noted that only 2 patients with abdominal discomfort had improved, and in both the results lasted for only a few months. Szur and Smith,[133] Greenberger et al.,[150] and Parmentier et al.[151] have confirmed beneficial results of splenic irradiation in a selected group of patients and for a limited period of time. As with

chemotherapy, the dose to cause splenic reduction is significantly lower than that needed to cause an effect in CGL.[150] A dose as low as 250 rad may be sufficient for response compared with 700 to 1200 rad for CGL. The radiation is given in small fractions at 15 to 25 rad per day to a port encompassing part or whole of the spleen. Counts are monitored daily because precipitous falls in WBC count or platelets may occur after just three or four treatments. Figure 19–10A illustrates the effect on spleen size and blood counts in a patient with hyperplastic MM-MF; Fig. 19–10B illustrates the results in a patient with pancytopenia and massive splenomegaly. The exact mechanism by which splenic irradiation works is unclear. Szur and Smith[133] have shown that splenic hematopoiesis is suppressed in the irradiated area, while splenic phagocytic activity is left unimpaired. The marked myelosuppression that occurs correlates well with the studies by Koeffler et al.[152] The splenic irradiation caused early and marked reduction of CFU-GM in the peripheral circulation.[152] These studies[150, 152] and others by Adler[153] appear to rationalize the anecdotal "abscopal effect," i.e., a systemic beneficial effect of splenic irradiation due to an inhibitory component released by the spleen. Radiation impairs proliferating myeloid progenitor cells that are located in or traveling through the spleen.[153] The irradiation effect, however, is transient; Fig. 19–10C illustrates the temporary results obtained with this therapy. The spleen returns to its previous size, and the pancytopenia simultaneously improves. Second courses of splenic irradiation are less effective, and beneficial results require higher doses. In a few cases, splenic irradiation has been effective in temporarily controlling splenic pain and pancytopenia in an inoperable patient, allowing an opportunity for that patient to be temporarily stabilized and then able to undergo splenectomy (see Fig. 19–10B). In summary, splenic irradiation offers temporary and brief therapeutic responses in symptomatic splenomegaly. Physiologic studies have not completely clarified the exact mechanism. A small number of patients who are unable to undergo surgery may be temporarily palliated by this technique.

Splenectomy has gone from being the least favorable alternative in managing symptomatic splenomegaly to the best. Hickling[154] in 1937 reviewed 27 patients who had under-

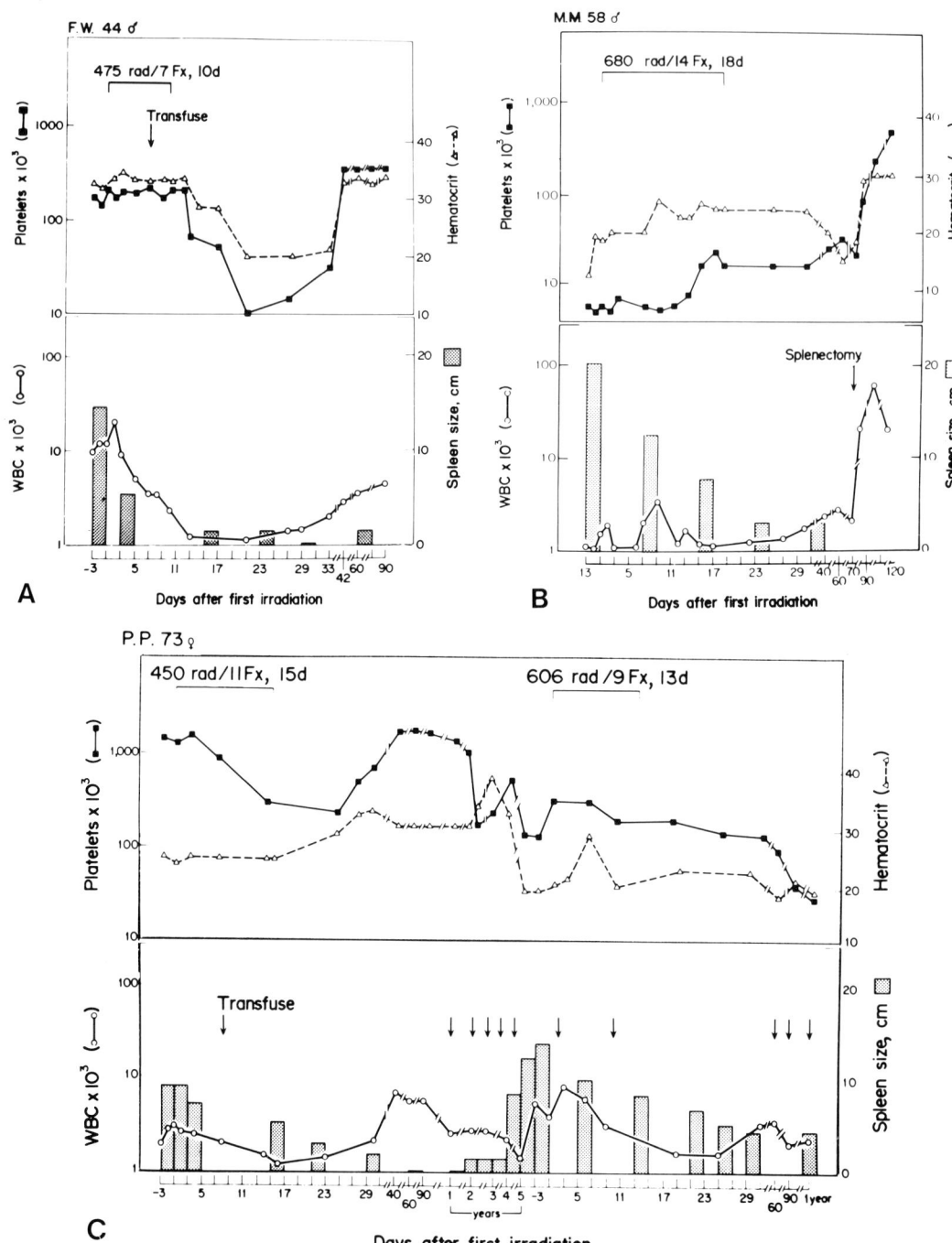

FIGURE 19–10. Results of splenic irradiation therapy in three different situations: (A) hyperplastic MM-MF, (B) hypoplastic MM-MF, and (C) repeated attempts at therapy. (Reprinted from Greenberger JS, et al: J Int Radiat: Oncol Biol Phys 2:1083–1090, 1977 with kind permission from Elsevier Science Ltd, The Boulevard, Langford Lane, Kidlington OX51GB, UK.)

gone splenectomy prior to that year. He concluded that the high postoperative mortality constituted a major contraindication for this form of therapy. Fifteen of the 27 died in the immediate postoperative period, and 6 others died within the year. Several other reports up to 1950 confirmed Hickling's observations.[147,148] In 1953, Green et al.[155] re-evaluated the procedure and noted that since Hickling's report, the morbidity and mortality were reduced but still quite significant (from 50 percent down to 20 percent). The major factors that have been considered indications for splenectomy are outlined in Table 19–12. Linman and Bethell[10] demonstrated effectiveness of the surgery in some patients who had hemolysis or life-threatening thrombocytopenia and were failures to medical management. Bouroncle and Doan[11] in 1962 reported many favorable outcomes and much reduced morbidity. Of 24 patients, 14 had a good hematologic or symptomatic response, 9 lost their transfusion requirement, and 5 had a decreased transfusion need. Complications were noted in 7 patients; none was fatal. These included a subphrenic abscess, postoperative bleeding, wound infections, and pneumonias. It was thus concluded that with better surgical techniques, splenectomy could be carried out safely. The types and frequency of postsplenectomy complications are listed in Table 19–13.

As it became evident that patients could undergo splenectomy safely, the attention of investigators then turned toward recognition of those patients who would best be managed by surgery. Crosby et al.[156] suggested that all patients should be splenectomized as soon as the diagnosis is made. This conclusion stemmed from a small number of patients who had either diagnostic splenectomies or else surgery with minimal symptoms. The postoperative morbidity was extremely low in this series, and patients so managed had a long survival. Unfortunately, this was not a controlled study, and because of the extreme variability of the disease, the results must remain anecdotal. Benbassat et al.,[157] however, reviewed 321 patients treated by splenectomy from 1939 through 1979 and concluded that survival time from diagnosis was not improved by splenectomy. Silverstein and ReMine[158] retrospectively compared the findings of 15 patients splenectomized between 1960 and 1965 for major hemolysis or massive splenomegaly and found that their

TABLE 19–12. INDICATIONS FOR SPLENECTOMY

Trauma
Spontaneous rupture
Hypersplenism
Painful spleen
Splenic abscess
Portal hypertension with GI bleeding
Severe thrombocytopenia

TABLE 19–13. POSTSPLENECTOMY COMPLICATIONS

Hemorrhage
Thrombotic event
Thrombocytosis
Hepatomegaly and hepatic coma
DIC
Infection

overall response and survival were better than a similar group of medically managed patients. Survival after splenectomy is extremely variable, and Rosenthal and Moloney[15] have suggested that shorter survival may be related to more advanced disease (myelofibrosis with hypoplasia or dysplasia). Wilson and colleagues[159] recently reported a series of 50 splenectomies in which 54 percent have survived greater than 2 years after splenectomy and 23 percent greater than 3 years.

Currently, massive splenomegaly, recurrent splenic infarctions, hypersplenism causing a significant transfusion requirement, and traumatic splenic rupture or hematoma are accepted indications for surgery. Portal hypertension secondary to EMH may be relieved in some patients by splenectomy with or without splenorenal shunts. Optimal results are obtained in patients with normal liver function tests, but the presence of cirrhosis may not be contradictory for a good result. Recently, large series of splenectomies have been reviewed by Wilson and Benbasset.[158–165] Mortality figures in the immediate or postoperative period range between 1 and 5 percent. The majority of patients have achieved symptomatic benefit, and many also have experienced improved hematologic studies (Fig. 19–11). Decreased morbidity is related to careful selection of the operative patient with respect to cardiac and renal function, improved surgical technique, improved blood bank support (especially with platelet transfusions), and early postoperative mobilization of the patient, preventing thrombophlebitis, pulmonary emboli, and left lower lobe pneumonia. According to Silverstein et al.,[166] women have a significantly lower postoperative complication rate than men. In retrospect, this may be related to a younger median age of the women in the study and more massive splenomegaly in the men.

Button et al.[88] and others[90, 113, 116] have attempted prospectively to evaluate the useful-

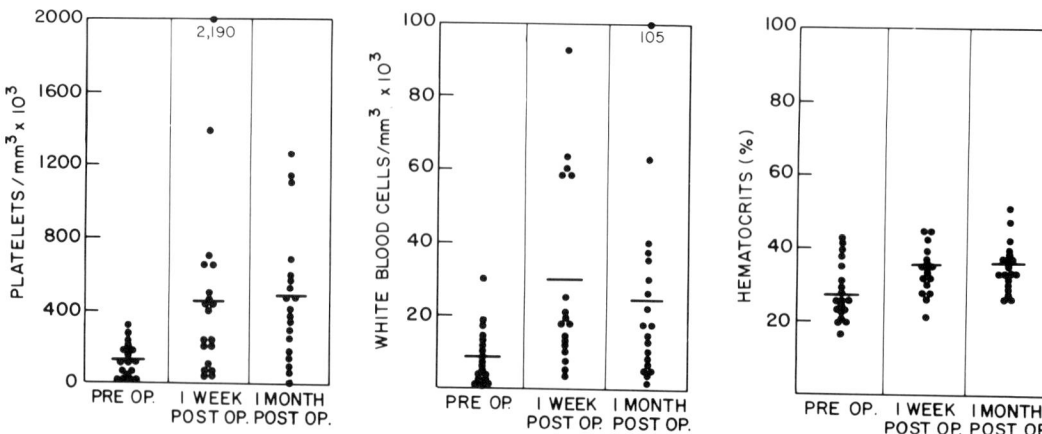

FIGURE 19–11. Hematologic response to splenectomy. *(Adapted with permission from Cabot EB, et al: Ann Surg 182:24–30, 1978.)*

ness of ferrokinetics and red cell survival studies in predicting response to splenectomy. However, these studies have not been any more helpful in selecting operative candidates than if the decision were based on clinical criteria alone, nor have they been of any help in predicting survival. The radioactive studies will aid in determining the degree of residual hematopoiesis and compensatory splenic hematopoiesis, thus differentiating early or minimal fibrosis from moderate to marked myelofibrosis, and may help in selecting out those patients who will become transfusion-dependent. However, in most cases when splenectomy is considered, the patient usually has significant hypersplenism, and isotope studies demonstrate that the spleen behaves more as a destructive organ than as a productive one.

The major postoperative complications in Table 19–13 are similar to those in patients with other diseases undergoing splenectomy. Most commonly, left-sided pleural effusion, atelectasis, bleeding, and thrombosis are seen. In Wilson's 50 cases, there was only 1 death within 30 days of surgery.[159] This death was due to postoperative hemorrhage in the subphrenic area. Others have reported increased thrombotic tendencies due to a marked postsplenectomy thrombocytosis[11, 16, 86, 160, 167] (see Fig. 19–11). Complications such as mesenteric or portal vein thrombosis have been reported if platelet counts are not well controlled.[168] Preoperative chemotherapy may be necessary to reduce the platelet level and the risk of thrombosis. Silverstein and ReMine,[158] on the other hand, reported that 14 of their 50 splenec-

tomized patients had significant bleeding in the immediate postoperative period and that of 8 requiring a repeat laparotomy, 3 died of bleeding and its complications. It was the investigators' opinion that a significant number of these bleeding complications were due to "inapparent" DIC that might have been evident preoperatively if studied. These authors require a full coagulation profile, including fibrin split products, in screening their potential splenectomy patients. The clinical efficacy of such studies, however, remains unproven.

In summary, accepted criteria for splenectomy are massive and symptomatic splenomegaly, severe thrombocytopenia, unacceptably high red cell transfusion rates, and portal hypertension. More recently, with better screening, better control of platelet counts, and awareness of potential postoperative problems, there is significant patient improvement with minimal immediate complications. Laboratory and isotopic studies are not helpful in selecting the patients and cannot predict the overall success of the procedure. Reviews have not shown that splenectomy has any effect on survival from diagnosis.[158, 159] The PVSG attempted to determine whether splenectomy or chemotherapy (Melphalan) was better in managing symptomatic splenomegaly. A randomized trial was approved, but in the 10 years following, only 8 patients were entered into study. Concerns about the protocol included the difficulty of a randomization between a medical and a surgical procedure and the presence of significant variables in degree of myelofibrosis and splenomegaly from one patient to another. Splenectomy does have an important therapeutic role in MM-MF and post-PV MM; consistency in selection and careful long-term follow-up will be helpful in determining its full impact on the disease. Recent trials of interferon in PV, with resultant shrinkage of spleen site, suggest a possible role in the treatment of MM-MF.

Hypermetabolic symptoms are as frequent with MM-MF as they are with CGL. They are usually associated with the "cellular" phase or the myelofibrosis with hyperplastic marrow. All blood counts are usually elevated, and the spleen is moderately enlarged. As mentioned earlier, in patients with symptomatic splenomegaly, alkylating agents were first shown to be beneficial by Dameshek et al.[141] Agents such as busulfan (Myleran) reduced spleen size, peripheral WBC count, and hypermetabolic symptoms. ^{32}P, alkylating agents, and more recently, hydroxyurea are all effective in reducing symptoms of the hyperplastic phase and controlling blood counts. Splenectomy may still be considered a therapeutic option in those patients with symptomatic splenomegaly, but as mentioned above, blood counts will have to be controlled with alkylating agents or hydroxyurea before splenectomy to minimize postoperative thrombocytosis and increased thrombosis. Just as with CGL, one chemotherapeutic agent has not been shown to be more effective than another. As will be noted below with therapy for thrombocytosis, all agents are effective, but some yield faster responses. In view of the experience with chemotherapy in PV, the recommended agent currently is hydroxyurea (PVSG). This agent, however, may cause a rapid decrease in blood counts in MM-MF, and repeat blood counts should be obtained within 7 days of initiating a starting oral dose of 10 to 15 mg/ kg per day.

Thrombocytosis with values greater than 800,000/mm^3 may occur in 15 to 25 percent of patients (see Fig. 19–6). Distinction from the thrombocytosis of other myeloproliferative disorders has been discussed elsewhere. In MM-MF, the most frequent morbid complication of thrombocytosis is a thrombotic episode. Thrombosis may be the clinical cause of death in 15 to 25 percent of patients, whereas at autopsy, 40 to 45 percent of patients will have thrombosis.[78–80] Although various qualitative platelet abnormalities have been noted, thrombocytosis has been

the presumptive cause.[77] However, as noted by Schafer,[77] the role of thrombocytosis in the pathogenesis of thrombosis is unclear. Recent PVSG studies,[169] as well as studies by Kessler et al.,[170] do not demonstrate a correlation between the incidence of thrombosis and the platelet number. Nevertheless, it has been shown that lowering the platelet count in a patient with an active or previous thrombotic problem may result in symptomatic improvement.[168, 171–175]

The treatment of thrombocytosis has included plateletpheresis, antiplatelet agents, chemotherapy, radiation (^{32}P), hydroxyurea, anagrelide, and interferon. Plateletpheresis has been used primarily to acutely lower the platelet count but is impractical as a prolonged means of control.[176] Pheresis may be quite helpful prior to emergency surgery, but immediate platelet rebound is quite likely.[174, 175] Myleran, Alkeran, and ^{32}P all have been used to control platelet elevations in an attempt to prevent thrombosis. There does not appear to be any difference in platelet control using these agents.[10, 13, 15, 16, 141, 177] Two PVSG protocols attempted to determine whether Alkeran or ^{32}P was more effective.[178] Both agents produced significant beneficial results in platelet control. Alkeran achieved platelet reduction to less than 600,000/mm^3 in 80 to 90 percent of patients within 3 months of therapy with minimal side effects and hematologic complications. Approximately 65 percent of patients treated with two ^{32}P schedules had a similar response, but a higher dose schedule (2.9 mCi/ m^2) had to be used to equal chemotherapy results. Although there was no statistical difference between the two programs, there did appear to be a faster platelet reduction with chemotherapy.

Concern about potentially leukemogenic therapy has led to efficacy trials of other agents such as hydroxyurea, anagrelide, and interferon-α. Hydroxyurea, an inhibitor of ribonucleoside reductase, does not induce mutations in vitro but does cause chromosome breaks and is teratogenic in animals.[178a] PVSG protocol 12 tested the efficacy of hydroxyurea in ET at 15 mg/kg per day by mouth.[179] Initial reports suggested a greater than 80 percent response rate, but it is still too early to assess long-term side effects. The finding of 3 cases of leukemia in 51 patients with PV similarly treated is discentering although not yet statistically significant.[179a] Discontinuation of the drug is associated with the rapid return of thrombocytosis, indicating that maintenance therapy is necessary.

Anagrelide (imidazole-2,1-b,quinazolin-2-one), considered as a potential anticoagulant, was found to cause thrombocytopenia. In a phase I trial, thrombocytosis, secondary to all chronic myeloproliferative disorders including MM-MF, responded well to doses of 1.5 to 2.5 mg every 6 hours.[179b] Maintenance doses of 0.5 mg were able to control the counts. The mechanism of action is unclear. Decreased marrow release of platelets may be the cause; marrow cellularity, megakaryocyte number and morphology, and response of megakaryocyte cultures and production of CFU-M are unaffected by the drug.[179c,179d] Toxicity includes nausea, headache, and mild hypotension. Red cells and white cells are not involved, but anagrelide inhibits platelet function and may cause increased bleeding.

Recombinant interferon-α, 3 million units SC three times per week, has shown promising results.[179e-179h] A 50 percent reduction in platelet count occurs by day 28, and symptoms of thrombocytosis resolve within 1 week. A maintenance program is required for continued control. Side effects such as an influenza-like illness caused about 20 percent of patients to withdraw from the trials. WBC counts do fall during therapy, and in some patients, spleen size has decreased. The obvious drawbacks of this therapy are the expense and the need for continued therapy.

Antiplatelet agent therapy remains controversial. Patients should be carefully selected for this therapy on the basis of clinical and laboratory data. The syndromes of digital and cerebral ischemia due to microvascular occlusion may be helped with antiplatelet agents.[77,171,180,181] More often, however, the use of aspirin or Persantine may be quiet hazardous.[181a] As mentioned in Chap. 15, a randomized trial by the PVSG to prevent thrombosis in PV resulted in an increased incidence of major bleeding problems without affecting the thrombotic tendency.[182] It appears that there can be no single approach to the use of antiplatelet agents. Schafer[77] has suggested an approach (Fig. 19–12) based on clinical and laboratory findings. Those patients with normal bleeding times and symptoms of digital or cerebral vascular ischemia may be helped by an aspirin dose of 80 to 325 mg/d. Patients with a prior history of thrombosis without laboratory abnormalities also may benefit from aspirin, but patients with a bleeding history or those with prolonged bleeding times and/or impaired aggregation may be at serious risk for increased and serious bleeding.

Significant advancements in the understanding of the pathogenesis of myelofibrosis has brought about three major possibilities to consider regarding the *therapy of myelofibrosis* (Table 19–14). Until recently, the major therapeutic modalities in MM-MF have been very limited and focused on the anemia and splenomegaly. With the increasing knowl-

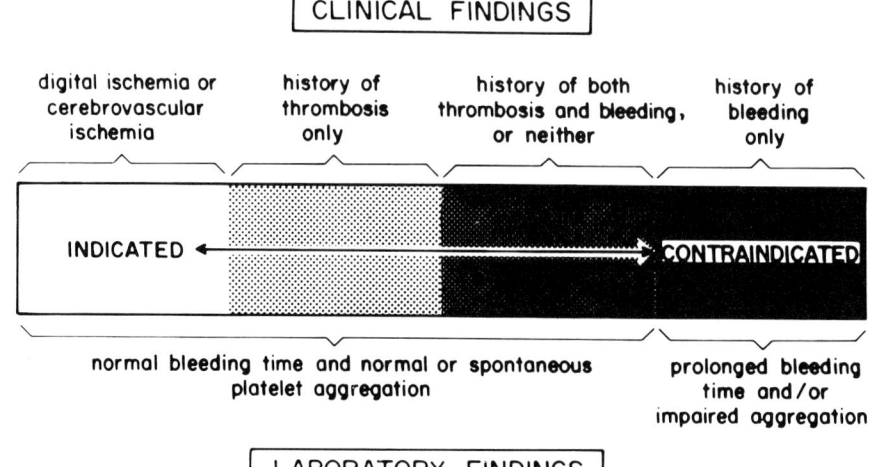

FIGURE 19–12. Rationale for the use of antiplatelet agents in thrombocytosis associated with myeloproliferative disorders. *(Adapted with permission from Schafer AI: Blood 64:1–12, 1984.)*

TABLE 19-14. THERAPY FOR MYELOFIBROSIS

Allogeneic marrow transplantation
Aggressive chemo- and irradiation therapy
Interference with collagen metabolism
  Hydroxyproline analogues
  Colchicine
  Vinblastine
  D-Penicillamine
Interference with fibroblast proliferation
  1,25(OH)$_2$ vitamin D

edge of collagen synthesis and the nature of fibrosis associated with other diseases such as scleroderma and cirrhosis, more rational approaches may be forthcoming.[183–185] As mentioned previously, it is now known that the fibrosis associated with MM-MF, other myeloproliferative disorders, and many malignancies such as Hodgkin's disease and breast cancer is a secondary phenomenon and not part of the malignant or myeloproliferative process.[17–19] It may be expected, therefore, that successful treatment of the underlying disorder might cause resolution of the fibrosis. In addition, the processes of collagen synthesis and degradation, recently reviewed by Prockop[185] and Krane,[186] suggest possible sites where collagen synthesis might be inhibited. The involvement of megakaryocyte PDGF and platelet factor IV in the development of myelofibrosis has led some investigators to study agents that might interfere with or modulate PDGF release or inhibit megakaryocyte production.[31, 67, 68] These approaches are reviewed below.

Table 19-15, adapted from Fruchtman,[187] illustrates the various sites of collagen formation and degradation that might be inhibited by various agents. The four major target sites are the hydroxylation process, collagen secretion by fibroblasts, the polymerization of collagen, and the enhancement of pro-

duction of tissue collagenase. The hydroxyproline moiety of the molecule appears to play a vital role in the stability of the complex collagen structure. Proline analogues have been used as substrate modifiers in experimental fibrosis.[188, 189] The agents listed in Table 19-15 have been shown to interfere with the three polypeptide chains of the triple collagen matrix. The resulting single chains remain nonfunctional. In addition, some analogues inhibit secretion of collagen from mammalian cells.[190] Very little in vivo activity has been demonstrated, but the proline analogues have been effective in inhibiting collagen synthesis in tendon injuries.[191] In in vitro studies, colchicine, vinblastine, and cytochalain B interfere with the microtubules and microfilaments of fibroblasts, causing impairment of collagen secretion.[192] In humans, these agents have been used to treat scleroderma and alcoholic cirrhosis.[193, 194] Rojkind et al.[195] demonstrated an improved clinical status of cirrhotic patients after 2 years of colchicine therapy with a dose of 5 mg/d 5 days a week. As noted below, colchicine also may accelerate or increase collagen degradation.[196] Minimal success has been noted in clinical trials with scleroderma patients.[194] Agents that will interfere with polymerization of collagen by blocking intermolecular bonds are best represented by D-penicillamine. As a copper chelator, it has several in vitro effects on collagen metabolism. Experimentally, it blocks aldehyde groups involved in the inter- and intramolecular cross-linkages of mature collagen.[197] In addition, it may accelerate collagen turnover by cleaving the intermolecular stabilizing collagen bonds.[197] In vitro animal trials have shown that the drug does interfere with experimentally induced hepatic and pulmonary fibrosis.[198, 199] Potassium p-aminobenzoate (POTABA), an agent that interferes with intermolecular linkages, has been studied by

TABLE 19-15. INTERFERENCE WITH COLLAGEN METABOLISM

TARGET	MECHANISM	AGENT
Hydroxylation	Substrate modification	Hydroxyproline analogues
Secretion	Microtubules	Colchicine
	Microfilaments	Vinblastine
		Cytochalasin B
Polymerization	Complexing chains	D-Penicillamine
	Cleaving cross-links	Potaba
	Lysyl oxidase inhibition	p-Aminoproprionitrile
Degradation	Increase collagenase	Colchicine

the PVSG in patients with post-PV MM and MM-MF.[200] A total of 34 patients with moderate to marked myelofibrosis were entered into study, and 11 have had sufficient follow-up to evaluate the drug result. Only one patient had a slight decrease in reticulin content. Of the 10 remaining patients, reticulin either increased or remained unchanged. The conclusions are either that the drug is not at all effective in reversing fibrosis or that in late stages of myelofibrosis the fibrosis is irreversible.

Another approach to collagen metabolism is to increase its catabolism by increasing levels of collagenase. Colchicine has a number of inhibitory effects on neutrophils, mononuclear cells, and mast cells but a stimulatory effect on mononuclear cells with respect to collagenase secretion.[186] Harris and Krane[196] demonstrated a 2- to 10-fold increase in collagenase activity by cultured rheumatoid synovium in the presence of the colchicine. Although there are some promising experimental data in CCl_4-induced cirrhosis, human studies are still quite preliminary.[195] Rojkind and his group[195] have randomized a large group of cirrhotics. Initially, there appears to be a significant improvement in the quality of life and in the stability of the cirrhosis in the treated group. Some of the beneficial results may be explained partially, however, by differences in the patient populations and follow-up. This agent is currently under study in myelofibrosis.

Since collagen deposition and fibrosis are secondary phenomena, it is unlikely that increased catabolism of the collagen will affect the underlying disease. Reversibility of myelofibrosis may occur spontaneously, secondary to successful treatment of the underlying disease, or with aggressive chemotherapy and total-body irradiation followed by marrow transplantation. There have been a sufficient number of anecdotal cases with spontaneous resolution of fibrosis to alert us to the fact that "fibrosis of the marrow is not cast in cement."[201] A significant number of patients who have transformed to acute nonlymphocytic leukemia or "blast crisis" have had their marrow fibrosis resolve and replaced with undifferentiated cells. In a series of 10 closely monitored patients with MM-MF who went into blast crisis, 5 lost all evidence of myelofibrosis.[21] Others have reported spontaneous regression of myelofibrosis without leukemic conversion and have demonstrated with marrow imaging techniques that the reversal was not a local phenomenon.[23] There are also reports of chemotherapy-induced reversal with agents such as hydroxyurea. This result is consistent with the experience of marrow fibrosis secondary to malignant disorders.[202] Myelofibrosis secondary to Hodgkin's disease, metastatic breast cancer, and acute lymphocytic and nonlymphocytic leukemia may resolve after successful remission-induction chemotherapy.[55, 203, 204] More recently, marrow transplantation following ablative chemoirradiation therapy has caused reversal of myelofibrosis in acute myelosclerosis, chronic granulocytic leukemia, hairy cell leukemia, and Gaucher's disease.[22, 24–26] The beneficial results imply that the fibrosis is reversible and that the cells secreting collagen are inhibited. Marrow transplantation (either allogeneic or autologous) may represent the treatment of choice for young patients with acute myelosclerosis, CGL with myelofibrosis, and MM-MF.

In 1966, an infant with rickets and myelofibrosis was treated with vitamin D with regression of the fibrosis.[53] Since then, 6 other children who presented with rickets and a classic peripheral blood and marrow picture of MM-MF have been treated with the vitamin.[205] All had hematologic and clinical improvement, with 4 returning totally to normal. In addition, 2 adults with fibrosis secondary to myeloproliferative malignancies apparently improved with 1,25-vitamin D therapy. From marrow culture studies, $1,25(OH)_2$ vitamin D_3, the active hormonal metabolite of vitamin D, inhibits the proliferation of megakaryocytes and apparently induces normal myeloid cell as well as leukemic cell to mature to mononuclear cells, such as monocytes and macrophages.[206, 207] The vitamin D_3 analogue may reduce myelofibrosis by inhibiting megakaryocyte growth and release of PDGF and thus fibroblast proliferation. At the same time, the vitamin might reduce megakaryocyte platelet factor IV production and promote mononuclear cell proliferation of collagenase-producing cells, resulting in increased degradation of the fibrosis.[208] These studies are preliminary, and prospective trials studying the therapeutic value of $1,25(OH)_2$ vitamin D_3 in patients with varying degrees of myelofibrosis are underway.

Acute leukemia is often the final pathway for all myeloproliferative disorders. MM-MF is not an exception. In combining two large series by Silverstein[36] and Rosenthal and Maloney,[21] there were 18 cases of acute leukemia in a total population of 367 patients followed over a 20-year span. The interval from diagnosis to leukemia ranged from 6 months to 9 years, with a median of 3 years. Preleukemia therapy included androgens, steroids, chemotherapy, and/or splenectomy. Neither study implicated any significant role for therapy in the transformation of MM-MF to acute leukemia. Although the preleukemic phase of the disease was measured in years, the duration of the leukemia phase was weeks to months. All 18 patients were dead within 6 months. The major morphologic type was myelogenous (M-1 or M-2) with monomyelocytic less frequent (M-4). The documentation of blast crisis may be difficult in many cases and in some patients only may be clarified by histologic examination at time of autopsy. Chemotherapy for the leukemic phase has been universally unsuccessful.[21] All types of acute leukemia have been described, including lymphocytic, megakaryocytic, and/or erythrocytic[21, 36, 209] In young patients, if a partial response or severe aplasia can be induced with aggressive therapy, a marrow transplant may be attempted.

This chapter has attempted to summarize the total information regarding MM-MF that has accrued over the past 100 years. At the present time, our therapies are primarily palliative. Future investigation directed at the recent knowledge linking megakaryocyte activity with fibroblast proliferation may produce new answers for preventing and reversing myelofibrosis.

REFERENCES

1. Heuck G: Zwei falle von leukamie mit eigenthumlichen blut-resp. Knochenmarksbefund. Arch Pathol Anat Physiol Virchows 78:475–496, 1879
2. Askanazy M: Uber extrauterine bildung von blutzellen in der leber. Verh Dtsch Ges Pathol 7:58–65, 1904
3. Assmann H: Beitrage zur osteosklerotischen anamie. Beitr Pathol Anat 41:565–595, 1907
4. Meyer E, Heineke A: Uber blutbildung bei schwere anamien und leukamien. Dtsch Arch Klin Med 88:435–492, 1907
5. Donhauser JL: The human spleen as an haematoplastic organ, as exemplified in a case of splenomegaly with sclerosis of the bone marrow. J Exp Med 10:559–574, 1908
6. Hirschfeld H: Die generalisierte aleukamische myelose und ihr stellung im system der leukamischen erkrankungen. Z Klin Med 80: 126–173, 1914
7. Vaughan JM, Harrison CV: Leuco-erythroblastic anaemia and myelosclerosis. J Pathol Bacteriol 48:339–352, 1939
8. Rawson R, Parker F Jr, Jackson H Jr: Industrial solvents as possible etiologic agents in myeloid metaplasia. Science 93:541–542, 1941
9. Dameshek W: Some speculations on the myeloproliferative disorders. Blood 6:372–375, 1951
10. Linman JW, Bethell FH: Agnogenic myeloid metaplasia: Its natural history and present day management. Am J Med 22:107–122, 1957
11. Bouroncle BA, Doan CA: Myelofibrosis: Clinical, hematologic and pathologic study of 110 patients. Am J Med Sci 243:697–715, 1962
12. Pitcock JA, Reinhard EH, Justus BW, Mendelsohn RS: A clinical and pathologic study of sixty cases of myelofibrosis. Ann Intern Med 57:73–84, 1962
13. Silverstein MN, Gomes MR, ReMine WH, et al: Agnogenic myeloid metaplasia: Natural history and treatment. Arch Intern Med 120: 546–550, 1967
14. Hickling RA: The natural history of chronic nonleukemic myelosis. Q J Med 37:267–279, 1968
15. Rosenthal DS, Moloney WC: Myeloid metaplasia: A study of 98 cases. Postgrad Med J 45:136–142, 1969
16. Ward HP, Block MH: The natural history of agnogenic myeloid metaplasia and a critical evaluation of its relationship with the myeloid proliferative disorders. Medicine 50:357–420, 1971
17. Maniatis AK, Amsel S, Mitus WJ, Coleman N: Chromosome pattern of bone marrow fibroblasts in patients with CGL. Nature 222: 1278–1279, 1969
18. Van Slyck EJ, Weiss L, Dully M: Chromosomal evidence for the secondary role of fibroblastic proliferation in acute myelofibrosis. Blood 36:729–735, 1970
19. Jacobson RJ, Salo A, Fialkow PJ: Agnogenic myeloid metaplasia: A clonal proliferation of hematopoietic cells with secondary myelofibrosis. Blood 51:189–194, 1978
20. Greenberg BR, Wilson FD, Woo L, Jenks HM: Cytogenetics of fibroblastic colonies in Ph'-positive chronic myelogenous leukemia. Blood 51:1039–1044, 1978
21. Rosenthal DS, Moloney WC: Occurrence of acute leukemia in myeloproliferative disorders. Br J Haematol 36:373–382, 1977
22. Rappeport JM, Parkman R, Belli J, et al: Reversibility of myelofibrosis after bone marrow transplantation. Blood 52(suppl 1):271, 1978
23. Pettit JE, Lewis SM, Goolden AW: Polycythemia vera: Transformation to myelofibrosis and subsequent reversal. Scand J Haematol 20: 63–69, 1978
24. Wolf JL, Spruce WE, Bearman RM, et al: Reversal of acute ("malignant") myelosclerosis by allogeneic bone marrow transplant. Blood 59:191–193, 1982
25. Oblon DJ, Elfenbeim GJ, Braylan RC, et al: The reversal of myelofibrosis associated with chronic myelogenous leukemia after allogeneic bone marrow transplantation. Exp Hematol 11:681–685, 1983

26. Mehfa AB, Baughan ASJ, Catovsky D, et al: Reversal of marrow fibrosis in acute megakaryoblastic leukaemia after remission induction and consolidation chemotherapy followed by bone marrow transplantation. Br J Haematol 53:445–449, 1983

27. Balk SD, Whitfield JF, Youdale T, Braun AC: Roles of calcium, serum, plasma and folic acid in the control of normal and Rous sarcoma virus–infected chicken fibroblasts. Proc Nat Acad Sci USA 70:675–679, 1973.

28. Ross R, Vogel A: The platelet-derived growth factor. Cell 14:203–210, 1978

29. Bentley SA, Herman CJ: Quantitation of myelofibrosis. Br J Haematol 42:51–59, 1979

30. Groopman JE: The pathogenesis of myelofibrosis in myeloproliferative disorders. Ann Intern Med 92:857–858, 1980

31. Castro-Malaspina M, Rabellino EM, Yen A, et al: Human megakaryocyte stimulation of proliferation of bone marrow fibroblasts. Blood 57:781–787, 1981

32. Bentley SA: Bone marrow connective tissue and the haematopoietic microenvironment. Br J Haematol 48:287–291, 1982

33. Hiti-Harper J, Wohl H, Harper E: Platelet factor IV: An inhibitor of collagenase. Science 199:991–992, 1978

34. Wolf BC, Luerano E, Neiman RS: Evidence to suggest that the human fetal spleen is not a hematopoietic organ. Am J Clin Pathol 80:140–144, 1983

35. Wolf BC, Neiman RS: Myelofibrosis with myeloid metaplasia: Pathophysiologic implications of the correlation between bone marrow changes and progression of splenomegaly. Blood (in press)

36. Silverstein MN: Agnogenic Myeloid Metaplasia. Acton, Mass, Publishing Sciences Group, 1975, pp 9–18

37. Selye H, Gabbiani G, Tuchweber B: An experimental model of osteomyelosclerosis. Acta Haematol (Basel) 29:51–62, 1963

38. Bunting CH: Experimental anaemia in the rabbit. J Exp Med 8:625–646, 1906

39. Mallory TB, Gall EA, Brickley WJ: Chronic exposure to benzene (Benzol): III. The pathologic results. J Indust Hyg 21:355–393, 1939

40. Rawson R, Parker F Jr, Jackson H Jr: Industrial solvents as possible etiologic agents in myeloid metaplasia. Science 93:541–542, 1941

41. Silberberg M, Silberberg R: Action of estrogen in skeletal tissues of immature guinea pigs. Arch Pathol 28:340–360, 1939

42. Upton AC, Furth J: A transmissable disease of mice characterized by anemia, leukopenia, splenomegaly and myelosclerosis. Acta Haematol (Basel) 13:65–76, 1955

43. Nettleship A: Bone marrow changes produced by specific antibodies. Am J Pathol 18:689–697, 1942

44. Stodtmeister R, Becker H, Cronkite EP, et al: Experimentelle knochen-markfibroses in ratten nach subletaler ganzkorper-rontgenbestrahlung und knochenmarktransfusionen als modell der mensschlichen myelofibrose. Schweiz Med Wochenschr 98:1671–1673, 1968

45. Donhauser JL: The human spleen as an hematopoietic organ, as exemplified in a case of splenomegaly with sclerosis of the bone marrow. J Exp Med 10:559–574, 1908

46. Werzberg A: Neue experimentelle beitxrage zur frage der myeloiden metaplasia. Virchows Arch [A] 204:272–338, 1911

47. Erf LA, Herbut PA: Primary and secondary myelofibrosis (a clinical and pathological study of 13 cases of fibrosis of the bone marrow). Ann Intern Med 21:863–889, 1944

48. Lang FJ: Myeloid metaplasia. In Downey H (ed): Handbook of Hematology. New York, Paul B Hoeber Inc, 1938, p 2104

49. Gulland GL, Goodall A: Pernicious anemia: A histologic study of seventeen cases. J Pathol Bacteriol 10:125–144, 1905

50. Brannan D: Extramedullary hematopoiesis in anemias. Bull Johns Hopkins Hosp 41:104–136, 1927

51. Rosenthal N, Erf LA: Clinical observations on osteopetrosis and myelofibrosis. Arch Intern Med 71:793–813, 1943

52. Carr WP Jr, Kyle RA, Bowie EJW: Hematologic changes in tuberculosis. Am J Med Sci 248:709–714, 1964

53. Cooperberg AA, Singer DP: Reversible myelofibrosis due to vitamin D deficiency rickets. Can Med Assoc J 94:392–395, 1966

54. Kiely JM, Silverstein MN: Metastatic carcinoma simulating agnogenic myeloid metaplasia. Cancer 24:1041–1044, 1969

55. Kiang DT, McKenna RW, Kennedy BJ: Reversal of myelofibrosis in advanced breast cancer. Am J Med 64:173–176, 1978

56. Editorial: Myelofibrosis. Lancet 1:127–129, 1980

57. Wyatt JP, Sommers SC: Chronic marrow failure, myelosclerosis and extramedullary hematopoiesis. Blood 5:329–347, 1950

58. Anderson RE, Hoshimo T, Yamamoto T: Myelofibrosis with myeloid metaplasia in survivors of the atomic bomb in Hiroshima. Ann Intern Med 60:1–18, 1964

59. Finch SC, Block MH: Personal communication, 1992

60. Rondeau E, Solal-Celigny P, Dhermy D, et al: Immune disorders in agnogenic myeloid metaplasia: Relations to myelofibrosis. Br J Haematol 53:467–475, 1983

61. Ben-Chetrit E, Gross DJ, Okan E, Levo Y: The association between autoimmunity and agnogenic myeloid metaplasia. Scand J Haematol 31:410–412, 1983

62. Gordon B: Immunologic abnormalities in myelofibrosis. In Berk PD, Castro-Malaspena H, Wasserman LR (eds): Myelofibrosis and the Biology of Connective Tissue. New York, Alan R Liss, 1984, pp 455–463

63. Waterfield MD, Scrace GT, Whittle N, et al: Platelet-derived growth factor is structurally related to the putative transforming protein p28^{sis} of simian sarcoma virus. Nature 304:35–39, 1983

64. Doolittle RF, Hunkapiller MW, Hood LE, et al: Simian sarcoma virus onc gene, v-sis, is derived from the gene (on genes) encoding a platelet-derived growth factor. Science 221:275–277, 1983

65. Castro-Malaspina H, Ebell W, Wang S: Human bone marrow fibroblast colony-forming units (CFU-F). In Berk PD, Castro-Malaspina H, Wasserman LR (eds): Myelofibrosis and the Bi-

ology of Connective Tissue. New York, Alan R Liss, 1984, pp 209–236

66. Ellis JT, Peterson P, Geller SA, Rappaport H: Studies of the bone marrow in polycythemia vera and the evolution of myelofibrosis and second hematologic malignancies. Semin Hematol 23:144–155, 1986

67. McCarthy DM: Annotation: Fibrosis of the bone marrow. Content and causes. Br J Haematol 59:1–7, 1985

68. Castro-Malaspina H: Pathogenesis of myelofibrosis: Role of ineffective megakaryopoiesis and megakaryocyte components. In Berk PD, Castro-Malaspina H, Wasserman LR (eds): Myelofibrosis and the Biology of Connective Tissue. New York, Alan R Liss, 1984, pp 427–454

69. Drouet L, Praloran V, Cywiner-Golenzer C, et al: Deficit congenital en alpha granules plaquetaires et fibrose reticulinique medullaire. Hypothese physiopathogenique. Nouv Rev Fr Hematol 23:95–100, 1981

70. Coller BS, Hultin MB, Nurden AT, et al: Isolated alpha-granule deficiency (gray platelet syndrome) with slight increase in bone marrow reticulin and possible glycoprotein and/or protease defect. Thromb Haemost 50:211, 1983

71. Marshall JB, Burnett DA, Anderson JC, Zefferman RK: Ascites progressing to an abdominal mass due to extramedullary hematopoiesis in a patient with agnogenic myeloid metaplasia. Dig Dis Sci 28:912–917, 1983

72. Martinelli G, Santini D, Bazzocchi F, et al: Myeloid metaplasia of the breast: A lesion which clinically mimics carcinoma. Virchows Arch [A] 401:203–207, 1983

73. Close AS, Taira Y, Cleveland DA: Spinal cord compression due to extramedullary hematopoiesis. Ann Intern Med 48:421–427, 1958

74. Ruebner B: Myelosclerosis with serosal myeloid metaplasia and fatal liver involvement. Ann Intern Med 53:1075–1088, 1960

75. Bubley G, Come P, MacDougall D, et al: Pericardial tamponade associated with myeloid metaplasia. Am J Hematol 14:185–188, 1983

76. Crawford DC, Nightingale S, Bates D, Tomlinson BE: Spinal cord compression by extramedullary hematopoiesis in myelofibrosis. Postgrad Med J 60:62–63, 1984

77. Schafer AI: Bleeding and thrombosis in the myeloproliferative disorders. Blood 64:1–12, 1984

78. Wu KK: Platelet hyperaggregability and thrombosis in patients with thrombocythemia. Ann Intern Med 88:7–11, 1978

79. Barbui T, Cortelazzo S, Viero P, et al: Thrombohemorrhagic complications in 101 cases of myeloproliferative disorders: relationship to platelet number and function. Eur J Cancer Clin Oncol 19:1593–1599, 1983

80. Silverstein MN, Linman JW: Causes of death in agnogenic myeloid metaplasia. Mayo Clin Proc 44:36–39, 1969

81. Manoharan A, Smart RC, Pitney WR: Prognostic factors in myelofibrosis. Pathology 14:455–461, 1982

82. Maldonado JE, Pintado T, Pierre RV: Dysplastic platelets and circulating megakaryocytes in chronic myeloproliferative disorders: I. The platelets: Ultrastructure and peroxidase reaction. Blood 43:797–809, 1974

83. Waddell CC, Brown JA, Repinecz YA: Abnormal platelet function in myeloproliferative disorders. Arch Pathol Lab Med 105:432–435, 1981

84. Cooper B, Schafer AI, Puchalsky D, Handin RI: Platelet resistance to prostaglandin D_2 in patients with myeloproliferative disorders. Blood 52:618–626, 1978

85. Silverstein MN, Brown AL Jr, Linman JW: Idiopathic myeloid metaplasia: its evolution into acute leukemia. Arch Intern Med 132:709–712, 1973

86. Lazlo J: Myeloproliferative disorders (MPD) myelofibrosis, myelosclerosis, extramedullary hematopoiesis, undifferentiated MPD, and hemorrhagic thrombocythemia. Sem Hematol 12:409–432, 1975

87. Huff RL, Elminger PJ, Garcia JF, et al: Ferrokinetics in normal persons and in patients having various erythropoietic disorders. J Clin Invest 30:1512–1526, 1951

88. Button LN, Rosenthal DS, Nathan DG, Moloney WC: Ferrokinetic and red cell sequestration studies as guides for splenectomy in myeloid metaplasia (abstract). American Society for Hematology 14th Annual Meeting. New York, Grune & Stratton, 1971, p 82

89. Brubaker LH, Briere J, Lazlo J, et al: Treatment of anemia in myeloproliferative disorders: A randomized study of fluoxymesterone versus transfusions only. Arch Intern Med 142:1533–1537, 1982

90. Najean Y, Caccione R, Castro-Malaspina H, Dresch C: Erythrokinetic studies in myelofibrosis: Their significance for prognosis. Br J Haematol 40:205–217, 1978

91. Dameshek W, Fudenberg H: Paroxysmal nocturnal hemoglobinuria: Atypical manifestations suggesting an immunologic disease. Arch Intern Med 99:202–208, 1957

92. Hansen NF, Killmann SA: Paroxysmal nocturnal hemoglobinuria in myelofibrosis. Blood 36:428–431, 1970

93. Kuo C, VanVoolen GA, Morrison AN: Primary and secondary myelofibrosis: Its relationship to "PNH-like defect." Blood 40:875–880, 1972

94. Gilbert HS, Wasserman LR: Hemorrhage in surgery in myelofibrosis, myelofibrosis, multiple myeloma, leukemia and lymphomas. Ann NY Acad Sci 115:169–178, 1964

95. Meytes D, Shacked N, Padeh B, et al: Immunoglobulin levels in polycythemia vera, erythrocytosis, secondary polycythemia and myelofibrosis. Isr J Med Sci 8:925–931, 1972

96. Herbert V: Diagnostic and prognostic values of measurement of serum vitamin B_{12}–binding proteins. Blood 32:305–312, 1968

97. Gilbert HS, Krauss S, Pasternack B, et al: Serum vitamin B_{12} content and unsaturated vitamin B_{12}–binding capacity in myeloproliferative disease. Ann Intern Med 71:719–729, 1969

98. Osserman EF, Lawlor DP: Serum and urine lysozyme in monocytic and monomyelocytic leukemia. J Exp Med 124:921–952, 1966

99. Skarin AT, Matsuo Y, Moloney WC: Muramidase in myeloproliferative disorders terminating in acute leukemia. Cancer 29:1336–1342, 1972

100. Rosenthal DS, Maglio R, Moloney WC: Muramidasuria and hyperkaluria in the chloro-

leukemic rat. Proc Soc Exp Biol Med 141: 499–500, 1972

101. Gilbert HS, Ginsberg H, Fagerstrom R, Brown WF: Characterization of hypocholesterolemia in myeloproliferative disease: Relation to disease manifestations and activity. Am J Med 71:595–602, 1981

102. Ginsberg H, Gilbert HS, Gibson JC, et al: Increased low density lipoprotein catabolism in myeloproliferative disorders. Ann Intern Med 96:311–316, 1982

103. Ginsberg H, Gilbert HS: Hypocholesterolemia in myeloproliferative diseases with myelofibrosis. In Berk PD, Casto-Malaspina H, Wasserman LR (eds): Myelofibrosis and the Biology of Connective Tissue. New York, Alan R Liss, 1984, pp 345–357

104. Whang-Peng J, Lee E, Knutsen T, et al: Cytogenetic studies in patients with myelofibrosis and myeloid metaplasia. Leuk Res 2:41–56, 1978

105. Pierre RV: Cytogenetics studies in hematologic disease. Am Soc Clin Pathol Syllabus, 1984

106. Westin A, Wahlstrom J, Swolin B: Chromosome studies in untreated polycythemia vera. Scand J Haematol 17:183–196, 1976

107. VanSlyck EJ, Weiss L, Dully M: Chromosomal evidence for the secondary role of fibroblastic proliferation in acute myelofibrosis. Blood 36:729–735, 1970

108. Sandberg AA: Myeloproliferative Disorders in the Chromosomes in Human Cancer and Leukemia. New York, Elsevier, 1980

109. Mitelman F, Levan G: Clustering of aberrations to specific chromosomes in human neoplasms: IV. Survey of 1871 cases. Hereditas 95:79–139, 1981

110. Geraedts JP, denOttolander GJ, Ploem JE, Muhtinghe OG: An identical translocation between chromosomes 1 and 7 in three patients with myelofibrosis and myeloid metaplasia. Br J Haematol 44:569–575, 1980

111. Cooper B, Tishler PV, Atkins L, Breg WR: Loss of Rh antigen associated with acquired Rh antibodies and a chromosome translocation in a patient with myeloid metaplasia. Blood 54:642–647, 1979

112. Pettigrew JD, Ward HP: Correlation of radiologic, histologic and clinical findings in agnogenic myeloid metaplasia. Radiology 93: 541–548, 1969

113. Bowdler AJ: Radioisotope investigations in primary myeloid metaplasia. J Clin Pathol 14: 595–602, 1961

114. Fordham EW, Ali A: Radionuclide imaging of bone marrow. Semin Hematol 18:222–239, 1981

115. McNeil BJ, Holman BL, Button LN, Rosenthal DS: Use of indium chloride scintigraphy in patients with myelofibrosis. J Nucl Med 8: 647–651, 1974

116. Button LN, Rosenthal DS, Nathan DG, Moloney WC: Computer evaluation of ferrokinetics and ^{51}Cr red cell survival, volume and sequestration in 37 patients with myeloid metaplasia. In Abstracts of the International Society for Haematology, 15th Congress, Israel, ISH, 1974, p 163

117. Sayle BA, Helmer RE III, Birdsong BA, et al: Bone marrow imaging with indium-111 chloride in aplastic anemia and myelofibrosis: Concise communication. J Nucl Med 23:121–125, 1982

118. Harnsberger HR, Daytz FL, Knochel JQ, Taylor AT: Failure to detect extramedullary hematopoiesis during bone marrow imaging with indium-111 or technetium-99 sulfur colloid. J Nucl Med 23:589–591, 1982

119. McNeil BJ, Rappeport JM, Nathan DG: Indium chloride scintigraphy: An index of severity in patients with aplastic anemia. Br J Haematol 34:599–604, 1976

120. Ruegsegger P, Elsasser U, Anliker M, et al: Quantification of bone mineralization using computed tomography. Radiology 121:93–97, 1976

121. Reich NE, Seidelman FE, Tubbs RR, et al: Determination of bone mineral content using CT scanning. AJR 127:593–594, 1976

122. Gilbert HS: Myelofibrosis revisited: Characterization and classification of myelofibrosis in the setting of myeloproliferative disease. In Berk PD, Casto-Malaspina H, Wasserman LR (eds): Myelofibrosis and the Biology of Connective Tissue. New York, Alan R Liss, 1984, pp 3–17

123. Lewis SM, Szur L: Malignant myelosclerosis. Br Med J 2:472–477, 1963

124. Bearman RM, Pangalis GA, Rappeport H: Acute (malignant) myelosclerosis. Cancer 43:279–293, 1979

125. Wood EE, Andrews CT: Subacute myelosclerosis: Report of 3 cases. Lancet 2:739–743, 1949

126. Esterez JM, Urueta EE, Moran TJ: Acute megakaryocytic myelofibrosis: Case report of an unusual myeloproliferative syndrome. Am J Clin Pathol 62:52–59, 1974

127. Bird T, Proctor SJ: Malignant myelosclerosis: myeloproliferative disorder or leukemia? Am J Clin Pathol 67:512–520, 1977

128. denOttolander GJ, teVelde J, Brederoo P, et al: Megakaryoblastic leukemia (acute myelofibrosis): A report of 3 cases. Br J Haematol 42:9–20, 1979

129. Bain BJ, Catovsky D, O'Brien M, et al: Megakaryoblastic leukemia presenting as acute myelofibrosis: A study of 4 cases with the platelet peroxidase reaction. Blood 58:206–213, 1981

129a. Koike T: Megakaryoblastic leukemia: The characterization and identification of megakaryoblasts. Blood 64:683–692, 1984

130. Hogan JA, Maniatis A, Moloney WC: The serum folate clearance test in various hematologic disorders. Blood 24:187–197, 1964

131. Lind I: Acute haemolytic anemia and hemorrhagic diathesis in the osteo myelofibrotic syndrome. Acta Haematol (Basel) 23:247–256, 1960

132. Khumbamonda M, Horowitz HI, Iyster ME: Coombs' positive hemolytic anemia in myelofibrosis with myeloid metaplasia. Am J Med Sci 258:89–93, 1969

133. Szur L, Smith MD: Red cell production and destruction in myelosclerosis. Br J Haematol 7:147–148, 1961

134. Nathan DG, Berlin NI: Studies of the production and life span of erythrocytes in myeloid metaplasia. Blood 14:668–682, 1959

135. Gardner F, Pringle JC Jr: Androgens and erythropoiesis: II. Treatment of myeloid metaplasia. N Engl J Med 264:103–111, 1961

136. Dexter TM, Allen TD, Lajtha LG: Conditions controlling the proliferation of haematopoietic stem cells in vitro. J Cell Physiol 91: 335–344, 1977

137. Juneja HS, Minguell JJ, Gardner FH, et al: The effect of dexamethasone on the growth of bone marrow fibroblasts in aplastic anemia. In Berk PD, Castro-Malaspina H, Wasserman LR (eds): Myelofibrosis and the Biology of Connective Tissue. New York, Alan R Liss, 1984, pp 265–274

138. Silver RT, Jenkins DE Jr, Engle RL Jr: Use of testosterone and busulfan in the treatment of myelofibrosis with myeloid metaplasia. Blood 23:341–353, 1964

139. Camitta BM, Thomas ED, Nathan DG, et al: A prospective study of androgens and bone marrow transplantation for treatment of severe aplastic anemia. Blood 53:504–514, 1979

140. Brubaker LH, for PVSG: Preliminary Results of Protocol 11. 1983

141. Dameshek W, Granville NB, Rubio F Jr: Therapy of the myeloproliferative disorders with Myleran. Ann NY Acad Sci 68:1001–1006, 1958

142. Oishi N, Swisher SN, Troup SB: Busulfan therapy in myeloid metaplasia. Blood 15:863–872, 1960

143. Berk PD, Goldberg JD, Silverstein MN, et al: Increased incidence of acute leukemia in polycythemia vera associated with chlorambucil therapy. N Engl J Med 304:441–447, 1981

144. Donovan PB, Berk PD, Goldberg JD, et al: Hydroxyurea, an effective agent for the treatment of polycythemia vera. Clin Res 30:315A, 1982

145. Hickling RA: Treatment of patients with myelosclerosis. Br Med J 2:411–414, 1953

146. Videback A: Unusual cases of osteomyelosclerosis. Acta Med Scand 153:459–465, 1956

147. Reich C, Rumsey W Jr: Agnogenic myeloid metaplasia of the spleen: report of 5 cases illustrating diagnostic difficulties and the danger of splenectomy and radiation therapy. JAMA 118:1200–1204, 1942

148. Block M, Jacobson LO: Myeloid metaplasia. JAMA 143:1390–1396, 1950

149. Beyreder J, Rieder H: Zur diagnostik und klinic der osteomyelosclklerose. Acta Haematol (Basel) 16:299–314, 1956

150. Greenberger JS, Chaffey JT, Rosenthal DS, Moloney WC: Irradiation for control of hypersplenism and painful splenomegaly in myeloid metaplasia. J Int Radiat Oncol Biol Phys. 2:1083–1090, 1977

151. Parmentier C, Charbord P, Tibi M, Tubiana M: Splenic irradiation in myelofibrosis: Clinical finding and ferrokinetics. J Int Radiat Oncol Biol Phys 2:1075–1081, 1977

152. Koeffler HP, Cline MJ, Golde DW: Splenic irradiation in myelofibrosis: Effect on circulating myeloid progenitor cells. Br J Haematol 43:69–77, 1979

153. Adler SS: Pathogenesis of spleen mediated phenomena in chronic myeloid leukaemia and agnogenic myeloid metaplasia: a non abscopal mechanism. Scand J Haematol 17:153–159, 1976

154. Hickling RA: Chronic non-leukaemic myelosis. Q J Med 6:253–275, 1937

155. Green TW, Conley CL, Ashburn LL, et al: Splenectomy for myeloid metaplasia of the spleen. N Engl J Med 248:211–219, 1953

156. Crosby WH, Whelan TJ, Heaton LD: Splenectomy in the elderly. Med Clin North Am 50:1533–1558, 1966

157. Benbassat J, Penchas S, Ligumski M: Splenectomy in patients with agnogenic myeloid metaplasia: An analysis of 321 published cases. Br J Haematol 42:207–214, 1979

158. Silverstein MN, ReMine WH: Splenectomy in myeloid metaplasia. Blood 53:515–518, 1979

159. Wilson RE, Rosenthal DS, Moloney WC, Osteen RT: Splenectomy for myeloproliferative disorders. World J Surg 9:431–436, 1985

160. Cabot EB, Brennan MF, Rosenthal DS, Wilson RE: Splenectomy in myeloid metaplasia. Ann Surg 182:24–30, 1978

161. Schwartz SI: Splenectomy for hematologic disease. Surg Clin North Am 61:117–125, 1981

162. Benbassat J, Penchas S: Early splenectomy and survival in agnogenic myeloid metaplasia: An analysis of 338 cases published since 1940. Acta Haematol (Basel) 65:189–192, 1981

163. Penchas J, Steinwel A, Sukenik S, Benbasset J: Splenectomy in agnogenic myeloid metaplasia: Factors of possible prognostic significance. Postgrad Med J 678:212–215, 1982

164. Bowdler AJ: Splenomegaly and hypersplenism. Clin Haematol 12:467–488, 1983

165. Goldman JM, Mulasco I: The spleen in myeloproliferative disorders. Clin Haematol 12:505–516, 1983

166. Silverstein MN, Romine WH: Sex, splenectomy and myeloid metaplasia. JAMA 227:424–425, 1974

167. Cartwright GE, Finch CA, Loeb V, et al: Panels in therapy: II. Splenectomy in myeloid metaplasia with myelosclerosis. Blood 10:550–554, 1955

168. Bensinger TA, Logue GL, Rundles RW: Hemorrhagic thrombocythaemia: Control of postsplenectomy thrombocytosis with melphalan. Blood 36:61–69, 1970

169. PVSG: Preliminary Report of Polycythemia Vera Study Group (PVSG). New York, 1983

170. Kessler CM, Klein HG, Harlik RJ: Uncontrolled thrombocytosis in chronic myeloproliferative disorders. Br J Haematol 50:157–167, 1982

171. Singh AK, Wetherly-Mein G: Microvascular occlusive lesions in primary primary thrombocythemia. Br J Hametol 36:553–564, 1977

172. Zucker S, Mielke CH: Classification of thrombocytosis based on platelet function test: Correlation with hemorrhagic and thrombotic complications. J Lab Clin Med 80:385–394, 1972

173. Hussain S, Schmitz JM, Friedman SA, Chua SN: Arterial thrombosis in essential thrombocythemia. Am Heart J 96:31–36, 1978

174. Orlin JB, Berkman EM: Improvement of platelet function following platelet pheresis in patients with myeloproliferative disease. Transfusion 20:540–545, 1980

175. Taft EG, Babcock RB, Scharfman WB, Tartaglia AP: Platelet pheresis in the management of thrombocytosis. Blood 50:927–933, 1977

176. Miller DS, Rundles RW, Silver CD: Hemorrhagic thrombocythemia; rapid plateletpheresis by continuous flow blood cell separation. Clin Res 19:426, 1971

177. Tubiana M, Buiron M: Le traitement des thrombocythemia par le phosphore radioactif. Sangre (Barce) 28:291–301, 1957

178. Murphy S, Rosenthal DS, Weinfeld A, et al: Essential thrombocythemia: Response during first year of therapy with melphalan and radioactive phosphorus: A PVSG report. Cancer Treat Rep 66:1495–1500, 1982

178a. Lofvenberg E, Wahlin A: Management of polycythemia vera, essential thrombocythemia and myelofibrosis with hydroxyurea. Eur J Haematol 41:375, 1988

179. Murphy S, Iland H, Rosenthal D, Laszlo J: Essential thrombocythemia: An interim report from the Polycythemia Vera Study Group. J Hematol 23:177, 1986

179a. Fruchtman SM, Kaplan MF, Peterson P, et al: Hydroxyurea in the management of polycythemia vera (PV): Analysis of long-term leukemogenic potential. Clin Res 1992

179b. Silverstein MN, Pettit RM, Sulberg LA Jr, et al: Anagrelide: A new drug for treating thrombocytosis. N Engl J Med 318:1292, 1988

179c. Solberg LA Jr, Oles KJ, Tarach J, et al: The effects of anagrelide on human megakaryocytopoiesis. Blood 74:32a, 1989

179d. Mazur EM, Sohl P, Newton J, et al: Mechanism of anagrelide induced thrombocytopenia. Blood 74:32a, 1989

179e. Giles EJ, Singer CRJ, Gray AG, et al: Alpha-interferon therapy for essential thrombocythemia. Lancet 2:70, 1988

179f. Gisslinger H, Ludwig H, Linkesch W, et al: Long-term interferon therapy for thrombocytosis in myeloproliferative diseases. Lancet 1:634, 1989

179g. Talpaz M, Kurzrock R, Kantarjian H, et al: Recombinant interferon-alpha therapy of Philadelphia chromosome–negative myeloproliferative disorders with thrombocytosis. Am J Med 86:554, 1989

179h. Tichelli A, Gratwohl A, Berger C, et al: Treatment of thrombocytosis in myeloproliferative disorders with interferon alpha-2. Blut 58:15, 1989

180. Preston FE: Aspirin, prostaglandins and peripheral gangrene. Am J Med 74(suppl):55–60, 1983

181. Jabaily J, Iland HJ, Lazlo J, et al: Neurological manifestations of essential thrombocytosis. Ann Intern Med 99:513–518, 1983

181a. Barbui T, Buell, M, Cortelazzo S, et al: Aspirin and risk of bleeding in patients with thrombocythemia. Am J Med 83:265, 1987

182. Tartaglia AP, Goldberg JD, Silverstein MN, et al: Aspirin and Persantine do not prevent thrombotic complications in patients with polycythemia vera treated with phlebotomy. Blood 58(suppl I):240a, 1981

183. Kuhn K, Templ R: Collagens: Molecular and antigenic structure. In Berk PD, Castro-Malaspina H, Wasserman LR (eds): Myelofibrosis and the Biology of Connective Tissue. New York, Alan R Liss, 1984, pp 45–49

184. Bernstein P, Horlein D. McPherson J: Regulation of collagen synthesis. In Berk PD, Castro-Malaspina H, Wasserman LR (eds): Myelofibrosis and the Biology of Connective Tissue. New York, Alan R Liss, 1984, pp 61–80

185. Prockop DJ: The synthesis of type I collagen fibers and potential inhibitors of the process. In Berk PD, Castro-Malaspina H, Wasserman LR (eds): Myelofibrosis and the Biology of Connective Tissue. New York, Alan R Liss, 1984, pp 81–88

186. Krane SM: Collagen degradation. In Berk PD, Castro-Malaspina H, Wasserman LR (eds): Myelofibrosis and the Biology of Connective Tissue. New York, Alan R Liss, 1984, pp 89–102

187. Fruchtman SM: Therapeutic implications of collagen metabolism in myelofibrosis. In Berk PD, Castro-Malaspina H, Wasserman LR (eds): Myelofibrosis and the Biology of Connective Tissue. New York, Alan R Liss, 1984, pp 467–474

188. Cardinale GJ, Udenfriend S: Prolylhydroxylase. Adv Enzymol 41:245–300, 1974

189. Uitto J, Prockop DJ: Incorporation of proline analogues into collagen polypeptides: Effects of extracellular procollagen and in the stability of the triple-helical structure of the molecule. Biochem Biophys Acta 336:234–251, 1974

190. Rosenbloom J, Prockop DJ: Incorporation of 3,4-dehydroproline into protocollagen and collagen: Limited hydroxylation of proline and lysine in the same polypeptide. J Biol Chem 245:3361–3368, 1970

191. Salvador RA, Tsai I, Marcel RJ, et al: The in vivo inhibition of collagen synthesis and the reduction of prolylhydroxylase activity by 3,4-dehydroproline. Arch Biochem Biophys 174:381–392, 1976

192. Bornstein P: The biosynthesis of collagen. Ann Rev Biochem 43:567–603, 1974

193. Tanner MS, Jackson D, Mowat AP: Hepatic collagen synthesis in a rat model of cirrhosis and its modification by colchicine. J Pathol 135:179–187, 1981

194. Alarcon-Segovia D, Ibanez G, Kershenobich D, Rajkind M: Treatment of scleroderma by modification of collagen metabolism: A double blind trial with colchicine and placebo. J Rheum 1(suppl):97, 1974

195. Rojkind M, Mourelle M, Kersherobich D: Anti-inflammatory and antifibrogenic activities of colchiase: treatment of liver cirrhosis. In Berk PD, Castro-Malaspina H, Wasserman LR (eds): Myelofibrosis and the Biology of Connective Tissue. New York, Alan R Liss, 1984, pp 475–489

196. Harris ED, Krane SM: Effect of colchicine on collagenase in cultures of rheumatoid synovium. Arthritis Rheum 14:669–684, 1971

197. Nimni ME: A defect in the intramolecular and intermolecular crosslinking of collagen caused by penicillamine: I. Metabolic and functional abnormalities in soft tissues. J Biol Chem 243:1457–1466, 1968

198. Nakagawa H, Ohkoshi K, Tsurufuji S: Selective inhibition of collagen synthesis by D-penicillamine in carrageenin-induced inflammation in rats. Biochem Pharmacol 28:1771–1775, 1979

199. Ward WF, Shih-Hoellwarth A, Tuttle RD: Collagen accumulation in irradiated rat lung: modification by D-penicillamine. Radiology 146:533–537, 1983

200. Protocol 07-PVSG: Potaba in treatment of myelofibrosis: Preliminary study. New York, Polycythemia Vera Study Group (PVSG), November 1983.

201. Crosby WC: Fibrosis of the marrow is not cast in cement. JAMA 246:1940–1941, 1981
202. Smith BR, Rosenthal DS: Successful management of acute myelofibrosis with hydroxyurea. Personal communication, 1992
203. Myers CE, Chabner BA, DeVita VT, Gralnik HR: Bone marrow involvement in Hodgkin's disease: Pathology and response to MOPP chemotherapy. Blood 44:197–204, 1974
204. Manoharan A, Hursley R, Pitney WR: The reticulin content of bone marrow in acute leukemia in adults. Br J Haematol 43:185–190, 1979
205. Yetgins S, Ozsoylo S: Myeloid metaplasia in vitamin D deficiency rickets. Scand J Haematol 28:180–185, 1982
206. McCarthy DM, San Miguel JF, Freake HC, et al: 1,25-Dihydroxyvitamin D_3 inhibits proliferation of human promyelocytic leukemia (HL60) cells and induces monocyte-macrophage differentiation in HL60 and normal human bone marrow cells. Leuk Res 7:51–55, 1984
207. Moore MAS, Gabrilove J, Sheridan AP: Induction of myeloid leukemia cell differentiation by endogenous cytokines and vitamin analogues. In Murphy SB, Gilbert JR (eds): Leukemia Research: Advances in Cell Biology and Treatment. Amsterdam, Elsevier Biomedical, 1983, pp 31–51
208. McCarthy DM, Hibbin JA, Goldman JM: A role for 1,25-dihydroxyvitamin D_3 in control of bone marrow collagen deposition. Lancet 1:78–80, 1984
209. Polliack A, Prokocimer M, Matzner Y: Lymphoblastic leukemic transformation in myelofibrosis and myeloid metaplasia. Am J Hematol 9:211–220, 1980

20

Essential Thrombocythemia

HARRY ILAND, JOHN LASZLO, *and* SCOTT MURPHY

HISTORICAL PERSPECTIVES

The foundations of our current understanding of the myeloproliferative disorders (MPDs) were originally laid over 100 years ago. In 1856, Virchow was able to distinguish between two forms of chronic leukemia on the basis of their differing clinical and morphologic features, referring to them as "splenic" leukemia (now known as *chronic granulocytic leukemia*) and "lymphatic" leukemia (*chronic lymphocytic leukemia*). The first description of myelofibrosis by Heuck appeared in 1879, that of polycythemia vera by Vaquez was in 1892, and di Guglielmo reported erythroleukemia in 1920, but it was not until 1934 that a disease resembling what we now refer to as *essential thrombocythemia* (ET) was first described by Epstein and Goedel.[1] Their patient had extreme thrombocytosis, megakaryocytic hyperplasia, splenic infarction and atrophy, thrombosis, and hemorrhage.

In 1951, Dameshek[2] immortalized his own ideas and those of several other workers when he published an editorial on the myeloproliferative syndromes in which he brought these disorders together under a common pathophysiologic process. He postulated that in response to some unrecognized stimulus, the myeloid, erythroid, megakaryocytic, and fibroblastic elements of the bone marrow proliferated en masse. He also suggested that dormant embryonal hematopoietic tissue in extramedullary sites became activated. While Dameshek's concept survives to this day, it has become necessary to adopt several modifications as a result of

evidence obtained from studies involving cytogenetics, heterozygosity for glucose-6-phosphate dehydrogenase (G-6-PD) isoenzymes, and cell culture techniques. For instance, it is now well established that the myelofibrosis is a reactive component of the myeloproliferative process, whereas the erythroid, myeloid, and megakaryocytic populations are clonally derived.[3] Furthermore, the extramedullary hematopoiesis is also part of the clonal proliferation which originates in the bone marrow. In vitro data suggest that the pathogenesis of the myelofibrosis is related to ineffective megakaryocytopoiesis, with excessive release of platelet-derived growth factor, transforming growth factor beta, platelet factor IV, and a platelet-derived collagenase inhibitor.[4] These compounds result in fibroblast proliferation and collagen secretion, together with inhibition of collagenase activity. The net effect is excessive deposition of collagen and bone marrow matrix.

More recent concepts of the MPDs encompass both acute and chronic varieties. The acute MPDs are synonymous with acute myeloblastic (nonlymphocytic) leukemia. Specific variants have been classified on the basis of morphology, cytochemistry, electron microscopy, and surface markers.[5] More recently, the classification has been refined through the use of cytogenetics and molecular genetics. The chronic MPDs are less easily categorized; although many cases have features that are distinct enough to fit one of the classic descriptions of these conditions, there are also many that have overlapping features. Regardless of where they fit within this group, chronic MPDs share certain features in common, *viz.*, panhyperplasia in the bone marrow, reactive myelofibrosis, extramedullary hematopoiesis, and a propensity for progressive myelofibrosis or evolution to acute leukemia.

ESSENTIAL THROMBOCYTHEMIA AS A DISTINCT ENTITY

Following Epstein and Goedel's original description of ET, increasing numbers of cases were reported in the literature.[6] However, there was considerable controversy as to whether this condition truly represented a distinct entity, and as recently as 1955, McCabe et al.[7] rejected this idea. They claimed that if patients with idiopathic thrombocytosis were followed for a sufficient length of time, some other underlying hematologic disorder would eventually emerge. It was not until the classic reviews of Gunz[8] and Ozer et al.[9] in 1960 that ET became widely accepted despite its lack of unique pathologic characteristics.

PREVIOUS DIAGNOSTIC CRITERIA

Thrombocytosis is the sine qua non of ET, but it also occurs in other MPDs, in myelodysplastic syndromes, and in certain reactive states.[10, 11] Despite its recognition over 50 years ago, and despite its eventual acceptance among the chronic MPDs, the early series demonstrated a notable lack of uniformity with respect to the diagnostic requirements for ET. Criteria have variably included the degree of thrombocytosis, spleen size, Philadelphia chromosome (Ph) status, leukocyte alkaline phosphatase (LAP) scores, and the presence or absence of thrombohemorrhagic phenomena, erythrocytosis, leukocytosis, and marrow fibrosis. Thrombotic and/or hemorrhagic phenomena have been required for diagnosis in some series,[8, 9, 12, 13] but not in all.[14, 15] Patients with splenic atrophy were excluded in at least two series,[9, 16] whereas other series included postsplenectomy patients.[8, 12, 17] Platelet counts were, by definition, greater than normal in all series, but exact levels were not always specified.[12] Only one series required LAP scores for inclusion.[16] Some series required a normal hemoglobin or red cell mass,[9, 13, 14, 16] while others interpreted erythrocytosis as a feature

of the disease.[8, 12, 18] Some authors have excluded chronic granulocytic leukemia (CGL) by the finding of marked leukocytosis[9] or by the presence of the Ph chromosome.[14–16] Finally, the presence of marrow fibrosis was acceptable in one series[8] but was considered sufficient grounds for exclusion by others.[13, 14, 16] Because of the inconsistent application of these criteria, ET has remained the least well-defined of the chronic MPDs.

PVSG CRITERIA FOR ESSENTIAL THROMBOCYTHEMIA

During the latter half of the 1970s, the myeloproliferative subcommittee of the Polycythemia Vera Study Group (PVSG) initiated a series of protocols dealing with the presenting manifestations, treatment, and course of ET and other MPDs characterized by marked thrombocytosis.[19–23] Strict diagnostic criteria were established for the identification of that subset of patients with ET; these criteria were directed primarily at the exclusion of PV, CGL, and idiopathic myelofibrosis (IMF), which is also known as agnogenic myeloid metaplasia (AMM). In addition to thrombocytosis (platelet count greater than or equal to 600×10^9/liter), megakaryocytic hyperplasia was an absolute requirement. For protocols involving myelosuppressive therapy, a platelet count of greater than or equal to 1000×10^9/liter was generally required. Patients were excluded if there was evidence of reactive thrombocytosis (e.g., carcinoma, previous splenectomy, sideroblastic anemia, etc.). A normal red cell mass or a hemoglobin less than 13 g/dl was required in order to exclude overt PV, and stainable marrow iron or no more than 1 g/dl increase in hemoglobin following 1 month of oral iron therapy was used to exclude masked PV. Only patients with a Ph-negative karyotype were included. Patients with collagen fibrosis involving more than one-third the cross-sectional area of the marrow biopsy were excluded, and patients with mild fibrosis (i.e., less than one-third the cross-sectional area of the biopsy) who also had splenomegaly and a leukoerythroblastic reaction also were excluded, since this triad of features may represent the cellular phase of IMF/AMM. This approach to the diagnosis of ET is schematically depicted in Fig. 20–1. Recently published studies of large numbers of

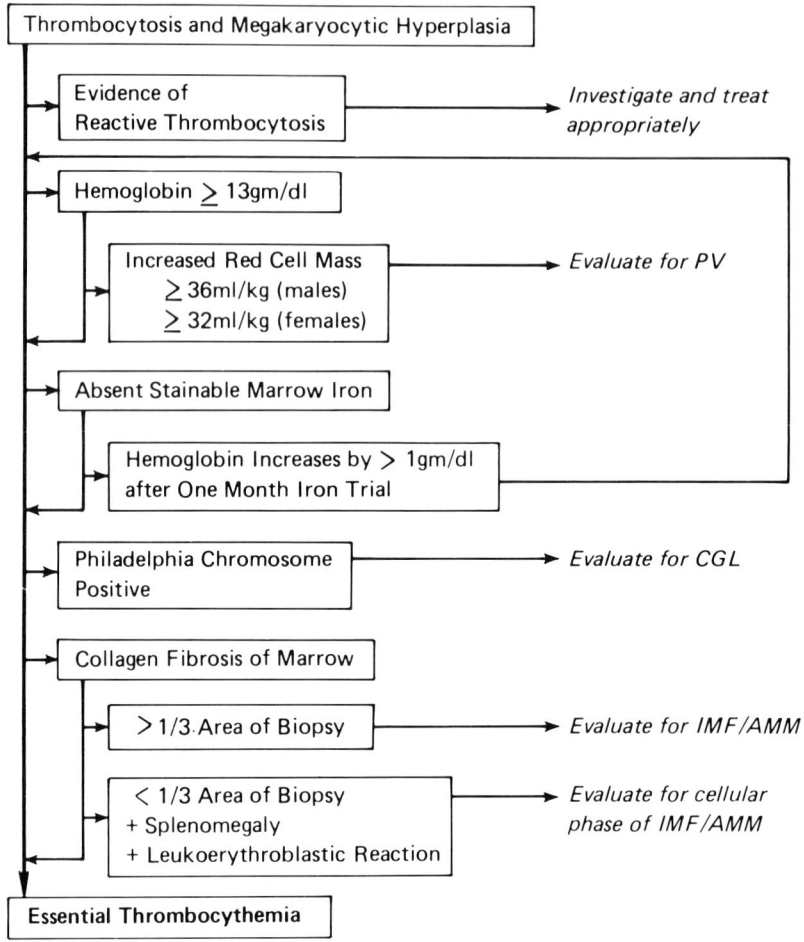

FIGURE 20-1. Schematic approach to the diagnosis of ET. *(Courtesy of the American Association of Physicians.)*

patients with ET have utilized diagnostic criteria that are very similar to, if not identical with, those promoted by the PVSG.[24-26]

ETIOLOGY

The etiology of ET remains unknown. Although exposure to ionizing radiation has been shown to cause some cases of chronic granulocytic leukemia (CGL) and idiopathic myelofibrosis/agnogenic myeloid metaplasia (IMF/AMM), such an association has not been observed for ET or polycythemia vera (PV). Reverse transcriptase (RNA-dependent DNA polymerase) activity and evidence of C-type retrovirus particles have been detected in the platelets of patients with a variety of MPDs including ET by one group of investigators.[27,28] Disappearance of the ret-

roviruses and reduction in aneuploidy were observed following initiation of myelosuppressive therapy,[29,30] but these observations have not been confirmed independently. Isolated case reports of the finding of the Ph chromosome in patients with ET have been published,[24,31-35] and the PVSG has collected six such patients. Five of these six patients have evolved to either an overt chronic phase of CGL or to acute leukemia, thus suggesting that ET may represent a "preleukemic" state of CGL in a small number of patients. Apart from the occasional occurrence of the Ph chromosome, and therefore presumably of c-*abl* and *bcr* gene rearrangements, ET has not been associated with amplification, rearrangement, or mutation of known oncogenes. Although the etiology of ET is unknown, it has repeatedly been shown to be a clonal hemopathy on the basis of G-6-PD isoenzyme distribution in heterozygotes,[36–39] as well as by the presence of a 1q+ cytogenetic abnormality in erythroid and granulocyte-monocyte progenitors in one patient.[40] Erythroid, myeloid, megakaryocytic, and multilineage progenitors are increased in some patients with ET,[41,42] and endogenous erythroid[41,43] and megakaryocytic[44] colony formation also has been observed, confirming the similarity of this disorder to PV.

EPIDEMIOLOGY

ET is a rare disorder. No accurate data on its incidence are available, but based on its frequency relative to PV, the number of newly diagnosed cases is probably less than 5 per 1 million per year. Most series have shown either no sex difference or a slight excess among women. The median age at diagnosis is approximately 60 years, although cases in childhood have been reported.[45–47] No racial predilection has been observed. Familial MPD associated with cases of ET has been reported but probably no more frequently than would have been expected by chance.[26,48–50]

CLINICAL FEATURES

The clinical syndromes seen in patients with ET are extremely varied.[1,6,8,9,12–18,21,24–26,46,51–97] Most manifestations can be grouped within the broad categories of thrombosis and hemorrhage, although a significant proportion of patients may be completely asymptomatic at the time of diagnosis. Indeed, the widespread use of automated platelet counters in routine diagnostic hematology laboratories is likely to facilitate the recognition of increasing numbers of such patients. Whereas the early reviews of ET emphasized hemorrhage as an essential diagnostic criterion, more recent studies suggest that hemorrhage is seen in only 35 percent of patients who satisfy currently accepted criteria for the diagnosis of ET.[24–26,97] When hemorrhage occurs, it is usually mucocutaneous in distribution, manifesting primarily as epistaxis and bruising. Life-threatening hemorrhage is infrequent and usually follows accidental or surgical trauma[77] or the use of platelet antiaggregating agents.[92] Deep tissue bleeding into joints,[66] muscles, and brain is rare. A

wide variety of thrombotic manifestations occurs in ET, and together they represent a more frequent problem than does hemorrhage. Large-vessel obstruction, both arterial and venous, as well as microvascular occlusion, may occur. Large-vessel obstruction may involve the cerebral,[62,82,87] coronary,[60,63,84] splenic,[8] renal,[67,74] mesenteric,[77] or femoral arteries,[86] the peripheral,[64,88] hepatic (Budd-Chiari syndrome),[71] or renal veins,[67] the sagittal[61] or longitudinal[81] sinuses, or the corpora cavernosa (priapism).[65,72] Microvascular obstruction[69,83] produces symptoms such as erythromelalgia,[91] peripheral ischemia and gangrene,[21,68,75,86,90] dysesthesias,[87] visual disturbances,[87] and metatarsalgia.[85] Neurologic manifestations are frequent[62,76,82,87] and include transient ischemic attacks, headache, stroke, dizziness, visual disturbance, dysesthesias, and seizures. Nonspecific symptoms of weakness and lethargy are common but not well understood,[21] and other features of chronic MPDs also may be present (e.g., fever, weight loss, peptic ulcers, pruritus, and gout).[21] Problems directly attributable to extramedullary hematopoiesis have been described (e.g., pericarditis).[70] Pyoderma gangrenosum[78] and fetal loss during pregnancy also have been reported.[84] Palpable splenomegaly is present in less than 50 percent of patients and, when present, rarely extends beyond 3 cm below the costal margin.[97] A proportion of patients with impalpable spleens can be shown to have mild splenomegaly by ultrasonography, computed axial tomography, or, if splenic area and volume are calculated, splenic scintigraphy. Hepatomegaly and lymphadenopathy are uncommon.

HEMATOLOGIC CHARACTERISTICS

Thrombocytosis is the most striking feature in the peripheral blood. Platelet morphology is frequently abnormal, and although the mean platelet volume remains normal, the distribution of platelet diameters is increased due to the presence of both microthrombocytes and macrothrombocytes.[98] Agranular platelets also may be seen. Mild anemia may occur in the absence of iron deficiency and blood loss[21,25] and is usually corrected when the myeloproliferative process is controlled with chemotherapy.[25] The red cells usually show normal morphology unless the following complications occur: iron deficiency secondary to blood loss, evolution to myelofibrosis, or splenic atrophy. An absolute reticulocytosis is present in one-third of patients.[21] Neutrophilic leukocytosis is present in approximately 50 percent of patients, but the white blood cell (WBC) count rarely exceeds 50×10^9/liter.[24,25,97] Mild basophilia and eosinophilia are present in over one-third of patients.[21] Occasional myeloid precursors, nucleated red blood cells, and circulating megakaryocytic fragments may be seen,[21,24,26] but less frequently than in myelofibrosis. Leukocyte alkaline phosphatase scores exhibit a wide range,[24,97] and a minority of patients have scores as low as is seen in CGL despite the absence of the Ph chromosome.[21] Overall marrow biopsy cellularity is increased in almost 90 percent of patients.[21,24] Megakaryocytic hyperplasia should always be present, and the megakaryocytes are often morphologically bizarre with varying degrees of cellular atypia, including nuclear pleomorphism.[21,24,25] As in PV, the megakaryocytes tend to be larger than normal, and clustering of megakaryocytes is almost invariable.[21] Erythroid and granulocytic elements are increased in the majority of patients, but the degree of hyperplasia is generally less than the degree of megakaryocytic hyperplasia.[21] In our experience, reticulin content is normal in greater than 80 percent of patients,[21] but others have reported increased reticulin in approximately 50 percent of patients.[24,26] Overt collagen fibrosis is usually associated with splenomegaly and a leukoerythroblastic reaction, and such patients should be regarded as having the cellular phase of agnogenic myeloid metaplasia rather than ET.[19–21] In our experience, such patients exhibit survival patterns more compatible with IMF/AMM than with ET (unpublished data). The likelihood of finding stainable marrow iron varies according to the criteria used to define ET. Patients with ET may have iron deficiency due to blood loss; however, if absence of iron deficiency is required for the diagnostic exclusion of PV, then stainable iron will be present in most cases.[97] In the absence of stainable iron, iron replacement therapy will not result in the rapid development of erythrocytosis if the diagnosis is ET, in contrast to PV. The iron stain is also useful in the recognition of myelodysplastic syndromes characterized by ringed sideroblasts and thrombocytosis.[99]

PLATELET FUNCTION STUDIES

A number of platelet function abnormalities have been described in the majority of patients with ET and MPD and have been reviewed extensively elsewhere.[98,100] Platelet abnormalities can be categorized under the following headings: platelet morphology, surface membrane, arachidonic acid metabolism, granules, and function.[98] Prolongation of skin bleeding time is uncommon,[52] whereas in vitro abnormalities indicative of impaired platelet function are frequent.[98,100] These include reduced platelet factor III activity,[101] reduced platelet adhesion,[102] defective platelet aggregation (particularly with epinephrine),[46,57,58,101] nucleotide[103] and 5-hydroxytryptamine[104] storage pool defects, decreased membrane glycoprotein I and increased glycoprotein IV,[105] abnormal thrombospondin (glycoprotein G),[106] defective glycosylation of platelet glycoproteins,[107] decreased α-adrenergic receptors,[108] reduced lipoxygenase activity[109,110] and malondialdehyde production,[56] defective mobilization of arachidonic acid from membrane phospholipid,[111] altered platelet membrane lipid composition[112,113] (which is partially reversed by aspirin),[113] decreased alpha and dense granules,[114] decreased platelet β-thromboglobulin content with increased plasma β-thromboglobulin that is reversible by aspirin,[115] defective platelet coagulant (factor X–activating) activity,[56] and increased levels of glyoxalase I.[116] Platelet hyperaggregability is also seen,[53,58] as shown by spontaneous platelet aggregation and "circulating" platelet aggregates. Platelet hyperaggregability in MPDs may be related in part to decreased prostaglandin D_2 receptors,[117] since prostaglandin D_2 normally inhibits platelet aggregation. Increased expression of Fc receptors on myeloproliferative platelets also may contribute to hyperaggregability.[118] In contrast, the vascular cyclooxygenase pathway remains intact in MPDs, as shown by normal prostacyclin generation.[119] Whether the platelet abnormalities associated with MPDs reflect primary defects in platelet precursors as part of the underlying clonal hemopathy or whether they are acquired in the circulation as a result of activation and release in vivo is controversial.[100] Finally, chronic low-grade disseminated intravascular coagulation (DIC) also may contribute to the hemostatic defects seen in ET and other

MPDs. Martinez et al.[120] have demonstrated increased prothrombin and fibrinogen catabolism in some patients, and Takahashi et al.[51] also have observed increased fibrin/fibrinogen degradation products, decreased antithrombin III, decreased plasminogen and α_2-plasmin inhibitor, and an increased VIIIRAg/VIIIC ratio. Conflicting data exist regarding the degree to which thrombocytosis and platelet dysfunction contribute to and interact in the genesis of thrombohemorrhagic phenomena in ET. This is partly because of the multitude of platelet function parameters that have been evaluated, partly because thrombosis and hemorrhage occur intermittently and asynchronously over time, and partly because both myelosuppressive and antiplatelet therapy produce inconsistent effects on platelet dysfunction. Therefore, categorical statements cannot be made, but the following observations reflect the balance of published data: (1) most studies have failed to show a clear relationship between the platelet count and platelet function abnormalities (see review by Schafer),[100] (2) the question of whether a causal relationship exists between hyperaggregability and thrombosis and between hypoaggregability and hemorrhage remains unanswered, numerous studies for[53,56,58,83,84,94,95,115,121] and against[52,55,56,79,101,122,123] such associations having been published, (3) clinically significant thrombohemorrhagic complications of myeloproliferative-related thrombocytosis respond, in most cases, to either myelosuppressive therapy[8,14,17,69,86,87,94] and/or plateletpheresis,[95,96] and (4) platelet antiaggregating agents also have produced clinical responses despite persistent thrombocytosis.[87,90] Unfortunately, none of the above-mentioned platelet function abnormalities are diagnostic of ET; they are often present in patients with IMF/AMM and, to a lesser extent, in patients with other MPDs. Their major value lies in their ability to differentiate myeloproliferative-related thrombocytosis from reactive thrombocytosis, since the latter is rarely associated with platelet dysfunction.[58,94,101,107,112,116,124,125]

BIOCHEMICAL FINDINGS

Biochemical abnormalities similar to those seen in PV also occur in ET.[21] The serum vitamin B_{12} level and the unbound B_{12}-binding capacity may be elevated because of increased levels of B_{12}-binding proteins in serum and leukocytes (transcobalamins I and III), but not to the same extent as in CGL. Hyperuricemia, increased lactate dehydrogenase,[126] and less frequently, hyperbilirubinemia also occur. Serum iron, total iron-binding capacity, and ferritin levels may reflect iron deficiency. Pseudohyperkalemia due to excessive release of intracellular potassium from platelets during collection of clotted serum samples may cause concern.[127] Simultaneous plasma and serum sampling will allow recognition of this artefact.

ULTRASTRUCTURAL AND KINETIC STUDIES

Ultrastructural studies of megakaryocytes in ET and other MPDs show several abnormalities, including increased megakaryocyte ploidy,[57,128,129] abnormal distribution of the demarcation membrane complex and granules,[57] and decreased dense bodies with increased intramembranous particles.[130] Emperipolesis, or "internal wandering of myeloid cells," is increased in ET and MPDs.[131] Electron microscopy has shown that the engulfed cells are not present inside megakaryocytes as a result of phagocytosis but rather are found inside the dilated cavities of the demarcation membranes. Their presence correlates positively with sites of thrombocytogenesis, and the frequency of emperipolesis is related to the height of the platelet count. Megakaryocyte area, number, and volume per microliter of bone marrow are increased in ET, the latter being 6.8 times normal megakaryocyte volume in one series.[129] This correlated with the platelet production rate, which was increased by a factor of 6.2 in that series. Platelet ultrastructure is also abnormal, with proliferation of the dense tubular system and deficiency of the surface-connected canalicular system.[57] There is an increased proportion of light-density platelets,[57,132] and platelet size distribution is abnormal, with an increased number of megathrombocytes and an increased breadth of the platelet volume distribution.[124,125]

Autologous platelet life span, assessed by ^{111}In-labeled platelets, is moderately decreased in ET[54,57] whether or not vascular occlusion has occurred. When the thrombocytosis is controlled by busulfan therapy, the shortened platelet survival persists.[54]

CYTOGENETICS

Nonstimulated metaphases obtained from marrow aspirates should be examined for cytogenetic abnormalities. Karyotypic analysis is primarily important in order to exclude the presence of the Ph chromosome, since in our experience the prognosis of patients with Ph-positive ET is similar to that of patients with Ph-positive CGL and unlike that of patients with Ph-negative ET (see Overlap with Chronic Granulocytic Leukemia, below).

Zaccaria and Tura[133] have observed a 21q− abnormality in G-banded metaphases from 5 consecutive patients with ET and have claimed that this abnormality may be uniquely associated with ET, but it has been suggested that some of these patients would not have met currently acceptable criteria for the diagnosis of ET.[134] This conclusion is supported by the absence of the 21q− abnormality in several recent series of strictly defined cases of ET.[21, 26, 134–136] Furthermore, a 21q− abnormality has subsequently been identified in patients with myeloproliferative-related thrombocytosis other than ET.[137] An elongation of the short arm of chromosome 21 also has been described in 6 of 8 patients with ET in one series,[14] but once again, this abnormality has not been confirmed in more recent studies using banded karyotypes. Isolated instances of a 20q− abnormality have been reported,[21, 26] although this is seen more commonly in patients with PV,[138] and 3 of 11 cases in a further study showed a 2q+ abnormality.[138] Despite these reports, the Third International Workshop on Chromosomes in Leukemia has concluded that only 5.3 percent of patients with ET show definite cytogenetic abnormalities.[139] Clonal evolution occasionally occurs in patients whose original karyotypes were normal, either with[49] or without[135] intervening chemotherapy, and particularly in association with blastic transformation.[26, 140]

THE CLONAL NATURE OF ESSENTIAL THROMBOCYTHEMIA

Evidence that ET is a clonal stem-cell disorder has been obtained from biochemical, cytogenetic, and clonogenic progenitor studies.[3] In patients heterozygous for G-6-PD variants, the erythrocytes, platelets, and granulocytes have been shown to express only one G-6-PD isoenzyme.[36–38] Involvement of B-lymphocytes in the clonal disorder has been shown in one patient by the demonstration of monotypic G-6-PD expression in Epstein-Barr virus–transformed B-lymphoblastoid lines.[39] The observation of a 1q+ abnormality in both erythroid and granulocyte-monocyte progenitors has provided cytogenetic confirmation of the clonal nature of ET.[40] Interestingly, monocytes and B-lymphocytes may not be part of the monoclonal proliferation in all patients with ET.[37] The use of molecular techniques involving X chromosome–linked probes and methylation-sensitive restriction enzymes is likely to further clarify the level of hematopoietic progenitor involvement in ET and other MPDs.[141]

HEMATOPOIETIC PROGENITORS IN ESSENTIAL THROMBOCYTHEMIA

A limited number of reports have examined hematopoietic progenitor levels and their responsiveness to growth factors in patients with ET. The majority of patients have increased levels of mixed (CFU-GEMM), erythroid (BFU-E), myeloid (CFU-GM), and megakaryocyte (CFU-M) progenitors, in both the peripheral blood and bone marrow.[41,42] The CFU-M pool is expanded in ET as part of the myeloproliferative process, and this is not due to increased levels of megakaryocyte colony-stimulating activity (Meg-CSA).[44] Although Meg-CSA–independent CFU-Ms are detectable in ET, CFU-Ms remain responsive to additional exogenous Meg-CSA, indicating that megakaryocytopoiesis is not entirely autonomous.[44] In contrast, the CFU-M pool in reactive thrombocytosis is normal quantitatively and in terms of its responsiveness to Meg-CSA.[44] Spontaneous erythroid colony formation is almost universal in ET, even in patients without overt evidence of erythroid involvement in the myeloproliferative process.[41,43] In the presence of exogenous erythropoietin, additional small increases in erythroid colony formation occur, consistent with the situation in PV.[43] In a detailed study of ET and other MPDs, several features correlated with incipient blastic transformation, including an increased proportion of abnormally light, buoyant-density colony-forming cells in peripheral blood and bone marrow, increased levels of urinary colony-stimulating factor, and low colony-forming capacity of bone marrow cells.[142]

DIFFERENTIAL DIAGNOSIS

Other Chronic Myeloproliferative Disorders

Although thrombocytosis is the sine qua non of ET, it also occurs in the other chronic MPDs, in myelodysplastic syndromes, and in many nonhematopoietic disorders.[11] Of the MPDs, PV most closely resembles ET,[97, 98] and the importance of iron replacement in excluding masked PV has already been stressed. CGL is usually easily differentiated from ET by the marked leukocytosis, the Ph chromosome, low or absent LAP activity, prominent splenomegaly, and predominant myeloid hyperplasia in the bone marrow. IMF/AMM is distinguished by the presence of marrow fibrosis, the marked red cell morphologic abnormalities, the more overt leukoerythroblastic reaction, and the prominent extramedullary hematopoiesis.

Myelodysplastic Syndromes

Of the myelodysplastic syndromes, the 5q− syndrome is most commonly associated with thrombocytosis, and cytogenetic analysis is helpful in identifying this disorder. Other features that differentiate this disorder from ET include macrocytic anemia and hypolobulated megakaryocytes.[143] Idiopathic refractory sideroblastic anemia also may exhibit thrombocytosis and can be recognized by the dimorphic peripheral blood red cells and the ringed sideroblasts in the marrow.[99]

Reactive Thrombocytosis

Reactive thrombocytosis is a common finding in a wide variety of clinical conditions.[11] In most situations, the underlying process is obvious, and investigations specifically directed at the thrombocytosis are not indicated. However, iron deficiency due to occult blood loss may cause difficulty in diagnosis, and underlying neoplasms should be excluded whether or not iron deficiency is pres-

ent. Bacterial infections and tumors are most likely to be accompanied by thrombocytosis when considerable tissue necrosis and suppuration are present. Hemolytic anemia is suggested by marked reticulocytosis and intense marrow erythroid hyperplasia; red cell changes characteristic of the underlying pathophysiologic process also may be apparent (immune hemolysis, Heinz body hemolysis, thalassemia, etc.). Permanent thrombocytosis may accompany splenectomy itself, or splenectomy may unmask an existing ET.[77] Postsplenectomy thrombocytosis also may coexist with other causes of secondary thrombocytosis, and their relative contributions to the thrombocytosis may be difficult to evaluate. We have recently observed a previously unreported association between tetracycline-induced benign intracranial hypertension and reactive thrombocytosis, which responded to tetracycline withdrawal and therapeutic spinal taps (unpublished observations). The features that are most helpful in distinguishing secondary thrombocytosis from ET include (1) the severity of the thrombocytosis parallels the activity of the underlying disorder and is often self-limited, (2) the platelet count rarely exceeds 1000×10^9/liter, and (3) platelet function abnormalities are not present. In addition, interleukin 6 (IL-6) assays may be helpful, since serum IL-6 levels are usually normal in myeloproliferative-related thrombocytosis but are frequently elevated in reactive thrombocytosis.[144] Table 20–1 lists the differential diagnosis of ET, and the bone marrow appearances in other conditions associated with thrombocytosis are summarized in Table 20–2.

THERAPEUTIC OPTIONS IN ESSENTIAL THROMBOCYTHEMIA

The therapeutic options for the treatment of ET are quite varied and include no therapy, plateletpheresis, platelet antiaggregating agents, myelosuppression with either ^{32}P or cytotoxic chemotherapeutic drugs, and new drugs such as interferon-α and anagrelide. In view of the many different ways in which ET manifests itself, the specific approach to be employed should be individualized to each patient. Several studies have emphasized the benign nature of ET and

TABLE 20-1. DIFFERENTIAL DIAGNOSIS OF THROMBOCYTOSIS

Chronic myeloproliferative disorders	Essential thrombocythemia Polycythemia vera Chronic granulocytic leukemia Idiopathic myelofibrosis/agnogenic myeloid metaplasia Overlap myeloproliferative disorders
Myelodysplastic syndromes associated with thrombocytosis	5q− syndrome Idiopathic refractory sideroblastic anemia
Reactive thrombocytosis	Blood loss and/or iron deficiency Splenectomy Hemolytic anemia Malignancy Myelophthisis Chronic inflammatory disorders Infection Drug-induced Rebound from thrombocytopenia Exercise Benign intracranial hypertension

myeloproliferative-related thrombocytosis in general,[92] particularly in the younger patient,[15] and have argued against active intervention. However, the disease is not benign in all young patients.[145] In a prospective study by the PVSG, age was not of prognostic value, with major thrombohemorrhagic complications occurring in both young and old patients.[21] However, age greater than 60 years has been correlated with reduced survival.[24] An increased incidence of arterial, but not venous, thrombosis in ET also has been linked to the presence of cardiovascular risk factors.[146] It seems reasonable, therefore, to withhold active intervention in patients who have mild thrombocytosis (platelets less than 1000×10^9/liter), are asymptomatic, and who have no underlying cardiovascular or neurologic diseases, particularly if they are less than 60 years of age.

Plateletpheresis allows rapid reduction in the circulating platelet count,[95,96,147,148] but the reduction is usually of short duration unless myelosuppressive therapy is initiated simultaneously.[147] Although long-term plateletpheresis can partially control thrombocytosis in some patients,[148] its major role lies in the acute management of thrombotic or hemorrhagic complications. Improvement in platelet function may accompany plateletpheresis, possibly due to the selective removal of larger-volume platelets.[95] While this may be beneficial for those with impaired platelet aggregation, patients with normal aggregation may develop hyperaggregability and ischemic symptoms after apheresis.[121]

The role and optimal dose of platelet antiaggregating agents have not been adequately clarified. Preston et al.[90] have demonstrated

TABLE 20-2. BONE MARROW APPEARANCES IN THROMBOCYTOSIS

Essential thrombocythemia	Panhyperplasia; markedly increased megakaryocytes with morphologic abnormalities; iron stores occasionally absent
Polycythemia vera	Similar to ET; iron stores almost always absent
Chronic granulocytic leukemia	Predominantly myeloid hyperplasia; megakaryocytes may be increased, but smaller in size than in ET or PV
Idiopathic myelofibrosis/agnogenic myeloid metaplasia	Typically a dry tap; marrow replaced by fibrosis; residual hematopoietic cells predominantly megakaryocytes
Idiopathic refractory sideroblastic anemia	Ringed sideroblasts; megaloblastoid dyserythropoiesis
5q− syndrome	Megakaryocytic hyperplasia with hypolobulation of megakaryocytes
Myelophthisis	Marrow replaced by tumor cells, granulomas, storage cells, or infarction-induced fibrosis
Other causes of reactive thrombocytosis	Megakaryocytes generally increased but morphologically normal; other features variable

the beneficial effects of aspirin in reversing incipient gangrene in patients with peripheral vascular disease associated with ET, and aspirin also reverses lower extremity pain associated with circulating platelet aggregates.[83] In the PVSG's review of the neurologic manifestations, aspirin appeared to be effective in some cases even when the thrombocytosis was not controlled by myelosuppression.[87] On the other hand, anti-inflammatory agents have been implicated in the genesis of hemorrhage associated with ET and other types of myeloproliferative-related thrombocytosis.[92] Aspirin and Persantine also were unsuccessful in reducing the increased thrombotic risk associated with phlebotomy in PV[149] and in fact produced an increased incidence of serious gastrointestinal hemorrhage. However, the dose of aspirin used in that study was significantly higher than that currently in vogue for inhibiting platelet function. Useful guidelines for the use of antiaggregating agents in myeloproliferative-related thrombocytosis have been published by Schafer.[100] He advocates this form of therapy for patients with thrombotic manifestations, particularly those due to peripheral vascular and neurologic complications. Evidence of platelet hyperaggregability is also an indication for this form of therapy. Patients with hemorrhagic manifestations and those with prominent platelet dysfunction, as manifest by significantly impaired platelet aggregation or a prolonged bleeding time, should not be treated with antiaggregant therapy.

The ability of myelosuppressive therapy to rapidly reduce platelet counts has been demonstrated in a number of reports. Most studies have utilized one or another form of alkylating agent therapy, such as busulfan,[29, 30, 150, 151] melphalan,[17, 20] CCNU,[151] thiotepa and chlorambucil,[25] and uracil mustard.[152] Virtually all these agents are capable of lowering the platelet count within 2 to 6 weeks, but their use in long-term maintenance regimens has fallen into disfavor because of their leukemogenic and, for chlorambucil at least, lymphomagenic potential.[153] [32]P, a major therapeutic alternative for polycythemia, also has been used in the treatment of ET,[20] but its leukemogenic potential also has been clearly demonstrated by the PVSG.[153] Antimetabolites such as 6-thioguanine[154] and hydroxyurea[23] also have been employed, and the PVSG currently recommends hydroxyurea for patients who require myelosuppression. Therapy should be initiated with 15 to 30 mg/kg per day for 1 week, depending on the urgency of the clinical situation, and then 15 mg/d until adequate control has been achieved (platelets less than 600×10^9/liter). Maintenance doses are variable and must be adjusted individually, since microvascular occlusive symptoms may persist until the platelet count falls below 400×10^9/liter. Isolated cases of acute leukemia following hydroxyurea therapy for ET have been reported,[26, 155] but convincing evidence of the leukemogenic potential of hydroxyurea has not yet been presented.

Based on its ability to control thrombocytosis in CGL,[156] interferon-α recently has been used in the treatment of ET. For most patients with ET, recombinant interferon-α_2, in doses of approximately 5 million units per day, is capable of reducing the platelet count to below 600×10^9/liter in 6 to 12 weeks.[157] Prolonged control of thrombocytosis can be achieved with even lower doses, but relapse will occur if the drug is stopped. Interferon mediates reduction in the platelet count primarily by reducing megakaryocyte size rather than megakaryocyte number,[158] resulting in decreased platelet production. Unfortunately, interferon toxicity remains a problem, particularly in the older age group, which is most at risk of ET. The flulike illness associated with short-term use is well recognized, and chronic use may be associated with an increased risk of autoimmune diseases[159] and significant depression.

Anagrelide[160] is a quinazolin derivative that was originally developed as an inhibitor of platelet function but which also produced thrombocytopenia in normal volunteers. Anagrelide appears to interfere with megakaryocyte maturation rather than reduce the megakaryocyte content of the bone marrow.[161] The experience of the Anagrelide Study Group with this drug in the treatment of 577 patients with myeloproliferative-related thrombocytosis has recently been reported.[162] The platelet count of the majority of patients fell to less than 600×10^9/liter in 2 to 4 weeks. Leukopenia did not occur, but mild anemia was common. However, 16 percent of patients discontinued the drug because of toxicity. Cardiac problems were the most significant, with frequent fluid retention, occasional congestive cardiac failure, and two instances of sudden death. Headaches and nausea also were common problems. The ability of anagrelide to prevent thrombohemorrhagic complications and its potential for long-term toxicity remain unknown.

THE PVSG'S EXPERIENCE WITH MYELOSUPPRESSIVE THERAPY

Two major prospective thrombocytosis trials have been conducted by the PVSG. The first study involved a randomized trial between ^{32}P and melphalan, and the first 12 months' experience has already been published by Murphy et al.[20] The original dose of ^{32}P was 2.3 mCi/m^2. However, this was subsequently increased to 2.9 mCi/m^2 because the lower dose appeared to be inadequate. Even after the dose was increased, patients treated with melphalan obtained a more rapid reduction in platelet count than those treated with ^{32}P. The median time to reach a platelet count less than 600×10^9/liter for patients treated with melphalan was 24 days, whereas the corresponding time for patients receiving ^{32}P was 44 days.[23] The second PVSG study was a single-arm phase II study of hydroxyurea.[23] The reduction in platelet counts was at least as rapid as that produced by melphalan, and the proportion of time from onset of treatment during which the platelet count remained below 600×10^9/liter also was significantly longer with both hydroxyurea and melphalan compared with ^{32}P. However, a disadvantage of hydroxyurea was the failure of this agent to achieve prolonged unmaintained remissions compared with both melphalan and ^{32}P. Since hydroxyurea has not yet been implicated as a leukemogenic agent, we currently recommend it as the treatment of choice for those patients who require myelosuppression, although ^{32}P is still useful in situations where frequent follow-up is difficult or poor patient compliance is a factor.

Whether all patients with ET actually need myelosuppression is still a controversial question. Myelosuppression, together with plateletpheresis, is clearly indicated in the presence of significant thrombohemorrhagic complications, as well as in patients who require major surgical intervention. Splenectomy should be avoided at all costs because of the risk of catastrophic thrombohemorrhagic complications which are likely to en-

sue.[77] If splenectomy cannot be avoided, the platelet count should be lowered aggressively, fresh-frozen plasma should be administered preoperatively, and consideration should be given to the use of heparin and/or aspirin, together with normal platelet transfusions.

If patients with ET are completely asymptomatic, we do not recommend myelosuppression. Decisions for patients who fall between these two extremes must be made on an individual basis. The multiplicity of useful agents now available for the treatment of ET (viz., hydroxyurea, interferon, anagrelide, and aspirin) and the equally reasonable alternative of observation alone have made treatment decisions difficult. There is clearly a need for randomized phase III studies of these agents, but these would require decades of follow-up to convincingly establish which agent(s) offered the greatest benefit for the least toxicity, and it is unlikely that such trials will ever be conducted.

OVERLAP MYELOPROLIFERATIVE SYNDROMES

When accepted diagnostic criteria are applied to patients with chronic MPDs, their categorization into the specific subgroups of PV, ET, CGL, and IMF/AMM cannot always be achieved. A proportion of patients with overlapping clinical and laboratory features remains, and reliable prognostic information about such patients is not available. In particular, overlap of ET with PV and with CGL have been problems in the PVSG series. We have therefore attempted to address this question, and the following subsections deal with this issue.

Overlap with Polycythemia Vera

In the PVSG trials of melphalan, ^{32}P, and hydroxyurea, 19 Ph-negative patients with platelet counts above 1000×10^9/liter were identified in whom the diagnosis of PV had not been adequately excluded either because a red cell mass determination was not performed or because iron deficiency had not been corrected prior to myelosuppressive therapy. Since patients who are not entered into multicenter trials are even less likely to be subjected to rigid exclusion of PV by these procedures, we have been interested in identifying simpler diagnostic criteria. We therefore compared the characteristics of 50 patients who satisfied all the PVSG criteria for ET with those of 27 patients who satisfied the PVSG criteria for PV and who also had marked thrombocytosis (platelet count in excess of 1000×10^9/liter).[97]

A univariate comparison of multiple clinical and laboratory features of the two groups revealed very few significant differences. For example, even though the two groups were originally classified on the basis of red cell mass, there was considerable overlap of the hematocrit values. We then employed logistic regression in an attempt to identify a pattern of variables that correlated better with the red cell mass–proven diagnosis than did any of the individual variables. Patients with low (less than 43 percent) or high (greater than 57 percent) hematocrits were invariably diagnosed correctly as having ET or PV, respectively, based on this criterion alone, whereas an algorithm based on the combination of hematocrit, spleen size, and WBC count resulted in a marked increase in diagnostic accuracy for patients with intermediate hematocrits (43 to 57 percent).[97] We also evaluated the algorithm (personal communication) by using it to predict the diagnosis of an independent sample of red cell mass–confirmed ET and PV patients,[25] and the algorithm's ability to correctly predict the diagnosis of patients with intermediate hematocrits was confirmed. When the algorithm was applied to the 19 PVSG patients in whom a diagnosis of PV had not been adequately excluded, 18 of 19 were predicted to have ET, and 1 was predicted to have PV. This patient's clinical and hematologic features were strongly suggestive of masked PV, thus supporting the reliability of the algorithm. The algorithm is recommended as an alternate method for differentiating ET from PV associated with marked thrombocytosis whenever the red cell mass is unavailable or iron deficiency cannot be excluded.

Overlap with Chronic Granulocytic Leukemia

The second overlap area that is of considerable interest is that of Ph-positive ET. Occasionally, patients with marked thrombocytosis and minimal leukocytosis, most suggestive of ET, are found to carry the Ph chromosome. Isolated case reports have appeared in the literature.[24, 31-35] In some cases the translocation was of the classic variety (t[9;21] [q34;q11]), whereas in others a complex variant translocation was found. A further six patients have now been identified by the PVSG.[163] These patients appeared to have ET according to the PVSG's rigid criteria but were all Ph-positive (Table 20–3). The main clue to the presence of the Ph chromosome was the degree of basophilia, which was significantly greater in the Ph-positive patients compared with the unequivocal (Ph-negative) ET patients ($p = 0.0001$, two-tailed Mann-Whitney U test). The range of LAP scores was not typical of CGL and was not significantly different from that seen in Ph-negative ET patients, and marrow morphology was not particularly suggestive of CGL in

TABLE 20–3. PHILADELPHIA CHROMOSOME–POSITIVE ESSENTIAL THROMBOCYTHEMIA

Hb[a]	WBC COUNT[b]	BASOPHILS[c]	IMMATURE[d]	PLATELETS[e]	LAP[f]	CLINICAL COURSE
12.2	15.3	0.77	4	2900	120	Blast transformation after 6 years
12.3	14.8	0.30	5	1400	78	Blast transformation after 7 years
13.7	8.0	0.72	0	1700	ND[g]	Accelerated phase of CGL after 4 years
14.4	32.6	1.96	0	2000	11	Blast transformation after 5 years
10.0	25.3	2.53	4	2800	66	Died after 5 years of unrelated causes
11.6	17.7	0.35	0	2600	16	Blast transformation after 4 years

a Hemoglobin (g/dl).
b White blood cell count ($\times 10^9$/liter).
c Absolute basophil count ($\times 10^9$/liter).
d Percent immature myeloid cells.
e Platelet count ($\times 10^9$/liter).
f Leukocyte alkaline phosphatase score.
g Not done.

most cases. Five patients entered an accelerated or blastic phase, and all died within
7 years of presentation. These data suggest
that the presence of the Ph chromosome con-
fers a poor prognosis on patients who are
thought to have ET by all other criteria. We
also have observed a similar sequence of
events in a patient with Ph-negative CGL.[164]

TRANSITIONAL PHENOMENA IN ESSENTIAL THROMBOCYTHEMIA

In 1955, McCabe et al.[7] claimed that all
patients with ET eventually exhibited features of other hematologic disorders and
thus argued that ET itself was not a distinct
entity. Three large series of patients with
ET have now been followed for several years,
and accurate data are available to examine
McCabe's claim.

Transition to Chronic Granulocytic Leukemia

Evolution to Ph-positive CGL has been observed only in patients who were Ph-positive
at the time of the original diagnosis of ET.[22]
No instances of development of the Ph chromosome have been recorded in patients
known to lack it at diagnosis. We also have
reported a single patient who developed Ph-
negative CGL following an illness that was
consistent with ET, but this remains an isolated observation.[164]

Transition to Acute Leukemia

Transition to acute leukemia occurs to a
varying extent in all the chronic MPDs, most
notably in CGL. In PV, the PVSG has clearly
demonstrated the influence of therapy on
the frequency of leukemic transformation.
Both chlorambucil and, to a lesser extent, ^{32}P
significantly increased the risk of leukemia
compared with treatment by phlebotomy
alone.[153] The role of therapy in leukemic
transformations of ET has not yet been determined, because the number of patients
studied for a sufficient length of time is still
relatively small. However, pooled data from
several studies suggest that the overall incidence of acute leukemia in ET is approximately 3 to 4 percent,[23–26,59] although this
figure may rise with longer follow-up. Acute
leukemia has been observed in patients
treated with alkylating agents,[25] ^{32}P,[9,18] alkylating agents with ^{32}P,[16,165] alkylating

agents with hydroxyurea,[23] and hydroxyurea alone,[26,166] as well as in patients who
have never received myelosuppressive therapy.[23,167] Transformation to acute leukemia
via a myelofibrotic phase, similar to the situation in CGL and PV, has been reported[18]
but does not seem frequent. Myeloblastic,[9,16,48,165,167] monoblastic,[168] myelomono-
blastic,[25] and megakaryoblastic[168] variants of
AML, as well as mixed-lineage leukemias,[165]
have been observed. The response to therapy of acute leukemia evolving on a background of ET has been universally disappointing.[165] No pretreatment characteristics
have been identified that are predictive of a
leukemic outcome, although the PVSG's experience suggests that patients who require
alkylating agents because of inadequate disease control with hydroxyurea alone may be at
increased risk of leukemic transformation.[169]

Transition to Myelofibrosis

Evolution to myelofibrosis has been reported in patients with ET, but its frequency
relative to leukemic transformation is controversial. Lewis et al.[18] described 5 patients
with ET, and 3 developed myelofibrosis after
^{32}P, including 1 who also progressed to acute
leukemia. Van de Pette et al.[24] observed
8 cases of myelofibrosis in 37 patients with
ET who were all treated with busulfan but
did not have any cases with acute leukemia.
In contrast, Bellucci et al.[26] noted 5 instances
of acute leukemia in 94 patients with myeloproliferative-related thrombocytosis (most
of whom had ET) and saw no cases of myelofibrosis despite a comparable period of follow-up. The PVSG[23] has seen an equal incidence of myelofibrosis and acute leukemia,
i.e., 2 each in 52 patients (4 percent). While
acute leukemia has followed a variety of therapies for ET, including no myelosuppression, virtually all published cases of myelofibrosis complicating ET have been
associated with ^{32}P and/or alkylating agent
therapy. However, very longterm followup of
French PV patients[170] suggests that myelofibrosis is more common in these treated
with ph lebotomy alone than in those
who received either ^{32}P or chlorambucil,
presumably as a result of uncontrolled
myeloproliferation.

Transition to Polycythemia Vera

In his classic description of ET, Gunz[8] emphasized the close relationship between ET

and PV and noted that polycythemic phases occurred in patients with ET, particularly when the thrombocytosis was controlled by myelosuppressive therapy. It might be argued that such patients actually represent cases in which the diagnosis of PV was not adequately excluded at the time of the initial evaluation. However, the PVSG has studied four patients with unequivocal ET at diagnosis, confirmed by red cell mass, who have subsequently had documented increases in red cell mass to polycythemic levels.[23] When the initial evaluation characteristics of these patients were reviewed, the only difference from the remainder of the unequivocal ET patients was that their initial red cell masses lay at the upper end of the normal range. It is therefore possible that many patients with ET exhibit rises in red cell mass during the course of their illness, but only those with high-normal red cell masses at presentation are likely to achieve frankly polycythemic levels.

Thus it would appear that McCabe's postulate that ET eventually evolves into one or another MPD cannot be sustained at the present time. The vast majority of ET patients do not evolve to either PV, myelofibrosis, CGL, or acute leukemia. While a specific diagnostic test for ET remains elusive, there appears to be sufficient clinical evidence that it represents a discrete member of the spectrum of MPDs.

SURVIVAL PATTERNS OF PATIENTS WITH ESSENTIAL THROMBOCYTHEMIA

The natural history of ET has not been well characterized, because early reports required hemorrhage as a diagnostic criterion and thus selected patients with a bad prognosis. Myelosuppressive therapy has been promoted on the basis of these early reports, and thus most survival data reflect such intervention. More recent reports which utilize broader diagnostic criteria have emphasized the benign nature of ET in many patients,[15, 92] and there is some evidence that young patients may tolerate marked thrombocytosis for years without active therapy.[15] A number of studies have now reported long-term follow-up of patients with ET.[23–26] Actuarial survival curves reveal 8-year survivals of 80 to 85 percent and median survivals of greater than 14 years. This contrasts with median survivals of approximately 10 years in PV, 5 years in IMF/AMM, and 3 to 4 years in CGL. A recent large age- and sex-matched Spanish review of life expectancy in chronic nonleukemic MPDs has reinforced the benign nature of ET and PV by demonstrating that patients with these conditions exhibited survival patterns no different from that of the control population.[171]

SUMMARY

In this chapter we have reviewed the current state of knowledge regarding ET. We have outlined its relationship to the other chronic MPDs and its distinction from reactive thrombocytosis. We have described the clinical and laboratory features of patients with ET as well as the therapeutic options that are available. We also have reviewed the data relating to clonality and hematopoietic progenitors in ET, and we have reviewed the literature concerning overlap syndromes, transitional phenomena, and survival in ET. Throughout the chapter, the contributions of the PVSG to our understanding of ET have been highlighted. In particular, the importance of strict and consistent diagnostic criteria has been emphasized. We recommend the adoption of the PVSG's criteria in future studies so that more can be learned of the natural history, response to therapy, and prognosis of patients with this disorder.

REFERENCES

1. Epstein E, Goedel A: Hämorrhagische thrombocythämie bei vasculärer Schrumpfmilz. 293:233–248, Virchows Arch [Pathol Anat] 1934
2. Dameshek W: Some speculations on the myeloproliferative syndromes. Blood 6:372–375, 1951
3. Adamson JW: Analysis of haemopoiesis: The use of cell markers and in vitro culture techniques in studies of clonal haemopathies in man. Clin Haematol 13:489–502, 1984
4. Castro-Malaspina H: Pathogenesis of myelofibrosis: Role of ineffective megakaryopoiesis and megakaryocyte components. Presented at the Myeloproliferative Disorder Symposium, XXI Congress of the International Society of Hematology, Sydney, Australia, May 16, 1986
5. Neame PB, Soamboonsrup P, Browman GP, et al: Classifying acute leukemia by immunophenotyping: A combined FAB-immunologic classification of AML. Blood 68:1355–1362, 1986

6. Fanger H, Cella LJ Jr, Litchman H: Thrombocythemia: Report of three cases and review of literature. N Engl J Med 250:456–461, 1954

7. McCabe WR, Bird RM, McLaughlin RA: Is primary hemorrhagic thrombocythemia a clinical myth? Ann Intern Med 43:182–190, 1955

8. Gunz FW: Hemorrhagic thrombocythemia: A critical review. Blood 15:706–723, 1960

9. Ozer FL, Truax WE, Miesch DC, et al: Primary hemorrhagic thrombocythemia. Am J Med 28:807–823, 1960

10. Weinfeld A, Branehog I, Kutti J: Platelets in the myeloproliferative syndrome. Clin Haematol 4:373–392, 1975

11. Iland H, Laszlo J: Myeloproliferative-related thrombocytosis: Clinical significance and comparison with other causes of thrombocytosis. Med Grand Rounds 3:225–238, 1984

12. Hardisty RM, Wolff HH: Haemorrhagic thrombocythaemia: A clinical and laboratory study. Br J Haematol 1:390–405, 1955

13. Silverstein MN: Primary or hemorrhagic thrombocythemia. Arch Intern Med 122:18–22, 1968

14. Frick PG: Primary thrombocythemia: Clinical, hematological and chromosomal studies of 13 patients. Helv Med Acta 35:20–29, 1969

15. Hoagland HC, Silverstein MN: Primary thrombocythemia in the young patient. Mayo Clin Proc 53:578–580, 1978

16. Herrmann RP, Gallon W, Jackson JM, et al: Idiopathic thrombocythaemia: A review of seven cases in western Australia. Aust NZ J Med 3:486–494, 1973

17. Bensinger TA, Logue GL, Rundles RW: Hemorrhagic thrombocythemia: Control of postsplenectomy thrombocytosis with melphalan. Blood 36:61–69, 1970

18. Lewis SM, Szur L, Hoffbrand AV: Thrombocythaemia. Clin Haematol 1:339–357, 1972

19. Laszlo J: Myeloproliferative disorders (MPD): Myelofibrosis, myelosclerosis, extramedullary hematopoiesis, undifferentiated MPD and hemorrhagic thrombocythaemia. Semin Hematol 12:409–432, 1975

20. Murphy S, Rosenthal DS, Weinfeld A, et al: Essential thrombocythemia: Response during the first year of therapy with melphalan and radioactive phosphorus: A Polycythemia Study Group Report. Cancer Treat Rep 66:1495–1500, 1982

21. Iland HJ, Laszlo J, Peterson P, et al: Essential thrombocythemia: Clinical and laboratory characteristics at presentation. Trans Assoc Am Physicians 96:165–174, 1983

22. Murphy S, Iland H, Rosenthal D, et al: Essential thrombocythemia: An interim report from the Polycythemia Vera Study Group. Semin Hematol 23:177–182, 1986

23. Iland HJ, Laszlo J, and the Myeloproliferative Subcommittee of the Polycythemia Vera Study Group: The Polycythemia Vera Study Group's experience with myelosuppressive therapy for essential thrombocythemia. Myeloproliferative Disorder Symposium, XXI Congress of the International Society of Hematology, Sydney, Australia, 1986

24. Van de Pette JEW, Prochazka AV, Pearson TC, et al: Primary thrombocythaemia treated with busulphan. Br J Haematol 62:229–237, 1986

25. Case DC Jr: Therapy of essential thrombocythemia with thiotepa and chlorambucil. Blood 63:51–54, 1984

26. Bellucci S, Janvier M, Tobelem G, et al: Essential thrombocythemia: Clinical evolutionary and biological data. Cancer 58:2440–2447, 1986

27. Brodsky I, Fuscaldo AA, Erlick BJ, et al: Analysis of platelets from patients with thrombocythemia for reverse transcriptase and virus-like particles. J Natl Cancer Inst 55:1069–1074, 1975

28. Strayer DR, Brodsky I, Caranfa MJ, et al: Quantitation of RNA-dependent DNA polymerase in patients with myeloproliferative disorders. Br J Haematol 50:521–530, 1982

29. Brodsky I, Fuscaldo AA, Erlick BJ, et al: Effect of busulfan on oncornavirus-like activity in platelets and chromosomes in polycythemia vera and essential thrombocythemia. J Natl Cancer Inst 59:61–67, 1977

30. Fuscaldo AA, Erlick BJ, Brodsky I, et al: Alteration of platelets and virus-like particles by busulfan in myeloproliferative disorders. Leuk Res 4:105–117, 1980

31. Ghosh ML: Primary haemorrhagic thrombocythaemia with Philadelphia chromosome. Postgrad Med J 48:686–688, 1972

32. Butoianu E, Colita A, Nicoara S, et al: LAP negative and Ph¹-positive hemorrhagic thrombocythemia. Med Interne 15:63–65, 1977

33. Fitzgerald PH, McEwan C, Fraser J, et al: A complex Ph¹ translocation in a patient with primary thrombocythaemia. Br J Haematol 47:571–575, 1981

34. Rajendra BR, Lee M, Nissenblatt MJ, et al: The occurrence of the Philadelphia chromosome in essential thrombocytosis. Hum Genet 56:287–291, 1981

35. Verhest A, Monsieur R: Philadelphia chromosome–positive thrombocythemia with leukemic transformation. N Engl J Med 308:1603, 1983

36. Fialkow PJ, Faguet GB, Jacobson RJ, et al: Evidence that essential thrombocythemia is a clonal disorder with origin in a multipotent stem cell. Blood 58:916–919, 1981

37. Gaetani GF, Ferraris AM, Galiano S, et al: Primary thrombocythemia: Clonal origin of platelets, erythrocytes, and granulocytes in a GdB/GdMediterranean subject. Blood 59:76–79, 1982

38. Singal U, Prasad AS, Halton DM, et al: Essential thrombocythemia: A clonal disorder of hematopoietic stem cell. Am J Hematol 14:193–196, 1983

39. Raskind WH, Jacobson R, Murphy S, et al: Evidence for the involvement of B-lymphoid cells in polycythemia vera and essential thrombocythemia. J Clin Invest 75:1388–1390, 1985

40. Knuutila S, Ruutu T, Partanen S, et al: Chromosome 1q+ in erythroid and granulocyte-monocyte precursors in a patient with essential thrombocythemia. Cancer Genet Cytogenet 9:245–249, 1983

41. Partanen S, Ruutu T, Vuopio P: Haematopoietic progenitors in essential thrombocythaemia. Scand J Haematol 30:130–134, 1983

42. Hibbin JA, Njoku OS, Matutes E, et al: Myeloid progenitor cells in the circulation of patients

with myelofibrosis and other myeloproliferative disorders. Br J Haematol 57:495–503, 1984

43. Eridani S, Batten E, Sawyer B: Erythroid colony formation in primary thrombocythaemia: Evidence of hypersensitivity to erythropoietin. Br J Haematol 56:157–161, 1984

44. Gewirtz AM, Bruno E, Elwell J, et al: In vitro studies of megakaryocytopoiesis in thrombocytotic disorders of man. Blood 61:384–389, 1983

45. Sceats DJ, Baitlon D: Primary thrombocythemia in a child. Clin Pediatr 19:298–300, 1980

46. Barnhart MI, Kim TH, Evatt BL, et al: Essential thrombocythemia in a child: Platelet ultrastructure and function. Am J Hematol 8:87–107, 1980

47. Linch DC, Hutton R, Cowan D, et al: Primary thrombocythaemia in childhood. Scand J Haematol 28:72–76, 1982

48. Fickers M, Speck B: Thrombocythemia: Familial occurrence and transition into blastic crisis. Acta Haematol (Basel) 51:257–265, 1974

49. Slee PH, van Everdingen JJ, Geraedts JP, et al: Familial myeloproliferative disease: Haematological and cytogenetic studies. Acta Med Scand 210:321–327, 1981

50. Dodsworth H: Primary thrombocythaemia in monozygotic twins. Br Med J 280:1506, 1980

51. Takahashi H, Hattori A, Shibata A: Profile of blood coagulation and fibrinolysis in chronic myeloproliferative disorders. Tohoku J Exp Med 138:71–80, 1982

52. Murphy S, Davis JL, Walsh PN, et al: Template bleeding time and clinical hemorrhage in myeloproliferative disease. Arch Intern Med 138:1251–1253, 1978

53. Wu KK: Platelet hyperaggregability in patients with thrombocythemia. Ann Intern Med 88:7–11, 1978

54. Bautista AP, Buckler PW, Towler HM, et al: Measurement of platelet life-span in normal subjects and patients with myeloproliferative disease with indium oxine labelled platelets. Br J Haematol 58:679–687, 1984

55. Najean Y, Poirier O, Lokiec F: The clinical significance of beta-thromboglobulin and platelet factor-4 in polycythaemic patients. Scand J Haematol 31:298–304, 1983

56. Cortelazzo S, Colucci M, Barbui T, et al: Reduced platelet factor-X activating activity: A possible contribution to bleeding complications in polycythaemia vera and essential thrombocythaemia. Haemostasis 10:37–50, 1981

57. Woodruff RK, Bell WR, Castaldi PA, et al: Essential thrombocythaemia. Haemostasis 9:105–125, 1980

58. Fabris F, Randi M, Sbrojavacca R, et al: The possible value of platelet aggregation studies in patients with increased platelet number. Blut 43:279–285, 1981

59. Brusamolino E, Canevari A, Salvaneschi L, et al: Efficacy trial of pipobraman in essential thrombocythemia: A study of 24 patients. Cancer Treat Rep 68:1339–1342, 1984

60. Pick RA, Glover MU, Nanfro JJ, et al: Acute myocardial infarction with essential thrombocythemia in a young man. Am Heart J 106:406–407, 1983

61. Murphy MF, Clarke CR, Brearley RL: Superior sagittal sinus thrombosis and essential thrombocythaemia. Br Med J 287:1344, 1983

62. Martin EA, Lavin PJ, Thompson AJ: Painful extremities and neurological disorder in essential thrombocythaemia. J R Soc Med 77:372–374, 1984

63. Douste-Blazy P, Taudou MJ, Delay M, et al: Essential thrombocythaemia and recurrent myocardial infarction. Lancet 2:992, 1984

64. Shattil SJ: Diagnosis and treatment of recurrent venous thromboembolism. Med Clin North Am 68:577–600, 1984

65. Welford C, Spies SM, Green D: Priapism in primary thrombocythaemia. Arch Intern Med 141:807–808, 1981

66. Siame JL, DuQuesnoy B, Thevenon A, et al: Hemarthrosis and thrombocythemia. J Rheumatol 8:521–522, 1981

67. Bello Nicolau I, Conde Zurita JM, Barrientos Guzman A, et al: Essential thrombocytosis with acute renal failure due to bilateral thrombosis of the renal arteries and veins. Nephron 32:73–74, 1982

68. Walden R, Zweig A, Adar R: Ischemia of toes as a presenting symptom in primary thrombosis: A case report. Angiology 29:779–781, 1978

69. Singh AK, Wetherley-Mein G: Microvascular occlusive lesions in primary thrombocythaemia. Br J Haematol 36:553–564, 1977

70. Averback P, Moinuddin M: Pericarditis as a manifestation of essential thrombocythemia. Can Med Assoc J 117:154–156, 1977

71. Thijs LG, Heidendal GA, Huijgens PC, et al: The use of nuclear medicine procedures in the diagnosis of Budd-Chiari syndrome. Clin Nucl Med 3:389–392, 1978

72. Leifer W, Leifer G: Priapism caused by primary thrombocythemia. J Urol 121:254–255, 1979

73. Pogrel MA: Thrombocythemia as a cause of oral hemorrhage. Oral Surg Oral Med Oral Pathol 44:535–538, 1977

74. Kirubakaran MG, Shastry JC, Date A, et al: Renal artery stenosis secondary to essential thrombocythemia. J Assoc Physicians India 23:213–216, 1975

75. Gillespie G: Peripheral gangrene as the presentation of myeloproliferative disorders. Br J Surg 60:377–380, 1973

76. Korenman G: Neurologic syndromes associated with primary thrombocythemia. J Mt Sinai Hosp 36:317–323, 1969

77. Ravich RBM, Gunz FW, Reed CS, et al: The dangers of surgery in uncontrolled haemorrhagic thrombocythaemia. Med J Aust 1:704–708, 1970

78. Shepherd P, Liddell K: Pyoderma gangrenosum associated with primary thrombocythaemia. Br Med J 285:837–838, 1982

79. Barbui T, Cortelazzo S, Viero P, et al: Thrombohaemorrhagic complications in 101 cases of myeloproliferative disorders: Relationship to platelet number and function. Eur J Cancer Clin Oncol 19:1593–1599, 1983

80. Tarocco RP, Faro G, Barile C, et al: Evaluation of platelet function and the frequency of vasculocutaneous lesions in primary thrombocythemia. Panminerva Med 25:79–83, 1983

81. Girolami A, Pardatscher K, Scanarini M, et al: Clotting changes in two patients with longitudi-

nal sinus thrombosis. Haemostasis 9:71–78, 1980

82. Delangre T, Mihout B, Borh JY, et al: Primary thrombocythemia in a patient with cerebellar infarction. Stroke 16:524–526, 1985

83. Salem HH, van der Weyden MB, Koutts J, et al: Leg pain and platelet aggregates in thrombocythemic myeloproliferative disease. JAMA 244:1122–1123, 1980

84. Okayasu N, Murata M, Ueda A, et al: Primary thrombocythemia and myocardial infarction in a 26-year-old woman with normal coronary arteriogram. Jpn Heart J 22:439–445, 1981

85. Rosenkranz L, Catalletto MM: Metatarsalgia caused by an increase in circulating platelets: A case report. Foot Ankle 4:216–217, 1984

86. Hussain S, Schwartz JM, Friedman SA, et al: Arterial thrombosis in essential thrombocythemia. Am Heart J 96:31–36, 1978

87. Jabaily J, Iland HJ, Laszlo J, et al: Neurologic manifestations of essential thrombocythemia. Ann Intern Med 99:513–518, 1983

88. Bjorkholm M, Mellstedt H, Sawe U: Essential thrombocythaemia and polycythaemia vera presenting with pulmonary embolism mimicking pneumonia: Case reports. Haematologica (Pavia) 66:667–672, 1981

89. Hehlmann R, Luderschmidt C, Goebel FD, et al: Relapsing acute febrile neutrophilic dermatosis and essential thrombocythemia. Blut 48:297–305, 1984

90. Preston FE, Emmanuel IG, Winfield DA, et al: Essential thrombocythaemia and peripheral gangrene. Br Med J 3:548–552, 1974

91. Michiels JJ, Abels J, Steketee J, et al: Erythromelalgia caused by platelet-mediated arteriolar inflammation and thrombosis in thrombocythemia. Ann Intern Med 102:466–471, 1985

92. Kessler CM, Klein HG, Havlik RJ: Uncontrolled thrombocytosis in chronic myeloproliferative disorders. Br J Haematol 50:157–167, 1982

93. Vera JC: Antiplatelet agents in the treatment of thrombotic complications of primary thrombocythemia. Can Med Assoc J 120:60–61, 1979

94. Zucker S, Mielke CH: Classification of thrombocytosis based on platelet function tests: Correlation with hemorrhagic and thrombotic complications. J Lab Clin Med 80:385–394, 1972

95. Orlin JB, Berkman EM: Improvement of platelet function following plateletpheresis in patients with myeloproliferative diseases. Transfusion 20:540–545, 1980

96. Younger J, Umlas J: Rapid reduction of platelet count in essential hemorrhagic thrombocythemia by discontinuous flow plateletpheresis. Am J Med 64:659–661, 1978

97. Iland HJ, Laszlo J, Case DC Jr, et al: Differentiation between essential thrombocythemia and polycythemia vera with marked thrombocytosis. Am J Hematol 25:191–207, 1987

98. Murphy S: Thrombocytosis and thrombocythaemia. Clin Haematol 12:89–106, 1983

99. Streeter RR, Presant CA, Reinhard E: Prognostic significance of thrombocytosis in idiopathic sideroblastic anemia. Blood 50:427–432, 1977

100. Schafer AI: Bleeding and thrombosis in the myeloproliferative disorders. Blood 64:1–12, 1984

101. Ginsburg AD: Platelet function in patients with high platelet counts. Ann Intern Med 82:506–511, 1975

102. Cronberg S, Nilsson IM, Gydell K: Haemorrhagic thrombocythaemia due to defective platelet adhesiveness. Scand J Haematol 2:208–219, 1965

103. Leoncini G, Maresca M, Balestrero F, et al: Some aspects of platelet glucose metabolism in thrombocytosis due to myeloproliferative disorders. Thromb Res 34:233–239, 1984

104. Cortelazzo S, Viero P, Buczko W, et al: Platelet 5-hydroxytryptamine transport and storage in myeloproliferative disorders. Scand J Haematol 34:146–151, 1985

105. Bolin RB, Okumura T, Jamieson GA: Changes in distribution of platelet membrane glycoproteins in patients with myeloproliferative disorders. Am J Hematol 3:63–71, 1977

106. Booth WJ, Berndt MC, Castaldi PA: An altered platelet granule glycoprotein in patients with essential thrombocythemia. J Clin Invest 73:291–297, 1984

107. Clezardin P, McGregor JL, Dechavanne M, et al: Platelet membrane glycoprotein abnormalities in patients with myeloproliferative disorders and secondary thrombocytosis. Br J Haematol 60:331–344, 1985

108. Kaywin P, McDonough M, Insel PA, et al: Platelet function in essential thrombocythemia: Decreased epinephrine responsiveness associated with a deficiency of platelet alpha-adrenergic receptors. N Engl J Med 299:505–509, 1978

109. Okuma M, Uchino H: Altered arachidonate metabolism by platelets in patients with myeloproliferative disorders. Blood 54:1258–1271, 1979

110. Schafer AI: Deficiency of platelet lipoxygenase activity in myeloproliferative disorders. N Engl J Med 306:381–386, 1982

111. Castaldi PA, Berndt MC, Booth W, et al: Evidence for a platelet membrane defect in the myeloproliferative syndromes. Thromb Res 27:601–609, 1982

112. Breuer JH, Harsanyi V, Solti V, et al: Platelet phospholipids in thrombocytosis due to myeloproliferative disorders. Haemostasis 10:134–140, 1981

113. Leoncini G, Maresca M, Balestrero F, et al: Platelet membrane fatty acids in thrombocytosis due to myeloproliferative disorders. Cell Biochem Funct 2:23–25, 1984

114. Maldonaldo JE, Pintado T, Pierre RV: Dysplastic platelet and circulating megakaryocytes in chronic myeloproliferative diseases: I. The platelets: Ultrastructure and peroxidase reaction. Blood 43:797–809, 1974

115. Boughton BJ, Allington MJ, King A: Platelet and plasma beta thromboglobulin in myeloproliferative syndromes and secondary thrombocytosis. Br J Haematol 40:125–132, 1978

116. Leoncini G, Maresca M, Balestrero F, et al: Platelet glyoxalases in thrombocytosis. Scand J Haematol 33:91–94, 1984

117. Cooper B, Schafer AI, Puchalsky D, et al: Platelet resistance to prostaglandin D_2 in patients with myeloproliferative disorders. Blood 52:618–626, 1978

118. Moore A, Nachman RL: Platelet Fc receptor: Increased expression in myeloproliferative disease. J Clin Invest 67:1064–1071, 1981

119. Cortelazzo S, Viero P, Morelli C, et al: Normal vascular prostacyclin generation in patients with chronic myeloproliferative disorders. Thromb Res 39:139–141, 1985

120. Martinez J, Shapiro SS, Holburn R: Metabolism of human prothrombin and fibrinogen in patients with thrombocytosis secondary to myeloproliferative states. Blood 42:35–46, 1973

121. Fabris F, Belloni M, Casonato A, et al: Improvement of platelet aggregation abnormalities in thrombocytosis after thrombocytopheresis. Folia Haematol (Leipz) 108:853–862, 1981

122. Walsh PN, Murphy S, Barry WE: The role of platelets in the pathogenesis of thrombosis and haemorrhage in patients with thrombocytosis. Thromb Haemost 38:1085–1096, 1977

123. Pareti FI, Gugliotta L, Mannucci L, et al: Biochemical and metabolic aspects of platelet dysfunction in chronic myeloproliferative disorders. Scand J Haematol 25:214–220, 1982

124. Hunt FA: A rapid method for assessing megathrombocytes: Its application to thrombocytotic and acquired thrombocytopenic states. Pathology 8:47–55, 1976

125. Small BM, Bettigole RE: Diagnosis of myeloproliferative disease by analysis of the platelet volume distribution. Am J Clin Pathol 76:685–691, 1981

126. Budman DR, Lackner H, Berczeller P, et al: The diagnostic value of the serum lactic dehydrogenase determination in the evaluation of unexplained thrombocytosis. Am J Clin Pathol 75:840–843, 1981

127. Parker NE, Jacobs P: Pseudohyperkalaemia: A cause of diagnostic confusion. S Afr Med J 60:973–974, 1981

128. Thiele J, Funke S, Holgado S, et al: Megakaryopoiesis in chronic myeloproliferative diseases: A morphometric evaluation with special emphasis on primary thrombocythemia. Anal Quant Cytol Histol 6:155–167, 1984

129. Branehog I, Ridell B, Swolin B, et al: Megakaryocyte quantifications in relation to thrombokinetics in primary thrombocythaemia and allied diseases. Scand J Haematol 15:321–332, 1975

130. Biagini G, Gugliotta L, Preda P, et al: Platelets in primary thrombocythemia: Electron microscopic study. Nouv Rev Fr Hematol 24:19–26, 1982

131. Thiele J, Krech R, Choritz H, et al: Emperipolesis: A peculiar feature of megakaryocytes as evaluated in chronic myeloproliferative diseases by morphometry and ultrastructure. Virchows Arch [B] 46:253–263, 1984

132. Boneu B, Nouvel C, Sie P, et al: Platelets in myeloproliferative disorders: I. A comparative evaluation with certain platelet function tests. Scand J Haematol 25:214–220, 1980

133. Zaccaria A, Tura S: A chromosomal abnormality in primary thrombocythemia. N Engl J Med 298:1422–1423, 1978

134. Case DC: Absence of a specific chromosomal marker in essential thrombocythemia. Cancer Genet Cytogenet 12:163–165, 1984

135. Kopf I, Swolin B, Weinfeld A: Cytogenetic studies on primary thrombocythaemia. Hereditas 97:217–220, 1982

136. Emilia G, Torelli G, Sacchi S, et al: Chromosomal abnormalities in essential thrombocythemia. Cancer Genet Cytogenet 18:91–93, 1985

137. Fuscaldo KE, Erlick BJ, Fuscaldo AA, et al: Correlation of a specific chromosomal marker, 21q−, and retroviral indicators in patients with thrombocythemia. Cancer Lett 6:51–56, 1979

138. Rowley JD: The role of cytogenetics in hematology. Blood 48:1–7, 1976

139. Third International Workshop on Chromosomes in Leukemia 1980: Report on essential thrombocythemia. Cancer Genet Cytogenet 4:136–142, 1981

140. Shah I, Lewkow LM, Koppitch F: Acute basophilic leukemia. Am J Med 76:1097–1099, 1984

141. Taylor KMcD, Shetta M, Talpaz M, et al: Myeloproliferative disorders: Usefulness of X-linked probes in diagnosis. Leukemia 3:419–422, 1989

142. Greenberg P, Mara B, Bax I, et al: The myeloproliferative disorders: Correlation between clinical evolution and alterations of granulopoiesis. Am J Med 61:878–891, 1976

143. Mahmood T, Robinson WA, Hamstra RD, et al: Macrocytic anemia, thrombocytosis and non-lobulated megakaryocytes. Am J Med 66:946–950, 1979

144. Hollen CW, Henthorn J, Koziol JA, et al: Elevated serum interleukin-6 levels in patients with reactive thrombocytosis. Br J Haematol 79:286–290, 1991

145. Millard FE, Hunter CS, Anderson M, et al: Clinical manifestations of essential thrombocythemia in young adults. Am J Hematol 33:27–31, 1990

146. Watson KV, Key N: Vascular complications of essential thrombocythaemia: A link to cardiovascular risk factors. Br J Haematol 83:198–203, 1993

147. Goldfinger D, Thompson R, Lowe C, et al: Long-term plateletpheresis in the management of primary thrombocytosis. Transfusion 19:336–338, 1979

148. Panlilio AL, Reiss RF: Therapeutic plateletpheresis in thrombocythemia. Transfusion 19:147–152, 1979

149. Tartaglia AP, Goldberg JD, Berk PD, et al: Adverse effects of antiaggregating platelet therapy in the treatment of polycythemia vera. Semin Hematol 23:172–176, 1986

150. Epstein IS: The treatment of polycythemia vera and thrombocythemia with Myleran (busulfan). Isr J Med Sci 1:797–799, 1965

151. Leoni F, Grossi A, Rossi Ferrini P: 1-(2-Chloroethyl)-cyclohexyl-nitrosourea–induced remission in essential thrombocythemia. Acta Haematol (Basel) 69:180–183, 1983

152. Shamasunder HK, Gregory SA, Knospe WH: Uracil mustard in the treatment of thrombocytosis. JAMA 244:1454–1455, 1980

153. Berk PD, Goldberg JD, Donovan PB, et al: Therapeutic recommendations in polycythemia vera based on Polycythemia Vera Study Group protocols. Semin Hematol 23:132–143, 1986

154. Delfini C, Porcellini A, Izzi T, et al: 6-Thioguanine treatment of uncontrolled thrombocytosis in polycythemia vera and essential throm-

bocythemia. Haematologica (Pavia) 69:766–767, 1984

155. Lofvenberg E, Nordenson I, Wahlin A: Cytogenetic abnormalities and leukemic transformation in hydroxyurea-treated patients with Philadelphia chromosome negative chronic myeloproliferative disease. Cancer Genet Cytogenet 49:57–67, 1990

156. Talpaz M, Mavligit G, Keating M, et al: Human leukocyte interferon to control thrombocytosis in chronic myelogenous leukemia. Ann Intern Med 99:789–792, 1983

157. Gisslinger H, Chott A, Scheithauer W, et al: Interferon in essential thrombocythaemia. Br J Haematol 79:42–47, 1991

158. Wadenvik H, Kutti J, Ridell B, et al: The effect of α-interferon on bone marrow megakaryocytes and platelet production rate in essential thrombocytemia. Blood 77:2103–2108, 1991

159. Ronnblom LE, Gunnar VA, Oberg KE: Autoimmunity after alpha-interferon therapy for malignant carcinoid tumors. Ann Intern Med 115:178–183, 1991

160. Silverstein MN, Petitt RM, Solberg LA Jr, et al: Anagrelide: A new drug for treating thrombocytosis. N Engl J Med 318:1292–1294, 1988

161. Mazur EM, Rosmarin AG, Sohl PA, et al: Analysis of the mechanism of anagrelide-induced thrombocytopenia in humans. Blood 79:1931–1937, 1992

162. Anagrelide Study Group: Anagrelide, a therapy for thrombocythemic states: Experience in 577 patients. Am J Med 92:69–76, 1992

163. Stoll DB, Peterson P, Exten R, et al: The clinical presentation and natural history of patients with essential thrombocythemia and the Philadelphia chromosome. Am J Hematol 27:77–83, 1988

164. Iland H, Chan W, Vincent PC: Myeloproliferative and lymphoproliferative disorders in the same patient. Aust NZ J Med 10:650–653, 1980

165. Frei-Lahr D, Barton JC, Hoffman R, et al: Blastic transformation of essential thrombocythemia: Dual expression of myelomonoblastic/megakaryoblastic phenotypes. Blood 63:866–872, 1984

166. Reiffers J, Dachary D, David B, et al: Megakaryoblastic transformation of primary thrombocythemia. Acta Haematol (Basel) 73:228–231, 1985

167. Geller SA, Shapiro E: Acute leukemia as a natural sequel to primary thrombocythemia. Am J Clin Pathol 77:353–356, 1982

168. Briere J, Bernheim A, Berger R, et al: Thrombocythemies primitives et leucemies aigues a propos de 2 cas. Nouv Rev Franc Hematol 22(suppl):C57, 1980

169. Murphy S, Peterson P, Iland HJ, et al: Hydroxyurea and other myelosuppressive agents in the treatment of essential thrombocythemia: Analysis of leukemogenic potential. In XIVth Congress of the International Society on Thrombosis and Haemostasis, New York, Schattaver, 1993

170. Najean Y, Dresch C, Rain J-D: The very-long term course of polycythemia: a complement to the previously published data of the Polycythemia Vera Study Group. Br J Haematol 86:233–235, 1994

171. Rozman C, Giralt M, Feliu E, et al: Life expectancy of patients with chronic nonleukemic myeloproliferative disorders. Cancer 67:2658–2663, 1991

ACKNOWLEDGEMENTS: The data relating to the PVSG patients could not have been obtained without the years of participation, dedication, and considerable cooperation of the members of the PVSG, to whom we are extremely indebted.

21

Chronic Myelocytic Leukemia

ANTHONY V. PISCIOTTA

HISTORY

Chronic myelocytic leukemia (CML) is a myeloproliferative disorder characterized by marked expansion of granulocyte precursor cells in the bone marrow. It results in increased delivery of mature and immature granulocytes to peripheral blood. It constitutes about 15 to 20 percent of all adult leukemias and has been estimated to affect 1 in 100,000 people per year.

Although not identified as a white blood cell (WBC) neoplasm at first, reports began to appear in 1827 when Velpeau[1] described a 64-year-old man with a huge liver and spleen. His blood was said to be as thick as gruel and to resemble red-colored pus. Similar descriptions were provided by Donne.[2] Most credit for the first description of CML was given to Craigie[3] and to Bennett,[4] who attributed death in their patient to suppuration of the blood associated with massive splenomegaly. At the same time, Virchow[5,6] named this condition *Weisses blut* (white blood, or leukemia).

In 1846, Fuller[7] described the first instance where an antemortem diagnosis was made. In 1870, Neumann,[8] aware that bone marrow was the origin of WBCs, felt that CML was due to overproduction of granulocytes.[9] In 1891, Ehrlich[10] stained blood cells with aniline dyes and thereby distinguished the various cell types. In this way, granulocytic and lymphocytic types were described. The advent of staining technology provided strong evidence that granulocytic leukemia was an overgrowth of myelocytes, basophils, and eosinophils.

The Philadelphia (Ph[1]) Chromosome: Pathogenesis and Mechanisms of CML

The discovery of the Philadelphia chromosome (Ph[1]) in 1960 was more than the development of a specific diagnostic procedure. It was a door opener in every sense of that word. Nowell and Hungerford[11] originally called attention to an abnormality in chromosome number 22 which they described as a minute structure in which a portion of the long (p) arm appeared to be broken off. Through that open door, Rowley[12] walked in and opened up one of her own in 1973. By Giemsa banding and DNA fluorescence, Rowley found that the missing portion of chromosome number 22 was adherent to the short arm (q) of chromosome number 9. The novel chromosomal rearrangement was designated as (t9;22) (q34;11). The so-called Ph[1] chromosome was considered to occur in 90 percent of CML but was not observed in fibroblasts or nonleukemic somatic cells. The Ph[1] chromosome was later observed in certain acute leukemias of children. In contrast to adult CML, it disappeared during remission, whereas it persisted in adult CML.[13,14] Furthermore, some doubt was expressed as to the identity of the childhood disease and adult CML.

The Ph[1] chromosome has been observed in granulocyte precursors, colony-forming units, erythroblasts, megakaryocytes, and some B cells.[15–18] It is not present in nonhematopoietic or somatic cells such as fibroblasts[19] or mitogen-stimulated lymphocytes. Because the Ph[1] chromosome is limited to

311

bone marrow–derived cells, it is considered to arise in a pluripotential hematopoietic stem cell.

During remission, the persisting Ph[1] chromosome continues to yield significant diagnostic evidence, even in a patient whose clinical and hematologic indicators of CML have been largely eradicated by treatment. Indeed, the abnormal chromosome continues to increase in numbers in marrow-derived cells. At the onset of disease, not all marrow cells have a Ph[1] chromosome. By 2 years, 100 percent of the myeloid cells manifest this abnormality.[20]

The breakpoint that characterizes the Ph[1] chromosome is known to be the point of origin of translocation of genetic material (t9:22) (q34.1:q11.21). It consistently occurred within the same chromosomal bands of different patients with CML[21] and resulted in the construction of a new chimeric oncogene, designated the *bcr-abl* gene.

Cellular oncogenes or protooncogenes are normal components of somatic cells, designated as three lowercase italic letters preceded by the letter *c*. These are potentially capable of being transformed to a cancer-related oncogene as mediated by a similar retrovirus corresponding to the *c-proto-oncogene*. It now becomes known as a *v-oncogene* and as such can give rise to the determinants of malignant transformation which regulate altered cell growth and proliferation. The original protooncogene (*c-abl*) was found by Abelson[22] to be localized to the long arm of chromosome 9 and was translocated to chromosome 22 in CML. The *c-abl* gene is homologous with the viral oncogene (*v-abl*), also known to be the active transforming sequence of the Maloney murine leukemic virus which causes leukemia in susceptible mice by transforming their lymphoid cells.

The corresponding cellular protoonco-gene found on chromosome 22 is *c-cis*, which also codes for the beta chain of platelet-derived growth factor but is not found as such in CML unless transformation takes place.

Loss of genetic material from chromosome 22 occurs at the breakpoint site, which is localized within an area encompassing 5 to 8 kilobases of DNA, known as the *breakpoint cluster region (bcr)*.[23] The fusion of the *bcr* region on chromosome 22 produces a chimeric gene with *c-abl* from chromosome 9 to produce a new protein identified by tyrosine kinase activities. Thus the *bcr/c-abl* fusion

gene result in an abnormal product that increases signal transduction and instructs stem cells to develop enhanced and uncontrolled proliferative events.

Activation of this novel chimeric oncogene is believed to derive primarily from a clone of stem cells which is later expressed as Ph[1] positivity.

A summary of steps[24] in the development of CML begins with translocation of a *c-abl* from chromosome 9 to chromosome 22. The fusion gene which results between 5'-*bcr* and *c-abl* gives rise to a hybrid 8-kb messenger RNA and then to a new *bcr c-abl* tyrosine kinase product[25] which plays a critical role in enhancing cellular proliferation.

McCarthy et al.[26] further described rearrangement of *c-myc*, the transforming agent of avian myelocytomatosis virus. It thus appears that interactions between marrow cellular oncogenes may precede development of CML. The definitive relationship between the abnormal protein and the development of CML remains unknown but is the subject of intensive investigation.

Abundant evidence now exists to show that CML develops from a single stem cell that proliferates to become a clone that eventually replaces a normal or nonneoplastic hematopoietic cell line. Kamada and Uchino[27] have shown that the Ph[1] chromosome antedates development of CML in atomic bomb victims who were followed closely after their exposure to ionizing radiation. The novel concepts of Fialkow et al.[28–30] clearly demonstrate the clonal nature of CML by an enzymatic marker in women who are heterozygous for a sex-linked mutant gene for glucose 6-phosphate dehydrogenase (G-6-PD). Autosomal nonhematogenous cells (e.g., fibroblasts) from these women show both the normal and the mutant forms of the enzyme, each derived from a separate Y chromosome and designated A and B. If such a person should fortuitously develop CML, peripheral blood granulocytes, bone marrow granulocyte, platelet, and erythrocyte precursors display only one or the other form of G-6-PD, either all A or all B. In the presence of both forms of the mutant enzyme in autosomal, nonhematogenous cells, the simultaneous occurrence of a single type of enzyme constitutes evidence for clonal expansion of a single pluripotential stem cell which ultimately replaces all the hematopoietic cells derived from marrow. Isolates of lymphocyte precursors have disclosed no Ph^1 chromosome in T cells, but that abnormality has been found in about half the B-lymphocytes. Similar observations made by Fialkow on B-lymphocytes from women who are heterozygous for G-6-PD disclose that over 70 percent of lymphocytes which are negative for the Ph^1 chromosome have a mutant enzyme pattern that is similar to that found in the Ph^1-positive leukemic cell line from the same patient. Since this figure exceeds that which would be ordinarily expected by chance, it suggests that the Ph^1 chromosome may appear in the neoplastic cells after they become malignant. Furthermore, it implies a survival or proliferative advantage of Ph^1-positive cells over those which are Ph^1-negative which eventually leads to a complete replacement of the negative clone with time.

Ph^1-positive leukemic transformation may occur in previously normal donor cells after they are transplanted to a Ph^1-positive CML subject.[31] Evidence for such a transformation was found in normal male marrow cells that were transplanted into the subject's sister, who had CML. While the donor cells retained the normal male Y chromosome, they also acquired Ph^1 positivity as they became leukemic. This observation suggests that the factor that initiated leukemia also produced leukemia in donor cells and that the 9:22 translocation predicts the onset.

ETIOLOGIC FACTORS

The etiologic factors that incite transformation of normal to neoplastic cells remain unknown. However, the defect is believed to be acquired rather than hereditary because no genetic predisposition has yet been found.[32] The disorder so far has occurred in a single twin but not in the concordant sibling.[33]

Although most cases of spontaneous CML seem to occur independently of exposure to environmental toxic or chemical factors,[32] there nevertheless appears to be a higher than coincidental occurrence in people who are exposed to irradiation.[34–37] For example, radiologists and radiotherapists have a higher than expected frequency of CML.[34] Those who have received therapeutic radiotherapy for ankylosing spondylitis[35] show a significant increment in the incidence of CML with increasing dosimetry. Published reports from Hiroshima and Nagasaki show

that people who were exposed to the atom bomb in 1945 manifested a clear-cut increase in CML that correlated with the amount of irradiation received and which occurred 5 to 15 years after exposure, independently of age at time of the bomb.[36–38] Exposure by inhalation to volatile solvents such as benzol, while associated with a higher incidence of acute leukemia, has not especially manifested transformation to typical CML.[39–41] Similarly, while specific viruses have been implicated in the pathogenesis of T-cell leukemias,[42] a similar relationship has yet to be established in CML. The large number of circulating polymorphonuclear leukocytes (PMNs) in CML is generated by a massive pool of stem cells, which nevertheless differentiate at a normal rate.[43] The large number of stem cells in equivalent volumes of bone marrow in CML results in a large yield of colony-forming units (CFU-GM) when such marrow is placed in tissue culture.[44] Furthermore, increased numbers of CFU-GMs develop during culture of peripheral blood from CML than from normal individuals, which indicates a higher number of circulating stem cells in CML. The circulating leukocytes in CML are capable of generating colony-stimulating factor (CSF) which is equivalent in amount to that generated by normal leukocytes.[45] However, WBCs in CML generate much less lactoferrin than do normal WBCs. Since this substance is believed to be involved in feedback control mechanisms, it is possible that an additional restraint has been removed in CML which results in increased numbers of stem cells. In addition, the proliferative advantage held by CML stem cells may be related to a loss or lack of IA-like antigens, which provides further regulatory effect.[46]

Cell Cycle Characteristics of CML[43, 47]

The cell cycle, or the time interval from mitosis to mitosis, is the same in CML and in normal marrow cells. Despite the greatly increased number of leukocytes, there is no evidence that CML granulocytes proliferate or are released from marrow at a more accelerated rate than normal. However, because of the larger number of cells, the number of uncommitted stem cells leading to CML granulocytes is believed to be four times greater than normal. CML leukocytes released from these stem cells are functionally normal in most measurable ways. Despite some evidence to the contrary, they seem fully capable of motility, migration, and bacterial killing and for these reasons have been used effectively as leukocyte transfusions to leukopenic patients. Occasionally, some leukocytes may be defective in phagocytic function.

Classification of CML

Clinical variants of CML are shown in Table 21–1. Most of these variants are Ph[1]-negative. Morphologic variants are designated by predominating cell type as eosinophilic, basophilic, monocytic, or myelomonocytic. Differences exist in clinical presentation, rapidity of development, and response to treatment.

Clinical Features[15, 48, 49]

Typical (Ph[1]-positive) CML

The onset of CML is insidious and cannot be dated accurately by the patient. Indeed, the diagnosis is frequently made by an incidental blood count during the course of a routine physical examination. Patients so affected are usually greatly astonished by the occurrence without warning of so serious a disorder.

If the patient has had no routine blood studies that would lead directly to the diagnosis, progressive symptoms and signs would sooner or later develop (Table 21–2). These may be grouped by categories into a number of clinical manifestations. Although anemia is mild, patients notice a lack of vigor, easy fatigue, diminished exercise tolerance,

TABLE 21–1. CLASSIFICATION OF CML

A. Clinical types
   1. Ph[1]-positive (typical) CML
   2. Ph[1]-negative (atypical) CML
   3. CML in infancy and childhood

B. Morphologic types
   1. Chronic eosinophilic leukemia
   2. Chronic basophilic leukemia
   3. Chronic neutrophilic leukemia
   4. Chronic monocytic leukemia
   5. Chronic myelomonocytic leukemia

C. Other similar myeloproliferative disorders
   1. Polycythemia vera
   2. Myelofibrosis

TABLE 21–2. CML SIGNS AND SYMPTOMS IN ORDER OF DECREASING FREQUENCY

A. Symptoms
   1. None detected by routine blood count
   2. Fatigue
   3. Weight loss
   4. Abdominal fullness or distress
   5. Pain in abdomen or left shoulder
   6. Ecchymoses or mucosal bleeding
   7. Poor appetite
   8. Night sweats

B. Signs
   1. Splenomegaly
   2. Hepatomegaly
   3. Sternal tenderness
   4. Purpura, petechiae, ecchymoses
   5. Retinal hemorrhagic
   6. Fever
   7. Lymphadenopathy

and shortness of breath which had not been there previously. With increase in metabolic rate, symptoms that suggest hyperthyroidism develop. These include unexplained weight loss despite good appetite, increased weariness, low-grade fever, irritability, heat intolerance, and diarrhea. Indeed, some of these patients may be erroneously treated for hyperthyroidism until the true situation is learned. Splenic enlargement constitutes the most prominent clinical feature and frequently reaches massive proportions even early in the course of illness. If this happens, splenic enlargement may be first perceived by the patient, who discovers a "lump" or mass on the left side or who becomes aware of a dull ache or dragging sensation across the upper abdomen. At times, the spleen may become massive enough to encroach on the capacity of the stomach, resulting in early satiation or inability to enjoy a full meal. Limited intake of food may further contribute to weight loss. Occasionally, asymptomatic enlargement of the liver occurs, or it also may produce upper abdominal discomfort. However, the lymph nodes are rarely enlarged, except as a very late manifestation of transformation to an acute disorder. In addition, hemorrhage into the skin or from the mucous membranes may be a late manifestation and is primarily associated with thrombocytopenia. Symptoms such as pruritus, urticaria, and peptic ulceration may occur because of increased proliferation of basophils and hyperhistaminemia.

Hyperuricemia is a regular feature of the increased WBC breakdown and purine catabolism. As such, it may result in gout with renal colic due to entrapment of uric acid calculi. In most advanced states, hyperuricemia may result in massive occlusion of renal or cerebral blood vessels because of precipitation of masses of uric acid crystals.

Since the mature PMNs retain their ability to phagocytize and kill bacteria, infection is rarely a problem unless the PMNs are eventually replaced by nonfunctioning blast cells.

LABORATORY FEATURES[50]

Chronic myelocytic leukemia is readily identified by ordinary hematologic examination. Unless altered by treatment, the leukocyte count is exceedingly high; frequently no less than 50×10^9/liter, it often plateaus to 100 to 500×10^9/liter. Leukocytes found in the smear consist mostly of neutrophilic mature polymorphonuclear and band leukocytes (PMNs) which appear normal (Fig. 21–1). In addition, increased numbers of eosinophils and basophils are present together with immature granulocyte precursors. The total aggregate of metamyelocytes, myelocytes, promyelocytes, and myeloblasts rarely exceeds 20 or 25 percent of the entire leukocyte population, and it is possible to trace the entire maturation sequence of the granulocyte series in a single slide. Lymphocytes and monocytes are normal in number and appearance, but a variant with consistent monocytosis is called chronic *mono-* or *myelomonocytic leukemia* and has been recognized as a variant of Ph^1-negative CML.[51] The hemoglobin (Hb), hematocrit (Hct), and erythrocyte values are frequently normal but with progression of disease become diminished. The moderate decline in red blood cell (RBC), Hb, and Hct values is proportionate, so the ensuing anemia is normocytic and normochromic. Hypochromic, microcytic indices are the eventual result of unrelated coincidental chronic blood loss that results in iron deficiency. Macrocytosis frequently accompanies treatment with hydroxyurea or methotrexate. The reticulocyte count is usually normal but may increase in the event of blood loss, rarely with hemolysis, or during recovery following cessation of myelosuppression therapy. The platelet count is frequently elevated but may be normal or low. Occasional coincidental elevations in RBC count and platelet count may be confused with polycythemia vera (PV) or essential thrombocythemia (ET). Bone marrow bi-

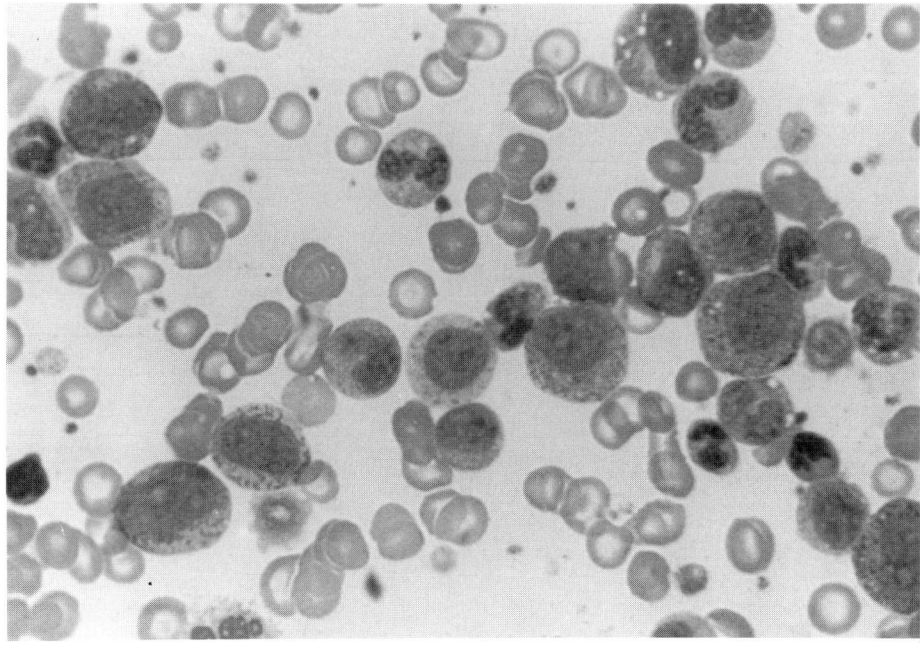

FIGURE 21–1. Peripheral blood smear, untreated chronic myelocytic leukemia.

opsy is rarely required for diagnosis of CML. Smears and biopsy confirm what is seen in peripheral blood (see Fig. 21–1). The bone marrow is entirely replaced with a collection of cells with little or no intervening fat spaces (Fig. 21–2). Since the marrow remains semifluid, it usually is easily aspirated. Occasionally, a dry tap may occur because of concomitant myelofibrosis or reticulin deposition. If this occurs, the peripheral blood shows fragmented red cells, teardrop-shaped erythrocytes, nucleated red cells, and small numbers of granulocyte precursors (leukoerythroblastosis). In addition, giant-sized platelets and megakaryocyte fragments may appear in myelofibrosis. The trephine biopsy indicates an increase in reticulin fibers.

Leukocyte alkaline phosphatase content of PMNs is characteristically depleted and may be scored by examining stained smears or by chemical analysis of WBC sonicates.[52,53] Indeed, a low leukocyte alkaline phosphatase activity constitutes a major objective way to distinguish CML from the other members of the myeloproliferative group because it is increased in PV, myelofibrosis, and ET. A low leukocyte alkaline phosphatase score is not necessarily unique to CML but has been observed in paroxysmal nocturnal hemoglobinuria (PNH), liver disease, and gout. Each

disorder is readily distinguished from CML by clinical criteria.

The elevated serum uric acid level derives from increased turnover rate of leukocytes, resulting in an increased yield of purines, some which are degraded to uric acid. The increased uric acid blood values may result in gout, uric acid nephrolithiasis, or in its most extreme degree, occlusion of renal and cerebral blood vessels by precipitated uric acid crystals. Breakdown of leukocytes in increased numbers also results in release of other intracellular substances to produce elevated blood values of lactate dehydrogenase (LDH).

The increase in leukocyte mass which occurs as a result of CGL and other members of the myeloproliferation group and, to a lesser extent, infectious leukocytosis is apt to lead to increased release of transcobalamin I,[54] which binds and transports B_{12}, leading to increase in serum B_{12} levels.[16]

DIFFERENTIAL DIAGNOSIS

CML is sometimes confused with infectious leukemoid reactions and the other members of the myeloproliferative group because of common hematologic features. A

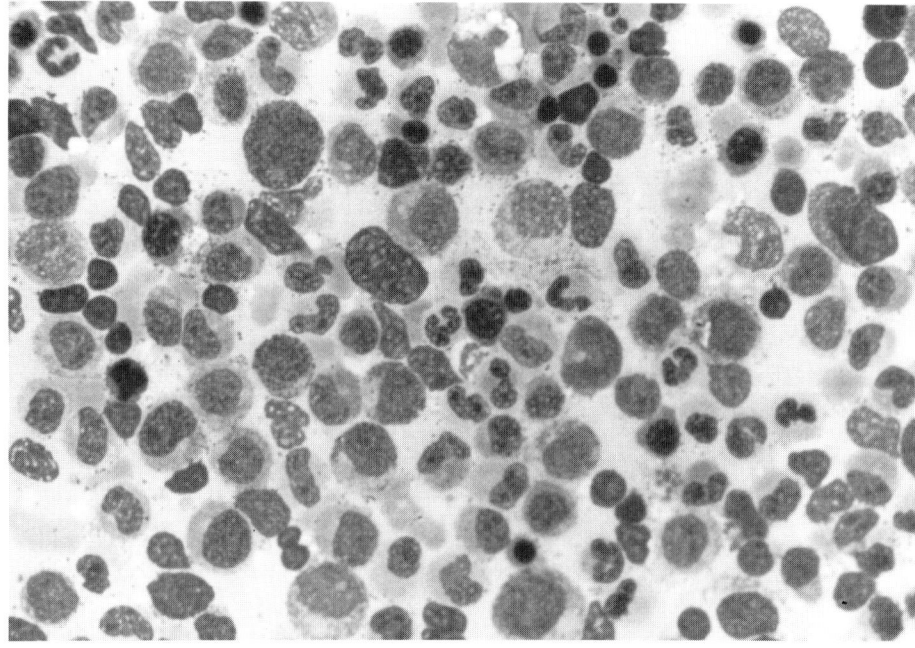

FIGURE 21–2. Bone marrow smear; untreated chronic myelocytic leukemia.

leukemoid reaction is characterized by an elevated leukocyte count with a small number of immature granulocyte precursors. It may result from overwhelming infection or from widely metastatic malignancy involving serosal cavities. Also, the bone marrow during recovery from drug-induced agranulocytosis may display marked overshoot of WBCs. These conditions are each readily differentiated from CML because of their characteristic clinical picture. Generally, patients with CML, despite a high WBC count, may be asymptomatic or ambulatory, whereas those with septic leukemoid reactions are seriously incapacitated with shaking, chills, fever, and infections or debilitated from far-advanced malignancy. In sepsis, if the spleen is enlarged at all, it rarely exceeds 2 or 3 cm below the costal margin and is soft in consistency. Leukemoid reactions characteristically are represented by high leukocyte counts which occasionally exceed 100×10^9/liter. In contrast to CML, relatively few immature granulocyte precursors are found in peripheral blood, rarely exceeding 5 or 6 percent leukocytes younger than metamyelocytes. Characteristically, leukocytes in sepsis show pronounced "toxic" granulation, vacuolization, and partial degranulation. Many of the PMNs display irregular areas of blue-gray staining in submembranous cytoplasmic locations—Doehle bodies. In leukemoid reactions, the leukocyte alkaline phosphatase (LAP) score is elevated rather than low. The Ph^1 chromosome is not present, but the serum B_{12} and B_{12}-binding capacity may be elevated, sometimes to the point of confusion. In common with CML, the bone marrow may show granulocytic hyperplasia, so the distinction must be made by criteria other than marrow biopsy. Occasionally, patients who have CML may coincidently develop overwhelming sepsis. In case of confusion brought about by similar hematologic features, the recent history, the size of the spleen, the LAP score, and the presence of the Ph^1 chromosome each offer an important means of differentiating between CML and leukemoid reactions.

The similarity between various MPDs has led to their inclusion into a group of myeloproliferative syndromes with common hematologic features and constitutes the general subject of this volume. Uncontrolled proliferation of precursor cell types[55] produces predominant overgrowth of megakaryocytes characteristic of ET, of fibroblasts and reticulin characterized by myelofibrosis, multipotent stem cells, and erythroblasts predominantly in PV, while granulocyte precursors dominate in CML. Criteria were developed which enabled distinction between the various members of this group. CML was the first disorder to be split off from the myeloproliferative group because of distinctive clinical and laboratory manifestations. Predominantly PMNs from CML show a low LAP score, whereas most patients with myelofibrosis, PV, and ET have an increased score. Moreover, the Ph^1 chromosome is unique to more than 90 percent of patients with CML, although this abnormality has been found occasionally in ET (see Table 21-1).

Philadelphia Chromosome–Negative Chronic Myelocytic Leukemia

About 10 percent of patients who have a blood picture resembling CML fail to show the Philadelphia (Ph^1) chromosome (Fig. 21-3) and hence are termed Ph^1-negative.[56,57] Why these patients maintain a normal cytogenetic pattern despite a peripheral blood and bone marrow picture that resembles CML remains puzzling. Many of these 10 percent have a translocation of c-abl to chromosome 22 which is not recognizable at the cytogenetic level.[58,59] However, important differences in clinical presentation serve to differentiate these variant disorders from more conventional Ph^1-positive CML. First, the clinical course is more aggressively downhill and frequently leads to death in a shorter time. Further, such patients remain refractory to conventional chemotherapy, which is more apt to provide a remission, if not a response, in Ph^1-positive CML. However, other differences may distinguish between both types. The serum muramidase level in Ph^1-negative patients is frequently increased, suggesting monocytic proliferation,[60] which indicates a major difference between some types of Ph^1-negative and the Ph^1-positive CML.

Travis et al.[61] critically studied 23 retrospectively selected Ph^1-negative CML patients. They generally presented at an older age, and all were anemic, had a lower leukocyte count without basophils, and failed to develop significant splenomegaly. None of these patients had absent or scant LAP

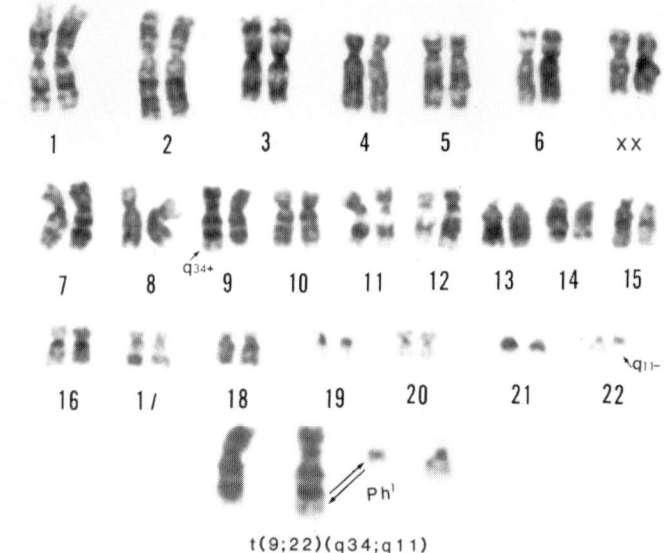

t(9;22)(q34;q11)

FIGURE 21-3. The Philadelphia (Ph¹) chromosome. *(Courtesy of Dr. J. Whang-Peng.)*

scores. The basic common denominator consisted of absence of the morphologic Ph¹ chromosome, but several others showed cytogenetic abnormalities in chromosomes other than 9 and 22.

In further contrast to Ph¹-positive subjects, dysplastic morphologic findings may be present in many Ph¹-negative patients. For example, morphologic abnormalities in granulocytes consisted of hypersegmented neutrophils, hypogranulation, pseudo-Pelger-Huet anomaly, and bizarre or dystrophic blasts. Dyserythropoiesis is expressed as normoblastic multinuclearity, impaired hemoglobin synthesis, megaloblastic changes, and ringed sideroblasts. Dysmegakaryocytopoiesis is expressed chiefly as micromegakaryocytosis and diminished numbers of megakaryocytes. These clinical and morphologic features permit a revision in diagnosis to chronic myelomonocytic leukemia, preleukemic syndrome, and undifferentiated chronic myeloproliferation syndrome.

The important points of distinction as defined by Mintz et al.[62] consist of the appearance of an elevated urine muramidase in response to chemotherapy and a shortened median survival time despite similarities in LAP scores, vitamin B₁₂ levels, and a peripheral blood and bone marrow picture. While Mintz et al. regard Ph¹-negative CML as a distinct entity, others regard it as part of a heterogeneous group of diseases other than CML with similar features.

On the other hand, most patients with Ph¹-negative CML also have translocation of c-*abl* to chromosome 22 without downstream translocation of *bcr*. This group differs from chronic myelomonocytic leukemia, which is not involved with *abl* or *bcr*.

Childhood Ph¹-Positive Leukemia

CML may occur in children as well as adults. When it does, it frequently presents a clinical picture indistinguishable from the adult variety except for the age of the patient. In a recent review of 39 children, Castro-Malaspina et al.[63] found a predominant incidence in girls over boys (24 versus 15) who exhibited a similar course and response to busulfan, eventual conversion to a blast crisis, and inevitable death from refractory acute leukemic transformation. Still another variant of Ph¹-positive leukemia has been observed. Peterson et al.[64] have reported a patient who had no history of previous CML but who presented with Ph¹-positive acute leukemia (Fig. 21–4). These patients were compared with 19 others who had a history of preceding chronic leukemia. The leukemias that seemed to arise de novo showed predominant lymphadenopathy and a febrile course. Those which followed chronic leukemia were morphologically indistinguishable from acute leukemia.

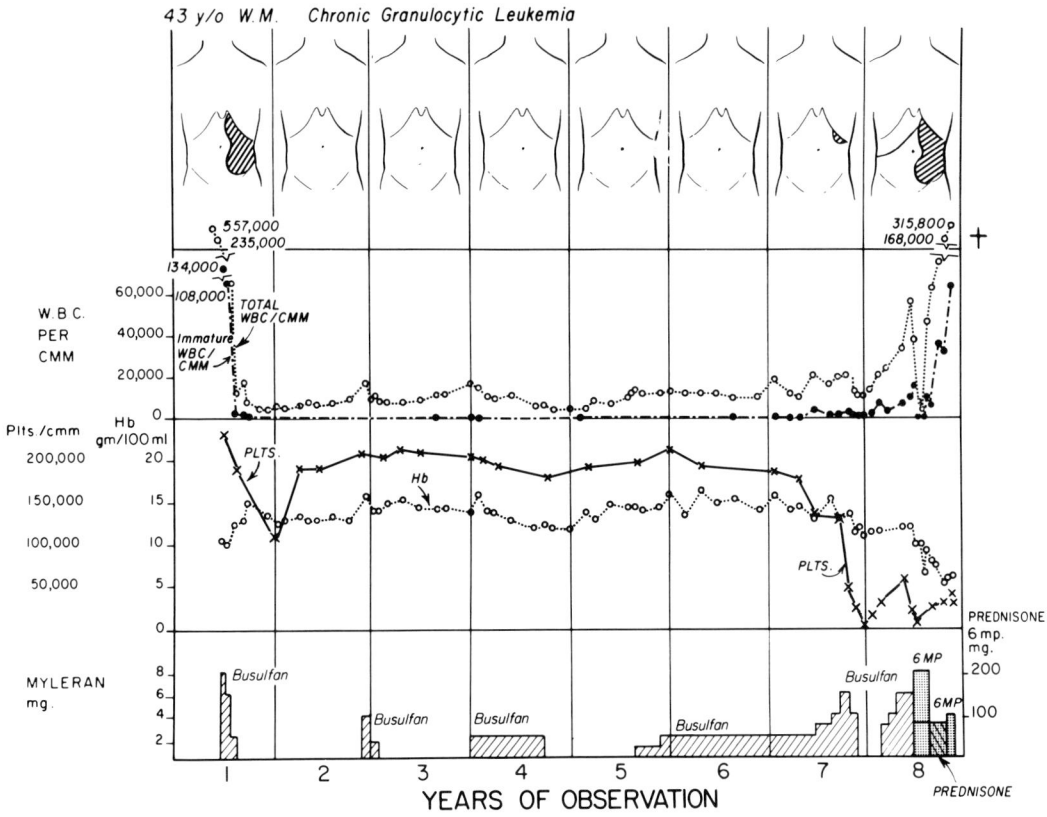

FIGURE 21-4. Course of CML in a 43-year-old man, over 8 years.

OTHER FORMS OF CML

Some patients characteristically manifest a progressively downhill course that is shorter than that of CML but longer than that of untreated AML. This so-called subacute granulocytic leukemia is characterized by more profound anemia, thrombocytopenia, and a lower leukocyte count. This variant manifests a greater number of myeloblasts in peripheral blood and bone marrow, some of which show Auer rods. The myeloblasts are encountered in peripheral blood together with mature PMNs but with few or no intermediate granulocyte precursors such as metamyelocytes, myelocytes, and promyelocytes. This so-called leukemic hiatus is frequently encountered in the subacute variant but not in CML, where one may observe the entire maturation sequence of the granulocyte precursors on a single peripheral blood and bone marrow smear.

An increased number of basophils and eosinophils is frequently encountered in late stages of CML. If these cells predominate early in the course of CML and then continue to increase progressively in number as time goes on, then the leukemia is referred to as *eosinophilic*[65, 66] or *basophilic*.[67] Rarely, a patient appears with hepatosplenomegaly, pleural effusions, massive eosinophilia in peripheral blood and bone marrow, and extensive infiltration into parenchymal organs. This unusual disorder is called the *hypereosinophilic syndrome*[68] and is believed to be a variant of chronic leukemia. These rare variants are often refractory to chemotherapy and bear a prognosis similar to that associated with the entrance of *ambiphils* into peripheral blood and bone marrow. Ambiphils are binucleated granulocyte precursors that bear both eosinophilic and basophilic granules in the same cell.[69] When they occur, they increase in number rapidly, become even more atypical in appearance, resist chemotherapy, and often result in death in short order.

Another more common variant that resembles CML is associated with myelofibrosis. The spleen is often very large, but the

RBC count and platelet count do not greatly deviate from normal. The extreme leukocytosis is characterized by a large proportion (i.e., over 20 percent) of metamyelocytes with myelocytes and blasts that manifest the Ph^1 chromosome. A low LAP score is present as well as an elevated serum B_{12}-binding capacity. In contrast to CML, anemia develops early in the course, together with teardrop deformities of erythrocytes, megakaryocytic fragments, and many nucleated red cells. The bone marrow is not aspirable through a biopsy needle. Instead, a trephine biopsy is necessary to obtain an adequate specimen, which is characterized by a heavy deposition of reticulin fibers and fibroblasts.

CHLOROMA–GRANULOCYTIC SARCOMA[70]

By definition, leukemia is widespread and diffuse. Its identity as a malignancy is emphasized by the appearance of localized and solid neoplastic growths composed of the same cell types as those seen in peripheral blood or bone marrow. This is known as *chloroma* or *granulocytic sarcoma*, a malignant tumor that consists of myeloblast and early myeloid precursors and which occasionally develops in chronic or acute granulocytic leukemia.

The lesion is called *chloroma* because of the green color of a freshly cut section that represents the green pigment of a large concentration of myeloperoxidase.[71] Chloroma provides prima facie evidence of a malignant neoplasm. The cells of which it consists are atypical, irregular in size and shape, and capable of metastasis and invasion to granules in contiguous sites.

Its identity with the granulocytic series is suggested by conventional histopathology as well as a positive peroxidase stain. Electron microscopy of ultrathin sections reveals primary granules similar to those seen in promyelocytes.

The chloroma that complicates late CML is accompanied by the characteristic peripheral blood and bone marrow picture of CML. Its clinical expression consists of the pressure of a rapidly growing tumor on adjacent sites. For example, unilateral exophthalmos is frequent because of the propensity of chloroma to attach to orbital periosteum and push the eyeball forward.[72] Other sites may be intra-thoracic or abdominal. It may be visualized by direct palpation, by computer-directed tomography (CT scan), or by conventional x-ray.

The prognosis following development of chloroma is very poor indeed. Irreparable damage may occur to the affected eye with blindness, infection, or hemorrhage. The course of disease is that of an uncontrolled malignant disorder: weight loss, cachexia, and profound weakness, all accompanied by enlargement of primary tumors or their metastasis to distant areas, plus uncontrolled leukemia. Death occurs within a relatively short time of development of chloroma.

COURSE

The average course of CML is divided into two well-marked phases and is largely determined by the presence or absence of the Ph^1 chromosome. The chronic phase is largely asymptomatic and ranges between 1 and 5 or more years in length. During this time, the patient remains mildly non- or asymptomatic and fully productive and responds readily to therapy. At the end of this apparently benign preliminary stage, the accelerated phase supervenes. In contrast, Ph^1-negative CML does not readily respond to conventional chemotherapy and progresses downhill more rapidly.

Accelerated Phase

The accelerated phase is characterized by the appearance of increasing numbers of immature and undifferentiated granulocytes and by deformities in mature PMNs with bilobed nuclei known as the *acquired Pelger-Huet anomaly*. An increased number of basophils or eosinophils may develop, frequently confusing the picture with eosinophilic or basophilic leukemia. From the clinical standpoint, the spleen enlarges rapidly with anemia and thrombocytopenia. During the accelerated phase, the patient becomes refractory to conventional therapy such as busulfan and hydroxyurea. In addition, patients in the accelerated phase do poorly with marrow transplantation. The development of the accelerated phase is not necessarily the same as the blast crisis, but both display an inexorable and rapidly downhill course.

The Blast Crisis

The blast crisis is characterized by the appearance of an increased number of phenotypic blast cells, which now exceed 30 percent in the peripheral blood and bone marrow as they replace more mature cellular populations. The factors that lead to the blast crisis are unknown, nor is it understood how the blast crisis may be delayed or prevented. Radiation therapy has been suspected to hasten development of the blast crisis,[73] which nevertheless continues to occur even if patients are treated solely with busulfan or hydroxyurea.

Despite the morphologic appearance of blast cells in converted CML,[74] it is clear that not all cases of accelerated CML are myeloid in origin.[64] About 25 percent of these patients show a peculiar form of DNA polymerase which is capable of adding nucleotide units to the ends of a DNA strand without the necessity of first adding primer DNA.[75, 76] This enzyme, termed *terminal deoxyribonucleotransferase*, was first isolated by Bollum[77] from thymic tissue and was believed to be peculiar to early thymocytes. Failure of these cells to mature results in persistence of the gene product terminal transferase. As such, it suggests that the blast cells in some cases of terminal CML are not myeloblast at all. Instead, they are believed to be undifferentiated derivatives of T cells.

This new information suggests that at least two different varieties of blast cells may exist in terminal CML. The first of these consists of stem cells that are incapable of maturing fully to normal granulocyte precursors. The second of these is characterized by increased terminal deoxyribonucleotide transferase (TdT) content which characterizes a T-cell–derived group of nucleolated cells that replace the myeloid cells and seem to convert the leukemia from a myelocytic to a lymphoblastic type.

These differences are associated with differences in response to chemotherapy. The myeloblastic type of blast crisis remains refractory to single-agent or combination chemotherapy and is characterized clinically by a rapidly downhill course and death within a few weeks or months of onset. On the other hand, the T-cell, TdT-positive form of blast crisis may respond temporarily to combinations of vincristine and prednisone and may even enter prolonged remission following treatment with these agents.

A clear-cut distinction between both types of blasts is not evident on morphologic grounds alone. Both are larger in size than myelocytes, are devoid of granules, have a deeply basophilic cytoplasm which may be punctuated by multiple vacuoles, and have an irregular, bizarre nucleus with diffuse chromatin pattern and many nucleoli. These cells generally show no Auer rods or primary granules, the peroxidase stain is negative, but a firm distinction between both is made in terms of TdT activity in one but not the other.

TREATMENT

In the many years that CML has been recognized, truly effective therapy remains unknown. Nevertheless, it has become possible to influence some of the early manifestations of this disease, especially during the chronic phase. Using a variety of therapeutic agents, the spleen may regress in size, the leukocyte count may be restored to normal, and the RBC count may increase to acceptable limits. Despite apparently successful treatments, the disease remains smoldering and frequently presents persisting basophilia, a few occasional immature granulocyte precursors in peripheral blood, and hyperplastic bone marrow. Eventually, nothing can be done to prevent or delay the inevitable conversion to the untreatable accelerated or blastic phase.

When chronic myelocytic leukemia was first recognized, any sort of therapy was unknown, and early patients were followed without treatment. This group of historical "controls" was reported by Minot and Buckman[78] to have a mean survival time of 31 months.

Arsenic in the form of Fowler's solution or neoarsphenamine was known to suppress output of bone marrow cells and was used as an early form of chemotherapy. Its toxicity and its failure to produce significant benefit eventually led to its abandonment.

Early therapeutic successes included irradiation and, later, chemotherapy in the form of urethane (ethyl carbamate). Although these agents alleviate a few manifestations of the disease, they remain toxic and are only temporarily, if at all, effective.

The diagnosis of CML remains in many ways a devastating psychological experience for both the patient and the family. It remains uncertain how soon treatment should be started after diagnosis. Like anything else for which definitive data do not exist, a number of debatable alternatives are possible. Some clinicians recommend that treatment be delayed until symptoms and signs are sufficient to interfere with ordinary activities. However, the extent to which weakness, weight loss, values of WBC and RBC counts, spleen size, etc. may reach before therapy is given is not adequately defined. The opposing viewpoint considers the serious psychological sequelae of coping with a disease that is deliberately left untreated until irreversible complications occur. For this reason, prompt treatment is usually recommended in order to produce psychological as well as medical support. The dilemma may be compromised in part by delaying treatment until the aggressiveness of the disease could be better evaluated by careful observation and baseline measurements of clinical, laboratory, morphologic, and cytogenetic changes. During the early phase of CML, peripheral blood and bone marrow samples may be collected and frozen in preparation for readministration by autotransplantation at a later date.

Irradiation

Irradiation was the first of the regularly employed forms of treatment found to be effective to prolong the length of the chronic phase. Unfortunately, it may be associated with a more rapid transition to the blast phase than chemotherapy.[73, 79] Nevertheless, irradiation regularly produces diminution in spleen size, a decline in leukocyte values, an increase in RBC count,[73] and a general increase in well-being.

Irradiation may be given locally to the splenic area (about 1000 rad) or as total-body irradiation if the WBC count is high but the spleen not too greatly enlarged. In similar clinical situations, ^{32}P, given intravenously, has the advantage that a single intravenous injection (2.3 mCi/m^2) may be followed by maximal clinical effect.[80] The clear disadvantage of ^{32}P is that an absolute therapeutic commitment is made from which retreat is not possible. Once radionuclides are given, their subsequent effects cannot be suppressed or attenuated in the event of overdose. Furthermore, this form of therapy is not designed to be interim or maintenance treatment.

A decline in the clinical and laboratory manifestations of CML may be evident with irradiation, but a convincing survival advantage of ^{32}P versus chemotherapy has not yet been observed. At the present time, irradiation remains useful to treat those who logistically cannot attend a clinic at sufficiently frequent intervals to be subjected to careful surveillance.

Irradiation also may be helpful to those people who cannot take chemotherapy because of individual intolerance. Extracorporeal irradiation has been used to minimize widespread exposure to x-rays. Irradiation and chemotherapy are not recommended to be used simultaneously because severe marrow hypoplasia may occur.

Busulfan

Busulfan (4-dimethanesulfonyloxybutane) is one of the first truly effective agents in the chemotherapy of malignant disease. It was first introduced in Great Britain by Haddow in 1953[81] and has been in continuous use ever since.[82] Like any other major therapeutic advance, its effectiveness is clouded by myelotoxicity, requiring that busulfan must be used with care. Unacceptably high doses, individual intolerant, and inadequate surveillance may result in permanent or even fatal marrow aplasia. Accordingly, several therapeutic strategies have been recommended. The first of these employs busulfan in small continuous maintenance dose (0.06 mg/kg per day), titrated against the leukocyte response. When a WBC count of 7 to 10 $\times$ 10^9/liter is reached, the dosage of busulfan is regulated by giving the smallest daily dosage to maintain a normal WBC count.

Alternatively, intermittent treatment is done with higher dose of busulfan than that listed above. Treatment must be discontinued when a normal WBC count is reached but would then be reinstituted whenever the WBC count or spleen size increases above arbitrary limits. A large bolus of busulfan, 50 to 150 mg, may be given once a month, based on the starting leukocyte count.

The choice of treatment regimens remains arbitrary, pending additional prospective clinical trials. It is possible that survival would be longer if the leukocyte count were maintained at normal levels, but this conclusion must await acquisition of more evidence.

The most serious side effect of busulfan consists of protracted, permanent, or fatal bone marrow suppression. This is more apt to occur during the use of exceptionally high doses. The fact that busulfan is metabolized and excreted slowly prolongs its toxic phase.

Related to its effect on inhibiting cell division, busulfan may produce temporary or permanent infertility. This is manifested in women by amenorrhea and hot flashes or fetal malformation if used in early pregnancy and in men as aspermia. Late in the course of treatment, a syndrome resembling Addison's disease may be produced. This consists primarily of skin pigmentation resembling localized spots of suntan. In contrast to Addison's disease, there is no pigmentation of mucous membranes or the folds of the skin and no alterations of blood levels of sodium and potassium. Weight loss, weakness, and occasionally hypotension may develop, but circulating glucocorticoid levels generally remain normal. A most serious late consequence of busulfan therapy may consist of pulmonary fibrosis and insufficiency with diminished vital capacity. This is manifested by shortness of breath, cough, and x-ray evidence of pulmonary infiltration. Histologic examination of the affected lung confirms the presence of interstitial pulmonary fibrosis.

Hydroxyurea

Hydroxyurea was originally developed in 1966 and soon thereafter found to be effective in CML.[83–85] This drug directly inhibits deoxyribonucleotide reductase and thereby suppresses DNA synthesis. In sufficient dosage it may produce a precipitous decline in WBCs and platelets. However, this effect is short-lived, since discontinuing the drug is quickly accompanied by restoration of leukocyte and platelet values.

Elsewhere in these pages (Chapters 15 and 20) will be found the beneficial effects of hydroxyurea in the treatment of PV and ET. A similar effectiveness is known in the treatment of CML.

Hydroxyurea is used in doses of 30 mg/kg to begin with and is reduced at weekly intervals until the desired decline in WBC count is achieved. It is accompanied by regression in spleen size. Precipitous leukopenia, which takes place with larger doses, will quickly reverse on cessation or reduction of treatment within a few days.

In present-day usage, some consider hydroxyurea to be superior to busulfan, chlorambucil, cytoxan, or irradiation as a second-line drug. It is especially useful if busulfan is ineffective or poorly tolerated. In cases of exceptionally high leukocyte counts, it may be used to advantage because its effects are so prompt. It is more difficult to achieve a steady control of WBCs with hydroxyurea than busulfan, and therefore, it requires meticulous surveillance. It is not expected to produce complete ablation of the Ph^1 chromosome and may not be as mutagenic or leukemogenic as busulfan.

Human Interferon-αA

Biologically derived or recombinant human interferon-αA has had limited use in the treatment of CML because of restricted experience. With the advent of recombinant DNA technology, production of this material in bacteria makes it possible to obtain greater quantities than ever before.

Several investigations on its potential usefulness has been reported. Talpez and associates[86] have successfully demonstrated the antiproliferative effect of bacterially synthesized interferon-αA in 51 patients. Reduction in leukocyte count and spleen size and suppression of Ph^1 chromosome were recorded in at least 41 patients (80 percent) during the chronic phase. Patients at high risk or with accelerated and blast transformation showed only a limited response, but the results are promising enough to encourage further investigation. Mild toxic effects include a flulike syndrome, muscular weakness, chills, and fever.

Other Drugs

Other drugs—either alone or in combination—have been used for treating CML in its early or late phases. These include dibromannitol,[87] melphalan,[88] 6-mercaptopurine,[89] and 6-thioguanine.[90] Such drugs are given chiefly if busulfan or hydroxyurea is ineffective or poorly tolerated. In later stages, they may be used in combination with other antileukemic drugs to control the blast or accelerated stage.

Early Aggressive Treatment of CML

In most patients, conventional treatment of early CML with radiotherapy or single agents will effectively influence the size of the spleen and restore most quantitative hematologic abnormalities to normal. However, basophilia may remain as the only manifestation of latent disease. Of course, the Ph[1] chromosome is not removed by conventional treatment. Therefore, the threat is constantly present that relapse or development of the accelerated phase or conversion to a blast crisis will sooner or later occur. As long as the Ph[1] chromosome remains, the disease continues to smolder and will eventually become out of control. In an attempt to eradicate the Ph[1] chromosome completely in order to restore normal hematopoiesis, aggressive therapeutic programs were explored.[91] One of these began with sufficient busulfan to produce a normal leukocyte count. Following this, splenic irradiation (800 rad) was given in order to remove a bulky mass of tumor cells. Next, the spleen was removed surgically, followed by sequential administration of cytosine arabinoside, 6-thioguanine, and L-asparaginase, finally followed by cyclical maintenance with methotrexate, daunorubicin, and lomustine CCNU. At Sloan-Kettering Institute, Cunningham et al.[91] treated 57 patients in this multidrug aggressive manner. Seven of these so treated eventually developed Ph[1]-negative marrow cells. Unfortunately, all relapsed in 1 to 43 months. Even this long survivor eventually succumbed to unrelated widespread malignancy. Thus no proof was produced that intensive treatment offered a survival advantage.

Marrow Transplantation[92–94]

In order to be effective, radical chemotherapy requires administration of lethal doses to provide any lasting benefit. It is clear that more intensive attempts at ablation must be supported by bone marrow replacements in suitable recipients. Bone marrow transplantation, therefore, is a potentially effective means of total eradication of CML as long as effective bone marrow ablation is first carried out. Complete marrow ablation with high-dose chemotherapy is combined with irradiation in lethal doses.

To prevent the hazards of graft rejection or serious graft-versus-host reaction (GVH), autologous transplantation is employed, where the patient's own marrow cells are infused. The procedure generally employed for autologous transplantation requires storage of peripheral blood and bone marrow in the frozen state. If the patient eventually transforms to an acute blast crisis, marrow ablation is carried out by chemotherapy and radiotherapy followed by intravenous administration of thawed and reconstituted marrow cells. This strategy effectively avoids complications such as graft-versus-host disease and minimizes failure to engraft because of immunologic rejection. However, the likelihood of permanent remission is lessened because Ph[1]-positive cells would have to be reinfused and may eventually produce a leukemic relapse. Furthermore, the blast cells that develop at the time of crisis may be resistant to irradiation and would not be completely ablated. To forestall this possibility, bone marrow purging in the autograft setting has been investigated.[95] Here, marrow is treated in vitro with interferon in an attempt to select Ph[1]-negative clones. Marrow from syngeneic identical twins is difficult to obtain. Therefore, allogenic marrow from HLA-identical siblings[92,93] provides a reasonable chance to replace marrow stem cells after a leukemic clone is eradicated. In the absence of a suitable donor, nonrelated HLA-matched donors may provide a potential source of cells, but this needs much more exploration. A major complication of allografting is the graft-versus-host reaction (GVH). This may offer an advantage in decreasing the number of leukemic cells by immunologic means.

T-cell depletion by in vitro means appears to diminish the threat of GVH.[94] Syngeneic or allogenic transplantation is feasible if suitable donors are available. The recipient must be prepared with high-dose cyclophosphamide and total-body irradiation with lethal dosimetry. Marrow is obtained from the donor by multiple punctures under general anesthesia. Following filtration and removal of fat from marrow, the remaining cells are given by intravenous infusion to the prepared recipient. Engraftment would be expected to result in eradication of Ph[1] chromosome and enhances the likelihood of survival for more than 5 years without recurrence.

A major consideration involves selection of patients most likely to be treated successfully by bone marrow transplantation. Recent experience confirms that successful marrow transplantation is best carried out during the chronic phase of CML on vigorous recipients aged less than 45 years.

A prime requirement, which further limits the frequency with which marrow transplantation may be carried out, has to do with the availability of a suitable donor. Identical twins are only rarely encountered. An HLA-identical sibling is only available in one of four potential donors. The potential usefulness and safety of nonrelated marrow donors are yet to be evaluated.

If a potential cure or prolonged remission is expected, then transplantation appears to offer promise. Those who tolerate the procedure well will experience prolonged survival in 80 percent of highly selected recipients.

Studies were reported on 198 patients with CML from Seattle by the group headed by Thomas,[93] who found that as many as 49 percent of these patients in the first chronic phase and 58 percent in the second chronic phase had a probability for long-term survival. Patients in the accelerated phase or blastic phase of disease were found to have the poorest chance for prolonged survival, since only about 15 percent were found to do so.

Prior splenectomy was deemed not to influence the eventual outcome. Those who survived remained free of the Ph^1 chromosome and of graft-versus-host disease for 1 to 3 years. Apparently no other form of therapy has been accompanied by so long a survival period free of objective evidence of activity. It appears that if CML is already transformed to a blastic phase, to myelofibrosis, or to accelerated CML, only 10 to 15 percent of patients will survive marrow transplant.

Treatment of Blast Transformation

Response to chemotherapy, hence prognosis, is largely determined by the type of blast transformation that has emerged. For this reason, therapy at the blast stage must be preceded by a careful search for markers that enable classification of the predominant cell type in the preterminal stage. The likelihood of response is variable because more than one cell type is involved in the terminal stage, even though the involved cells resemble each other. The most favorable cell type from a therapeutic and prognostic point of view is derived from undifferentiated early T cells of the lymphoblastic series as identified by the presence of TdT. These cells are not sufficiently differentiated to show the common lymphocytic leukemia antigen (CALLA) or the IA antigen. In addition, despite their apparent origin from a myeloid clone, these cells are negative for peroxidase, Sudan black, and nonspecific esterase. The presence of TdT is associated with response to treatment with vincristine and prednisone. While this simple therapy is by no means curative, it does offer a few weeks or months of salvage and time.

The more conventional precursors of granulocytic stem cells are negative for TdT but positive for peroxidase, Sudan black, and nonspecific esterase. These early myeloblasts retain the Ph^1 chromosome. Occasionally, in the blast crisis, multiple Ph^1 chromosomes are seen per cell. In addition, miscellaneous nonspecific chromosomal abnormalities, breaks, reduplication, ring formation, etc. may be present. These findings suggest a reversion to an early form of myeloid rather than lymphoblastic leukemia and offer a more serious prognosis.

In these cases, administration of drugs ordinarily used to treat acute leukemia or increased doses of busulfan or hydroxyurea have been given, frequently without avail. In contrast to TdT-positive leukemia, vincristine and prednisone are usually ineffective. Equally futile have been daunorubicin for 3 days, cytosine arabinoside for 7 days, 6-thioguanine, 6-mercaptopurine, methotrexate, VP-16, etc., despite their usefulness in the treatment of adult acute leukemia.

Other groups of drugs have been explored. Koller and Miller[96] used a combination of plicamycin (mithromycin) and hydroxyurea. Eight patients in the blastic phase of CML were so treated. During the course of treatment of one of these for hypercalcemia, it was found that the blastic leukemia had reverted back to its chronic phase.

Six patients with myeloid acute leukemia responded to the combination of plicamycin and hydroxyurea; the two with lymphoblastic morphology did not. If confirmed, these data may promise possible effectiveness in the myeloid blast phase of CML.

The observation that a clinical effect is possible without a preliminary aplastic phase suggests that this therapeutic effort produces differentiation of existing blast cells rather than ablation. Furthermore, this therapy seems to be effective only if given continuously.

The final stages of blast transformation may be characterized by proliferation of massive numbers of blasts which result in exceedingly high leukocyte counts, which stick together and occlude cerebral blood vessels, and which release large amounts of lactic acid to produce lactic acidosis. This is a truly life-threatening emergency and requires prompt treatment by leukopheresis,[97,98] in which large numbers of leukocytes are removed mechanically to increase patency of smaller blood vessels. This procedure cannot be expected to prolong life significantly, but it may buy sufficient time to enable additional chemotherapy to take effect.

REFERENCES

1. Velpeau A: Sur la resorption du pusaet sur l'alteration dusang dans les maladies clinique de persection nenemant premier observation. Rev Med 2:216, 1827
2. Donne A: De l'origine des globules du sang, de leur mode deformation, de leur fin. C R Acad Sci. 14:366, 1842
3. Craigie D: Case of disease of the spleen in which death took place in consequence of the presence of purulent matter in the blood. Edinburgh Med Surg J 64:400, 1845
4. Bennett JH: Case of hypertrophy of the spleen and liver in which death took place from suppuration of the blood. Edinburgh Med Surg J 64:413, 1845
5. Virchow R: Weisses blut. Froieps Notizen 36:151, 1845
6. Virchow R: Weiss blut und milztumoren. Med Z 15:157, 1846
7. Fuller H: Particulars of a case in which enormous enlargement of the spleen and liver, together with dilation of all the blood vessels of the body, were found coincident with a peculiarly altered condition of the blood. Lancet 2:43, 1846
8. Neumann E: Ein fall von leukamie mit erkrankung desknockenmarkes. Arch Heilk 11:1, 1870
9. Neumann E: Uber myelogene leukamie. Berl Klin Wochenschr 15:69, 1878
10. Ehrlich P: Parbenanalytische Untersuchungen zur Histologie und Klinic des Blutes. Berlin, Hirschwald, 1891
11. Nowell PC, Hungerford DA: A minute chromosome in human chronic granulocytic leukemia. J Natl Cancer Inst 25:85, 1960
12. Rowley JD: A new consistent chromosomal abnormality in chronic myelogenous leukaemia identified by quinacrine fluorescence and giemsa bonding. Nature 243:290, 1973
13. Chessells JM, Janossy A, Lawler SD, et al: The Ph[1] chromosome in childhood leukaemia. Br J Haematol 41:25, 1979
14. Sandberg AA: The Chromosomes in Human Cancer and Leukemia. New York, Elsevier, 1980
15. Canellos GP: Diagnosis and treatment of chronic granulocytic leukemia from neoplastic diseases of the blood. In Wiernik PH, Canellos GP, Kyle RA, Schiffer CA (eds): Neoplastic Diseases of the Blood. New York, Churchill Livingstone, 1985

16. Chikkappa G, Corcino J, Greenberg ML, et al: Correlation between various blood white cell pools and the serum B_{12} binding capacities. Blood 37:142, 1971
17. Lawler SD: The cytogenetics of chronic granulocytic leukaemia. Clin Haematol 6:55, 1977
18. Rastrick JM, Fitzgerald PH, Gunz FW: Direct evidence for presence of Ph[1] in erythroid cells. Br Med J 1:96, 1968
19. Maniatis AK, Amsel S, Mitus WJ: Chromosomal pattern of bone marrow fibroblasts in patient with chronic granulocytic leukaemia. Nature 222:1278, 1969
20. Chervenick PA, Boggs DR: Granulocytic kinetics in chronic myelocytic leukaemia. Semin Hematol 1:24, 1968
21. Silver RT, Gale RP: Chronic myeloid leukemia. Am J Med 80:1137, 1986
22. Abelson HT, Rabstein LS: Lymphosarcoma virus induced thymic independent disease in mice. Cancer Res 30:2213, 1970
23. Groffen J, Stephenson JR, Heistercamp N, et al: Philadelphia chromosome breakpoints are clustered within a limited region, bcv, on chromosome 22. Cell 36:93, 1984
24. Champlin RE, Golde DW: Chronic myelogenous leukemia: Recent advances. Blood 65:1039, 1985
25. Wang JYF, Queen C, Baltimore D: Expression of an Abelson leukemia virus, enclosed protein in Escherichia coli causes extensive phosphorylation of tyrosine residues. J Biol Chem 257:13181, 1982
26. McCarthy DM, Rassool FV, Goldman JM, et al: Genomic alternations involving the c-myc proto-oncogene locus during evaluation of a case of chronic granulocytic leukaemia. Lancet 1:1362, 1984
27. Kamada N, Uchino H: Chronologic sequence in appearance of clinical and laboratory findings characteristic of chronic myelocytic leukemia. Blood 51:843, 1978
28. Fialkow PJ, Gartler SM, Yoshida A: Clonal origin of chronic myelocytic leukemia in man. Proc Nat Acad Sci USA 58:1468, 1967
29. Barr RD, Fialkow PJ: Clonal origin of chronic myelocytic leukemia. N Engl J Med 289:307, 1973
30. Fialkow PJ, Jacobson RJ, Papayannopoulou T: Chronic myelocytic leukemia: Clonal origin in a stem cell common to the granulocyte, erythrocyte, platelet and monocyte/macrophage. Am J Med 63:125, 1977
31. Marmont A, Frassoni F, Baciagalupo A, et al: Recurrence of Ph[1]-positive leukemia in donor cells after marrow transplantation for chronic granulocytic leukemia. N Engl J Med 310:903, 1984
32. Gunz F: The epidemiology and genetics of the chronic leukemias. Clin Haematol 6:3, 1977
33. Goh KO, Swisher SN, Herman EC: Chronic myelocytic leukemia and identical twins: Additional evidence of the Philadelphia chromosome as a post-zygotic abnormality. Arch Intern Med 120:214, 1967
34. Lewis EB: Leukemia, multiple myeloma and aplastic anemia in American radiologists. Science 142:1492, 1963
35. Court-Brown WM, Doll R: Mortality from cancer and other causes after radiotherapy for ankylosing spondylitis. Br Med J 2:1327, 1965

36. Beebe GW, Kato H, Land CE: Studies on the mortality of A-bomb survivors, mortality and radiation dose, 1950–1974. Radiat Res 75:138, 1978

37. Bizzozero OJ, Johnson KG, Ciocco A, et al: Radiation related leukemia in Hiroshima and Nagasaki, 1946–1964: II. Observations on type-specific leukemia, survivorship and clinical behavior. Ann Intern Med 66:522, 1967

38. Ichimaru M, Ishimaru T, Belsky JL: Incidence of leukemia in atomic bomb survivors, belonging to a fixed cohort in Hiroshima and Nagasaki, 1950–71: Radiation dose, years after exposure, age at exposure and type of leukemia. Radiat Res 19:262, 1978

39. Nigiani EC, Saita G: Benzene and leukemia. N Engl J Med 271:872, 1964

40. Infante PF, Wagoner JK, Rinsy RA, et al: Leukemia in benzene workers. Lancet 2:76, 1977

41. Aksoy M, Erdem S: Follow-up study on the mortality and development of leukemia in 44 pancytopenic patients with chronic exposure to benzene. Blood 52:285, 1978

42. Gallo RC, Reitz MS Jr: Human retroviruses and adult T-cell leukemia-lymphoma. J Natl Cancer Inst 69:1209, 1982

43. Galbraith PR, Abu-Zahra HT: Granulopoiesis in chronic granulocytic leukemia. Br J Haematol 22:135, 1972

44. Broxmeyer HE, Grossbard E, Jacobsen N, Moore MAS: Evidence for a proliferative advantage of human leukemia colony-forming cells (CFU-C) in vitro. J Natl Cancer Inst 60:513, 1970

45. Burgess AW, Metcalf P: The nature and action of granulocyte-macrophage colony stimulating factors. Blood 56:947, 1980

46. Fitchen JH, Ferrone S, Quaranta V, et al: Monoclonal antibodies to HLA-A1B and Ia-like antigens inhibit colony formation by human myeloid progenitor cells. J Immunol 125:2004, 1980

47. Moore MAS, Williams M, Metcalf D: In vitro colony formulation by normal and leukemic human hematopoietic cells: Characterization of the colony forming cells. J Natl Cancer Inst 5:63, 1973

48. Spiers ASP: The clinical features of chronic granulocytic leukaemia. Clin Haematol 6:77, 1977

49. Gunz FW, Henderson ES: Leukemia, 4th ed. New York, Grune & Stratton, 1983

50. Lee GR, Bithel TL, Foerster J, et al: Wintrobe's Clinical Hematology, 9th ed. Philadelphia, Lea & Febiger, 1993

51. Ezdinli EA, Sokal JE, Crosswhite L, et al: Philadelphia chromosome positive and negative chronic myelocytic leukemia. Ann Intern Med 72:175, 1970

52. DeChatelet LR, et al: Absence of measurable leukocyte alkaline phosphatase from leukocytes of patient with chronic granulocytic leukaemia. Clin Chem 16:798, 1970

53. Rosner F, Schreiber ZR, Parise F: Leukocyte alkaline phosphatase. Arch Intern Med 130:892, 1972

54. Corcino J, Krauss S, Waxman S, et al: Release of vitamin B_{12}-binding protein by human leukocytes in vitro. J Clin Invest 49:2250, 1970

55. Dameshek W: Some speculations on the myeloproliferative syndromes. Blood 6:322, 1951

56. Canellos GP, Whang-Peng J, DeVita VT: Chronic granulocytic leukemia without the Philadelphia chromosome. Am J Clin Pathol 65:467, 1976

57. Kohno SL, Abe S, Sandberg AA: The chromosomes and causation of human cancer and leukemia: XXXVIII. Cytogenetic experience in Ph¹-negative chronic myelocytic leukemia (CML). Am J Hematol 7:281, 1979

58. Morris CM, Reeve AE, Fitzgerald PH, et al: Genourich diversity correlates with clinical diversity in Ph¹-negative chronic myeloid leukemia. Nature 320:281, 1986

59. Kurzrock NM, Blick MB, Talpaz M, et al: Rearrangement of the breakpoint cluster region in Philadelphia-negative chronic myelogenous leukemia. Ann Intern Med 105:673, 1986

60. Perillie PE, Finch SC: Muramidase studies in Philadelphia chromosome positive and chromosome negative chronic granulocytic leukemia. N Engl J Med 283:456, 1970

61. Travis LB, Pierre RV, Dewald GW: Ph¹-negative chronic granulocytic leukemia: A nonentity. Ann J Clin Pathol 85:186, 1986

62. Mintz V, Varmidian J, Golomb H, Rowley JD: Evolution of karyotypes in Philadelphia (Ph¹) chromosome negative chronic myelogenous leukemia. Cancer 43:411, 1979

63. Castro-Malaspina H, Schaison G, Briere J, et al: Philadelphia chromosome positive chronic myelocytic leukemia in children. Cancer 52:721, 1983

64. Peterson LC, Bloomfield CP, Brunning RB: Blast crisis as an initial or terminal manifestation of chronic myeloid leukemia: A study of twenty-eight patients. Am J Med 60:209, 1976

65. Kauer GL, Engle RL Jr: Eosinophilic leukemia with Ph¹-positive cells. Lancet 2:1340, 1964

66. Benvenisti DS, Ultmann JE: Eosinophilic leukemia: Report of five cases and review of literature. Ann Intern Med 71:731, 1969

67. Kyle RA, Pease GL: Basophilic leukemia. Arch Intern Med 118:205, 1966

68. Chusid MJ, Dale DC, West BC, Wolff SM: The hypereosinophilic syndrome: Analysis of fourteen cases with review of the literature. Medicine 54:1, 1975

69. Doan CA, Reinhart HL: The basophil granulocyte, basophilocytosis, and myeloid leukemia basophil and "mixed granule" types: An experimental clinical pathologic study with the report of a new syndrome. Am J Clin Pathol 11:1, 1941

70. Ross RR: Chloroma and chloroleukemia. Am J Med 28:671, 1955

71. Schultz J, Schwartz S: The chemistry of experimental chloroma. Cancer Res 16:565, 1959

72. Edgerton AE: Chloroma: Report of a case and review of the literature. J Am Ophthalmol Soc 45:376, 1947

73. Conrad FG: Survival in chronic granulocytic leukemia. Splenic irradiation vs busulfan. Arch Intern Med 131:684, 1973

74. Bakhshi A, Minowada J, Arnold A, et al: Lymphoid blast crises of chronic myelogenous leukemia represent stages in the development of B-cell precursors. N Engl J Med 309:826, 1983

75. Bollum EJ: Terminal deoxynucleotidyl transferase as a hematopoietic cell marker (review). Blood 54, 1203, 1979

76. McMaffrey R, Harrison TA, Parkman R, Baltimore D: Terminal deoxyribonucleotidyl transferase activity in human leukemic cells and in

normal human thymocytes. N Engl J Med 292:775, 1975

77. Bollum GT: Methods enzymology. *In* Boyer EA (ed): The Enzymes. New York, Academic Press, 1974, p 145

78. Minot GR, Buckman TE, Isaacs R: Chronic myelogenous leukemia. JAMA 82:1489, 1924

79. Report of Medical Research Council's Working Party for Therapeutic Trials in Leukemia: Chronic granulocytic leukemia: A comparison of radiotherapy and busulfan therapy. Br Med J 1:201, 1968

80. Lawrence JH, Dobson RL, Low-Beer BVA, et al: Chronic myelocytic leukemia: Study of 129 cases in which treatment was with radioactive phosphorus. JAMA 136:672, 1948

81. Haddow A, Timmis GM: Myleran in chronic myeloid leukemia: Chemical constitution and biological action. Lancet 1:207, 1953

82. Galton DAG: Myleran in chronic myeloid leukemia. Lancet 1:208, 1953

83. Kennedy BJ, Yarbro JW: Metabolic and therapeutic effects of hydroxyurea in chronic myelogenous leukemia. Trans Assoc Am Physicians 78:391, 1965

84. Bolin RW, Robinson WA, Sutherland T, Hamman RF: Busulfan versus hydroxyurea in long term therapy of chronic myelogenous leukemia. Cancer 50:1683, 1982

85. Tanzer J, Briere J, Auclerc A, et al: Long term results for 47 patients with Ph[1] + chronic myelocytic leukemia given hydroxyurea as major treatment (abstract). Blood 54:212a, 1979

86. Talpez M, Kantarjian HM, McCredie K, et al: Hematologic remission and cytogenetic improvement induced by recombinant human interferon-alpha in chronic myelogenous leukemia. N Engl J Med 314:1065, 1986

87. Dibromomannitol Cooperative Study Group: Survival of chronic myeloid leukaemic patients treated by dibromomannitol. Eur J Cancer 9:583, 1974

88. Hauch T, Logue G, Laszlo J, et al: Treatment of chronic granulocytic leukemia with melphalan. Blood 51:571, 1978

89. Huguley CM, Grizzle J, Rundles RW, et al: Comparison of 6-mercaptopurine and busulfan in chronic granulocytic leukemia. Blood 21:89, 1963

90. Souers AS, Spiers AS, Galton DA, Kaur J, et al: Thioguanine as primary treatment for chronic granulocytic leukemia. Lancet 1:892, 1975

91. Cunningham I, Gee T, Dowling M, et al: Results of treatment of Ph[1] chronic myelogenous leukemia with an intensive treatment regimen (L-S protocol). Blood 55:375, 1979

92. Fefer A, Cheever MA, Thomas ED, et al: Disappearance of Ph[1]-positive cells in four patients with chronic granulocytic leukemia after chemotherapy, irradiation and marrow transplantation from an identical twin. N Engl J Med 300:333, 1979

93. Thomas ED, Clift RA, Fefer A, et al: Bone marrow transplantation for the treatment of chronic myelogenous leukemia. Ann Intern Med 104:155, 1986

94. Goldman JM, Gale RP, Horowitz MM, et al: Bone marrow transplantation for chronic myelogenous leukemia in chronic phase: Increased risk of relapse associated with T cell depletion. Ann Intern Med (submitted)

95. Champlin R: Preparative regimens for autologous marrow transplantation. Blood 8:277, 1993

96. Koller CA, Miller DM: Preliminary observations on the therapy of the myeloid blast phase of chronic granulocytic leukemia with plicamycin and hydroxyurea. N Engl J Med 3115:1433, 1986

97. Vallejos CG, McCredie KR, Britten GM, Freireich EN: Biological effects of repeated leukopheresis of patient with chronic myelogenous leukemia. Blood 42:925, 1973

98. Hadlock DC, Fortuny IE, McCullough J, Kennedy BJ: Continuous flow centrifuge leukopheresis in the management of chronic myelogenous leukemia. Br J Haematol 29:443, 1975

22

Anagrelide in Myeloproliferative Diseases

MURRAY N. SILVERSTEIN

Anagrelide is a member of the imidazo(2,
1-b)quinazolin-2-one series of compounds
(Fig. 22–1). This family of drugs has been
demonstrated to have a powerful antiaggregating effect on platelets in laboratory animals.[1] During studies in humans, unexpectedly and interestingly, anagrelide in small
doses has been found to produce profound
thrombocytopenia. My interest in thrombocythemic states led the drug producers to a
series of discussions as to the possible efficacy
of anagrelide in thrombocythemic states. My
colleagues and I therefore evaluated anagrelide in the treatment of thrombocytosis
and initially observed platelet levels in 15 of
17 patients with primary thrombocythemia,
2 patients with polycythemia and thrombocytosis, and 1 patient with chronic granulocytic
leukemia and thrombocytosis and noted
platelet counts to return to normal and be
well controlled with the use of this agent.[2]
After our initial favorable experience with
anagrelide, we formed an Anagrelide Study
Group to generate more data on the efficacy
of this agent on the thrombocythemia of
various myeloproliferative states. The Anagrelide Study Group members are listed in
Appendix 22A. Studies were undertaken on
577 patients with thrombocythemia, and the
data therefrom were reported.[3]

OVERALL CLINICAL EXPERIENCE

To date, over 1300 patients with thrombocythemia have been treated with anagrelide. For purposes of the overall clinical
experience, only patients seen between Sep-
tember of 1985 and August of 1991 will be
discussed. Patients with thrombocythemia
secondary to four classes of disease have
been treated. These patients have had essential thrombocythemia, polycythemia vera,
chronic myelogenous leukemia, and other
myeloproliferative diseases including agnogenic myeloid metaplasia.

Demography

Demographic information is available on
817 patients. Of these patients, 59 percent
were female. The mean age of the patients at
initiation of therapy was 58 years, and the
median age was 62 years. The racial distribution is 91 percent white, 6 percent black,
1 percent Oriental, and 1 percent other races
(Table 22–1).

Prior Therapy

Of 607 patients for whom information on
previous treatment was available, 607 (91
percent) had received prior treatment for
thrombocythemia before starting treatment
with anagrelide. Of these 607 patients, 518
had received hydroxyurea, 126 received
busulphan, 71 received interferon, and 50
received radiophosphorus. Some patients received more than one form of treatment
prior to starting on anagrelide. Of the 607
previously treated patients, 110 received
more than one form of treatment with some
agent prior to beginning anagrelide. Ana-

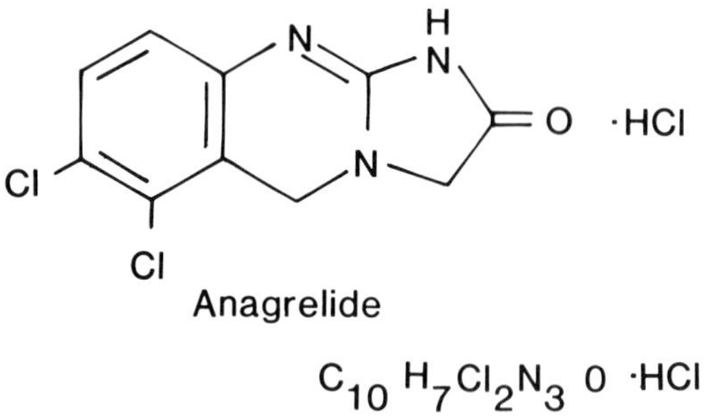

FIGURE 22-1. The molecular structure of anagrelide.

Anagrelide

$$C_{10} H_7 Cl_2 N_3 O \cdot HCl$$

grelide was used only in those patients who either failed to have an effective lowering of their platelet counts or had toxicity from the previous agent (Table 22–2).

Efficacy of Response

In 577 patients in whom efficacy of response has been fully documented, the overall response rate to anagrelide is 93 percent (Table 22–3). Patients with essential thrombocythemia and chronic granulocytic leukemia appear to have a somewhat better response rate than patients with polycythemia vera. A patient was considered to be a responder if he or she was on treatment for at least 1 month and if his or her platelet count, usually in the range of 1 million or above, had dropped within 1 month's time to below 650,000/mm^3.

Dosage

The average dose of anagrelide required to control platelet counts is approximately 2 mg/d, and the dose does not change appreciably over time. The mean dose for 698 evaluable people during the first month of therapy was 2.4 mg/d, and the median dose was 2.0 mg/d. Through 36 months of therapy, the mean daily dose for evaluable patients remained between 2.3 and 2.6 mg, while the median dose stayed at 2.0 mg (Table 22–4).

Anagrelide Treatment Duration

For 700 evaluable patients, the average length of time on therapy for which data were currently available was 304 days, and the median was 206 days. For these patients, the range of treatment duration was between 1 and 1828 days (Table 22–5).

Symptoms

All patients were monitored for pretreatment symptoms and on-treatment symptoms associated with thrombocythemia. Symptoms occurring at any time prior to the start of anagrelide therapy were defined as pretreatment symptoms. In the data base, 337 of 871 patients (41.2 percent) reported symptoms during pretreatment. Of 707 evaluable patients, 193 (27.3 percent) reported symp-

TABLE 22-1.   DEMOGRAPHY BY DIAGNOSIS: ALL PATIENTS

DIAGNOSIS	NUMBER OF PATIENTS	AGE (YEARS)			SEX		NUMBER OF PATIENTS BY RACE			
		Mean	Median	Range	M (%)	F(%)	White	Black	Oriental	Other
ET	490	58	61	11–92	195 (40)	295 (60)	441	39	5	5
PV	91	60	61	23–83	35 (38)	56 (62)	89	0	1	1
CML	165	55	58	12–90	69 (42)	96 (58)	152	9	1	2
OMPD	71	63	66	24–87	36 (51)	35 (49)	64	5	0	2
TOTAL	817	58	62	11–92	335 (41)	482 (59)	746	53	7	10

TABLE 22-2.   PRIOR THERAPY: ALL PATIENTS

STUDY	NUMBER OF PATIENTS	PRIOR THERAPY FOR THROMBOCYTHEMIA				NUMBER OF PATIENTS RECEIVING			
		Yes (%)	No (%)	Prior Therapy ≤2 Weeks	Prior Therapy >2 Weeks	Hydroxyurea	Busulfan	Interferon	32P
12	37	26 (70)	11 (30)	8	18	17	2	0	1
13	4	4 (100)	0 (0)	2	2	4	2	1	0
14	307	270 (88)	37 (12)	42	228	223	52	18	25
15	4	2 (50)	2 (50)	1	1	0	0	0	0
999	318	305 (96)	13 (4)	57	248	274	70	52	24
TOTAL	670	607 (91)	63 (9)	110	497	518	126	71	50

TABLE 22-3. RESPONSE TO ANAGRELIDE THERAPY

	NUMBER ENTERED	NUMBER (%*) EVALUABLE	NUMBER (%†) RESPONDING
PV			
All patients	68	47 (69)	40 (85)
No prior treatment	8	8 (100)	7 (88)
Prior myelosuppressive agents	41	27 (66)	24 (89)
Prior IFN + myelosuppressive agents	6	3 (50)	2 (67)
Treatment data missing	2	2 (100)	2 (100)
ET			
All patients	335	262 (78)	247 (94)
No prior treatment	44	34 (77)	33 (97)
Prior myelosuppressive agents	219	169 (77)	157 (93)
Prior IFN + myelosuppressive agents	16	13 (81)	23 (92)
Treatment data missing	13	11 (85)	11 (100)
CGL			
All patients	114	73 (64)	70 (96)
No prior treatment	0	0	0
Prior myelosuppressive agents	78	52 (67)	50 (96)
Prior IFN + myelosuppressive agents	35	21 (60)	20 (95)
Treatment data missing	0	0	0
Other			
All patients	60	42 (70)	39 (93)
No prior treatment	6	5 (83)	5 (100)
Prior myelosuppressive agents	43	30 (70)	27 (90)
Prior IFN + myelosuppressive agents	4	1 (25)	1 (100)
Treatment data missing	0	0	0
Overall	577	424 (73)	396 (93)

* Percent of patients entered.
† Percent of patients evaluable.

toms in the first 3 months of anagrelide treatment, a drop of 34 percent from pretreatment. From 4 to 6 months, 82 of 485 evaluable patients (16.9 percent) reported symptoms, a decrease of 59 percent from pretreatment. By 16 to 18 months, there were only 17 patients (9.4 percent) reporting symptoms in that 3-month period, a drop of 77 percent from pretreatment. Thus anagrelide effectively suppresses the symptoms normally associated with thrombocythemia. There were a total of 540 occurrences of

TABLE 22-4. DOSAGE: ALL PATIENTS

MONTHS ON THERAPY	NUMBER OF PATIENTS	MILLIGRAMS PER DAY	
		Mean	Median
1	698	2.35	2.02
2	619	2.51	2.00
3	540	2.55	2.00
4	465	2.48	2.00
5	428	2.43	2.00
6	390	2.44	2.00
7	362	2.40	2.00
8	335	2.42	2.00
9	305	2.44	2.00
10	279	2.40	2.00
11	251	2.38	2.00
12	234	2.37	2.00
13–15	216	2.34	2.00
16–18	167	2.40	2.00
19–21	125	2.45	2.00
22–24	97	2.46	2.00
25–30	76	2.48	2.03
31–36	41	2.57	2.00

TABLE 22-5. TREATMENT DURATION: ALL PATIENTS

MONTHS TREATED	NUMBER OF PATIENTS
1–3	222
4–6	104
7–9	82
10–12	67
13–15	52
16–18	44
19–21	29
22–24	23
25–30	35
31–36	24
37–42	12
43–48	0
49–54	4
55–60	1
61–66	1
TOTAL	700

pretreatment symptoms. The total number of pretreatment symptoms probably would have been higher if prior therapy had not been given to so many patients. The most common pretreatment symptoms reported were 51 transient ischemic attacks, 42 occurrences of acral paresthesias, and 41 instances of bruising. An average of 0.66 total occurrences of all symptoms per patient occurred during pretreatment. In the first 3 months of anagrelide therapy, the number of occurrences per patient decreased to 0.5, with acral paresthesias reported the most frequently. The number of transient ischemic attacks during this period declined to 18, a decrease of 65 percent from pretreatment. Both the number of symptoms reported and the number of occurrences per patient continued to decline with time on therapy. In the case of venous thrombosis, there were 20 occurrences in the pretreatment period, 7 in the first 3 months of therapy (a drop of 65 percent), and none in all the remaining time on therapy. After 6 months of treatment, there were less than 0.2 occurrences of all symptoms per patient during any 3-month period. From 28 to 30 months on anagrelide therapy, there were only 4 occurrences of symptoms, or 0.07 occurrences per patient (Table 22–6 and Fig. 22–2).

Selectivity for Platelets

Hematocrit, hemoglobin, and white blood cell count were measured at baseline and

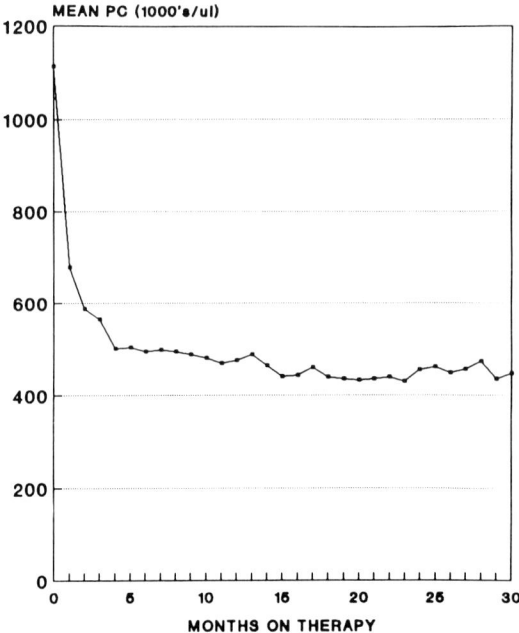

FIGURE 22-2. Mean platelet count vs. months on therapy—essential thrombocythemia patients.

throughout anagrelide therapy. Slight overall decreases in mean and median hematocrit and hemoglobin occurring during therapy are apparent. Mean and median white blood cell counts were variable over time but within normal limits. These data indicate that anagrelide affects platelets selectively (Table 22–7).

TABLE 22-6. SYMPTOMS BY MONTHS ON THERAPY: ALL PATIENTS

	NUMBER OF OCCURRENCES PER TIME PERIOD											
SYMPTOM	Pretreatment	1–3 mos	4–6 mos	7–9 mos	10–12 mos	13–15 mos	16–18 mos	19–21 mos	22–24 mos	25–27 mos	28–30 mos	>30 mos
TIA	51	18	6	2	4	3	3	1	0	1	1	1
Acral paresthesia	42	45	8	5	3	1	1	0	1	0	1	1
Bruising	41	20	5	1	1	2	2	2	1	0	0	2
Digital ischemia	32	24	10	6	3	1	0	0	0	0	1	0
Erythromelalgia	27	25	3	1	0	1	1	0	1	0	0	3
GI bleeding	25	18	8	0	2	2	2	1	0	0	0	0
Epistaxis	25	14	12	7	2	3	4	1	0	3	0	5
Venous thrombosis	20	7	0	0	0	0	0	0	0	0	0	0
Other bleeding	16	10	6	3	1	0	1	0	2	0	0	0
Ischemic ulcers	13	10	1	3	0	0	1	0	2	0	0	0
Angina	10	7	0	0	0	0	0	0	0	0	0	0
Pulmonary embolus	7	4	0	1	0	1	0	0	0	0	0	0
Intestinal ischemia	6	2	2	0	0	0	0	0	0	0	0	0
Arterial thrombosis	5	2	0	0	2	1	0	0	0	0	0	0
Hemoptysis	4	0	0	0	1	0	0	0	0	0	0	0
Other	216	151	58	45	29	14	14	7	5	2	1	8
Total	540	357	119	74	48	29	29	12	12	6	4	20
Number of patients	817	707	485	381	299	232	180	136	107	84	60	49
Number of occurrences per patient	0.66	0.50	0.25	0.19	0.16	0.12	0.16	0.09	0.11	0.07	0.07	0.41

TABLE 22-7. LAB PROFILE: ALL PATIENTS

MONTHS ON THERAPY	NUMBER OF PATIENTS	HEMATOCRIT (in percent)		
		Mean	Median	95% Confidence Limits
0	683	37.303	37.750	36.803–37.803
1	659	35.972	36.020	35.529–36.415
4–6	465	35.731	35.800	35.188–36.274
10–12	278	35.264	35.200	34.533–35.995
16–18	174	34.874	34.575	33.958–35.791
29–30	36	34.800	35.013	33.018–36.582

MONTHS ON THERAPY	NUMBER OF PATIENTS	HEMOGLOBIN (in g/dl)		
		Mean	Median	95% Confidence Limits
0	682	12.368	12.500	12.202–12.535
1	664	11.911	11.971	11.762–12.060
4–6	480	11.819	11.900	11.638–11.999
10–12	290	11.686	11.700	11.453–11.919
16–18	175	11.554	11.500	11.254–11.855
29–30	37	11.602	11.750	11.005–12.200

MONTHS ON THERAPY	NUMBER OF PATIENTS	WHITE BLOOD CELL COUNT (in 10^9 per liter)		
		Mean	Median	95% Confidence Limits
0	689	11.801	9.000	10.999–12.603
1	675	15.095	10.025	13.636–16.554
4–6	486	16.280	9.850	14.736–17.824
10–12	291	14.775	9.925	13.061–16.488
16–18	181	13.796	9.700	11.964–15.629
29–30	39	11.672	9.600	9.661–13.682

Adverse Reactions

The adverse reactions reported included all those in the data base that were observed during the course of anagrelide therapy, whether or not the event is believed to be related to anagrelide. The adverse reaction that occurred in the greatest number of patients was headache, which was reported at least once in 27 percent of 707 evaluable patients. The other most frequent adverse reactions, by number of patients, were fluid retention (20 percent), diarrhea (20 percent), nausea (19 percent), abdominal pain (18 percent), and dizzyness (11 percent). As to severity of these various adverse reactions, over 92 percent were classified as either mild or moderate. In only 19 patients were adverse reactions classified as life-threatening. Of these 19 life-threatening reactions, only 3 were judged to be due to anagrelide therapy. Two of the events were congestive heart failure in older patients who had previous severe cardiac incompetence and pulmonary effusions in 1 patient.

Deaths

Table 22–8 lists 37 patients who died while on therapy with anagrelide or within 15 days of therapy discontinuation. Of the 37 deaths,

11 were due to cardiac events, 11 were pulmonary, 5 were neurologic, 5 were hematologic, and 2 were due to infection. One was due to complications of the patient's myeloproliferative disease, and one was a sudden death, the cause of which was unknown. Of the 37 deaths, 32 were determined to be unrelated to anagrelide therapy. In the other 5 deaths, the possible relationship to anagrelide therapy is not known at the present time.

Life-Threatening Symptoms and Anagrelide Therapy

During study of this huge cohort of patients treated with anagrelide who had thrombocythemia, it was of great interest to us to review patients with life-threatening symptoms. We considered a patient to have a life-threatening symptom if two criteria were met. First, the patient had to have one or more of the following eight symptoms prior to treatment with anagrelide:

1. Gastrointestinal bleeding
2. Arterial thrombosis
3. Preinfarction angina
4. Recurrent pulmonary embolus

TABLE 22-8. DEATHS: ALL PATIENTS

STUDY	INVEST.	PATIENT	CAUSE OF DEATH	DAYS ON	DAYS OFF	RELATED?
12	1	10	Cardiac arrest	96	12	No
14	1	31	Pneumonia	542	13	No
14	1	58	CVA	147	0	Not known
14	1	67	Complications of illness	169	10	No
14	4	47	Cardiac arrest	305	1	No
14	5	7	MI	304	10	No
14	5	34	Pneumonia	208	0	No
14	10	2	Cardiac arrhythmia	43	0	Not known
15	8	2	MI	72	1	No
999	6	1	CVA	356	1	No
999	9	1	Sudden death	64	0	Not known
999	14	1	Pneumonia	513	0	Not known
999	15	1	Sepsis	33	12	No
999	17	1	Pulmonary hypertension	176	0	No
999	23	1	Acute leukemia	189	0	No
999	29	1	Resp. failure	40	2	No
999	39	1	CVA	36	2	No
999	63	1	Not known	244	0	Not known
999	66	1	Cardiac arrhythmia	115	0	No
999	70	1	Cardiac arrest	113	0	No
999	98	1	Pneumonia	35	4	No
999	113	1	Pneumonia	15	2	No
999	132	1	Acute leukemia	276	8	No
999	170	1	Pneumonia	287	0	No
999	177	1	Spontaneous tension pneumothorax	506	0	No
999	178	1	CHF	137	0	No
999	186	1	Acute leukemia	300	1	No
999	192	1	CVA	23	1	No
999	235	1	Pneumonia	353	0	No
999	274	1	MI	118	0	No
999	282	1	Thrombocytosis	16	0	No
999	296	1	Sepsis	271	0	No
999	322	1	CVA	286	0	No
999	339	1	Cardiac arrest	16	0	No
999	368	1	MI	69	0	No
999	407	1	Acute leukemia	73	0	No
999	417	1	Pneumonia	58	0	No

Note: Of the 37 deaths, 11 were due to cardiac events, 11 were pulmonary, 5 were neurologic, 5 were hematologic, 2 were due to infection, 1 was due to complications of the patient's myeloproliferative disease, 1 was a sudden death, and the cause of 1 is not known at this time. Thirty-two of the 37 deaths were determined to be unrelated to anagrelide therapy. In the other 5 deaths, the possible relationship to anagrelide treatment is not known at the present time. The study investigators for these 5 patients have been contacted and an investigation is underway to ascertain whether anagrelide played a role in any of these deaths.

5. Transient ischemic attacks
6. Recurrent venous thrombosis
7. Cerebrovascular accident
8. Myocardial infarction

Second, the severity of the symptoms must have been such that there was a reasonable likelihood that death would have occurred within a matter of months or that premature death was likely to occur without expeditious therapy.

Demographically, of 717 patients analyzed, 111 patients were found to have life-threatening symptoms. Of these, 65 percent were female. The mean age at initiation of therapy was 62 years, and the median age was 66 years. The racial distribution was 94 percent white, 4 percent black, 0 percent Oriental, and 3 percent other races. In this cohort studied, of 106 patients with evaluable life-threatening symptoms for whom information was available, prior therapy was given in 93 percent prior to treatment with anagrelide. Anagrelide was used only if the patient's count would not come down with the prior therapy or if the patient had side effects with the prior therapy. Of 99 patients, 76 had received hydroxyurea, 20 busulfan, 8 interferon, and 8 radiophosphorus. Again, the dosage of anagrelide was 2.3 mg/d, with a median of 2.0 mg/d orally. Mean doses through 36 months of study were 2.2 mg, while the median dose was around 2.0 mg. Again, in 93 percent of these patients, a complete response to anagrelide occurred within 1 month's time. Interestingly, the life-threatening symptoms dropped to 22 percent within the first 3 months of anagrelide therapy to 15 percent from 4 to 6 months after anagrelide, and only one patient reported a life-threatening symptom 19 to 21 months after anagrelide therapy. As was noted in the cohort, adverse reactions occurred. These were mainly headache, abdominal pain, nausea, and diarrhea, and over 90 percent of these reactions were mild to moderate.

DISCUSSION

Anagrelide was originally synthesized as a potent platelet antiaggregating agent. This phenomenon had been demonstrated repeatedly in laboratory animals. When the drug was given to humans, interestingly and unexpectedly, there was a precipitous drop in the platelet count. With the extensive experience that has been encountered with anagrelide, the drug has been found to be extremely efficacious in controlling thrombocythemia in patients with chronic myeloproliferative diseases, i.e., essential thrombocythemia, polycythemia vera, and chronic granulocytic leukemia. The drug, given orally, has an effect usually in 6 to 10 days. Invariably, within 1 month's time, all patients' platelet counts have dropped to a level of 650,000/mm^3 or below. The dosages of anagrelide to achieve these responses have been quite low, approximately 2.0 to 2.3 mg/d. Over time, the dosages of anagrelide have remained stable; thus no patient has been found to become fast to this agent. Adverse reactions to anagrelide have included primarily headache, fluid retention, nausea, diarrhea, and abdominal pain. These adverse reactions have tended to be quite mild, and headaches are usually controlled with Tylenol. I have ascertained that those patients with nausea, diarrhea, and abdominal pain are usually lactase-deficient, and the use of Lact-Aid has abolished this group of symptoms. Anagrelide has a potent vasodilator and inotropic effect, and it may decrease renal blood flow. The inotropic effect may lead to a sense of palpitations, but no severe life-threatening arrhythmias have occurred with the use of the drug. The decrease in renal blood flow may be operative in fluid retention that some patients develop. I suspect that in older people with severely incapacitated hearts, anagrelide conceivably may precipitate congestive heart failure. This appears to be the only group of patients in whom the drug should be withheld.

The mechanism whereby anagrelide produces a decrease in the platelet count is not known, but data generated by Solberg[4] and confirmed by others now suggest that the drug acts primarily by inhibiting megakaryocyte maturation. Megakaryocytes are inhibited to a level effecting subsequent platelet release.

Overall, it appears that anagrelide should revolutionize the approach to patients with thrombocythemic states complicating myeloproliferative diseases. The drug's major action appears to be that of inhibiting megakaryocyte maturation, and no chromosomal damaging issues have been related to anagrelide. A leukemogenic effect by this drug, under these circumstances, would not be anticipated. I would suggest that anagrelide will become the drug of choice for the treatment of thrombocythemic states complicating myeloproliferative disease.

One additional issue has developed relating to anagrelide which is quite fascinating. I have observed that the anticipated conversion in a huge cohort of patients with primary thrombocythemia to postthrombocythemic myelofibrosis has not occurred over an 8-year period of time. I have intensively studied 6 patients who had well-demonstrable fibrosis while on anagrelide for a period of a year or more, and it now appears that the fibrosis in these patients has diminished. I am prospectively now looking at a study to determine the influence of anagrelide in myelofibrosis. If the key issue to myelofibrosis is a mutation of megakaryocytes which, in turn, causes leaking of transforming growth factor beta and platelet-derived growth factors, it may well be that anagrelide, in inhibiting megakaryocyte maturation, may seal off membranes, thus preventing the leakage of these fibrogenic substances. I am currently studying this issue.

REFERENCES

1. Fleming JS, Buyniski JP: Anagrelide. *In* Scriabine A (ed): New Drugs Annual: Cardiovascular Drugs, vol 1. New York, Raven Press, 1983, p 277
2. Silverstein MN, Petitt RM, Solberg LA Jr, et al: Ana-

grelide: A new drug for treating thrombocytosis. N Engl J Med 318:1292–1294, 1988
3. Anagrelide Study Group: Anagrelide, a therapy for thrombocythemic states: Experience in 577 patients. Am J Med 92:69–76, 1992
4. Solberg LA Jr, Oles KJ, Tarach J, et al: The effects of anagrelide on human megakaryocytopoiesis (abstract). Blood 74(Suppl 1):20a, 1989

Appendix 22A: Anagrelide Study Group Members

Murray N. Silverstein, M.D., Ph.D., Mayo Clinic, Rochester, Minnesota; Robert M. Petitt, M.D., Mayo Clinic, Rochester, Minnesota; Lawrence A. Solberg, Jr., M.D., Ph.D., Mayo Clinic Jacksonville, Jacksonville, Florida; Barry Rosenbloom, M.D., Cedars-Sinai Medical Center, Los Angeles, California; Richard T. Silver, M.D., New York Hospital–Cornell Medical Center, New York, New York; William Knospe, M.D., Rush Presbyterian–St. Luke's Medical Center, Chicago, Illinois; Thomas Fitch, M.D., Mayo Clinic Scottsdale, Scottsdale, Arizona; Gerardo Colon-Oterno, M.D., Mayo Clinic Jacksonville, Jacksonville, Florida; Eric Mazur, M.D., Miriam Hospital, Providence, Rhode Island; Gary J. Doyle, B.S., Bristol-Myers Squibb Company, Wallingford, Connecticut; Steven L. Allen, M.D., North Shore University Hospital–Cornell University Medical College, Manhasset, New York; Harriet S. Gilbert, M.D., Albert Einstein College of Medicine, The Bronx, New York; Janet Cuttner, M.D., Mount Sinai Medical Center, New York, New York; James Weick, M.D., The Cleveland Clinic, Cleveland, Ohio; Eugene P. Frenkel, M.D., Southwestern Medical Center, Dallas, Texas; William Miller, M.D., Scripps Clinic, La Jolla, California; Nehemiah C. Cherng, Ph.D., Bristol-Myers Squibb Company, Wallingford, Connecticut; James N. Burroughs, Bristol-Myers Squibb Company, Wallingford, Connecticut; Nancy L. Yovan, B.A., Bristol-Myers Squibb Company, Wallingford, Connecticut; Majid Khoory, M.D., Bryn Mawr Hospital, Bryn Mawr, Pennsylvania; Janis L. Grechko, Ph.D., Bristol-Myers Squibb Company, Wallingford, Connecticut; Lee P. Schacter, Ph.D., M.D., Bristol-Myers Squibb Company, Wallingford, Connecticut; Ted P. Szatrowski, M.D., New York Hospital–Cornell Medical Center, New York, New York.; Christopher C. Chapman, M.D., Roberts Pharmaceutical Corporation, Eatontown, New Jersey; Michael Petrone, M.D., Roberts Pharmaceutical Corporation, Eatontown, New Jersey.

23

Therapeutic Recommendations for Polycythemia Vera

Steven M. Fruchtman *and* Louis R. Wasserman

The pathogenesis of polycythemia vera (PV) is not known. Therefore, like other diseases whose etiology remains obscure, the optimal management leading to longevity and well-being for patients with PV is unclear and controversial. However, as our conceptual understanding of this disease grows, our ability to manage these patients improves. As will be discussed, treatment strategy for patients with PV demands careful attention to diagnostic classification and familiarity with the natural history of the disease.

PV is a chronic, slowly progressive disorder characterized by panhyperplasia of the bone marrow involving the erythroid, myeloid, and megakaryocytic series.[1] The hyperplastic marrow leads to elevation of the red cell mass, considered essential for the diagnosis of the disease, and varying degrees of leukocytosis and thrombocytosis.[2] It is believed that the hemorrhagic and thrombotic complications of the disease are secondary to the hyperplastic marrow and increased number of circulating elements on both a mechanical and perhaps a humoral basis.

Although the onset of the disease may be insidious and its course chronic, PV is a hematologic malignancy involving an abnormal clone of the pluripotent marrow stem cell. The fact that PV is a neoplastic process was demonstrated by Adamson and coworkers,[3] who studied female patients with PV heterozygous at the X chromosome–linked locus for glucose-6-phosphate dehydrogenase (G-6-PD). In nonhematopoietic tissue, such as skin fibroblasts, as predicted by Lyon's hypothesis of random inactivation of one X chromosome, equal amounts of type A and type B isoenzymes are found. If, however, a neoplasm represents the progeny (clone) derived from a single cell, all cells derived from that clone will have the same isoenzyme. In patients with PV, when peripheral blood red cells, granulocytes, and platelets are studied, only one G-6-PD isoenzyme is found, either type A or type B. This suggests the presence of an abnormality in the pluripotent stem cell giving rise to a clone with proliferative advantage and replacement of the marrow and peripheral blood elements with this abnormal clone resulting in PV.

In vitro culture studies of bone marrow and peripheral blood from patients with PV also have shown that in contrast to normal individuals, stem cells from these patients are capable of forming erythroid colonies without the addition of erythropoietin to the culture system.[4,5] These "endogenous" erythroid colonies arise from progenitor cells which are part of the abnormal clone, and their ability to proliferate in vitro in the absence of demonstrable erythropoietin may be taken as additional evidence for autonomous cell growth. Experimental manipulation of these hematopoietic precursors in cell culture systems has shown that presumably normal stem cells do exist as well in patients with PV. Why their differentiation and maturation are suppressed in the host is not known.[6]

Clinical observation also has helped to confirm the biochemical findings that PV can behave as a malignant process. Patients with PV left untreated do very poorly; 50 percent are reported to die within 18 months after the onset of the first symptom or sign.[7] Untreated PV patients are at an especially high risk of developing both thrombotic and hemorrhagic complications, with death due to thrombosis of the cerebral, coronary, and pulmonary circulation. Unusual sites for thrombosis, such as the hepatic veins and femoral artery or vein, and mesenteric thrombosis are also seen.

The pathogenesis of the increased risk from thrombosis in these patients is unclear. Several recent studies[8] using xenon-133 clearance techniques have shown that cerebral blood flow is decreased in individuals with hematocrits above 53 percent and returns to normal by hematocrit control to normal levels. Furthermore, cerebral function is impaired at high hematocrit values and is improved by reduction of the hematocrit to levels below 45 percent, when cerebral blood flow is improved.[9] By studying whole-blood viscosity in vitro before and after venesection, it has been shown that the increase in cerebral blood flow is mainly due to the fall in blood viscosity that occurs when the hematocrit is reduced.[10] Indeed, the Framingham Study identified the hemoglobin value as an important risk factor for cerebral infarction in the general population.[11] A postmortem study also demonstrated a greater incidence of cerebral infarction in patients with packed red cell volume levels above 46 percent than in those with lower values.[12] The degree of hematocrit elevation also may influence the size of a cerebral infarct in both animals and humans.[13] Thus the propensity for thrombosis and infarction in PV may be related to a reversible impairment of blood flow.

Hemorrhage is another frequent cause of early mortality. Epistaxis, ecchymosis, and menorrhagia are frequent problems. The gastrointestinal tract is the most common site of severe bleeding, and cerebral hemorrhage may be fatal. Although blood fluidity is important in influencing the thrombotic and hemorrhagic tendencies seen in PV, even when the blood volume is normalized by phlebotomy, these patients are still prone to thrombotic and hemorrhagic complications. In addition to whole-blood viscosity, abnormalities of the circulating elements and the vascular endothelium may play a role. A multitude of platelet abnormalities are found in PV, and the platelet has been incriminated in the thrombohemorrhagic complications of PV with respect to both increased numbers and abnormal function (see Chap. 9). Typically, patients with PV have elevated platelet counts and a multitude of in vitro abnormalities in platelet aggregation, and these platelets may undergo in vivo degranulation.[14,15] Qualitative platelet defects that have been described include lipooxygenase deficiency, loss of response or increased sensitivity to aggregating agents, decreased numbers of α-adrenergic and prostaglandin D receptors, increased expression of Fc receptors, acquired storage-pool disease, and abnormal platelet-membrane glycoprotein patterns.[16-19] However, the association between these quantitative platelet defects and clinical bleeding or thrombotic sequelae has generally been questionable.

Because of the potential malignant nature of the disease, close monitoring and appropriate therapy for these patients are of great importance. With therapy, a dramatic improvement in survival has been reported, with recent studies citing median survival of 8 to 15 years.[20] However, before appropriate therapy can be instituted, one must be able to recognize and identify the spectrum of clinical conditions that have in common an increase above normal in the concentration of packed red cells per unit volume of peripheral blood. Relative or spurious polycythemia must be differentiated from absolute polycythemia and secondary erythrocytosis from the primary variety. Therapeutic modalities designed to suppress the bone marrow would be inappropriate in situations where increased erythropoietic activity reflects the marrow's physiologic response to a hypoxemic state. In secondary polycythemia, one must find the underlying cause and attempt to correct it. It is essential, therefore, that the clinician understand the mechanism of erythrocytosis before initiating therapy.

The Polycythemia Vera Study Group (PVSG) was founded in 1967 to help determine the optimal treatment for PV. It was clear to the group that rigorous, although widely available, diagnostic criteria would have to be met before a diagnosis of PV could be established. This would ensure that patients with the same category of disease were being studied and compared. These criteria have been discussed in detail elsewhere (see Chap. 3).

PRINCIPLES OF MANAGEMENT

The optimal management of PV remains elusive, although the findings of the PVSG make appropriate therapy more rational and suggest areas for continued study. It is clear that one cannot simply measure the level of hemoglobin and initiate therapy. An accurate diagnosis must be established in patients with an elevated hematocrit to avoid inappropriate therapy. Measurement of the ^{51}Cr-labeled erythrocyte mass is essential in determining the existence of true erythrocytosis. A hematocrit above 60 percent usually predicts an elevated erythrocyte mass, but at hematocrits below 60 percent, the erythrocyte mass may be normal or even low.[21] Once the diagnosis of PV is established by using the criteria of the PVSG, attention must be given to the level of the circulating platelets and white cells, the stage of immaturity of the white cell series, the size of the spleen, the history of bleeding or thrombosis, and the clinical or performance status of the patient. Other important factors must be taken into account before the treatment modality is decided on, i.e., the age of the patient and the presence of diabetes, arteriosclerosis, cardiopulmonary disease, and venous access. Before specific treatment approaches are discussed, guidelines for managing these patients are offered in Table 23–1. The management of patients with secondary polycythemia and relative polycythemia is discussed elsewhere (see Chaps. 16 and 18).

Phlebotomy

The benefits resulting from reduction of an expanded blood volume were recorded as early as 1899 by Cabot,[22] who noted the symptomatic improvement that occurred in a polycythemic patient following tooth extraction with copious bleeding. Osler[23] used bleeding as an effective measure for relieving headaches and vertigo. Hookworm infestation also had been used as a therapeutic modality in the past to produce a state of iron deficiency, thus interfering with erythropoiesis.[24] Today, venesection is considered a more palatable method to reduce the blood volume and create a state of iron deficiency for long-term control.

TABLE 23–1. GENERAL PRINCIPLES IN THE MANAGEMENT OF POLYCYTHEMIA VERA

1. Therapy must be tailored to suit the clinical needs of the patient. Status of the formed elements of the blood, marrow morphology, and complications of hepatosplenomegaly must be considered.
2. The blood volume should be normalized with phlebotomy as rapidly as clinically possible (250 to 500 cc every other day). The elderly or patients with cardiovascular disease should be phlebotomized cautiously and with reduced amounts.
3. Suppression of the panmyelosis with ^{32}P or chemotherapy is to be used in most patients over age 50 and in all patients over age 70. In patients with (a) a thrombotic tendency and a normal red cell volume following phlebotomy or (b) the development of thrombocythemia following phlebotomy, marrow suppression may have to be instituted earlier.
4. Blood values should be maintained at normal levels by regular examination and treatment.
5. Overtreatment and toxicity should be avoided by careful and judicious use of chemotherapy and radiation. Supplemental phlebotomy rather than excess bone marrow suppression is preferred.
6. Elective surgery should be postponed until long-term control of the disease is established.
7. Women of child-bearing age are to treated only with phlebotomies. In young males, myelosuppressive therapy may produce aspermia, and treatment should be evaluated carefully before any chemotherapy or radiotherapy is used.
8. The PVSG no longer recommends the use of alkylating agents due to the increased incidence of leukemia and certain types of cancer associated with their use.
9. Hyperuricemia should be treated with allopurinol (100 to 300 mg/d) until remission has been attained. For acute gouty attacks, colchicine or other antiinflammatory agents are indicated (see Chap. 13).

Once the diagnosis of PV is established, relatively rapid reduction in the blood volume may prevent serious hemorrhagic and/or thromboembolic episodes in those patients susceptible to such complications. Phlebotomy therapy is particularly useful in indolent cases of PV where occasional venesections (500 cc every few months) will be sufficient to control the erythrocytosis. Initially, phlebotomies of 250 to 500 cc should be performed until a hematocrit of between 40 and 45 percent is obtained. In the elderly or those with a compromised cardiovascular system, smaller amounts of blood (200 to 300 cc) should be withdrawn twice weekly. Once normalization of the hematocrit has been obtained, blood counts at regular intervals (every 4 to 8 weeks) will establish the frequency of future phlebotomies. Sufficient blood should be removed to maintain the hematocrit at the lower limit of normal (40 to 45 percent).

With the development of iron deficiency, small, hypochromic cells become prominent. While following the patient, the hematocrit may begin to rise slowly, and if values above or equal to 45 percent are reached, one to two phlebotomies at intervals of 2 to 3 days should be performed. Iron is not given because it may cause the hematocrit and red cell mass to increase rapidly. An obvious question is whether the state of chronic iron deficiency is in any way harmful to the patient. Controversy exists as to whether there is a correlation between whole-blood viscosity at a fixed hemoglobin level and mean cell hemoglobin (MCH). It has been reported[25] that iron-deficient red cells, as indicated by a low MCH value, resulted in a relative increase in whole-blood viscosity, particularly at the low shear rates that may exist in patients with concomitant circulatory disease. These findings are in contrast to those of others,[26,27] who found no difference in viscosity due to hypochromic, microcytic red cell changes. Debate in the literature on methodological aspects has not resolved the conflict,[28] and the role of hypochromic, microcytic red cells in influencing red cell deformability is likely to be a matter for further investigation. However, the current belief is that if microcytic, hypochromic red cells have altered red cell deformability, these changes are insufficient to change whole-blood viscosity at a given hematocrit because the influence of other factors, including plasma proteins, plays an important role (see Chap. 10).

Iron deficiency is reported to produce symptoms that are unrelated to anemia, such as dysphagia, soreness or burning of the tongue, fissures at the corners of the mouth, koilonychia, and pica, although in practice these findings are seen rarely. Chronic fatigue and muscular weakness have been attributed to iron depletion even in the absence of anemia. Iron deficiency not accompanied by anemia may represent a physiologic liability. Finch and coworkers[29] have reported that striated muscle dysfunction occurs in nonanemic iron deficiency due to a decrease in mitochondrial α-glycerophosphate–mediated phosphorylation. This biochemical defect may help to explain some of the nonhematologic symptoms of iron deficiency, such as anorexia and malaise, that may complicate phlebotomy therapy. Despite this theoretical problem, patients invariably feel better once adjustment to their lower red cell mass has occurred, and the rarity of the expected signs and symptoms of iron deficiency in clinical practice is noteworthy.[30]

We recommend that in the clinical management of PV the venous hematocrit should be maintained at or below the lower end of the normal range. Based on the observation that there are fewer vascular occlusive episodes in these patients when the hematocrit is maintained below 45 percent than when the hematocrit is in the higher-normal range,[31] the value of 45 percent is a reasonable therapeutic objective. A scheme for managing PV patients with phlebotomy is presented in Fig. 23–1.

Phlebotomy should be considered the treatment of choice in young patients, in whom one may fear the sequelae of the long-term use of myelosuppressive therapy or radioactive agents. It is recommended that patients below age 50 and all women in the child-bearing years should be managed with phlebotomy. Phlebotomy is also indicated in the rare case of a patient with PV who is pregnant, although in such patients the hematocrit often declines to normal or anemic levels due to changes in blood volume and/or hormonal effects associated with pregnancy, followed by a progressive increase in the hematocrit postpartum.

In patients who require myelosuppressive therapy, phlebotomy must be used initially to bring the hematocrit into the therapeutic range (40 to 45 percent) so that the morbidity and potential mortality of an elevated red cell mass can be avoided before the effects of bone marrow suppression become evident in the peripheral blood. In these patients, intermittent phlebotomy should be used when the hematocrit is above 45 percent to help minimize the amount of myelosuppression that must be employed.

Myelosuppression

Phlebotomy as the sole form of therapy in PV is advocated by those who believe that morbidity and mortality are primarily reduced by correcting the increased blood volume. However, it will not control thrombocytosis, leukocytosis, the painfully enlarging

Induction

Maintenance

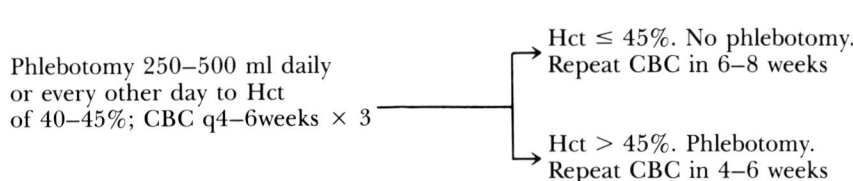

Phlebotomy 250–500 ml daily
or every other day to Hct
of 40–45%; CBC q4–6weeks × 3

Hct ≤ 45%. No phlebotomy.
Repeat CBC in 6–8 weeks

Hct > 45%. Phlebotomy.
Repeat CBC in 4–6 weeks

Comments

1. The Hct is to be maintained between 40 and 45%.
2. Supplemental iron therapy should not be given.

FIGURE 23–1. Management of polycythemia vera with phlebotomy.

spleen, hyperuricemia and its complications, or pruritus. In addition, patients treated with phlebotomy alone, especially early in the course of their disease, have a high incidence of thrombotic events which may prove to be fatal or disabling. Thrombosis is the cause of death in patients treated with phlebotomy in 47 percent of cases as compared with 28 percent in a chlorambucil-treated group and 31 percent in patients treated with radioactive phosphorus. Thrombosis is especially common in the elderly, in patients with a prior history of thrombosis, and in those with a high phlebotomy requirement.[32]

Thus, although phlebotomy is the treatment of choice for certain patients with PV, it does not control all the ramifications of the disease, and these patients remain susceptible to potentially fatal thrombotic events. Myelosuppression with either ^{32}P or cytostatic agents will help to control the thrombocytosis, leukocytosis, splenomegaly, and hyperuricemia that are found in association with this disorder. Weight gain and improved performance status and sense of well-being, with relief from pruritus and the potential for hyperuricemia and its complications, accompany marrow suppression and hematologic remission. In a majority of patients there is reduction in spleen size. The myelosuppressive agent used must be predictable in its action, have a minimum of side effects, and should lend itself to continued or repeated use over the many years during which marrow suppression may be required. The use of agents that produce profound hematopoietic suppression and life-threatening side effects has no place in the management of PV.

Chlorambucil (Leukeran) was a commonly used alkylating agent for the treatment of PV due to an extensive experience with this drug. However, as a result of the PVSG's first protocol, which showed that the risk of developing acute leukemia in patients given chlorambucil was 2 to 3 times that in patients given radioactive phosphorus and 13 times that in patients treated with phlebotomy alone, the PVSG no longer recommends the use of chlorambucil in the treatment of PV.[32] Other trials have used melphalan, cyclophosphamide, and busulfan as cytostatic agents. These alkylating drugs are effective in reducing the hematocrit, the platelet count, and the white cell count in patients with PV.[33] In the doses studied, a reduction in platelet count typically followed a decrease in the white cell count and was produced most regularly by busulfan. Thrombocytosis was corrected in all cases by busulfan and chlorambucil, whereas cyclosphamide tends to be more platelet sparing. Busulfan has a more marked effect on megakaryocytes and may more frequently induce long-standing thrombocytopenia. However, as has been shown with chlorambucil in long-term management of PV, the fear is that no alkylating agent has been absolved from leukemogenic potential, and there are numerous reports of the association of alkylating agent therapy and leukemia in both hematologic[34,35] and nonhematologic disorders.[35,36] Some workers[37] have suggested that busulfan's mechanism of action is significantly different from that of the classic alkylating agents and therefore warrants continued study in patients with PV to see if the tendency to leukemic transformation that is seen with other alkylating agents can be avoided.[38] However, because of the effect of busulfan on thrombopoiesis, these patients require frequent monitoring to detect a tendency toward thrombocytopenia; failure to do so can lead to severe and potentially life-threatening thrombocytopenia as well as marrow aplasia in sensitive patients.

Pulmonary fibrosis also has been noted in patients receiving chronic busulfan therapy. As cases of diffuse pulmonary disease associated with busulfan treatment were reported, the syndrome of "busulfan lung" was recognized as a distinct clinical entity.[39] An insidious onset of cough, dyspnea, and low-grade fever may occur. These symptoms can appear 8 months to 10 years after initiation of therapy, with an average of 4 years. Chest roentgenograms typically demonstrate diffuse interstitial and alveolar infiltrates. Pulmonary function studies reveal diminished diffusing capacity, as well as changes of restrictive lung disease. Because of the chronic course of PV and the potential need for long-term therapy when myelosuppression is indicated, busulfan may be a hazardous agent when used for the management of PV.

Antimetabolites such as 6-thioguanine[40] and azaribine,[41] alkaloids such as harringtonine[42] and pipobroman,[43] and dibromomannitol[44] have been used effectively to treat patients with PV; the long-term consequences are unknown, and these agents cannot be recommended as initial therapy.

The possible beneficial effect of the pyrimidine analogue azaribine in PV was suggested by the selective suppression of erythropoiesis observed in patients with psoriasis during treatment with this agent. In PV, this toxic manifestation was used to therapeutic advantage, and when azaribine was administered orally at a dosage of 270 mg/kg per day in three divided doses every 8 hours for 6 to 12 weeks, as governed by clinical and hematologic response, suppression of erythropoiesis was achieved without leukopenia or thrombocytopenia. The effects of the drug are gradual and are reversed by discontinuation of therapy.

Myelobromol (1,6-dibromo-1,6-dideoxy-D-mannitol) is effective in controlling the erythrocytosis, splenomegaly, and clinical symptoms in patients with and without prior cytostatic therapy. When 250 mg is given orally daily, the average length of time for achieving remission is 40 days, and the drug may be stopped without the need for maintenance doses. Remissions may last for greater than 1 year. Pipobroman, a piperazine derivative, has been used for the treatment of PV, and hematologic remission is reported in 92 percent of patients.[45] Maintenance therapy is required to avoid recurrence of an increase in the circulating blood elements. The risk of the development of acute leukemia is still significant.

Radioactive Phosphorus

Radioactive phosphorus has been used for the treatment of PV for more than 50 years. Lawrence and associates[46] in 1939 published the first report of therapeutic results obtained with radioactive phosphorus in leukemia and PV. Since then, many observers have recorded additional experience in a wide range of neoplastic disorders, principally PV.[47–50]

To prepare radioactive phosphorus, stable phosphorus is exposed to high-speed deuterons (nuclei of heavy hydrogen) emitted by a cyclotron. As a result of this bombardment, a neutron enters the nucleus of a small fraction of the phosphorus atoms. Stable phosphorus (^{32}P) has an atomic mass of 31. When a neutron enters the phosphorus nucleus, the resulting nucleus has a mass of 32; this nucleus is unstable, and the atom is radioactive. Eventually, an atom of ^{32}P emits a beta ray (an electron), and these beta rays have energies as high as 1.8 million electronvolts; their average energy is approximately 0.6 million electronvolts. The maximum range of penetration of these rays through the body tissues is approximately 0.7 cm, and the half-life of ^{32}P is 14.3 days. This rate of decay is short enough that the radiation effects can be controlled, and yet it is sufficiently long that a given tissue can be subjected to relatively prolonged low-grade radiation. Since ^{32}P emits beta rays that produce their ionization in the immediate vicinity of the deposited phosphorus atoms, this material offers a method of giving localized irradiation in diseases of the bone marrow. The isotope is initially selectively concentrated in the mitotically active cells of the bone marrow and within a few days is incorporated in the calcium phosphate of the bone lying adjacent to the endosteum, from which further radiation of the marrow results. ^{32}P maintains the chemical characteristics of its naturally occurring relative and undergoes the same chemical reactions in the body as does naturally occurring phosphorus. This explains its minimal toxicity and its normal metabolism.

Bone has a high inorganic phosphorus content, and it takes up a significant amount of the radioactive isotope. Neoplastic tissue invariably takes up a great deal more phosphorus than does the same type of tissue in a normal state of growth, and since the radioactive isotope is built into nucleoprotein just as is naturally occurring ^{32}P, those cells which are multiplying at the fastest rate use proportionately more of the ^{32}P than do cells that are being produced more slowly. As a result, relatively high concentrations of radioactivity are reached in the organs principally involved in PV: the bone marrow and sites of extramedullary hematopoiesis. However, enough of the material is deposited in normal tissues and cells to limit the total dose that can be given without the potential for toxic manifestations.

The beta particle released by ^{32}P produces sufficient radiation effects to the hyperplastic marrow that the peripheral blood is normalized in 1 to 2 months in about 80 percent of patients.[51] Radioactive phosphorus is an effective agent for controlling the clinical symptoms of PV. Fatigability, headache, bone pain, pruritus, and visual disturbances are relieved.[52] Radioactive phosphorus also ameliorates abnormal physical findings in a majority of patients. The bright red color of the skin and mucous membranes, the cyanosis, and the distended retinal venules disappeared after treatment in practically all patients. About two-thirds of the enlarged spleens and livers become nonpalpable after treatment.

There is no doubt that it is the most convenient method for the patient. There is no radiation sickness associated with its use, and the patient does not have to take a drug whose dosage must be regulated constantly with care or inconvenience himself or herself with repeated phlebotomies. Easily produced remissions may be maintained without further therapy for many months or years.

The dosage schedule (Figs. 23–2 and 23–4) recommended by the PVSG is as follows: 2.3 mCi/m² of body surface area administered intravenously for the first dose, not to exceed 5 mCi. This usually will produce a satisfactory remission with normal peripheral blood counts, but if it is found to be suboptimal in 3 months, the dose may be increased by 25 percent. If at the expiration of an additional 3 months, remission is still not satisfactory, a further 25 percent increase in the second dose may be administered, not to exceed 7 mCi. Retreatment

should be restricted to 6-month intervals thereafter (total yearly dose of 15 mCi), and supplemental phlebotomies should be used as necessary before and during ^{32}P therapy. Complete blood counts are required every 2 to 3 months.[53] Of course, if there is no response or a minimal effect is produced, other forms of therapy must be considered. Administering the same inadequate dose of ^{32}P repeatedly accomplishes nothing.[54]

It has been suggested that radiation in patients with PV increases the risk of developing malignant disease. Landaw[55] has reviewed the results of more than 25 large studies which suggested that the treatment of PV with radiation, whether in the form of x-rays of ^{32}P, was associated with an increased incidence of acute leukemic transformation. Lawrence and associates[56] have argued that the increased incidence of leukemic transformation was explained by the longer survival in ^{32}P-treated patients, thereby permitting the natural history of the disease to express itself. However, in patients followed on the PVSG protocols, median survival from entry until death is 11.8 years for ^{32}P-treated patients, 8.9 years for chlorambucil-treated patients, and 13.9 years for the phlebotomy-treated group. During this follow-up period, a sufficient number of cases of acute leukemia have accumulated in the ^{32}P arm of the study to confirm the suspicion that, like chlorambucil, this agent is leukemogenic. Of 134 patients managed with phlebotomy, 2 patients developed acute leukemia; of 141 patients managed with chlorambucil, 24 have developed leukemia or lymphoma; and of the 156 patients managed with ^{32}P, 16 have developed leukemia, although the peak incidence of developing acute leukemia in patients treated with ^{32}P occurred later than in those treated with chlorambucil. It appears that treatment with ^{32}P increases the likelihood of the development of acute leukemia many years after exposure to the drug. Therefore, based on the results of this study to date, it is considered that the best treatment for PV in the elderly (patients over age 70), due to the increased risk of thrombosis associated with age, appears to be ^{32}P and supplemental phlebotomy rather than phlebotomy alone. The agent of choice in younger patients (between the ages of 50 to 70) with a history of thrombotic tendencies or those with a high phlebotomy requirement (since these patients are prone to thrombosis)

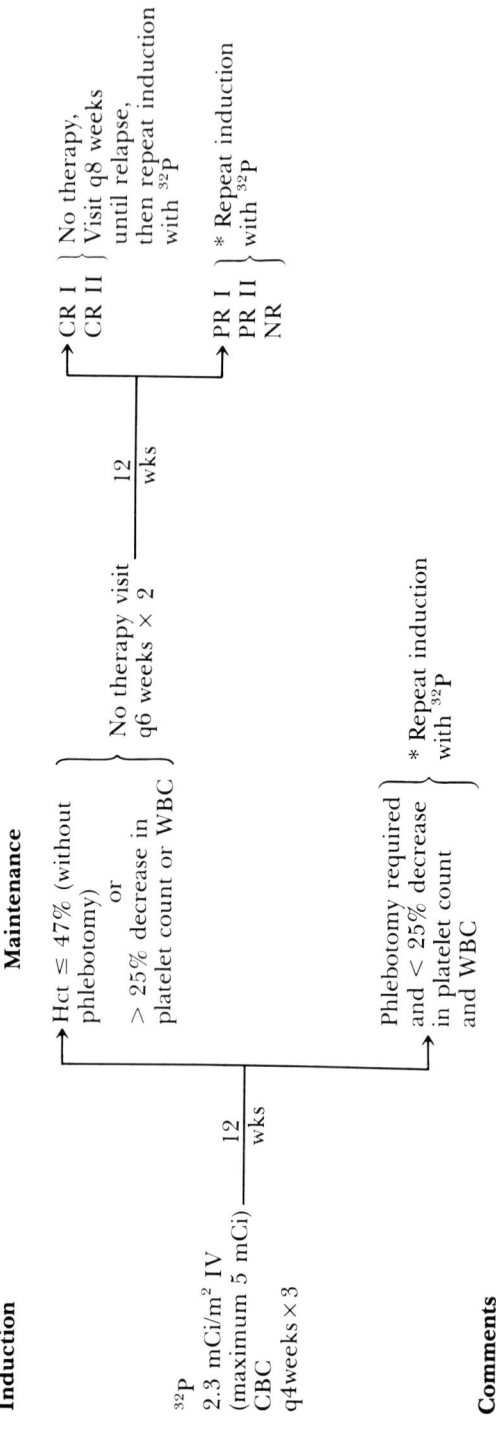

FIGURE 23-2. Management of polycythemia vera with radioactive phosphorus (^{32}P).

Comments

1. Hct to be maintained between 40 and 45% by supplemental phlebotomy if necessary.
2. Minimum interval between ^{32}P doses is 12 weeks.
3. Second and subsequent doses of ^{32}P may be increased by 25% of preceding dose (limit 7 mCi).
4. If after 1 year of incremental doses of ^{32}P, response is inadequate, control with phlebotomy alone or hydroxyurea.

may well be hydroxyurea. In patients between the ages of 50 and 70 who need myelosuppressive therapy due to a high phlebotomy requirement, history of thrombosis or ischemia, intractable pruritus, or painful splenic enlargement but who cannot be managed successfully with hydroxyurea, ^{32}P may have to be utilized.

Recombinant Interferon-α

Silver[57] has reported on the efficacy of recombinant interferon-α (rIFN-α) in the management of PV. rIFN-α is a biologic response modifier with myelosuppressive activity that has been used predominately for the treatment of chronic myelocytic leukemia.[58] The precise mechanisms by which the interferons affect the bone marrow remain unknown. Interferons suppress myeloid colony formation, B-cell proliferation, and myeloid differentiation.

Typically, patients are started on 3.0×10^6 U/m^2 three times a week subcutaneously. The need for phlebotomy can be reduced, thrombocytosis is controlled, and the spleen regresses in size. Dosages must be adjusted depending on response. Although recombinant interferon-α appears to be an interesting new agent for the management of PV, further studies are warranted to determine its role and long-term safety.

Hydroxyurea

The need for a safe myelosuppressive agent in patients with PV in whom phlebotomy is not ideal therapy prompted the study of hydroxyurea.[59] Hydroxyurea has been used primarily in the treatment of chronic myelocytic leukemia,[60] psoriasis,[61] and less frequently, other malignant conditions. It is a nonalkylating myelosuppressive agent specific for the inhibition of cells in the synthetic phase of the cell cycle. It decreases DNA synthesis by inhibiting ribonucleoside diphosphate reductase[62] and has been shown to adequately control the hematocrit and platelet levels in between 80 and 90 percent of patients so treated within 12 weeks of initiation of therapy.[68] When initially studied, patients were given a loading dose of 30 mg/kg per day for 1 week, which was then reduced to 15 mg/kg per day. The drug is well tolerated; however, because of the development of transient cytopenias at this dosage, it

is recommended that hydroxyurea be administered initially at a dose of 15 to 20 mg/kg per day following normalization of the hematocrit with phlebotomy (Figs. 23–3 and 23–4). The patient is followed with weekly blood counts. When a steady state is achieved, the interval between blood counts is lengthened to 2 weeks and then to 4 weeks. If the WBC falls below 3500/mm^3 or the platelet count falls to less than 100,000/mm^3, hydroxyurea is withheld and reinstituted at 50 percent of the dose when the blood count normalizes. For poorly controlled patients who require frequent phlebotomies or are thrombocythemic (platelet counts greater than 600,000/mm^3), the dose can be increased by 5 mg/kg per day at monthly intervals with frequent monitoring until control is achieved. Acute toxicity is rare; occasionally, patients may develop a rash, gastrointestinal complaints, oral ulcers, or fever. To date, hydroxyurea has not been shown to be leukemogenic; further study is required to be certain that this form of long-term myelosuppression will not be mutagenic.

Adjuvant Therapy

As part of the total comprehensive care of the patient with PV, it is often necessary to provide relief of symptoms that may be associated with active disease. Complications of hyperuricemia, such as acute gout and nephrolithiasis, due to increased nucleoprotein breakdown secondary to the accelerated hematopoiesis, usually can be controlled by effective myelosuppressive therapy. However, if the patient is being managed by phlebotomy alone, allopurinol 300 mg/d given orally will usually control the hyperuricemia. Acute attacks of gout can be managed with colchicine or nonsteroidal anti-inflammatory agents such as naproxen as required.

Pruritis, present in about 50 percent of patients with PV, is frequently generalized and may be made worse by bathing or showering and by brisk rubbing with a towel. The skin should be patted gently dry and not rubbed. In extreme cases, starch baths (a half box of Linet starch) in a tub of lukewarm water followed by gentle drying may be effective. If myelosuppressive therapy is used, as the peripheral blood normalizes, itching frequently subsides. Antihistamines may prove helpful, and both H$_1$ antagonists (cyproheptadine 4 mg orally three times daily) or H$_2$

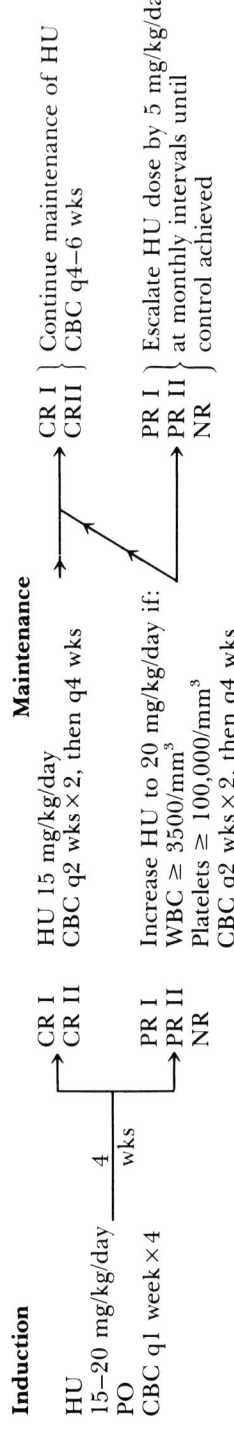

Induction

HU
15–20 mg/kg/day
PO
CBC q1 week ×4
—— 4 wks ——

→ CR I
  CR II

→ PR I
  PR II
  NR

Maintenance

CR I / CR II   HU 15 mg/kg/day
                CBC q2 wks × 2, then q4 wks

PR I / PR II / NR   Increase HU to 20 mg/kg/day if:
                     WBC ≥ 3500/mm³
                     Platelets ≥ 100,000/mm³
                     CBC q2 wks × 2, then q4 wks

→ CR I / CRII   Continue maintenance of HU
                 CBC q4–6 wks

→ PR I / PR II / NR   Escalate HU dose by 5 mg/kg/day
                       at monthly intervals until
                       control achieved

Comments

1. Hct to be maintained between 40 and 45% by supplementary phlebotomy if necessary.
2. If WBC < 3500/mm³ and/or platelet count < 100,000/mm³, stop therapy. Patient to be managed with phlebotomy alone. When WBC > 3500/mm³ and/or platelets > 100,000/mm³, HU can be restarted at 50% of maintenance dose.
3. After dose of HU is increased, obtain CBC q2 wks × 2, then q4–6 wks during maintenance.
4. Patients unable to achieve CR I or CR II despite escalation of HU dose due to WBC < 3500/mm³ or platelets < 100,000/mm³ should be placed on optimum HU dose and phlebotomized.

FIGURE 23–3. Management of polycythemia vera with hydroxyurea (HU).

Hct (%)	Platelets/cu mm	Classification
42–47	≤600,000	CR I
<42	≤600,000	CR II
42–47	>600,000	PR I
<42	>600,000	PR II
>47	>600,000	NR

Comments
CR = Complete Remission
PR = Partial Remission
NR = No Response

FIGURE 23–4. Classification of response to therapy.

antagonists (cimetidine 300 mg orally four times daily) have been used either singly or in combination.[64] The response to histamine antagonists in patients with pruritus has suggested a role of hyperhistaminemia or some derangement of histamine metabolism in these patients.[65] Cholestyramine has been reported to offer relief to patients with intractable pruritus[66]; however, the basis for its use is unclear, since bile acids have not been reported to be elevated in this disorder.

SURGERY IN PATIENTS WITH POLYCYTHEMIA VERA

Since the majority of patients with PV are middle-aged or elderly, the need for surgical and dental intervention in these patients becomes commonplace. However, the performance of such procedures is fraught with danger and accompanied by an excessively high morbidity and mortality. Because of the expanded blood volume and platelet abnormalities, the difficulties in obtaining effective hemostasis are understandable. Rigby and Leavell[67] reported a surgical complication rate of over 30 percent and mortality of 7 percent in these patients. In a series of more than 81 operative procedures performed on 68 patients with PV (average age 58 years), Wasserman and Gilbert[68] noted a postoperative morbidity of almost 50 percent and a postoperative mortality of 16 percent. The mortality rate in patients after major surgery is reported to be 2 percent in patients under age 60 and 5 percent in those over 60 years of age.[69] As expected, the majority of these complications were related to uncontrolled hemorrhage or vascular thrombosis.

The tendency for adverse complications is directly related to the level of elevation of the hematocrit. The postoperative mortality was seven times greater in uncontrolled patients (hematocrit ≥ 52 percent) than in those in whom hematocrit control was achieved (Fig. 23–5). In addition, the duration of hematologic control is an important factor in determining the frequency of postoperative complications. The complication rate was more than five times greater when hematologic control was maintained for less than 4 months than when patients were well controlled for greater than 4 months. The number of deaths was decreased from 15 percent in patients in whom short-term control was achieved to zero in the group whose disease was controlled for more than 4 months before surgery (Fig. 23–6).

Because of these observations, in patients with PV, elective surgery should not be contemplated unless the hematologic values have been normalized for several months. The better the hematologic control and the longer control has been achieved, the lower is the incidence of postoperative complications and death. If emergency surgery is necessary, the patient should be phlebotomized rapidly until a normal hematocrit is achieved. The intravascular volume should be maintained with fluids. As part of good general postoperative care, these patients should be mobilized as rapidly as possible postoperatively to avoid thrombotic complications. Until ambulation is achieved, low-dose subcutaneous heparin (5000 units SC every

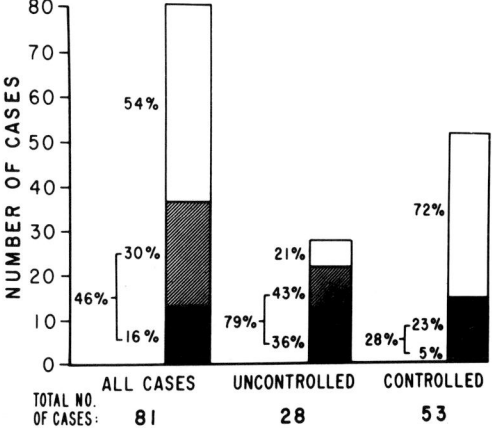

FIGURE 23–5. Complications of surgery in "controlled" and uncontrolled patients with polycythemia vera. Incidence of fatal and nonfatal complications after major surgery in hematologically "controlled" and uncontrolled patients with polycythemia vera. □ = uncomplicated; ▨ = complicated; ■ = death. (From Wasserman LR, Gilbert HS: Ann NY Acad Sci 115:125, 1964.)

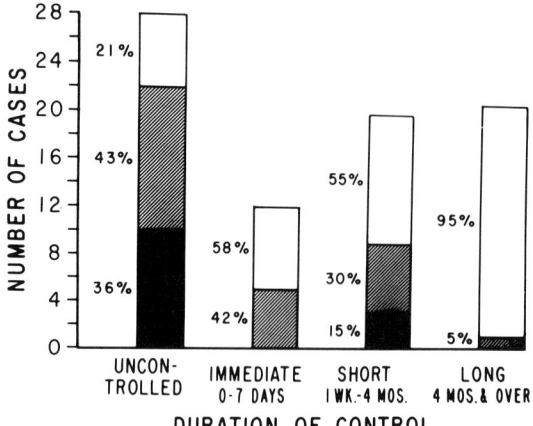

FIGURE 23–6. Duration of hematologic "control" and incidence of complications following surgery in polycythemia vera. □ = uncomplicated; ▨ = complicated; ■ = death. *(From Wasserman LR, Gilbert HS: Ann NY Acad Sci 115:127, 1964.)*

12 hours) can be efficacious in preventing the thrombotic complications postoperatively in these patients and should not exacerbate an underlying hemorrhagic tendency at these doses. Dental extractions also can cause excessive bleeding and, if possible, should be delayed until good hematologic control has been achieved.

REFERENCES

1. Kurnick JE, Ward HP, Block MH: Bone marrow sections in the differential diagnosis of polycythemia. Arch Pathol 94:489–499, 1972
2. Wasserman LR: Polycythemia vera: Its course and treatment. Relation to myeloid metaplasia and leukemia. Bull NY Acad Med 3:343–375, 1954
3. Adamson JW, Fialkow PJ, Murphy S, et al: Polycythemia vera: Stem-cell and probable clonal origin of the disease. N Engl J Med 295:913–916, 1976
4. Zanjani ED, Lutton JD, Hoffman R, Wasserman LR: Erythroid colony formation by polycythemia vera bone marrow in vitro. J Clin Invest 59:841–848, 1977
5. Horland A, Ludman S, Murphy MJ, Moore MAS: Proliferation of erythroid colonies in semi-solid agar. Br J Haematol 36:495–499, 1977
6. Prchal JF, Adamson JW, Murphy S, et al: Polycythemia vera: The in vitro response of normal and abnormal stem cell lines to erythropoietin. J Clin Invest 61:1044–1047, 1978
7. Chievitz E, Thiede T: Complication and causes of death in polycythemia vera. Acta Med Scand 172:513–523, 1962
8. Thomas DJ, DuBoulay GH, Marshall J, et al: Cerebral blood flow in polycythemia. Lancet 2:1161–1165, 1977
9. Willison JR, Thomas DJ, Boulay GH, et al: Effect of high haematocrit on alertness. Lancet 1:846–848, 1980
10. Humphrey PRD, Marshall J, Ross-Russel RW, et al: Cerebral blood flow and viscosity in relative polycythemia. Lancet 2:873–876, 1979
11. Kannel WB, Gordon T, Wolf PA, McNamara P: Hemoglobin and the risk of cerebral infarction: The Framingham Study. Stroke 3:409–420, 1972
12. Tohgi H, Yamanouchi H, Murakami M, Kameyama M: Importance of the hematocrit as a risk factor in cerebral infarction. Stroke 9:369–374, 1978
13. Harrison MJG, Pollock S, Kendall BE, Marshall J: Effect of haematocrit on carotid stenosis and cerebral infarction. Lancet 2:114–115, 1981
14. Berger S, Aldort LM, Gilbert HS, et al: Abnormalities of platelet function in patients with polycythemia vera. Cancer Res 33:2683–2687, 1973
15. Viero P, Cortelazzo S, Bassan R, Barbui T: Effect of aspirin on platelet 5-hydroxytryptamine and B-thromboglobulin plasma levels in patients with myeloproliferative diseases. Thromb Haemost 48:125–126, 1982
16. Schafer AJ: Deficiency of platelet lipoxygenase activity in myeloproliferative disorders. N Engl J Med 306:381–386, 1982
17. Zucker S, Mielke CH: Classification of thrombocytosis based on platelet function tests: Correlation with hemorrhagic and thrombotic complications. J Lab Clin Med 80:385–394, 1972
18. Cooper B, Schafer AJ, Puchalsky D, Handin RI: Platelet resistance to prostaglandin D₂ in patients with myeloproliferative disorders. Blood 52:618–626, 1978
19. Bolin RB, Okumura T, Jamieson GA: Changes in distribution of platelet membrane glycoproteins in patients with myeloproliferative disorders. Am J Hematol 3:63–72, 1977
20. Wasserman LR, Balcerzak SP, Berk PD, et al: Influence of therapy on causes of death in polycythemia vera. Trans Assoc Am Physicians 1104:30–38, 1981
21. Berlin NI: Diagnosis and classification of the polycythemias. Semin Hematol 12:339–351, 1975
22. Cabot RC: Case of chronic cyanosis without discoverable cause, ending in cerebral hemorrhage. Boston Med Surg J 141:574–581, 1899
23. Osler W: A clinical lecture on erythraemia (polycythemia with cyanosis, maladie de Vaquez). Lancet 1:143–160, 1908
24. Myhre J, Wallace F: Hookworm treatment of polycythemia vera. Minn Med 39:99, 1956
25. Milligan DW, MacNamee R, Roberts BE, Davies JA: The influence of iron deficient indices on whole blood viscosity in polycythemia. Br J Haematol 50:467–473, 1982
26. Pearson TC, Ring CP, Wetherley-Mein G: Plasma and whole blood viscosity in treated primary polycythemia. Clin Lab Haematol 2:73–82, 1980
27. Birgegard G, Carlsson M, Sandhagen B, Mannting F: Does iron deficiency in treated polycythemia vera affect whole blood viscosity? Acta Med Scand 216:165–169, 1984
28. Milligan DW, Roberts BE, Davies JA: Iron deficiency and whole blood viscosity in polycythemia (letter). Br J Haematol 51:501–503, 1982
29. Finch CA, Miller LR, Inamdar AR, et al: Iron deficiency in rat. J Clin Invest 58:447–461, 1976
30. Rector WG, Fortuin NJ, Conley CL: Nonhematologic effects of chronic iron deficiency: A

study of patients with polycythemia vera treated solely with venesections. Medicine 61:382–389, 1982

31. Pearson TC, Wetherley-Mein G: Vascular occlusive episodes and venous haematocrit in primary proliferative polycythemia. Lancet 2:1219–1222, 1978

32. Berk PD, Goldberg JD, Silverstein MN, et al: Increased incidence of acute leukemia in polycythemia vera associated with chlorambucil therapy. N Engl J Med 304:441–447, 1981

33. Gilbert HS: Problems relating to control of polycythemia vera: The use of alkylating agents. Blood 32:500–505, 1968

34. Weinfeld A, Westin J, Ridell B, et al: Polycythemia vera terminating in acute leukemia: A clinical, cytogenetic and morphologic study in 8 patients treated with alkylating agents. J Scand Haematol 19:255–272, 1977

35. Casciato DA, Scott JL: Acute leukemia following prolonged cytotoxic agent therapy. Medicine 58:32–47, 1979

36. Reimer RR, Hoover R, Fraumeni J, et al: Acute leukemia after alkylating agent therapy of ovarian cancer. N Engl J Med 297:177–181, 1977

37. Brodsky I: Busulphan treatment of polycythemia vera. Br J Haematol 52:1–6, 1982

38. Haanan L, Mathe G, Hayat M: Treatment of polycythemia vera by radiophosphorus or busulphan: A randomized trial. Br J Cancer 44:75–80, 1981

39. Feingold ML, Kass LG: Effects of long term administration of busulfan. Arch Intern Med 124:66–72, 1969

40. Milligan DW, Thein SL, Roberts BE: Secondary treatment of polycythemia rubra vera with 6-thioguanine. Cancer 50:836–839, 1982

41. Deconti RC, Calabresi P: Treatment of polycythemia vera with azauridine and azaribine. Ann Intern Med 73:575–580, 1970

42. Lian-Huang Lu, Shu-ping L, Yu-ying L: Harringtonine in treatment of polycythemia vera. Chin Med J 96:533–535, 1983

43. Council on Drugs: Evaluation of two antineoplastic agents. JAMA 200:139–140, 1967

44. Szentklaray J, Hartmann E: Treatment of polycythemia vera with myelobromol. Ther Hung 14:143–148, 1966

45. Brusamolino E, Salvaneschi L, Canevari A, et al: Efficacy trial of pipobroman in polycythemia vera and incidence of acute leukemia. J Clin Oncol 2:558–561, 1984

46. Lawrence JH, Scott KG, Tuttle LW: Studies of leukemia with the aid of radioactive phosphorus. Int Clin 3:33–58, 1939

47. Lawrence JH: Nuclear physics and therapy: Preliminary report on a new method of treatment of leukemia and polycythemia. Radiology 35:51–60, 1940

48. Fitz-Hugh T Jr, Hodes PJ: Clinical experience with radiophosphorus in the treatment of certain blood dyscrasias. Am J Med Sci 204:662–683, 1942

49. Najean Y, Triebel F, Dresch C: ^{32}P therapy of polycythemia: A review and reappraisal. Clin Nucl Med 5:275–280, 1980

50. Tubiana M, Flamant R, Attie E, et al: A study of hematological complications occurring in patients with polycythemia vera treated with ^{32}P. Blood 32:536–542, 1968

51. Lawrence JH: Polycythemia: Physiology, Diagnosis, and Treatment. New York, Grune and Stratton, 1955

52. Reinhard EH, Moore CV, Bierbaum OS, Moore S: Radioactive phosphorus as a therapeutic agent: A review of the literature and analysis of the results of treatment of 155 patients with various blood dyscrasias, lymphomas and other malignant neoplastic diseases. J Lab Clin Med 31:107–189, 1946

53. Wasserman LR: The treatment of polycythemia vera. Semin Hematol 13:57–78, 1976

54. Osgood EE: The threshold dose of ^{32}P for leukemia cells of the lymphocytic and granulocytic series. Blood 16:1102–1110, 1960

55. Landaw SA: Acute leukemia in polycythemia vera. Semin Hematol 13:33–48, 1976

56. Lawrence JH, Winchell HS, Donald WG: Leukemia in polycythemia vera: Relationship to splenic myeloid metaplasia and therapeutic radiation dose. Ann Intern Med 70:763–771, 1969

57. Silver RT: A new treatment for polycythemia vera: Recombinant interferon-alpha. Blood 76:664–665, 1990

58. Talpaz M, Kantarjian HM, McCrediek, et al: Hematologic remission and cytogenetic improvement induced by recombinant human interferon alpha in chronic myelogenous leukemia. N Engl J Med 314:1065–1069, 1986

59. West WO, Ruff DJ, Yarbo JW: Response of polycythemia to treatment with a new agent: Hydroxyurea. J Lab Clin Med 74:1022–1023, 1969

60. Kennedy BJ: Hydroxyurea therapy in chronic myelogenous leukemia. Cancer 29:1052–1059, 1972

61. Dahl MGC, Comaish JS: Long-term effects of hydroxyurea in psoriasis. Br Med J 4:585–587, 1972

62. Krakoff IGH, Brown NC, Reichard P: Inhibition of ribonucleoside diphosphatase reductase by hydroxyurea. Cancer Res 28:1559–1565, 1968

63. Donovan PB, Kaplan ME, Goldberg JD, et al: Treatment of polycythemia vera with hydroxyurea. Am J Hematol 17:329–334, 1984

64. Easton P, Galbraith PR: Cimetidine treatment of pruritus in polycythemia vera (letter). N Engl J Med 299:1134, 1978

65. Gilbert HS, Warner RP, Wasserman LR: A study of histamine in myeloproliferative disease. Blood 28:795–799, 1966

66. Chanarin I, Szur L: Relief of intractable pruritus in polycythemia rubra vera with cholestyramine. Br J Haematol 29:669–670, 1975

67. Rigby PG, Leavell BS: Polycythemia vera. Arch Intern Med 106:622–631, 1960

68. Wasserman LR, Gilbert HS: Surgical bleeding in polycythemia vera. Ann NY Acad Sci 115:122–138, 1964

69. Cole WH: Operability in the young and aged. Ann Surg 138:145–157, 1953

ACKNOWLEDGMENTS: This work was supported by Grant CA-10728 from the National Cancer Institute to the Polycythemia Vera Study Group and aided by the Jack Martin Fund, the Polly Annenberg Levee Charitable Trust, and the Cavallo Family Philanthropic Fund of the Jewish Communal Fund.

INDEX

Note: Page numbers in *italics* refer to illustrations;
page numbers followed by t refer to tables

ISBN 0-7216-4213-6

90038